MEDICINAL PLANTS : UTILISATION AND CONSERVATION

Prof. Pravin Chandra Trivedi (b. 3 March 1953), Ph.D., Post-Doct. (U.S.A.), F.L.S. (London), F.B.S., F.P.S.I., F.B.R.S., F.M.A., F.E.S., F.N.R.S., F.I.A.T., Professor, Department of Botany, has a brilliant academic career standing first in all examinations. Prof. Trivedi served as Head, Department of Botany and Co-ordinator, P.G. Course in Biotechnology (2003-06); Director, College Development Council (2001-04); Vice-Principal, Maharaja's College (2000-03) and is Member of Senate Academic Council and Convenor of BOS Botany in the University of Rajasthan.

He worked as Post-Doctoral Fellow at the Department of Plant Pathology, North Carolina State University, Raleigh, U.S.A. in 1983-84. Prof. Trivedi has 34 years of teaching and research experience in the University of Rajasthan, Jaipur. He has published more than 250 research papers and review articles in journals of repute. He has edited and written more than 100 books and guided 35 Ph.D. students. He has been the Principal Investigator of 20 major research projects funded by national organisations. He is an elected Fellow of nine reputed academic bodies. Dr. Trivedi visited several major research laboratories and delivered invited talks in many international conferences held in the U.S.A., Canada, the U.K., Germany, the Netherlands, Italy, Japan, Denmark, Switzerland, Luxembourg, Malaysia, Singapore, Austria and Belgium.

Prof. Trivedi is an elected Secretary of the Indian Botanical Society (2005-2010); Council Member of Indian Science Congress Association, Kolkata (2007-09) and a member of the editorial and advisory boards of eight reputed journals. For his research contribution he was awarded Scientist of the Year Award (2001); M. J. Narsimhan Award (2004), Bioved Fellowship Award (2005) and Birbal Sahni Foundation Honour (2007).

MEDICINAL PLANTS
Utilisation and Conservation

2nd Revised and Enlarged Edition

Editor

Prof. Pravin Chandra Trivedi

Ph.D., Post-Doct. (U.S.A.), F.L.S. (London), F.B.S., F.P.S.I., F.N.S.I., F.B.R.S., F.M.A., F.E.S., F.I.A.A.T.

Department of Botany
University of Rajasthan
Jaipur-302 004, India

Aavishkar Publishers, Distributors
Jaipur 302 003 (Raj) India

Published by
Prem C. Bakliwal
Aavishkar Publishers, Distributors
807, Vyas Building, Chaura Rasta
Jaipur 302 003 (Raj) India
Phone : 0141-2578159
e-mail : aavishkarbooks@hotmail.com

ISBN 978-81-7910-228-2

First Published in 2004
Second Revised and Enlarged Edition 2009

Printed at
Sheetal Printers
Jaipur 302 003 (Raj) India

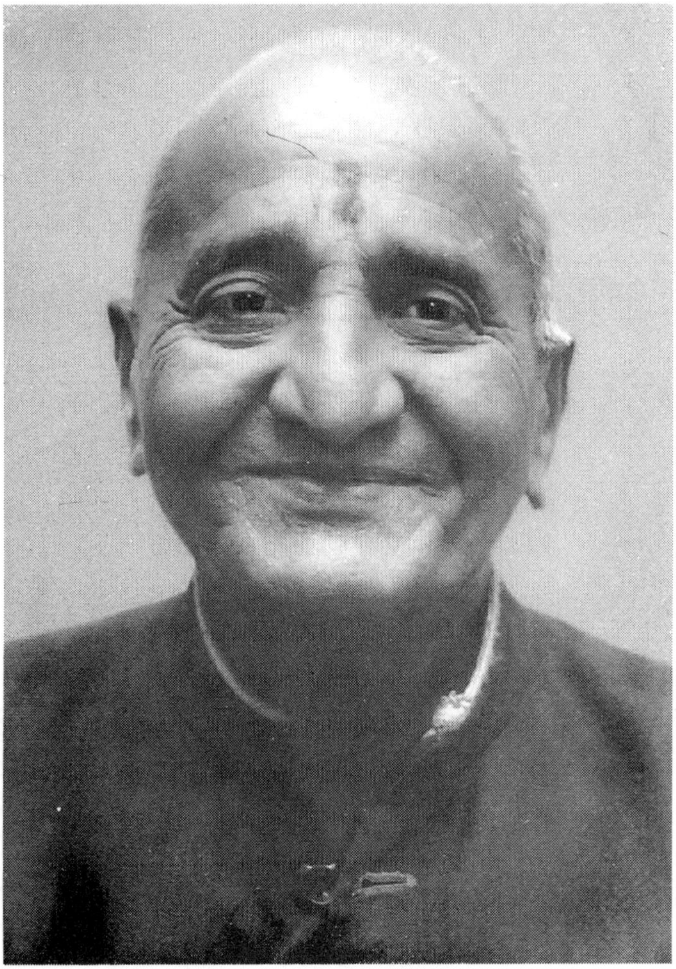

Dedicated to my father

Late Shri D. S. Trivedi

who was a strong supporter of Indian traditional drugs

PREFACE

THE quest for good health and immortality has been a continuous human endeavour since the beginning of civilisation throughout the world. In India, it may be through 'yoga' (a technique by which the physical and mental status of an individual can be elevated to the highest level and his spirit is united with divinity), 'tantra' (a spiritual prescription for an orderly life according to the laws of nature, exhaling everything, discarding nothing, relegating everything to its rightful place and accepting the world as it is, spread to save), or "oushadha" (commonly referred to as "Ayurveda" in which a number of medicaments are prescribed for maintenance of health, vitality, youthfulness and longevity).

Plants have been used as a source of medicine by man from ancient times. Initially, these formed the bulk of folk or ethnomedicine, practised in India and some other parts of the world like China, the Middle East, Africa and South America. Later, a considerable part of this indigenous knowledge was formulated, documented and eventually passed into the organised systems of medicine, such as Ayurveda, Unani, Siddha or some other systems outside India. Subsequently, with the advance in techniques of phytochemistry and pharmacology, a number of active principles of medicinal plants were isolated and introduced as valuable drugs in modern medicine. Hence, it is accepted that plants are useful in their crude or advanced forms as drugs. The medicinal plants are now defined as "All higher plants that have been identified to possess medicinal properties, that is, effects that relate to health or which contain constituents that are used directly as drugs, or as medicaments in different indigenous systems and practices or which have been proven to be useful as drugs by Western standards."

According to an estimate of the World Health Organisation (WHO), approximately 80 per cent of the people in developing countries rely chiefly on traditional medicines for primary health care needs; a major portion of these involves the use of medicinal plants. It is assumed that 20,000-30,000 species of higher plants are used as medicines in various cultures of the world. In India, the contributions made during the last one hundred years have meticulously brought into focus much of the diverse information on a large number of medicinal plants. These medicinal plants can be placed in the following three categories:

1. **Plants of Codified Knowledge**—1,500: Those which are used in organised systems of medicine like Ayurveda, Unani and Sidha.
2. **Plants of Empirical Knowledge**—3,000: Those which are used in ethnomedicine or folk medicine based on oral information from generation to generation. Recent ethnobotanical researches have revealed unknown uses of many unrecorded plants.
3. **Plants of Scientific Knowledge**—700: Those which have been investigated pharmacologically and chemically and their active principles are used in modern medicine or are providing valuable leads for partial or total synthesis of new drugs.

It is noteworthy that some of the most important drugs of the last 50 years for some serious diseases, which did not have suitable remedies in the modern system, have been developed from plants. Though a majority of these 'wonder drugs' have been discovered in Western countries, they are from such plants as had been used in primitive societies or in indigenous medicine. These include the anti-hypertensive reserpine from *Rauvolfia serpentina,* the anti-cancer vinblastine and vincristine from *Catharanthus roseus*; the anti-malarial quinine from *Cinchona ladgeriana*; the anti-glaucoma pilocarpine from *Pilocarpus jaborandi*; the topical anaesthetic cocaine from *Erythroxylon coca*; the pain killer morphine and the anti-cough codeine from *Papaver somniferum;* the anti-asthmatic and cold medicine atropine from *Atropa belladonna* and *Hyoscymus niger*, etc. Evidently, the experimental investigations of medicinal plants used in folk or indigenous systems can lead to many novel useful drugs, but modern and traditional uses may be entirely different.

The present work, *Medicinal Plants: Conservation and Utilisation* is a well-documented comprehensive review of significant investigations on medicinal plants. This volume contains 20 chapters covering holistic information on medicinal plants, their utilisation, conservation, cultivation and diseases with special reference to the Indian scenario. In addition, articles on cultivation and propagation of medicinal plants, medicinal pteridophytes and diseases of medicinal and aromatic plants and their management have been included. A comprehensive account of "current advances in herbal-based contraceptive research" and plants with anti-oxidative properties in radio-protection have added to the value of the book. Excellent account of Intellectual Property Rights, growth and competitiveness of Indian pharmaceutical industries have been given in the book.

In 20 chapters, prepared by specialists who have devoted long years to teaching and research, almost all areas of medicinal plants are discussed. The gaps in our present knowledge have been highlighted, and a programme of future investigations has been emphasised to fill up the gaps and to keep pace with international progress in the 21st century.

This book provides adequate background and current information on medicinal plants. It will be very useful for a variety of scholars—historians and practitioners of medicine, researchers in botany, phytochemistry and pharmacology, and also phytogeographers and conservationists.

I am grateful to my colleagues all over the country for writing authoritative and informative articles for this volume. While dealing with such a voluminous work, errors are likely to occur, despite my best efforts. However, the onus of the technical content rests with the contributors.

This book is dedicated to the sacred memory of my father, late Shri D. S. Trivedi, (2nd Jan 1925 – 14th Jan 2003) who was a strong supporter of herbal Indian traditional drugs for the cure of various ailments.

I also wish to record the encouragement from my wife, Kusum, my daughter, Priyanka and son Rohit during the preparation of this book. I appreciate the cooperation and support of Mr. Akshay Jain of Aavishkar Publishers, Distributors for publishing this book with patience, care and interest. I am confident that the book will be widely accepted by all students, teachers and researchers in the field of medicine.

Jaipur **Prof. P. C. Trivedi**

Preface to the Second Enlarged Edition

APPLICATION of medicinal plants and related research continues to progress rapidly each year with the aid of new techniques, new research findings and new insights into the plant world. The present second edition of "Medicinal Plants—Utilisation and Conservation" update the first edition of the book by weaving the current information as and where required besides adding four new chapters. Present edition contains 24 chapters. New chapters added includes articles on "Medicinal plant solutions to Asthmatic Problems; Biotechnological advances in some Ethnomedicinal plant species; *Catharanthus roseus* a potential drug source for cancer chemotherapy and Biotechnological interventions and role of secondary metabolites in defense mechanism of plants." Hopefully, the second revised edition will meet out the demand of readers.

Helps and critical suggestions rendered by the students, scientist, teachers, colleagues and friends are gratefully acknowledged.

I am confident that the users will find the book more useful and apprise of their critical views for further improvement of the book. My sincere thanks are due to Mr. Akshay Jain of Aavishkar Publishers, Distributors for publishing second edition of this book with keen interest.

Jaipur

—**Prof. P.C. Trivedi**

CONTENTS

Contributors

Agarwal, Mala
Government College, Chimanpura (Rajasthan).

Agnihotri, A.K.
Central Institute of Medicinal and Aromatic Plants, Lucknow 226 015 (Uttar Pradesh).

Ansari, A. S.
Department of Zoology, University of Rajasthan, Jaipur 302 004 (Rajasthan).

Audichya, K. C.
M. S. Central Research Institute (Ay), Jaipur (Rajasthan).

Bhandari, M. M.
Emeritus Professor of Botany, J. N. V. University, Jodhpur 302 001 (Rajasthan).

Bhatia, A. L.
Department of Zoology, University of Rajasthan, Jaipur 302 002 (Rajasthan).

Braganza sj, Vincent J.
Loyola Centre for Research & Development, St. Xavier's College Campus, Ahmedabad 380 009 (Gujarat).

D'Souza, Kirti
Loyola Centre for Research & Development, St. Xavier's College Campus, Ahmedabad 380 009 (Gujarat).

Dayal, Narsinha
Department of Botany, Ranchi University, Ranchi 834 008 (Jharkhand).

Dixit, A. M.
Gujarat Institute of Desert Ecology, Bhuj (Kachchh) 370 001 (Gujarat).

Dixit, R. D.
Botanical Survey of India, Central Circle, Allahabad (Uttar Pradesh).

Giri, Archana
Centre for Biotechnology, Institute of Science & Technology (IST), Jawaharlal Nehru Technological University, Kukatpally, Hyderabad 500 085 (A.P.).

Giri, C. C.
Centre for Plant Molecular Biology (CPMB), Department of Genetics, Osmania University, Hyderabad 500 007 (A.P.).

Gupta, Leena
Gujarat Institute of Desert Ecology, Bhuj (Kachchh) 370 001 (Gujarat).

Jain, Manish
P. G. T., Biotechnology, Subodh Public School, Jaipur (Rajasthan).

Jakhar, M. L.
SKN College of Agriculture (Rajasthan Agricultural University), Jobner (Rajasthan).

Joshi, S. C.
Department of Zoology, University of Rajasthan, Jaipur 302 004 (Rajasthan).

Kakralya, B. L.
SKN College of Agriculture (Rajasthan Agricultural University), Jobner (Rajasthan).

Kasera, Pawan K.
Laboratory of Plant Ecology, Department of Botany, Jai Narain Vyas University, Jodhpur 302 001 (Rajasthan).

Khanuja, S. P. S.
Central Institute of Medicinal and Aromatic Plants, Lucknow 226 015 (Uttar Pradesh).

Kumar, Padma
Laboratory of Plant Tissue Culture and Secondary Metabolities, Department of Botany, University of Rajasthan, Jaipur 302 004 (Rajasthan).

Lal, R. K.
Central Institute of Medicinal and Aromatic Plants, Lucknow 226 015 (Uttar Pradesh).

Malik, C. P.
Director, Life Sciences, SADTM, Jaipur (Rajasthan).

Mistry, Nisha
Gujarat Institute of Desert Ecology, Bhuj (Kachchh) 370 001 (Gujarat).

Mohammed, Sher
Government Lohia (PG) College, Churu 331 001 (Rajasthan).

Mukherjee, Tapan
National Institute of Science Communication and Information Resources (NISCAIR), CSIR, New Delhi 110012.

Narasu, M. Lakshmi
Centre for Biotechnology, Institute of Science & Technology (IST), Jawaharlal Nehru Technological University, Kukatpally, Hyderabad 500 085 (A.P.).

Nehra, Sampat
Department of Botany, University of Rajasthan, Jaipur 302 004 (Rajasthan).

Pandey, Rakesh
Central Institute of Medicinal and Aromatic Plants, Lucknow 226 015 (Uttar Pradesh).

Sarin, Renu
Department of Botany, University of Rajasthan, Jaipur 302 004 (Rajasthan).

Saxena, V. S.
Ex-Chief Conservator of Forests, Jaipur 302 018 (Rajasthan).

Sharma, Satish Kumar
Range Forest Officer, Phulwari Wildlife Sanctuary, Kotra, District Udaipur 307 025 (Rajasthan)

Sharma, Vinita
Department of Botany, Mohan Lal Sukhadia University, Udaipur 313 002 (Rajasthan).

Shukla, Jitentra K.
Laboratory of Plant Ecology, Department of Botany, Jai Narain Vyas University, Jodhpur 302 001 (Rajasthan).

Silori, C. S.
TERI, Forestry and Biodiversity Group, New Delhi 110 003.

Singh, Anand
National Botanical Research Institute, Lucknow 226 001 (Uttar Pradesh).

Singh, B. P.
Formerly Principal Scientist and Head, Division of Germplasm Exchange, NBPGR (ICAR), New Delhi.

Singh, H. B.
Central Institute of Medicinal and Aromatic Plants, Lucknow 226015 (Uttar Pradesh).

Singh, Karan
Agricultural Research Station, Durgapura, Jaipur 302 018 (Rajasthan).

Singh, S. J.
Agricultural Research Station, Durgapura, Jaipur 302 018 (Rajasthan).

Singh, Shweta
Botanical Survey of India, Central Circle, Allahabad (Uttar Pradesh).

Siyol, U. R.
Officer in Charge, Forest Research Farm, Banki, Udaipur (Rajasthan).

Trivedi, P. C.
Department of Botany, University of Rajasthan, Jaipur 302 004 (Rajasthan).

Tyagi, Sandhya
Department of Botany, Mohan Lal Sukhadia University, Udaipur 313 002 (Rajasthan).

Vaidya, Gayatri K.
Loyola Centre for Research & Development, St. Xavier's College campus, Ahmedabad 380 009 (Gujarat).

1

Germplasm Introduction, Exchange, Collection/Evaluation and Conservation of Medicinal and Aromatic Plants—Their Export Potential

B. P. Singh

THE Indian subcontinent is one of the mega-centres of crop-plant diversity. A wide spectrum of agro-climatic and regional topography ranging from humid tropical to semi-arid, temperate to alpine, makes it to grow all types of crop plants. The country also possesses cultural and ethnic diversity, including 550 tribal communities of 227 ethnic groups, spread over 5,000 forested villages who have further contributed significantly over the millennia to the diversification of agro-biodiversity. The Indian subcontinent is a centre for domestication and diversification of plants. India has about 15,000 species of higher plants occurring in 16 major vegetation types. About 33 per cent of species are endemic. It is a treasure house of wild economic plants, which are largely under-utilised, particularly wild edible and medicinal and aromatic plants (Arora, 1996).

Fast erosion of PGR due to fast-growing population pressure causing excessive collection and exploitation has depleted the forest wealth, where most of the indigenous plant genetic resources of medicinal and aromatic plants existed/and are still prevalent—therefore there is priority needs for their exploration, collection, maintenance, evaluation and their conservation for their use for the present and the future.

India possesses about 166 species of agri-horticultural crop plants and about 324 species of wild relatives of crop plants. The World Health Organisation (WHO) has compiled a list of 20,000 medicinal plants used in different parts of the globe (Gupta and Chadha, 1995).

In all, over 7,000 plants are known to be used for medicinal and aromatic purposes in India. The heritage of medicinal plants use in India has an ancient history dating back to the pre-Vedic culture, at least 4,000 years. Today it is estimated that at least 70 per cent of the country's population rely on herbal medicines for primary health care, and many others make use of such treatments in conjunction with other forms of medical therapy. The estimates concentrate mainly on well-documented systems such as Ayurveda, Siddha and Unani as well as Homeopathy and Allopathy.

INTRODUCTION (EXCHANGE) OF PLANT GENETIC RESOURCES OF M & AP THROUGH NBPGR (ICAR), NEW DELHI

The National Bureau of Plant Genetic Resources (NBPGR) is a nodal institution in India, which has a mandate of germplasm exchange of agrihorticultural and agri-silvicultural crops/plants for research purposes, strictly under phytosanitary conditions. It has been undertaking exchange of plant genetic resources (PGR) with about 102 countries. The NBPGR has also developed strong partnership for PGR exchange with International Agricultural Research Centres (IARCs). The Bureau introduces PGR on the basis of specific requests from scientists across the country and also on the initiative of scientists of its own organisation particularly from the Division of Germplasm Exchange, who scan world literature to identify useful genetic stocks, improved cultivars recently developed as well as other useful plant genetic resources from foreign countries. It exchanges PGR with IARCs and other Plant Introduction Agencies/Organisations/Botanical gardens/ Arboretums, particularly, with which India has joint Protocols/Memoranda of Understanding (MOUs), on reciprocal basis. The main focus has been on introducing new crops, elite strains, promising genetic stocks, improved cultivars, including wild relatives of crop plants. With the enactment of the New Policy on Seed Development (1988) the Government of India has made it obligatory for all plant breeders and researchers intending to import seed/planting materials to fulfil the following two mandatory requirements of the Plants, Fruits and Seeds (Regulation of Import into India) Order 1989:

(a). "Import permit" before importing of any seed plant material.

(b). "Phytosanitary certificate" from the country of origin.

These two documents must accompany every seed/planting material consignments coming from foreign countries. The Director, NBPGR, has been authorised to issue import permits for seed plant material meant for research purposes in small quantities.

Imported seed/ plant material consignments meant for research must be addressed to the Director, NBPGR, New Delhi, only, well in advance of their sowing/planting time, etc. and should be accompanied by a "Phytosanitary Certificate" from the country of origin along with "Import Permit". The Director, NBPGR, in turn, arranges release of such consignments from concerned airlines, their Customs clearance and their quarantine examination at the point of entry. These material consignments are then again examined critically in the Plant Quarantine Division (PQ) of the NBPGR and only disease/pest-free materials are the accessioned (EC number) and repacked and forwarded to the indentor/user organisation in the country by air freight/airmail, speed post or courier service depending on the size of the consignment as well as based on urgency.

In recent years major events that have influenced germplasm exchange of PGR across the world are the Convention on Biological Diversity (CBD), agreed in 1993; and the establishment of the World Trade Organisation (WTO) in 1995. PGR, a "Heritage of mankind," has become "Sovereign rights of States." Further, the WTO recognises the Intellectual Property Rights (IPR) over the PGR. Therefore, Material Transfer Agreements (MTAs) have come to the forefront and MOUs have become essential components for germplasm exchange (Table 1).

TABLE 1
Exchange (Import/Export) of PGR of Medicinal and Aromatic Plants Through NBPGR (1976–March 2001)

Import of PGR of M&AP			Export of PGR of M&AP Plants No. of Accessions	National Supplies of PGR of M&AP No. of Accessions
No. of Accessions	No. of Genera	No. of Species		
3,809	117	361	403	1,710

(Refer: Dhillon, B. S. *et al* (Eds.). 2001 National Bureau of Plant Genetic Resources: *A Compendium of Achievements.* New Delhi: NBPGR: xvi + 329)

EXPLORATION AND COLLECTION OF PGR OF MEDICINAL AND AROMATIC PLANTS

- During the period 1975-1996, over 1,500 germplasm collections of medicinal and aromatic plants had been collected through plant explorations in some of the prominent medicinal and aromatic plants by the NBPGR, namely, Isabgol (*Plantago ovata*)—80 collections from Gujarat; opium poppy (*Papavar somniferum*)—140 collections from Gujarat, Madhya Pradesh and Uttar Pradesh; Palmarosa (*Cymbopogon martinii*)—62 collections from Maharashtra and Madhya Pradesh; Vetiver (*Vetiveria zizanioides*)—115 collections from Rajasthan and Utter Pradesh. In addition, over 550 germplasm accessions from Uttaranchal hills, and from Kerala and over 100 accessions from Kanger valley, 'Keshkal', Kanker reserve forest areas in Bastar (Chattisgarh) were also made.
- In addition to the above, 264 germplasm accessions of M&AP were also collected from Katarmiaghat, Nishangarh, Lakhimpur, Rishikesh/Haridwar, in Uttar Pradesh, Uttaranchal and Chattisgarh (reserve forest in Bastar) under G-15 collaborative project. The details have already been highlighted (Gautam *et al*, 2000, *20 Glorious Years of NBPGR 1976-1996*). These collections have been grown, maintained/ evaluated for various economic characters. Also chemical and biochemical evaluation had been carried out in case of selected accessions of over 221, particularly in case of neem (*Azadirachta indica*) and other groups of medicinal and aromatic plants.

Under Jai Vigyan National Science and Technology Mission on Conservation of Agro-biodiversity (Plant Genetic Resources), National Agricultural Technology Project (NATP) on sustainable management of plant biodiversity launched in July 1999 by NBPGR, New Delhi, in collaboration with various cooperators. Plant explorations were undertaken in various areas and over 8,300 germplasm accessions of medicinal and aromatic plants were made (during July 1999 to February 2003). Many of them are rare and endangered ones and are listed in Table 2.

EVALUATION AND UTILISATION OF GERMPLASM COLLECTIONS OF MEDICINAL AND AROMATIC PLANTS (IMPORTED AND COLLECTED WITHIN INDIA)

The main recipients of medicinal and aromatic plants germplasm introduced/collected by the NBPGR were the network of All India Co-ordinated Project on Medicinal and Aromatic Plants and

TABLE 2
Areas Explored and Major Medicinal and Aromatic Plants Collected

Areas Explored	Major Collections of Medicinal and Aromatic Plants
Moist deciduous forest of Gujarat	*Aegle, Asparagus, Bacopa, Solanum, Commiphora, Tribulus,* etc.
Simlipal reserve forest of Orissa	*Chlorophytum, Mucuna, Urgenia, Withania, Curculigo, Costus,* etc.
Northwestern Himalayan region	*Angelica, Picrorrhiza, Podophyllum, Rheum, Orchis, Taxus, Nardostachys,* etc.
Western Ghats and southern regions	*Andrographics, Chlorophytum, Gloriosa, Piper, Rauwolfia, Tylophora,* etc.

Source: Anonymous. Agro-biodiversity (PGR)-35 Technical Progress Report, NBPGR, New Delhi, 2003.

scientists handling medicinal and aromatic plants in Agricultural Universities and other centres. Besides, the Bureau too evaluated and conducted performance trials of such materials at its headquarters and some of its regional stations.

The entire range of exotic medicinal and aromatic plant materials imported was not used and conserved by any single agency. Collections were maintained to the extent possible at different institutions and locations by the specialists/scientists concerned with these crops throughout the country. The pharmaceutical industries have been dependent on the collection of raw materials from wild sources, both in India as well as abroad. As such, several of the plant collections under cultivation in India were introduced from countries like the U. S. A., USSR, Hungary, Germany, Japan, Poland, the United Kingdom, Bulgaria, Portugal, Czechoslovakia, France, Italy and Australia. Some of the important plant genetic resources introduced included *Anethum graveolens, Atropa* sp., *Glaucium flavum, Lavandula vera, Lavandula angustifolia, Matricaria chamomila, Pyrethrum* sp. and *Salvia sclarea* from Bulgaria; *Acontirum nepallus, Chrysanthemum cinerarifolium, Glycyrrhiza glabra* and *Plantago* sp. from Czechoslovakia; *Papavar bracteatum* (2n = 14), *Papavar orientale* (2n = 28) and *Papavar somniferum* (2n = 22) from Finland; *Pogostemon cablin* from Indonesia and *Apium graveolens, Artemisia annua, Datura* sp., *Glycyrrhiza glabra, Gentiana* sp., *Hypericumperforatum, Hyssopus officinalis, Lavandula angustifolia, Mentha* sp., *Ocimum* sp., *Plantago (psyllium), Salvia officinalis, Satureja holensis, Silybum marianum, Solanum laciniatum* and *Valeriana, officinalis* from Hungary and Germany.

Promising Introductions of Importance

Introduction activities resulted in selection of promising material in different medicinal and aromatic plants. The details of some of the promising introductions have been highlighted (Singh, 1988; Singh *et al*, 1989; Gupta, 1993; Gupta and Chadha, 1995; Pareek, 1998). Evaluation of these materials resulted in identification of some promising introductions in *Artemisia annua*, a native of Indo-China, with the active constituent artemisinine. This drug could be used for controlling malaria where existing anti-malarial drugs failed; leaves of EC 172510 (U. S. A.) at the flowering stage yielded artemisinine content of 0. 02 per cent. Artemisine and Arteannium are used for cerebral thrombosis in China. *Catharanthus roseus*. G. Don (syn. *Vinca rosea*), a native of Caribbean Islands in the West Indies, and naturalised all over the tropics was found to grow wild along the coastal area of Tamil Nadu, Andhra Pradesh, Karnataka, Assam and West Bengal. The leaves, rich in vincristine (VCR) and vincaleuco-blastine (VLB) could be used in the treatment of cancer. Ajmalicine and serpentine from roots are used for controlling high blood pressure. There are two other constituents, namely, vindoline and catharanthine in leaves, which could be used in synthesis of VLB analogues.

An exotic introduction, EC 120837 (USSR), rich in alkaloids was identified as promising at the NBPGR, rich in alkaloid content (Mandal and Maheshwari, 1987). In pyrethrum (*Chrysanthemum cinerarifolium*), promising introductions were EC 138836-37 (Malawi) with white and pink flowers and several accessions procured from Kenya, particularly EC 145650 was a promising type with prolific flowering. EC 115996 of foxglove (*Digitalis lanata*) from Poland was selected for higher content of glycoside in the foliage of Solan in 1983. Seventeen accessions of *Glycyrrhiza glabra* and other related species were received from various countries. Though no significant differences among accessions were recorded for root yield, EC 128587 (Pakistan) and EC 114304 (USSR) gave significantly higher glycyrrhizic acid percentage than others. *Glycyrrhiza foetidissima* (EC 144048, ex. USSR) contained a very high amount of glycyrrhizic acid (14. 87 per cent). In *Hyoscyamus muticus*, among others, EC 93928 (Germany) showed high alkaloid content of 0. 122–59 per cent.

Hyoscyamus albus, EC 85759 (Germany), showed high herbage yield of 400-500 g/plant on a fresh weight basis and 0.0850-0.1065 per cent alkaloid content (Saxena *et al,* 1979). Among *Lavandula* sp., *Lavandula stoechas* ssp. *luisieri* (EC 120176) from Portugal and *Lavandula angustifolia* (EC 165432) and (EC 154023) from the U. K. were found to establish well at Kodaikanal and flowering twigs gave an oil yield of 0.30 per cent on distillation. In *Mentha piperita*, EC 41911 (USSR) showed promise for higher herbage yield, essential oil content (0.5 per cent) and menthol (60 per cent). This accession was recommended for release for cultivation. Thirteen accessions in *Matricaria chamomila* gave promising results at Kodaikanal centre and were put for multiplication.

In anise (*Pimpinella anisum*) anethole rich collection, EC 22091 (France) was evaluated and one plant was identified best which is rich in anethole content (Pareek *et al*, 1980). *Ocimum* oil is used in perfumery and food flavouring industry. *Ocimum basilicum* (EC 176934 from France) with the highest percentage of oil (0.43 per cent) and linalool (76.86 per cent), *Papavar somniferum* (EC 196249) containing considerable amount of morphine (0. 40-0.82 per cent) and noscapine (0.12-0.27 per cent) were promising. EC 196430 with high percentage of morphine (0. 33-0.77 pr cent); papavarine (0.00-0.20 per cent), moscapine (0.33-0.04 per cent), EC 196433, morphine (0.31-0.67 per cent) and papavarine (0. 06-0.19 per cent) were introduced from Finland. In *Papavar bracteatum*, EC 196437 and EC 196438 were chemotypes varying in thebaine-alpinigenine and rich in thebaine content of 30.50 per cent and 0.48 per cent. In hops (*Humulus lupulus* L.), promising varieties like Late cluster (EC 38868, U. S. A.), *Tardifde bourgigyne* (EC 38804, Japan), Hybrid-2 (EC 3496, South Africa) and F51 (EC 39993, South Africa) were identified promising in trials conducted at Shimla. Other promising materials were *Rosemarinus* sp., EC 154021 from the U. K. with 0.10 per cent essential oil, *Solanum khasianum* and *Solanum laciniatum* (EC 113464, U. S. A.) with high solasidine content in aerial parts (0.05 per cent) and in dry berries (6.6 per cent). Some of the significant improved cultivars identified from exotic as well indigenous materials are listed in Table 3.

CONSERVATION OF PLANT DIVERSITY OF MEDICINAL AND AROMATIC PLANTS

Strategies for Conservation of Plant Genetic Resources

At present, there are 8 Government departments dealing with PGR conservation programmes in India.

1. Department of Agriculture and Cooperation (DAC), Government of India.
2. Ministry of Agriculture, Department of Agricultural Research and Education (DARE) including ICAR, Ministry of Agriculture, Government of India.
3. Department of Environment and Forest (DoE&F), Ministry of Environment and Forest, Government of India.
4. Department of Commerce (DoC), Ministry of Commerce, Government of India.
5. Ministry of Health and Family Welfare, Government of India.
6. Ministry of Textiles, Government of India.
7. Council of Scientific and Industrial Research (CSIR), Ministry of Science and Technology, Government of India.
8. Department of Biotechnology, Ministry of Science and Technology, Government of India.

Conservation of plant genetic resources involves two basic strategies, the *in-situ* and the *ex-situ*.

(a) *In-situ* conservation is the continued maintenance of plant population within its ecosystem to which it is adapted. This strategy has the potential to conserve wild relatives of crop plant species, their land races and traditional cultivars and also allow the natural forces of evolution to play their role in generating further variability for natural or conscious selection in favourable combination over generations. It allows genetic shifts to a sizeable extent giving rise to new plants. Literally 'in place', for example, conservation in natural habitat. The Ministry of Environment and Forest, Government of India, is implementing *in situ* conservation of biodiversity. The most commonly referred *in situ* conservation methods are highlighted below:

1. **Biosphere Reserves:** The Ministry of Environment and Forest, Government ofl India, had identified 14 biosphere reserves based on survey data and 7 of them have already been made operational by now (Table 4).
2. **National Parks:** Out of a total of 91 National Parks in the country, 2 have been established in Himachal Pradesh, that is, Pin Valley National Park and Great Himalayan Park in the districts of Lahaul-Spiti and Kulu, respectively.
3. In addition to the above wildlife sanctuaries (448), there are World Heritage sites (5), Wetlands (19, including 6 Ramsagar sites), Mangroves (15), Coral Reefs (4) and other areas such as sacred groves, natural monuments, ethno-biological reserves, etc. These will definitely

TABLE 3
Improved Cultivars Identified, Developed/Superior Selections Made in Medicinal and Aromatic Plants

Local Name	Botanical Name	Improved Cultivars/Superior Selection
Isabgol	*Plantago ovata*	Gujarat Isabgol-1, Gujarat Isabgol-2
Opium poppy	*Papavar somniferum*	Jawahar Aphium-16 (JA-16), Trishna(I.C. 402), Shaktiman, Kirtiman, Chetak=Aphium, E.C. 179777, E.C. 196430 (Finland), E.C. 196433 (Hungary), Sujata (Opium less and alkaloid free poppy)
Senna	*Cassia angustifolia*	ALFT 2
Periwinkle	*Catharanthus roseus*	E.C. 120837 (Russia), I.C. 49581
Liquorice	*Glycyrrhiza glabra*	E.C. 114304 (Russia), E.C. 41911 E.C. 128587 (Pakistan)
Asgandh	*Withania somnifera*	R.S.I. Jawahar Asgand-20 (WS-20)
Jasmine	*Jasminum grandiflorum*	Pitchi (Co.)
Palmarosa	*Cymbopogan martini* var. *motia*	I.W. 31245
Vetiver/khus	*Vetiveria zizanioides*	For root yield: Hyb. 9, Hyb. 8, Hyb. 26, NC. 66403, NC 66404, NC 66415. For oil yield: Hyb. 8, NC 66403, NC 66416
Lemon grass	*Cymbopogon flexuosus*	O.D. 15, O.D. 19, Pragati
Rose geranium	*Pelargonium graveolens*	NIC 23414—an Algerian type
Patchouli	*Pogostemon patchouli*	
Introductory Crops		
Henbane	*Hyoscymus muticus,* *H. niger*	E.C. 93928 I.C. 66
Chamomilla	*Matricaria chamomilla*	E.C. 217012 (Romania)
Sage	*Salvia officinalis*	E.C. 314321
Basil/Tulsi	*Ocimum basilicum*	I.C. 75730, E.C. 176934 (France)
Lavender	*Lavendula officinalis*	E.C. 120176 (Portugal), E.C. 16543, E.C. 15023 (U. K.)
Rosemary	*Rosemarinus officinalis* *Melissa officinalis*	E.C. 273873 E.C. 273873
Mints	*Mentha* sp.	*M. piperita:* E.C. 41911 (Russia), E.C. 41912, Siwalik *M. longifolia:* E.C.390182 (U. S. A.), *M. spicata* - PBVPBY

Continued...

...Continued

Local Name	Botanical Name	Improved Cultivars/Superior Selection
Native Species		
Mucuna/kawanch	*Mucuna pruriens*	
Gwarpatha/Aloe	*Aloe barbedensis*	
Giloe	*Tinospora cordifolia*	I.C. 281970, I.C. 281959, I.C. 281872
Celastrus	*Celastrus paniculatus*	
Piplamool	*Piper longum*	Cheemathippali
Satwari	*Asparagus racemosus*	
Guggal	*Commiphora wightii*	
Babchi/Psoralea	*Psoralea cordifolia*	I.C. 111249, I.C. 111238, I.C. 11246
Safed musli	*Chlorophytum borivillianum*	
Annis	*Pimpinella anisum*	E.C. 22091
Sarpagandha	*Rauwolfia serpentina*	R.S. 1
Steroidal yarns	*Dioscorea floribunda*	PB(c) 1, Arka Upkar
Khasi kateli	*Solanum viarum*	Arka Sanjeevani
Kangaroo Keali	*Solanum laciniatum*	E.C. 113465

serve in conserving biodiversity in their respective regions (Chauhan, 2001; Singh, 2002).

The other complementary methods of *in-situ* conservation are:

4. **On-Farm Conservation:** On-Farm Conservation involves the maintenance of traditional crop cultivars (land races) or farming systems by farmers within the traditional agricultural system (Hodgkin *et al*, 1993; Ramanatha Rao, 1997). Traditional farmers use land races, which are developed by the farmer and well adapted to the local environment (Harlan, 1992). This method of conservation has been gaining importance in recent years, though farmers have used it for centuries. In case of agrobiodiversity, the effects of growers practices are of paramount importance. Systemic documentation of farmers' knowledge of diversity and usages is needed.
5. **Home Gardens:** Home garden conservation is very similar to on-farm conservation, however scale is much smaller. In rural situations, home gardens tend to contain a wide spectrum of species such as vegetables, fruits, medicinal and spice plants.
6. Zero energy input based concept of parafrost conservation in the Himalayan region which remains covered with snow.

TABLE 4
Identified and Operational Biosphere Reserves

Biographic Region	Biosphere Reserve	Area (sq. km)	States Involved
Operational			
Himalayan highlands	Nanda Devi	1,560	Uttaranchal (Garhwal Hills)
Indo-Myanmar	Nokrek	80	Meghalaya Region, N-E
Monsoon Bengalian	Manas	2,837	Assam
Rain Forest Zone	Sunderbans	9,630	West Bengal
Corromandal Regions	Gulf of Mannar	555	Tamil Nadu
Malabar (Western Ghats)	Neelgiri	5,520	Karnataka, Kerala, T. Nadu
Andaman & Nicobar Islands	Great Nicobar	885	Andaman & Nicobar Islands
Identified Sites			
North-Eastern Hills	Namdapha	4,500	Arunachal Pradesh
Uttaranchal	Valley of Flowers	2,000	Uttaranchal
North-Eastern Hills	Kaziranga	760	Assam
Rajputana	Thar Desert	760	Rajasthan
Central India	Kanha	760	Madhya Pradesh
Western India	Rann of Kutch	5,000	Gujarat

Source: Country Report on Status of Plant Genetic Resources: India. In process of demarcation and delineation.

(b). Ex-situ Conservation

It refers to when conservation of PGR is attempted outside or away from their natural habitat such as

I. Seed storage in gene banks;
2. Cryo preservation (in liquid nitrogen –165°C to –196°C) of seeds, pollen, shoot tips, etc.;
3. *In vitro* (tissue culture) technology/repository;
4. Conservation of DNA at –20°C;
5. Botanical gardens/Arboreta; and
6. Field gene bank (field repository/clonal repository).

(i). Gene Bank: Storage in the form of seed (Base collection at –20°C; Active collection at +4°C to 10°C). The three national gene banks have been established in India for *ex situ* conservation of medicinal and aromatic plants.

(a) National Bureau of Plants Genetic Resources (NBPGR), New Delhi, under ICAR.

(b) Central Institute of Medicinal and Aromatic Plants (CIMAP), Lucknow, Uttar Pradesh, under the Council of Scientific Industrial Research (CSIR), Ministry of Science and Technology, Government of India.

(c) Tropical Botanical Gardens Research Institute, (TBGRI), Palode, Thiruvananthapuram (Kerala).

The conservation of genetic variability of cultivated plants and their wild relatives is the sole responsibility of the National Bureau of Plant Genetic Resources (NBPGR) that operates under the Indian Council of Agricultural Research (ICAR), Department of Agricultural Research and Education (DARE).

THE NATIONAL GENE BANK (NGB) AT NBPGR, NEW DELHI

i. Seed Gene Bank

Germplasm conservation in Seed Gene Bank is more economical. The NBPGR, New Delhi, houses National Gene Bank (NGB) which is primarily responsible for conservation of germplasm of agri-horticultural crops and their wild relatives for long-term seed storage for posterity. These are referred to as "Base Collection" stored in modules maintained at –20°C. The seeds are dried to attain 4-6 per cent moisture content and hermetically sealed in moisture proof aluminium foil packets. These stored seeds remain viable for 50 to 100 years. In most crops, seeds samples with more than 85 per cent seed viability are only processed. The seeds in gene bank are stored preferably as per the gene bank standards recommended by FAO/IPGRI.

The Indian NGB has 12 modules with a capacity to hold around one million accessions. The present base collection holdings in the NGB on December 31, 2001, are 209,493 accessions (Table 5).

National Active Germplasm Sites

The national active germplasm sites (NAGS) are the integral component of the network. There are presently 40 NAGS, which are based at ICAR institutes, (crop-based institutes for a specific crop or a group of crops) and SAUs. These are integral part of national plant biodiversity conservation network. The NAGS are entrusted with the responsibility of multiplication, evaluation, maintenance and the conservation of active collection and their distribution to bonafide users both at the national and international levels. These active/working collections are stored in modules maintained at +4°C and 35-40 per cent relative humidity (RH). Under these temperatures, seeds are expected to remain viable for 15 to 50 years. For medium term storage, seed moisture content is brought down to 8 to 10 per cent. The NBPGR has a network of 11 regional stations located in different agroclimatic zones of the country to support the active germplasm conservation activities of the regions. The total holdings of these 40 National Active Germplasm sites (NAGS) as on 31st December 2001 are listed in Table 6.

ii. Cryopreservation (in liquid nitrogen at –165°C to –196°C)

Cyropreservation or freeze preservation under liquid nitrogen.

(a). **Seed Preservation:** The seeds have been grouped broadly into two categories, based on their response to dehydration (Roberts, 1972). A majority of them are

TABLE 5
Plant Germplasm Holdings in the Indian National Seed Genebank at National Bureau of Plant Genetic Resources, New Delhi (as on December 31, 2001)

Crop Group	Species (No.)	Accessions (No.)
Cereals	7	96,915
Millets and forages	11	17,448
Pseudo cereals	4	2,546
Grain legumes	24	33,393
Oilseeds	9	26,099
Fibre crops	6	6,755
Vegetables	28	10,324
Fruits	6	139
Medicinal and aromatic plants	82	814
Narcotics	1	778
Spices and condiments	5	2,126
Genetic stocks	43+	194
Released varieties	89	1,770
Duplicate safety samples	22++	10,192
Total	199	209,493

\+ Thirty-eight species are common with those listed under various crops; only five are additional.

++ Species are included in the respective crops/crop groups.

desiccation tolerant, called 'Orthodox' and hence can be stored for longer durations. The second group of plant species are called 'Recalcitrant', whose seeds suffer injury on their drying and therefore cannot be stored at subzero temperatures. In the 'Cryobank' of NBPGR, New Delhi, so far 365 species of 140 genera have been cryopreserved (as on 31st March 2001). The details are given in Table 7.

(b) **Pollen Preservation:** Pollen storage was mainly developed as a tool for controlled pollination of synchronous flowering in plants, especially in fruit tree species. In addition, pollen storage has also been considered as an emerging technology for genetic conservation (Harrington, 1970; Robert, 1975; Withers, 1991). Pollen can easily be collected and cryopreserved in large quantities in relatively small spaces. Exchange of germplasm through pollen poses fewer plant quarantine problems. In recent years, cryopreservation techniques have been developed for pollen in a large number of species (Towil, 1985) and cryobank of pollen has been established for fruit-tree species in several countries (Alexander and Ganeshan, 1993).

iii. *In vitro* (on Tissue Culture) Conservation

The essential prerequisites for an *in vitro* conservation programme are creation of special

TABLE 6
Crop Germplasm Holdings of 40 National Active Germplasm Sites (NAGS)

Crop(s)	Institute	Accessions (No.)
Field Crops		
Cotton	Central Institute of Cotton Research Nagpur[4]	8,768
Crops of N-E Region	ICAR, Research Complex, Northest Hill Region, Shillong	–
Fodder Crops	Indian Grassland and Fodder Research Institute, Jhansi[4]	6,267
Groundnut	NRC[1] on Groundnut, Junagarh[4]	6,437
Jute and Allied Fibres	Central Research Institute for Jute and Allied Fibres, Barrackpore (W. B.)	3,226
Maize	Project Directorate on Maize, IARI, New Delhi	2,500
Oilseeds	Directorate of Oilseeds Research, Hyderabad[4]	10,550
Pearlmillet	AICRIP[2] on Pearlmillet, Jodhpur	2,794
Pulses	Indian Institute of Pulses Research, Kanpur[4]	5,021
Rapeseed and Mustard	NRC on Rapeseed and Mustard, Bharatpur	8,082
Rice	Central Rice Research Institute, Cuttack[4]	24,000
Rice and Lathyrus	Indira Gandhi Krishi Viswavidyalaya, Raipur	15,000
Small millets	AICRP on Small Millets, Bangalore[4]	8,572
Sorghum	NRC on Sorghum, Hyderabad	7,366
Soybean	NRC on Soybean, Indore	2,500
Sugarcane	Sugarcane Breeding Institute, Coimbatore	5,861
Tobacco	Central Tobacco Research Institute, Rajahmundry	1,500
Under-utilised crops	NBPGR Headquarters, New Delhi[4]	199
Wheat and Barley	Dirctorate of Wheat Research, Karnal[4]	7,000
Horticultural/Agroforestry Crops		
Agroforestry sp.	NRC on Agroforestry, Jhansi	40
Arid fruits	NRC on Arid Horticulture, Bikaner	1,923
Banana	NRC on Banana, Tiruchrapalli	907
Cashew	NRC on Cashew, Puttur, Dakshin Kannada	433
Citrus species	NRC on Citrus, Nagpur	51
Grapes	NRC on Grapes, Pune	660
Leechi, Bael, Aonla, Jackfruit and other horticultural crops[3]	Central Horticultural Experimental Station, Ranchi Indian Institute of Horticulture Research, Bangalore 560089	2,426
Medicinal and Aromatic Plants	NRC on Medicinal and Aromatic Plants, Anand	120

Continued...

...*Continued*

Crop(s)	Institute	Accessions (No.)
Mango	Central Institute for Sub-tropical Horticulture, Lucknow	587
Mulberry	Central Silk and Mulberry Genetic Resources Centre, Hosur	
Oil Palm	NRC on Oil Palm, Eluru	119
Onion and Garlic	NRC on Onion and Garlic, Nasik	1,066
Orchids	NRC for Orchids, Gangtok	225
Ornamentals and Non-traditional crops[3]	National Botanical Research Institute, Lucknow	
Plantation crops	Central Plantation Crops Research Institute, Kesargod	522
Potato	Central Potato Research Institute, Shimla	2,500
Spices	Indian Institute of Spices Research, Calicut	6,055
Temperate horticultural crops[3]	Central Institute of Temperate Horticulture, Srinagar/NBPGR Regional Station, Shimla	
Tropical fruits	Indian Institute of Horticulture Research, Bangalore	11,467
Tuber Crops	Central Tuber Crops Research Institute, Thiruvanthapuram	3,871
Vegetables	Indian Institute of Vegetables Research, Varanasi[4]	16,139

[1] AICRIP (All India Coordinated Research Project.

[2] NRC (National Research Centre).

[3] Figures not available.

[4] With medium term storage facility.

facilities (culture rooms with controlled environment, artificial lights, laminar airflow cabinets, autoclave, etc.) and trained scientists and technicians. Information on the *in vitro* multiplication and/or conservation protocols of those plant species is also desirable. Any *in vitro* conservation programme primarily comprises two stages: (i). *in-vitro* multiplication to build up a large number of plants, and (ii) *in vitro* storage. The material stored *in vitro* may be in the form of meristems, shoot tips, axillary buds, embryos, and even callus and cell suspension. *In vitro* gene banks are easy to maintain and often inexpensive provided effective storage systems are developed.

Development of Conservation Protocols

Various slow growth strategies such as low temperature incubation, use of osmotic agents, growth retardant, nutritional or hormonal manipulations were evaluated for different crop species at NBPGR. The status of *in vitro* conserved germplasm at NBPGR (as on 31st March 2001) is listed in Table 8.

TABLE 7
Status of Cryopreserved Germplasm at National Cryobank (–196°C) at NBPGR, New Delhi (as on March 31, 2001)

Crop Groups	Accessions* (No.)
Cereals and pseudocereals	190
Millets	151
Grain legumes	419
Oilseeds	211
Vegetables	246
Fruits and nuts	269
Spices and condiments	51
Narcotics	4
Medicinal plants	320
Fibre crops	17
Fodder crops	2
Plantation crops	4
Aromatic crops	109
Wild crops	98
Agro-forestry species	985
Total	3,076

* Total number of species 365.

iv. DNA Storage (Conservation at –20°C)

Storage of DNA is, in principle, simple to carry out and widely applicable. The storage of DNA seems to be relatively easy and cheap. In recent years genetic engineering has resulted in breaking down the species and genus barriers for transferring genes. Transgenic plants have been produced with genes transferred from viruses, bacteria and fungi and even mice. These efforts have led to the establishment of DNA Libraries (Mattick *et al*, 1992). Necessary strategies and procedures have to be developed on how to use the material stored in the form of DNA.

v. Botanical Gardens/Arboreta

A botanical garden is an institution holding documented collection of living plants for the purpose of scientific research, conservation, display and education (Jackson, 1999). They serve as repositories of germplasm collections, specially rare and endangered ones of indigenous and exotic origin (Sharma and Goel, 1994). Botanic Garden Conservation International (BGCI), an international organisation with its headquarters in London (U. K.) was established in 1987 for global co-operation and monitoring the conservation programmes of the botanical gardens. The BGCI has 500 member botanical gardens in 111 countries all over the world (Jackson, 2000). There are about 1,846 botanical gardens worldwide as per the BGCI database. About 4 million accessions are currently held by botanical gardens worldwide (Roy, 2001).

TABLE 8
Status of *in vitro* Conserved Germplasm at NBPGR, New Delhi
(as on March 31, 2001)

Crop	Storage Temp. (°C)	Optimum (months) Subculture Interval	Accessions (No.)
Tuber and Bulb Crops			
Allium sativum	25,4	16-20	97
Allium sp.	25,10,4	12-22	14
Alocasia sp.	25	10	1
Colocasia esculenta	25	8-10	49
Dioscorea sp.	25	8-12	44
Ipomoea batatas	25	8-12	260
Xanthosoma sagittifolium	25	10	3
Spices and Industrial Plants			
Curcuma sp.	25	6-10	53
Elettaria sp.	25	15	5
Fagara schinifolia	25	6	1
Humulus lupulus	25	–	8
Piper sp.	25	10-22	7
Vanilla planifolia	25	6	5
Simmondsia chinensis	25	6	12
Zingiber sp.	25	8-24	160
Fruits			
Actinidia chinensis	25	8	3
Musa sp.	25	8-12	350
Fragaria sp.	25	8-10	20
Prunus sp.	25	4	2
Rubus sp.	25	8-10	5
Malus sp.	25	3-4	3
Medicinal and Aromatic Plants			
Bacopa monneieri	25	6	1
Coleus forskohlii	25	12	7
Digitalis sp.	4	11	5
Eremostachys superba	25	6	2
Gentiana kuroo	4	12	1
Mentha sp.	25	12	22
Picrorrhiza kurroa	4	12	4

Continued...

...Continued

Crop	Storage Temp. (ºC)	Optimum (months) Subculture Interval	Accessions (No.)
Pogostemon patchouli	25	12	1
Pyncnanthemum sp.	25	6	4
Rauwolfia serpentina	25	22	6
Rauwolfia canescens	25	22	1
Rheum moorcroftianum	4	12	1
Saussurea lappa	4	11	2
Swertia chirayta	4	6	2
Tylophora indica	25	12	2
Valeriana wallichii	4	12	4
Total			1,138

Source: Dhillon, B. S., Varaprasad, K. S., Kalyani Srinivasan, Mahendra Singh, Sunil Archak, Umesh Srivastava and Sharma, G. D. (Eds.). National Bureau of Plant Genetic Resources, New Delhi, pp. xvi+329..

vi. Field Gene Bank (FGB)/Field Repository/Clonal Repository

Plant genetic resources of perennial fruit plants/many ornamentals and forestry plants are maintained by vegetative propagation in order to maintain their genetic makeup true to the type. In cases of fruit germplasm collections, usually conservation is done in field gene bank, which were known as varietal collections, living collections or clonal repositories. FGBs may run a risk of being damaged by natural calamities, infections, neglect or abuse. The field gene bank in tree species requires a substantial number of plants per germplasm collection and are relatively expensive to maintain. However, FGBs provide easy and ready access to conserve material for research as well as for their use.

This country needs to develop such field gene banks on the pattern of clonal germplasm repositories in the U. S. A.

6. EXPORT OF MEDICINAL AND AROMATIC PLANTS—INDIAN PERSPECTIVE

EXIM (Export/Import) Policy of the Government of India 1997-2002 and revised 2002-2007 (effective from April 1, 2003).

1. The export and import of seeds/planting materials (of agri horticultural/forestry plants, etc.) are governed by the provisions of the Export and Import Policy of the Government of India; 56 plant species including some medicinal plants are prohibited from export. However, if they are cultivated, a certificate from the designated forest authorities in this regard is essential to export either in raw form or as value added formulations/extraction or derivatives. These species covered under the EXIM policy, include 6 species of Appendix 1 and 15 of Appendix of CITES (Conservation of International Trade in Endangered Species) permit, besides

a certificate of cultivation, origin from the designated forest authorities.

2. The export of all other species of wild origin not covered under the Wildlife Protection Act 1992 and EXIM policy is permitted only upon furnishing of legal procurement certificate from the designated forest authorities.

- 1995: WTO came into force, quarantine concerns in trade started, sanitary and Phytosanitary (SPS) agreement of WTO signed.

- Sanitary and Phytosanitary measures

The phytosanitation aspects of PGR needs to be properly addressed. The National Plant Quarantine System needs strengthening on a priority basis.

Elements of the SPS Agreement

Transparency: members are required to

(a). publish their SPS regulations;

(b). to notify WTO if there are significant changes in regulations; and

(c). to use scientific data in preparation of risk analysis.

Developing Pest Risk Analysis and Identifying Pest Free Areas

For the successful implementation of SPS, each member country has to undertake Pest Risk Analysis (PRA) for all the export and import of agricultural commodities (including medicinal and aromatic plants).

The burden of demonstration of disease-free areas rests on the exporting member. India may not be able to compete in export of agriculture commodities, unless it meets the standards in the near future. We have to develop not only national standards for SPS, but also a system for their notification, particularly to promote export. We must also examine various possibilities for information dissemination. This will help in monitoring the SPS measures.

SPS measures need to be modified from time to time, as the new scientific facts become available and conditions change both for inclusion of provisions for new pests or removal of those found to be redundant. In the exercise for developing PRA, pest-free areas need to be identified whenever it is possible. This will be of great help in policy decisions for optimum utilisation of diminishing land resources. The developed countries such as the U. S. A., Australia and New Zealand have already geared up their activities to develop and furnish PRA for their exports. It is high time that India should not lag behind in developing PRA, otherwise its agricultural trade will be adversely affected leading to a huge loss in export earnings and would lag behind our competitions in market penetration. Besides such an eventuality may drag the country into their trade disputes and in litigation at WTO (Gupta *et al*, 2002).

Fixing of Maximum Residue Limits

Pesticide residues in commodities have become a major concern for exports and imports and it is necessary to minimise risk to human health due to pesticides. Maximum Residue Limited (MRLs) are applied to domestic and imported produce. These residue limits and unauthorised pesticides are the most common cause of refusal of consignments in the country. The MRLs vary from country to country. These create impediments to trade. India needs to develop its standards, which should be based on the extent necessary to protect our plant and animal health based on scientific data and international standards.

Consideration for Planting Material and Germplasm

SPS measures are supposed to be developed for export and import of commodities, and not for the exchange of planting material and/or germplasm. One should be equally vigilant, sometimes commodities may, intentionally or unintentionally, find their way to agriculture land. We should also look into the requirements of exchange of germplasm and planting material and the end product of which may ultimately assume the form of commodities.

Networking

There is an urgent need to develop an information network through:

(a). Linkage with codex committees, OIE, IPPC, FAO, WHO, WTO, ISO, etc.;

(b). Coordination mechanism involving planning and network system; and

(c). Dissemination of information on standards and codes of practices.

Harmonisation

The Indian SPS measures should be in harmony with international standards and followed by neighbouring and other countries, which have a similar agricultural system. This can be done only when we have our well-defined SPS agreement.

Upgradation of the National Quarantine Set-Up

It is difficult to have an ideal quarantine system. We have to strive hard to get the best and act fast to face the emerging problems. For this, we have to look at our National Plant Protection Organisation in totality. We have to upgrade its manpower and infrastructure to bring it up to the international standard. A National Plant Quarantine Information System (NPQIS) should be established to develop a national data base on RPA, quarantine methodologies, policies and related issues (Khetarpal and Rajan, 1999).

The export of seeds requires advance planning and intensive marketing efforts. The present export policy is designed, based on the exigencies of domestic requirements and supply situation. Under the EXIM policy, plants, fruits and seeds are placed in the restricted items for import. However, import of seeds is regularised through New Policy on Seed Development, 1988.

Export of Indian Medicinal Plant Products

According to World Health Organisation (WHO) estimates, the present demand for medicinal plants is about US $ 14 billion a year, and projected demand by the year 2050 is likely to be US dollars 5 trillion. Medicinal plant related trade in India is estimated to be around Rs. 550 crore/year, while the value of global trade in medicinal plants has been put at over US $ 60 billion per year. India's total turnover of Rs. 2,300 crore of Ayurvedic and herbal products, major over-the-counter (OTC) products contribute around Rs. 1,200 crore. Other formulations fetch around Rs. 650 crore, and classical Ayurvedic formulations contribute the remaining Rs. 450 crore. With world demand growing at 1 per cent annually, the export market for medicinal plants appears to be growing faster than the Indian domestic market.

According to a UNIDO study, the following constraints are associated with the use of the traditional medicine sector in developing countries including India.

- Poor agricultural practices.
- Poor harvesting and post-harvest practices.
- Lack of research on development of high-yielding varieties in many medicinal and aromatic plants.
- Poor propagation methods.
- Inefficient processing techniques leading to low yields and poor quality products.
- Poor quality control procedures.
- High energy losses during processing.
- Lack of current good manufacturing practices.
- Difficulties in marketing.
- Lack of local market for primary processed products.
- Lack of trained personnel and equipment.
- Lack of facilities to fabricate equipment locally.
- Lack of access to latest technological and market information.

Exports of finished products, rather than of crude material should be encouraged. The cosmetics industry as well as aromatherapy are two important areas where Indian medicinal plants or the value added extracts or essential oil can contribute a lot globally. India will have to develop its marketing skills with suitable strategies. Integrated approach to promote export of medicinal and aromatic plants from India right from the state of research, cultivation, collection, storage, processing and proper packaging and marketing, in a well-organised manner, which requires help from leading pharmaceutical companies/Apeda. India has not able to capitalise on its herbal wealth by promoting its use in the developed countries, despite their renewed interests in herbal medicines. This can by achieved by judicious product identification based on diseases found or prevalent in the developed world for which no medicines are available. Such herbal medicine will find steady access into those countries. Indian embassies located in these foreign countries could play an important role.

The Basic Requirements for gaining entry or access into developed countries include:

i. Well documented traditional use;

ii. Single plant medicines;

iii. Medicinal plants free from pesticides/diseases, etc.

iv. Standardisation based on chemical activity profiles; and

v. Safety and stability.

TABLE 9
Some Medicinal Plants Exported from India

No.	Plant Species	Part Exported
1.	*Plantago ovata*	Seed, husk
2.	*Cassia angustifolia*	Leaf, pod
3.	*Rheum australe*	Rhizome
4.	*Inula racemosa*	Rhizome
5.	*Rauwolfia serpentina*	Root
6.	*Hedychium spicatum*	Rhizome
7.	*Zingiber officinale*	Rhizome
8.	*Colchicum luteum*	Rhizome, seed
9.	*Valeriana wallichii*	Rhizome
10.	*Acorus calamus*	Rhizome
11.	*Adhatoda vasica*	Whole plant
12.	*Juglans regia*	Bark
13.	*Punica granatum*	Flower, root, bark
14.	*Barberis aristata*	Root
15.	*Juniperus communis*	Fruit
16.	*Juniperus macropoda*	Fruit
17.	*Heracleum candicans*	Rhizome
18.	*Picrorrhiza kurroa*	Root
19.	*Aconitum* sp.	Root
20.	*Saussurea lappa*	Rhizome
21.	*Swertia chirayita*	Whole plant
22.	*Podophyllum emodi*	Rhizome

Source: Srivastava, J. J., Lambert and Vietmeryer, N (1995). *Medicinal Plants: A Growing Role in Development.* The World Bank, Washington DC., U. S. A.: Department of Agriculture and Forestry Systems.

In conclusion, the other important points which need priority attention are:

1. Cultivation practices/cropping system of medicinal and aromatic plants: Efforts should be made to introduce these crops in the cropping system, as an inter-crop, catch crop, border crop, under crop, in partial shade in orchards and developing suitable cultivation practices for such conditions.

2. Quality Control: Post-harvest processing for quality procedure, storage, proper handling of harvested produce and their proper storage becomes very important in order to maintain quality produce. Proper stage conditions in order to check the losses in potency of M&AP, including optimum stage for harvest, drying condition, moisture content, grading, packaging and transportation.

TABLE 10
Threatened Medicinal Plants of India

No.	Name	Family	Present Status
1.	*Aconitum deinorrhizum*	Ranunculaceae	Almost extinct
2.	*Aconitum heterophyllum*	Ranunculaceae	Greatly threatened
3.	*Angelica glauca*	Umbelliferae (Apiaceae)	Threatened
4.	*Arnebia benthemii*	Boraginaceae	Threatened
5.	*Artemisia brevifolia*	Compositae (Asteraceae)	Likely to be threatened
6.	*Artemisia meritima*	Compositae (Asteraceae)	Threatened
7.	*Atropa acuminata*	Solanaceae	Threatened
8.	*Berberis aristata*	Berberidaceae	Greatly threatened
9.	*Bunium persicum*	Umbelliferae (Apiaceae)	Threatened
10.	*Colchicum luteum*	Liliaceae	Threatened
11.	*Corydalis govaniana*	Papavaraceae	Likely to be threatened
12.	*Dactrylorhiza hatagirea*		Threatened
13.	*Dioscorea deltoidea*	Dioscoreaeaceac	Threatened
14.	*Ephedra gerardiana*	Gnetaceae	Likely to be threatened
15.	*Ferula jaeschkeana*	Umbelliferae (Apiaceae)	Threatened
16.	*Gentiana kurroa*	Gentianaceae	Threatened
17.	*Hedychium spicatum*	Zingiberaceae	Likely to be threatened
18.	*Jurinea dolomiaea*	Compositae (Asteraceae)	Likely to be threatened
19.	*Nardostachys jatamansi*	Valerianaceae	Threatened
20.	*Orchis latifolia*	Orchidaceae	Threatened
21.	*Picrorrhiza kurroa*	Scrophulariaceae	Likely to be threatened
22.	*Podophyllum emodi*	Berberidaceae	Threatened
23.	*Rheum emodi*	Polygonaceae	Threatened
24.	*Swertia chirayita*	Gentianaceae	Threatened
25.	*Valeriana wallichii*	Valerianaceae	Likely to be threatened
26.	*Xanthoxylum alatum*	Polygonaceae	Likely to be threatened

Source: Nayar, M. P., and Shastry, A. R. K. (1960). *Red Data Book of Indian Plants.* Vol. 3, Botanical Survey of India.

3. Chemistry of raw material and development of proper analytical procedures and reliable equipment and their servicing facilities.

4. Seed production in ideal areas, free from pests and diseases.

5. Emerging new plant drugs.

6. Certificate of raw materials: A valid methodology for certification of M&AP.

TABLE 11
List of Priority Species Identified by the Ministry of Health and Family Welfare, Government of India

No.	Botanical Name	Common Name
1.	*Acontium chasmanthum*	Vatsnabh
2.	*Aconitum heterophyllum*	Ativisha
3.	*Aconitum napellus*	Monk's Hood
4.	*Aegle marmelos*	Bilva
5.	*Anacyclus pyrethrum*	Akarkarha
6.	*Arnica montena*	Leopard's Bane
7.	*Asparagus racemosus*	Shatavari
8.	*Asparagus adscandens*	Safed Musli
9.	*Carum carvi*	Krishnajirak
10.	*Celastrus paniculatus*	Jyotishmati
11.	*Commiphora mukul*	Guggulu
12.	*Convolvulus scammonia*	Saqmonia
13.	*Coptis teeta*	Mamiran
14.	*Crocus sativus*	Kesara
15.	*Desmodium gangeticum*	Salparni
16.	*Glycyrrhiza glabra*	Yastimadhu
17.	*Gmelina aroborea*	Gambhari
18.	*Hemidesmus indicus*	Anantmool
19.	*Hydrastis canadensis*	Golden Seal
20.	*Illicium verum*	Badiyan Khatai
21.	*Mesua ferrea*	Nagkesar
22.	*Myristica fragrans*	Jatiphyala
23.	*Nardostachys grandiflora*	Jatamansi
24.	*Onosma bracteatum*	Gaozaban
25.	*Oroxylum indicum*	Syonak
26.	*Picrorrhiza kurroa*	Kukti
27.	*Pilocarpus jaborandi*	Jaborandi
28.	*Piper longum*	Pippali
29.	*Pistacia lentiscus*	Mastagi Roomi
30.	*Pluchea lanceolata*	Rasna
31.	*Plumbago zelyanica*	Chitrak

Continued...

...*Continued*

No.	Botanical Name	Common Name
32.	a. *Premna integrifolia*	Agnimanth
	b. *Premna micronata*	Agnimanth
33.	*Saraca indica*	Ashoka
34.	*Saussurea lappa*	Kushtha
35.	*Senecio cinerraria*	Dusti Miller
36.	*Smilax china*	Chobchini
37.	*Stereospermum suaveolens*	Patola
38.	*Swertiya chirayita*	Chirayatha
39.	*Terminalia arjuna*	Arjuna
40.	*Tinospora sinensis*	Guduchi
41.	*Uraria picta*	Prishniparni
42.	*Valeriana jatamansi*	Tagar
43.	*Viburnum opulus*	Grandberry Highbush
44.	*Viola serens*	Banafsha
45.	*Zizyphus sativa*	Unnab

7. Proper policies, incentives, regulatory framework, research support, market support and market information.

8. Export credit, export promotion activities, tax rebate, brand building are some of the activities required to be taken on priority to promote medicinal plant product export.

9. Developing the export market will require innovative measures. There is need to consolidate, mobilise and organise the medicinal plant sector.

The world would look to India as a source of supply, and for India, global market is almost given. While India has the knowledge, skill and resources, it has neglected the opportunities in the global market. We have to gear up to face the challenges given by China and Korea in this sector. Industry needs to focus on exportable packages and services.

India mainly exports parts of 22 plant species (Table 9) but the quantitative information on these exports is not available.

The recent thrust on reverting to natural products, most of which have been over-exploited with little or no regard to the future and increasing consumer demand and indiscriminate harvest of wild growing plants mostly from forest areas has led to the situation wherein a number of these plants have appeared in the endangered list of plants (Red Data Book) published by the Botanical survey of India (1990). There are about 26 medicinal plants which are threatened with extinction and have become rare or endangered which have been listed in Table 10.

The Department of Indian System of Medicine and Homeopathy of the Ministry of Health and Family Welfare, Government of India, has a Central Scheme for the Cultivation and Development of Medicinal Plants in which 45 species of medicinal plants (enumerated in Table 11) have been identified for promoting their cultivation in order to reduce pressure on their natural habitat and to meet the shortage in their demand by the industry involved in producing the ISM and Homeopathy medicines.

REFERENCES

Alexander, M. P. and Ganeshan, S. 'Pollen storage'. In: *Advances in Horticulture.* Vol. 1. *Fruit Crops*-part 1. (Eds.). Chadha, K. L. and Pareek, O. P. New Delhi: Malhotra Publishing House, pp. 481-496, 1993.

Anonymous. *Agro Biodiversity (PGR).* 35th Technical Progress Report, NBPGR, New Delhi, 2003.

Arora, R. K. 'Indian region provides treasure house of wild plant resources'. *Diversity* 12(3): 22-23, 1996.

Chauhan, N. S. 'Genetic diversity of medicinal and aromatic plants of Himalayan region (Himachal Pradesh) and its conservation'. *Indian J. Plant Genet Resour.* 14(2): 318-322, 2001.

Dhillon, B. S., Varaprasad, K. S., Srinivasan, Kalyani; Singh, Mahendra; Archak, Sunil; Srivastava, Umesh and Sharma, G. D. (Eds.). *A Compendium of Achievements.* New Delhi: National Bureau of Plant Genetic Resources, pp. xxi, 329, 2001.

Gautam, P. L., Sharma, G. D., Umesh Srivastava; Singh, B. M., Kumar, Ashok; Saxena, R. K. and Srinivasan, Kalyani (Eds.). *20 Glorious Years of NBPGR (1976-1996).* New Delhi: NBPGR, 2000.

Gupta, Kavita; Pandey, B. M. and Khetrapal, 'Pest risk analysis and its significance in India under WTO regime'. *Seed Tech. News* 32(2 & 3): 266-269, 2002.

Gupta, R. 'Medicinal and aromatic plants in India'. In: *Proceedings of the Regional Expert Consultation on Breeding and Improvement of Medicinal and Aromatic Plants in Asia.* (Eds.). Chom-Chalow, Norong and Henie, Hans V. Bangkok: FAO Regional Office for Asia Pacific (RAPA), pp. 117-130, 1993.

Gupta, R. and Chadha, K. L. 'Medicinal and aromatic plants in India'. In: *Advances in Horticulture*, vol. 11, *Medicinal and Aromatic Plants.* (Eds.). Chadha, K. L. and Gupta, R. New Delhi: Malhotra Publishing House, pp. 199-222, 1995.

Harlan, J. R. *Crops and Man 1992.* Madison, U. S. A.: American Society of Agronomy and Crop Science Society of America, 1993.

Harrington, J. F. 'Seed and pollen storage for conservation of plant genetic resources'. In: *Genetic Resources in Plants, Their Exploration and Conservation.* (Eds.). Frankel, O. H. and Bennet, E. Edinburgh, U. K: Blackwell, pp. 501-521, 1970.

Harrington, J. F. 'Seed storage and longevity'. In: *Seed Biology*, vol. 13. (Ed.). Koslowski, T. T. Academic Press, pp. 145-245, 1972.

Hodgkin, T. H., Rao, V. Ramanatha and Riley, K. W. 'Current issues in conserving crop land races'. Presented at the FAO-IBPGR On-Farm Conservation Workshop, 6-8 December, 1993, Bogor, Indonesia, 1993.

Jackson, W. P. 'Launch of the new international agenda for botanic gardens, Asheville'. *BGCI News* 23-25, 2000.

Jackson, W. P. 'Plenary address, BGCI. 4th International Congress on Education in Botanic Gardens held in Thiruvanthapuram, Kerala, 1999.

Mandal, S. and Maheshwari, M. L. 'High pressure liquid chromatic determination of vindoline, catharanthene vinca-leukoblastine and vincristine in periwinkle leaf'. *Indian J. Pharm. Sci.* 49(6): 205-209, 1989.

Mattick, J. S., Albett, E. M. and Edmonson, D. L. 'The gene library—preservation and analysis of genetic diversity in Australia'. In: *Conservation of Plant Genes, DNA Banking and In-situ Biotechnology*. (Eds.). Adams, R. P. and Adams, J. E. San Diego, U. S. A.: Academic Press, pp. 15-35, 1972.

Pareek, S. K. 'Medicinal plants in India: Present status and future prospects'. In: *Prospects of Medicinal Plants*. (Eds.). Gautam, P. L., Raina, R., Srivastava, Umesh; Rai Choudhari, S. P. and Singh, B. B. New Delhi: Indian Society of Plant Genetic Resources, pp. 1-4, 1998.

Pareek, S. K., Maheshwari, M. L. and Gupta, R. 'Domestication studies on *Ocimum sanctum* oil and eugenol content'. *Indian Perfumer* 24(2): 93-100, 1980.

Pareek, S. K., Singh S., Srivastava, V. K., Mandal, S., Maheshwari, M. L. and Gupta, R. 'Effect of nitrogen application and age on yield and alkaloid content of periwinkle'. Proc. National Seminar on Medicinal and Aromatic Plants, Tamilnadu Agriculture University, Coimbatore. (Ed.). Muthukrishnan, C. R., pp. 40-44, 1982.

Ramanatha Rao, V. 'Complementary conservation strategy presented to IPGRI-ICAR-UTFANET Regional Training Course on the conservation and use of germplasm of tropical fruits in Asia, held at IIHR, Bangalore, 18-31 May, 1997.

Roberts, E. H. 'Problems of long-term storage and seed and pollen of genetic resources conservation'. In: *Crop Genetic Resources for Today and Tomorrow*. (Eds.). Frankel, O. H. and Hawks, J. G. Cambridge, U. K.: Cambridge University Press, pp. 226-296, 1975.

Roberts, E. H. *Viability of Seeds*. London: Chapman and Hall, 1972.

Roy, R. K. '*Ex-situ* conservation and sustainable utilisation of plant genetic resources of India: The role of botanic gardens in the new millennium'. *Indian J. Plant Genet. Resour.* 14: 316-318, 2001.

Saxena, R. K., Kidwai, M. A. and Hardas, M. W. 'Plant introduction experiments with henbane—new raw material for Indian drug industry'. *Indian Drugs* 16(5): 102-104, 1979.

Sharma, S. C. and Goel, A. K. 'Role of botanic gardens in modern times'. *Indian J. Forestry* 17: 230-238, 1994.

Singh, A. K. 'Management of plant genetic resources: An Indian perspective'. *Science Letters*, 25(3 & 4): 74-87, 2002.

Singh, B. P. 'Germplasm exchange: Priorities, achievements and problems'. In: *Plant Genetic Resources—Indian Perspective*. (Eds.). Paroda, R. S., Arora, R. K. and Chandel, K. P. S. New Delhi: National Bureau of Plant Genetic Resources, pp. 95-120, 1998.

Singh, B. P., Deep Chand, Singh, R. V. and Saxena, R. K. 'Introduction and collection of plant genetic resources of medicinal and aromatic plants and their utilisation'. *Indian J. Plant Genet. Resour.* 2(1): 91-94, 1989.

Tcwill, L. E. 'Genetic considerations for germplasm preservation of clonal materials'. *Hort. Sci.* 23: 91-97, 1998.

Towill, L. E. 'Low temperature and freeze/vacuum-drying preservation of pollen'. In: *Cryopreservation of Plant Cells and Organs*. (Ed.). Kartha, K. K. Boca Raton, Florida, U. S. A.: CRC Press, pp. 171-198, 1985.

Withers, L. A. 'Biotechnology and plant genetic resources conservation'. In: *Plant Genetic Resources Conservation and Management*. (Eds.). Paroda, R. S. and Arora, R. K. New Delhi: IBPGR Regional Office, pp. 273-297, 1991.

—oo(O)oo—

2

Intellectual Property Rights, Growth and Competitiveness of Indian Pharmaceutical Industries

C. P. Malik

It is generally stated that 'necessity is the mother of invention' and most human endeavour results in monetary gain, which can be converted into material possessions. In brief, man works hard, uses his inventiveness and ingenuity and talent to convert them into money. The State(s) has devised various ways to evolve methods to protect and reward inventors. Some States award exclusive rights to the artisan. It was in 1474 when the first law on patents was passed in Venice, which awarded monopoly rights to artisans for their inventions. Subsequently, the House of Commons in the United Kingdom, in 1623, passed the Act of Proprietorship. The condition was that the invention is useful to society. In India, novel techniques and inventions were retained within the family, for example, craftsmanship, carving, artisans.

In any case, no system was available to protect talent. Based on the British Law of 1852, the then Government of India introduced the Act of Protection of Invention in 1883 and subsequently changed it to the Inventions and Designs Act in 1888. And on August 15, 1947, Indian patents and designs came to be managed by the Controller of Patents and Designs. In 1970, the Indian Patents Act was passed. Over the years, sublime and novel ideas, a design or an invention or a manuscript were defined as 'intellectual property'. But in any case, these properties led to useful products/applications. The tragedy is that most intellectual properties can be copied or imitated, thus lowering returns to the original inventor. The above account recognises the right of an inventor to accrue economic gains from his inventions. This right is called Intellectual Property Right (IPR). The stipulation is that the inventions are not detrimental to society.

The IPR is protected in several ways: trade secrets, patents, plant breeders' right and copyright. It may be stated that patents have only territorial validity, are expensive and time consuming. Further, IPR protection in different countries necessitates patents to be secured in those countries. This involves high cost and long periods for approval since patent laws vary from country to country. Of late, developed countries are endeavouring to harmonise the patent laws of different countries. The Paris Convention (1983) established equal protection of industrial IPR. This stipulated that inventions claim priority in all member States by filing a patent application in one member country. This convention had 100 members initially and India joined it in December 1998. In 1978, the European Patent Convention came into being and had 17 member States. Incidentally, provisions for biotechnology inventions were introduced. In January 1995, the Trade Related Intellectual Property Rights (TRIPs) agreement, pertinent to IPR, came into force. This is enforced and administered by the World Trade Organisation (WTO), Geneva. Each member country has the option to frame its patent laws as defined in the GATT agreement.

On a complaint by the U. S. A. in 1997, India is required to modify its patent laws by 2004.

Incidentally, biotechnological inventions demand huge financial inputs and, therefore, developed countries have a superior position to register high technology patents. Consequently, most patents have been registered from Europe, Japan and the U. S. A. from where nearly 90 per cent of the applications for patents were filed. The Indian scenario is slightly different where only 3,500 applications were filed during 1974-94, which went up to 5,000 in 1995. Most patents were filed by CIBA, Colgate, Hindustan Lever, Pfizer and Lucas. Recently, Dr. Reddy's Lab, Ranbaxy and Lupin Lab, BASF, Englehart and Eli Lily have also filed patents.

It appears India needs to undertake several drastic changes rapidly in order to withstand the economic stringency imposed by the changing IPR scenario.

The management of IPR and the benefits accruing from it are numerous. The former includes transfer of IPR, establishment of collaborative linkages and monitoring non-compliance of the IPR renewal.

Renewal of patents needs attention periodically as well as quantitative evaluation of such factors as R&D investment to economic ratio. There are several benefits from the IPR regime, for example, it encourages and safeguards intellectual and artisan creations, helps in spreading new ideas, encourages added investment in R&D and furnishes consumers with data on new creations.

The fast alterations in the IPR scenario in India have taken the scientific community and technologists by surprise. This is partly due to the fact that Indians believe in heritage, tradition and benefits to society at the cost of individual interest. In the expanding domain of IPR, it is essential to make systematic and continued efforts for survival.

A news item (*The Hindustan Times,* July 7, 2003) highlights recent relaxation announced by the U. S. A.. FDA in the generic segment. Consequently, Indian pharma majors are in for a big bonanza. For instance, several blockbuster drugs are going off patent and this will help Indian companies to venture into the world's biggest lucrative market. In recent years, Indian companies have built world class facilities and have inherent cost advantages, a large pool of human resources and superior process engineering skills. So the time needed for approval of generic drugs will be less. Some companies have made a good beginning in biopharma and blockbuster drugs, which have a market of $ 82 billion.

In this article, IPR and the growth and competitiveness of the Indian pharmaceutical industry have been evaluated.

Intellectual Property Rights (IPR) is a very vital issue for India's future and for the future of the developing world. How protection of IPR can promote economic growth, provide incentives for innovation and attract investment that will ultimately create new jobs and opportunities for India demands careful analysis.

Everyone is eagerly looking forward to the day when India fully exploits its incredible potential and occupies its rightful place in the global economy. Hence, India's own interest and the well being of the Indian people are at stake. Reacting to the challenges of development will benefit India and set an example of leadership for other developing economies of the world. The Indian and foreign governments and the private sectors of these countries, working together, can help India initiate the steps it requires to leap forward and exploit its full economic potential.

In a democratic set up, all sectors must make an effort to create ripples. It is especially desired of forward-looking sectors having a vision of the future and are endeavouring to make that vision a reality. In fact, Intellectual Property Protection (IPP) is the key to such a vision.

Amongst the developing countries, India has the building blocks in order to raise a vibrant, knowledge-based economy. But firm action is required to raise a legal system, infrastructure and enforcement systems to glue those building blocks together so that they may be used to their greatest advantage.

In 2002, the Indian Parliament amended IP protection and took a positive lead. This was done for the second time, the first being the 1970 Patent Law. However, more is desired to bring Indian IPP to the world class level, by initiating steps for economic growth across all facets of the knowledge-based economy.

In this context, it will be helpful to recall and discuss the Jordanian experience.

A strong IPR regime can affect economic development. Some years ago, the Kingdom of Jordan had a pharmaceutical sector which created generic drugs at low prices employing reverse engineering. However, these generic companies had to compete with several generics throughout the developing world, as well as those in the developed world. Facing severe economic adversity, the Jordanian Government enforced an economic development plan implementing strong Intellectual Property Rights to promote research, development and expansion of the knowledge-based economy.

The Jordanian Government evolved a world class patent system through legislation, infrastructure development and strict enforcement. The outcome was a dramatic increase in foreign investments from major pharmaceutical companies who have now opened offices or expanded their commercial and research activities in Jordan. Consequently, Jordanian exports of pharmaceuticals jumped from $ 150 million (1999) to $ 200 million (2001), a significant increase for a country with a population of just five million.

The most significant fear, however, is that the concern for a strong Patent Protection regime would increase drug prices have been unfounded. In fact, prices for new, patent-protected medicines have not exceeded pre-patent prices and have actually come down in the market. The generic industry has also gained from patenting, since foreign investment has increased and R&D trebled in Japan and Mexico after they improved their patent laws. On the other hand, several developing countries lacking strong IPR regimes remain trapped in economic stagnation and have suffered the negative effect of 'brain drain'. Talented scientists, engineers, entrepreneurs and inventors leave their countries where work is unprotected and migrate to those countries where it is.

INDIA—A GLOBAL PLAYER

It is satisfying that India is the fourth leading supplier of bulk pharmaceutical drugs and active ingredients globally. Having some $ 2 billion in exports, India's pharmaceutical industry is recognised as a global player. It is impressive that India has the world's third largest pool of scientifically and technically trained personnel. Even though we lack pharmaceutical patent protection, a small research and development sector is emerging.

One may note that Indian pharmaceutical companies have started benefiting from IPP on their products. Further, a strong product patent protection protocol will encourage this development. Ranbaxy, an Indian company, which has developed a new drug delivery system (DDS) for ciprofloxacin and has licensed it to Bayer for $ 65 million plus royalties, is a glaring instance. Other Indian research-based companies have also earned nearly $ 70 million from milestone R&D payments.

For increased benefits, the following three steps are essential:

STEP ONE: LEGISLATION

With product patent protection, imagine how strong the pharmaceutical industry could be. Due to lack of patent protection, India's highly trained scientists have not been able to employ their skills in India and this has drastically suppressed the incentive for India's best scientific minds to remain in the country. According to one study, it is estimated that more than 15 per cent of the scientists engaged in pharmaceutical R&D in the U. S. A. are of Indian origin. Had their creative work been adequately protected in India, these scientists would not have emigrated. In turn, this would have led to a more innovative pharmaceutical sector, opening up more jobs and more products for export.

The second amendment to the 1970 Patent Law, which was passed in May 2002, includes extension of pharmaceutical patent protection from seven to 20 years. This is a positive step and fulfils part of India's commitment to the international community on protecting intellectual property. However, there are some glaring concerns and these are:

- Transition to a Product Patent regime has been excluded until 2005.
- The Bill envisages a broad, ambiguous allowance for compulsory licensing.
- It is ambiguous regarding patent protection for imports.

The Indian pharmaceutical industry will gain the most from patent legislation and should it realise its resources and press for the passage of the Product Patent legislation before the 2005 deadline. India is a strong democratic society, and hence the people engaged in day-to-day economic activity, must make their voice heard by those who regulate and monitor that activity.

The former Commerce Minister, while introducing the Patent Bill in Parliament, said: "The Indian pharma industry is emerging as the new leader of the knowledge-based drug industry in the world, following software and IT. Now is the time for the rest of the industry to come out of its reverse engineering mode and move forward into the era of innovative R&D mode, clinching the opportunities."

STEP TWO: DATA EXCLUSIVITY

It has been repeatedly found that data exclusivity is the key to the protection of public health and the pharmaceutical sector's hard work. And it is pertinent to the foreign investment in the pharma sector. Protection of test data is the key to company decisions on location of clinical trials. According to the U. S. National Institute of Health (NIH), the lack of data exclusivity in India is the major factor why it ranks ninth (compared to China which ranks second), in funding given by the NIH outside the U. S. A. American pharmaceutical companies spent $ 30 billion on R&D last year. If only a fraction of that amount was channelled into India, it would broaden U. S.-Indian scientific ties, increase the demand for Indian scientists and ultimately benefit the health and lives of millions of people. Indian pharmaceutical companies and researchers, especially in the biotechnological sector, would benefit enormously from the enhanced diffusion of knowledge that flows from international partnerships and increased integration.

It may be remembered that data exclusivity is an administrative protection which can be enforced without the intervention of Parliament. One of the effective methods of providing protection for the creative work of scientists, while legislators draft laws to complete the legal IP framework, requires the Government to treat data as the exclusive property of the firm that generated it for a specific time. Data exclusivity requires each company to fully test its products. Reverse engineered drugs do not always compare with the original, since different manufacturing processes can alter the drug and impact public health. Relying on another company's data is not only business malpractice, but it also discourages R&D investment and poses potential public health dangers.

Some of the arguments against patent legislation and data exclusivity anticipate price increase and depriving the poor from the availability of essential drugs. While introducing the Patents Bill, the former Commerce Minister pointed out that not a single drug in the Indian essential drug list is patented and hence prices of these drugs will be unaffected. Further, Product Patent protection will apply to new drugs introduced after the law is enacted; a small percentage of the total market—estimated to peak at 20-22 per cent of the total market, 10 years from now.

STEP THREE: IMPROVING IPR INFRASTRUCTURE AND ENFORCEMENT

Knowledge-based industries will help in creating thousands of jobs for Indian workers, generate enormous revenues for the Government and lead to substantial increase in India's exports. But to harness these benefits, IPR must be enforced seriously. This calls for political will from the top and additional resources to improve the institutions and train the personnel required to carry out IPR protection. The Government of the day must designate this as a priority area. A close linkage between industry, Government and the law enforcement officials is essential. Concomitantly, industry must make its needs explicit in order to cause an impetus for a change.

The Indian Patent Office is faced with a growing backing of approximately 5,000 unexamined patent applications in its Delhi, Mumbai and Kolkata offices. Enforcement of IP protection is seriously lacking. Judicial delays mean that cases can take up to 10 years to see resolution and payment of damages on IPR violations. In Japan, 400,000 cases are cleared every year. In China, 40 per cent cases are cleared annually. Familiarity with new IPR laws is also an important issue for lawyers, the courts and the police. The Indian Government is fast responding to the need for the development of IPR infrastructure.

RESULTS AND BENEFITS

A strong pharmaceutical patent regime would strengthen India's research and development sector, will attract more foreign investments and provide a basis for Indian pharmaceutical firms to begin tackling diseases that have a serious effect on the Indian population. Local pharmaceutical companies have the high advantage of being acquainted with prevalent disease patterns especially indigenous communicable diseases and hence can develop drugs by exploiting local R and D. Diseases such as tuberculosis, malaria, leprosy, plague and dengue fever continue to pose serious health problems in India and take millions of lives each year. Talented Indian scientists, attracted by adequate patent laws, are urgently needed in the country to conquer these endemic diseases.

As India's knowledge based economy grows, it will benefit not only India, but the rest of the world as well, especially the developing world. This is India's big challenge, and one in which developed countries, for example, the U. S. A., would like to co-operate. With Indo-U.S. relations improving with strides Indian business is becoming increasingly global. It is high time for 'new link' to prevail in the IPR debate.

I strongly believe that if a country wishes to increase its wealth she must enact a strong patent system. Shall I say that patent systems are actually one of the good inventions of the new world. However, they are viewed over time with different perspectives. Currently, patent systems are popular in the U. S. A., Europe and most interestingly even in Japan.

The Japanese view that it is in their own interest to have a strong patent system. Interestingly, their educational system pertaining to law and technology in relation with IP is being revamped. Concomitantly, they are revamping their judicial system as well. Most significantly, they plan to award and contemplating to award real damages for IPR violations.

India should have adopted a strong patent system long back. Even then, it is not too late now to enact these laws. Let us accept that mistakes have already been committed. In India, the worst mistake is by way of self-inflicted wounds. One such blunder was the amendment of the patent system in 1970, where the decision was intended to drop Products Patent. Now the time has come that decision should be undone because an international quality patent regime is in the larger interest of India. A strong patent regime contemplates a system that will provide full protection to inventions across the range of technologies in this country.

NO PATENT PROTECTION, NO NEW INVENTIONS

A patent system in place is essential because without it capitalism does not work. Capitalism permits copying of other people's intellectual creations and in a free market, copying is easy. Such a step will discourage inventors who have a potential for developing a new product. The derogatory steps will preclude new creations. This, thus necessitated, a patent system to stop exploitation of weakness in the developed world. In a way, IPR seems to be a great invention and it is one of the few governmental interventions which tends to improve situations. It is proposed to raise wealth and permit everyone to have a fair share of it.

In the U. S. A., a patent system exists for all technologies in all the industries. It implies that industries cannot afford to copy the creations or inventions of others. Indeed, the creator of the newly invented product is protected for the next two decades or so against copying/plagiarisng and has the exclusive right to do business from it. At the end of two decades, the next generation and the generations thereafter are awarded the right free of charge. That is an enormous gift to the future generations. For instance, antibiotics are great inventions—they keep millions of people alive and without the supporting patent system, many of us would be travelling to the next world.

Clearly everyone in this country is a beneficiary of the Patent system and those Antibiotics. Take, for instance, all the patents on semi-synthetic penicillin, developed in the United Kingdom; the technology was superb and involved some vital key discoveries. With the advent of time, all that is in the public domain. Consequently, we all use it.

Another drug, Cipro, that will hit the public domain in the U. S. A. next year is one of the greatest antibiotics discovered totally by chance. Unbelievable story, pure luck led to its discovery. The chemist who was developing this molecule felt failure of its working. Under extreme stress of his work, he had a heart attack and this led to the discovery of Ciprofloxin.

Cipro has kept the Bayer Company going up and strong but concomitantly saved several precious lives and has kept many people alive. It is a great antibiotic. It is a fine example of the equality in the system. The patent system encourages creations and inventions and helps exploitation of inventions as well. Somebody actually owns it and has the commercial incentive to develop the technology at great investment. It encourages industry to innovate, invest money in new inventions and thus serve humanity.

It is highly desirable to evolve a positive patent system. Unfortunately, India even now does not have one. Even though she has the technical manpower to run a functional patent office which is a vital part of the whole procedure. Let me argue that India is far ahead of China in judicial systems. So we need to develop the patent offices and train officials to evoke a positive patent regime.

Let us not forget that by 2006 India has to comply with their WTO-TRIPs agreement for product production in the area of pharmaceuticals. So this country has to do much more about patent protection especially for biotech products. There is another controversy over data exclusivity in India. It is an entirely separate issue and should not be confused with patent issues. Let us assume that somebody does clinical studies in India at enormous cost and produces tremendous amount of crucial data. This clinical data has to be submitted to the health regulatory authority to secure permission to market the antibiotic. It may be noted that the investor company's competitor in the trade can use this exclusive data.

The competitor, after access to the data can manufacture a competitive product that has legal sanctions and is cheaper because having spent nothing on the invention or clinical trials. This is absolutely unfair to the inventor under the garb of providing vital drugs at cheaper price.

There is a general agreement of five and 10 years as a fair period for data protection. The U. S. A. has agreed for five years, because the pharmaceutical company which turns over the information to the U. S. authorities has to be provided data exclusivity protection. India must come forward with an assurance for data exclusivity and invite the big MNCs to contract local pharmaceutical companies for clinical trials.

By strengthening the patent regime, Indian scientists and Indian pharmaceutical manufacturers are absolute gainers without losing anything. Seemingly, it is a win-win situation for the people and the country as a whole.

INDIA'S MEAGRE R & D BUDGET

India's total R & D budget is 3.5 billion dollars, which is nearly half than Pfizer's (5.5 billion dollars). The latter is less than that of General Motors which is 9 billion dollars. Even with such financial constraints, India has several scientific achievements to her credit. For instance, India has demonstrated the capability to design, fabricate and launch our own satellites. Furthermore, we launch not only our satellites but those of Germany and Korea as well.

In Genomics, we have the unique advantage to work and understand the vast and diverse Indian genetic pool. This provides a unique opportunity to discover functional significance of human genome sequence of hitherto unknown functions through analysis. Interestingly, Nicholas Piramal and CSIR have forged the partnership and have created Genomate in Centre for Biochemical Technology at Delhi. It is named as Institute of Genomics and Integrated Biology. The emergence of this will set an interesting example for the future in terms of fast results and new vistas.

COMPARABLE ADVANTAGE

Two things are vital. One was to identify the areas where our comparative advantage lies basically, for example, the human genetic diversity and second, to build a close relationship with industry and academic institutions. This is in contrast to previous functioning where public institutions existed on their own resources and manpower. In the context of changing scenario, functional plasmodesmatal links between academicia, industry and research institutions is desired. The point to note is Genomate, which is actually an enterprise of Swati Piramal, has established strong links within the heart of CSIR laboratory. Such type of mutual trust and confidence are beneficial economically and will take India on the road to economic prosperity.

In the post-Genomic era, of late, the BT industries are partly depending for the growth on the traditional development and production of recombinant proteins in microbial, animal and plant sectors to more areas of therapeutic modalities, including gene therapy and customised product development based on Pharmacogenomics and Proteconomics. The potential to target specific genes for drugs thus assisting the development of tailor made therapies. The recent developments of SMPs and DNA chip technology have made it possible to detect errors in gene expression and genetic disorders in individuals, groups of individuals or families and a whole new field of regenerative medicine is opening up.

At a point in time when we were ill we took antibiotic, it was curative. When we wanted to protect ourselves from getting a disease, we had preventive medicine, which was vaccination, and now we are talking in terms of predictive medicine. When one develops schizophrenia, a drop of blood can be tested and predicted as to whether a cure is possible or not. Then corrective medicine is possible through gene therapy. Scientists are actively engaged in regenerating organs. That means, now BT has moved from being curative to preventive to predictive and corrective to regenerative process.

There are several vital issues that impinge on the future of cell research which are not only scientific or technical in nature, but are pertinent to ethical and moral issues on the use of human embryonic or adult cells, IPR and the sharing of the accompanying reward systems.

Ultimately, when it comes to manufacturing the drugs for the poor, modern Biotechnology is going to be a key factor and India is going to play a major role backed by the wherewithal that we have in this country.

REFERENCES

Ganguli, P. 'Patenting innovation: New demands in emerging contents'. *Curr. Sci.* 75:433-439, 1998.

Ganguli, P. *Gearing up for Patents—The Indian Scenario.* Hyderabad: University Press, 1998.

Gupta, P. K. 'Transgenic plants: Some current issues'. *Current Sci.* 70: 654-660, 1996.

Mashelkar, R. A. 'Biotechnology—Solution to India's future'. *Intellectual Capital* 1: 1-3, 2002.

Mashelkar, R. A. 'Intellectual property rights and the Third World'. *Curr. Sci.* 81:955-965, 2001.

Narayan, P. *Patent Law.* 2nd edn. Kolkata: Eastern Law House Pvt. Ltd., 1985.

Sahai, S. 'India's plant variety protection and farmer's rights Act, 2001'. *Current Sci.* 84: 407, 2003.

—oo(O)oo—

3

Enhancing the Export Potential of Medicinal Plants Through Biodiversity Conservation and Development Under Multi-Adversity Environment

M. L. Jakhar, B. L. Kakralya, S. J. Singh and Karan Singh

ANY plant which harbours curative elements or properties in one or more of its organs may be termed as medicinal plant and plant-based medicaments have been employed since the dawn of civilisation for prolonging the life of man by combating various ailments (Singh and Kumar, 1984; Kumar, 1986; Padulosi *et al,* 2002). Ancient ethnic communities around the world have learnt to utilise their neighbourhood herbal wealth for curative as well as offensive purposes. Amongst the ancient civilisations, India has been known to be a rich repository of medicinal plants. The *Rig Veda* (5,000 BC) mentioned 67 medicinal plants, the *Yajur Veda* 81 and the *Atharva Veda* (4,500–2,500 BC), 290 species. Later on, the *Charaka Samhita* (700 BC) and the *Sushruta Samhita* (200 BC) described the properties and uses of 1,100 and 1,270 plants respectively, in compounding of drugs and these are still used in classical formulations in the Ayurvedic system of medicine.

The World Health Organisation (WHO) has compiled a list of 20,000 medicinal plants used in different parts of the globe. A large number of these species have local uses within the country or spread over several countries in a region. Amongst these over 100 botanicals are reported to have consistently large demand and are traded in major drug markets in the world. The medicinal virtues of these raw materials including chemical contents and composition of these species have been well worked out to have merited inclusion in National Pharmacopoeias and official formularies in different countries (Govil *et al,* 2002).

In the present context of 'back to nature' in health care, it is very relevant that these valuable plant species should not only be preserved but also their cultivation should be developed in order to meet the entire demand of the domestic industries as also to exploit the bright prospects for export and providing higher returns to the farmers. Shift from collection to cultivation of medicinal and aromatic plants will ensure purity, authenticity and sustainable supply of raw materials required for herbal drugs. The international market of medicinal plants is over US$ 60 billion per year, which is growing at the rate of 7 per cent. India at present exports herbal material and medicines to the tune of Rs. 446.3 crores only which can be raised to Rs. 3,000 crores by 2005. China and India are two great producers of medicinal plants having more than 40 per cent of global biodiversity. China besides meeting its domestic requirement is earning US$ 5 billion per year from herbal trade. There is, thus, an enormous scope for India also to emerge as a major player in the global herbal product based medicines. However, this requires a grand strategic plan, which takes a holistic view of the entire situation to boost the export of Rs. 10,000 crores by 2010 and minimising the import (Anonymous, 2000).

The biological variation in nature over time and space constitutes the basis of organic evolution. This biodiversity constitutes the foundation of development of different taxonomic groups of plants and animals both in micro-organisms and higher forms of life. Hence, this biodiversity has attracted the attention of not only the scientific community but also politicians, planners and administrators (Conner, 2001). Our awareness of conservation and further development of biodiversity has rapidly increased during the recent past. One of the most important reasons for such an awareness has been the new emerging threats to quantitative and qualitative spectra of biodiversity (Edwards and Hilbek, 2001). India is rich in medicinal plant diversity. All known types of agroclimatic, ecological and edaphic conditions are met within India. The biogeographic position of India is so unique that all known types of ecosystems ranging from the coldest place like the Nubra valley with –57°C, dry cold deserts of Ladakh, temperate and alpine and subtropical regions of North-West and trans-Himalayas, rain forests with the world's highest rainfall in Cheerapunji in Meghalaya, wet evergreen humid tropics of Western Ghats, arid and semi-arid conditions of peninsular India, dry desert conditions of Rajasthan and Gujarat to the tidal mangroves of the Sunderbans, India is rich in all the three levels of medicinal biodiversity such as species diversity, genetic diversity and habitat diversity. There are about 426 biomes representing different habitat diversities that give rise to one of the richest centres in the world for plant genetic resources. The total number of flowering plant species, although only 17,000, the intra-specific variability found in them make it one of the highest in the world (Janick, 2001).

However, experiences have amply demonstrated that in a densely populated developing country like India, where a sizeable population is living in close proximity to forests, declaring protected areas will not entirely be sufficient to ensure conservation on the fast eroding biological diversity. The success of any conservation programme vests solely on the efficient management of protected areas. The involvement of local communities in conservation activities has now been increasingly realised. A people-nature oriented approach thus, becomes highly imperative. This will help to generate a sense of responsibility among the local people about the values of biodiversity and the need to use it in a sustainable manner. for their own prosperity and the maintenance of ecosystem resilience (Anonymous, 2000).

Plant biodiversity is vital to the development and welfare of human society. Plant genetic resources constitute enormously valuable assets for achieving global objectives of food security, poverty alleviation, environment protection and subsequently, sustainable development. The International Plant Genetic Resources Institute Rome, Italy (IPGRI), has been the pivotal organisation for making equilibrated and scientific efforts for plant biodiversity conservation at the global level. Concerted efforts in this regard have focused on eight priority areas of work, namely, strengthening the national systems or programmes, promoting regional crop and thematic networks, improving conservation and strategies and technologies, increasing the use of plant genetic resources, managing and communicating the relevant information, addressing socio economic and policy issues, conserving and using specific crops and also conserving and judiciously utilising the forest resources (Anonymous, 2000). Recently IPGRI has focused its attention on *in situ* conservation of agro biodiversity, giving appropriate weightage to farmers participation in such efforts (Nosberger *et al,* 2001; Deb, 2002). This focus of IPGRI is based on the fact that *in situ* conservation of plant genetic resources has the advantage of continuing evolution and adaptation of genetic material and conserving the wider range of biodiversity and development. It is imperative to pinpoint some basic aspects of plant biodiversity.

DISTRIBUTION OF MEDICINAL FLORA

Medicinal plants are distributed across diverse habitats and landscape. Around 70 per cent of India's medicinal plants are found in tropical areas mostly in the various forest types spread across the Western and Eastern ghats, the Vindhyas, Chhota Nagpur plateau, Aravallis and Himalayas. Although less than 30 per cent of the medicinal plants are found in the temperate and alpine areas and higher altitudes they include species of high medicinal value. Macro studies show that a larger percentage of the known medicinal plants occur in the dry and moist deciduous vegetation as compared to the evergreen or temperate habitats. Analysis of habits of medicinal plants indicate that they are distributed across various habitats. One third are trees and an equal portion includes shrubs and the remaining one third are herbs, grasses and climbers (Table 1). Of the 386 families and 2,200 genera in which medicinal plants are recorded, the families like Asteraceae, Euphorbiaceae, Lamiaceae, Fabaceae and Rubiaceae share the larger proportion of medicinal plant species with the highest number of species (419) falling under Asteraceae (Table 2). About 90 per cent of medicinal plants used by the industries are collected from the wild. While over 800 species are used in drug production by industry, less than 20 species of plants are under commercial cultivation. Over 70 per cent of the plant collections involve destructive harvesting because of the use of parts like roots, bark, wood, stem and the whole plant in the case of herbs (Table 3).

TYPES OF BIODIVERSITY

1. Generic Diversity

This includes variability in different genera of the same family. For example, family Leguminosae has great biodiversity and three sub-families (now elevated to the rank of families) Papilionaceae (Fabaceae), Mimosaceae and Caesalpiniaceae have genera of herbs, shrubs, tree climber and tree habit. In Papilionaceae, *Glycyrrhiza glabra* is a perennial herb, kulthi (*Dolichos biflorus)* is

TABLE 1
Distribution of Medicinal Plants by Habits

No.	Plant Type	Share
1.	Trees	33%
2.	Shrubs	20%
3.	Climbers	12%
4.	Herbs	32%
5.	Others	3%

TABLE 2
Distribution of Medicinal Plants by Families

No.	Family	Genera
1.	Asteraceae	419
2.	Euphorbiaceae	214
3.	Lamiaceae	214
4.	Fabaceae	214
5.	Rubiaceae	208
6.	Poaceae	168
7.	Acanthaceae	141
8.	Rosaceae	129
9.	Apiaceae	118

TABLE 3
Breakup of Medicinal Plants by Their Parts Utilised

No.	Plant Part	Share
1.	Root	29%
2.	Stem	6%
3.	Flower	5%
4.	Fruit	10%
5.	Leaf	6%
6.	Seed	7%
7.	Bark	14%
8.	Wood	3%
9.	Rhizome	4%
10.	Whole part	16%

a herb whereas several medicinal plants of this family are trees. Similar biodiversity exists in other families of medicinal plants.

2. Species Diversity

This is the diversity existing in different species of the same genus. This variation may be due to phytogeographical distribution of some genera. For example, Pinus genus have 100 species, a great diversity exists in respect of growth habit (Tables 4 and 5). This biodiversity is reflected in growth habit, phenology, reproductive behaviour, distribution and wild species of cultivated plants which are good source of such biodiversity and are immensely valuable for scientific exploration and exploitation of plants.

TABLE 4
Important Medicinal Plants from Indian Forests Showing Biodiversity at Species Level

No.	Botanical Name	Family	Part Used	Uses
1.	*Acontium* sp. (24 species) *A. nepellus* *A. deinorrhizum* *A. ferox* *A. heterophyllum* *A. palmatum* *A. violaceum*	Ranunculaceae	Roots	Astringent, Stomachic, debility combater
2.	*Asparagus* sp. (6 species) *A. adscendus* *A. gonoclodus* *A. officinalis* *A. plumosus* *A. racemosus* *A. sarmentosus* *A. sprengeri*	Liliaceae	Root	Diarrhoea, dysentery, general debility
3.	*Berberis* sp (13 species) *B. aristata* *B. vulgaris* *B. asiatica* *B. lycium*	Berbidaceae	Root, bark	Opthalmic problems
4.	*Cephaelis ipecacuha* = *Ipecae ipecacuha*	Rubiaceae	Roots	Emetic, diuretic, amoebic dystentery. Now cultivated in India
5.	*Colchicum luteum*	*Liliaceae*	Corns	Carminative, laxative, aphrodisiac

Continued...

...*Continued*

No.	Botanical Name	Family	Part Used	Uses
6.	*Discorea* sp. (8 species)	Dioscoreaceae	Roots, tubers	Detoxication, steroids (diosgenis)
	D. alata			
	D. bulbifera			
	D. deldtoidia			
	D. hookeri			
	D. pentaphylla			
	D. prazeri			
	D. tometosa			
7.	*Glycirrhiza glabra*	Papilionaceae	Roots	Tonic, expectorant
8.	*Rauwolfia serpentina*	Rubiaceae	Roots	Blood pressure
9.	*Altonia scholaris*	Apocynaceae	Bark	Tonic
10.	*Cassia* sp. (15 species)	Caesalpiniaceae	Variable effects	
	C. absus			
	C. alata			
	C. angustifolia		Leaves, fruts	
	C. obtusifolia=C. tora			
	C. occidentalis			
	C. artemissoiden			
	C. auriculata			
	C. fistula			
	C. grandis			
	C. javanica			
	C. nodos			
	C. renigera			
	C. sophera			
	C. suratensis			

Continued...

...Continued...

No.	Botanical Name	Family	Part Used	Uses
11.	*Ephedra* (6 species)	Ephedraceae	Wood	Source of ephedrine, a very useful alkaloid for cough, asthma, fever, etc.
	E. foliata *E. genordiano* *E. intermedia* *E. major*			
12.	*Atropa* *A. accuminata* *A. pelladon*	Solanaceae	Leaves	Eye trouble
13.	*Datura* (4 species)	Solanaceae	Leaves, seeds flowring tops	In smal doses for bronchial problems
	D. innoxia *D. alba=D. metel* *D. stramonium* *D. suavaolus*			
14.	*Swertia chirato*	Gentianaceae	Dried plants	Tonia, stomachic, bronchial ashtma
15.	*Artemisia* (4 species)		Flowers	Stimulant, vermifuge, etc.
	A. brevifolia *A. maritima* *A. absinthium* *A. vulgaris*	Compositae	Flowers, leaves	Stimulant, vermifuge, etc.
16.	*Aegle marmelos*	Rutaceae	Fruit, pulp	Digestive problems
17.	*Withania somnifera*	Solanaceae	Leaves, fruits, roots	Many ailments, anti-inflammatory, anti-tumour, anti-stress, antioxidants, immunomodulatory, homoeopathic, revuvenating nervous system, cardiopulmonary

TABLE 5
Species Biodiversity in Pinus Genus

No.	Species	Common Name	Uses
1.	*Pinus edulis*	Mutpine	Treatment of syphilis
2.	*Pinus elliotii*	Slash pine	Treatment of gonorrhea, chronic inflammation
3.	*Pinus palustris*	Pitch pine	Tapeworm, colic
4.	*Pinus roxburghii*	Chir	Cure and chronic bronchitis
5.	*Pinus silvestris*	Pine	Rheumatism and gout
6.	*Pinus strobes*	Black pine	Skin diseases
7.	*Pinus wallichiana*	Kail	Sizing paper and cloth

3. Ecosystem Diversity

Depending upon abiotic component of an ecosystem, the biotic components exhibit great diversity. This is evident from the study of fauna and flora of forest, crop land, aquatic and desert ecosystems of the world. Amongst forests, tropical, sub-tropical and temperate forests are having a great deal of plant biodiversity due to variability of ecological niche. In India, ample biodiversity prevails in medicinal plants component of forests. The records of ICFRE, Dehradun, enunciate this situation (Table 6).

4. Agro Biodiversity

When wild plants are brought under cultivation, tremendous biodiversity is depicted and developed in varieties, hybrids, clones and wild relatives. Among agroecosystem, cropland, forage land, orchard, ornamental ecosystems are important. Cassman (2001) emphasised that research priorities for scientific exploitation of plant genetic resources in these ecosystems will depend upon several factors. However, the research-derived technologies to increase productivity of such ecosystems must be investigated with long-term effects on wild life habitat, biodiversity and social conservation (Wilkings, 2001), Oag and Rao (2001) with agroforestry ecosystem, Edwards and Hilbeck (2001) with cropland ecosystems and Janick (2001) with potential of domestication of new crop species have also advocated on the conservation of biodiversity keeping in view the sustainability concept. Development of agro biodiversity by new varieties is well exemplified in *Withania somnifera, Papavar somniferum, Plantago ovata, Ocimum sanctum, Cassia angustifolia, Cephaelis ipecacuanha, Glycirrhiza glabra, Eucalyptus* species, *Cinchona, Dioscorea,* etc. Similar biodiversity also exists in herbs collected from different ecosystems in terms of active principles (Table 7).

LEVELS OF BIODIVERSITY

With a broader perspective, biodiversity is also studied at various levels:

I. Global Biodiversity

Over 5-30 million species of living form exist but only 1.5 million have been identified so far (Nosberger *et al,* 2001). Out of these, about 300,000 are green plants and fungi, 800,000 are

TABLE 6
Medicinal Plants of Indian Forests' Ecosystem

Botanical Name	Common or Trade Name	Family	Parts Used	Complaints Against Which Used
Abroma augusta	–	Sterculiaceae	Root, bark	Emmen., uterine tonic, in dysmen.
Abrus precatorius	Bead tree, Indian liquorice	Leguminosae	Seed Root	Purg., emetic, tonic, aphrodis. Emetic, alexiteric.
Abutilon indicum	Indian mallow	Malvaceae	Leaf Bark Seed	Demulc. Astrin., diru. Aphrodis. laxt., demulc.
Acacia nilotica sp. *indica*	Babul	Leguminosae	Bark	Astrin., demulc.
Acacia catechu	Catechu	Leguminosae	Bark	Astrin.
Acacia concinna	Shigakai	Leguminosae	Pod Leaf	Aper., expect., emetic, Cath.
Acorus calamus	Sweet flag	Araceae	Rhizome	Emetic, stomch., nervice tonic in snake bite.
Adansonia digitata	Baob tree	Bombacaceae	Fruit pulp Leaf	Aper., demulc., astrin. Diaphor.
Adhatoda vasica	–	Acanthaceae	Leaf Root	Cough, chr. broncht., insecticidal, rheumatism Ashtma, phthisis.
Aegle marmelos	Bael	Rutaceae	Pulp of ripe fruit Half ripe frt. Root bark	Arom., cooling, laxt. Astrin., digest., stomch. Intermittent fever, fish.

Continued...

...Continued

Botanical Name	Common or Trade Name	Family	Parts Used	Complaints Against Which Used
Ailanthus excelsa	Maharukh	Simarubiaceae	Bark	Arom. tonic, febge., expect., antisp., astrin.
Ailanthus excelsa	Maharukh	Simarubiaceae	Bark	Arom., tonic, febge.,expect., antisp., astrin.
Ailanthus triphysa (*A. malabarica*)	Maharukh	Simarubiaceae	Bark	Carmin., tonic, febge.
Alangium salviifolium (*A. lamarckii*)	–	Alangiaceae	Root bark	Purg., anthelm.
Albizia lebbeck	Siris	Leguminosae	Bark, seed	Astrin., tonic, restor.
Allinia galanga	Greater galanga	Scitaminacea	Rhizome	Stomch., stiml, aphrodis.
Alstonia scholaris	Chatian	Apocynaceae	Bark	Tonic, alter., febge.
Anamirta cocculus	–	Menispermaceae	Berry Seed	Fish poison, used in night sweats of phthisis.
Annona squamosa	Custard apple	Annonaceae	Root Seed Fruit Leaf Seed	Purg. Insecticide, fish poison Insecticide, fish poison Insecticide, fish poison Irrit., abortif.
Aristolochia bracteata	Wormkiller	Aristolochiaceae	Plant	Purg., anthelm., emmen.
Artemisia absinthium	Absinthe	Compositae	Flower	Vermifuge, tonic in intermittent fever
Artemisia maritima	Wormwood	Compositae	Flower head Decoction of leaves	Anthelm Ague fevers

Continued...

...Continued

Botanical Name	Common or Trade Name	Family	Parts Used	Complaints Against Which Used
Artemisia vulgaris	–	Compositae	Herb	Emmen., Anthelm., antisp., stomch.
			Root	Tonic, antisp.
			Infusion of leaves	Asthma, nervous affections.
Azadirachta indica	Neem	Meliaceae	Bark	Tonic, astrin., antiper.
			Bark, root bark and young fruit	Tonic, antiper., alter.
			Decoc. of leaf	Antisep.
			Gum	Demulc., tonic.
			Dry flower	Tonic, stomch.
			Oil	Stim., antisep., alter
			Berries	Purg., emul., anthelm.
Barringtonia acutangula	Hijal	Lecythidaceae	Powdered seed	Emetic, expect.
			Bark, root and seed	Fish poison
			Root	Cooling, aper.
			Juice of leaf	In diar.
Bauhinia variegata	–	Leguminosae	Bark	Alter., tonic, astrin.
			Decoc. of root	In dyspep.
			Root	Antidote to snake poison
Boerhaavia diffusa	Hogweed	Nyctaginaceae	Root	Diru., laxt., expect., in ashtma, stomch., in oedema, anaemia, jaundice, scanty urine and internal inflam., antid. to snake venom

Continued...

...Continued

Botanical Name	Common or Trade Name	Family	Parts Used	Complaints Against Which Used
Boswellia serrata	Indian olibanum tree, Salai	Bursecraceae	Gum	Diaphor., diur., astrin., emmen.
Butea monosperma	Flame of the Forest, Palas	Leguminosae	Seed	Anthelm.
			Gum	Astrin.
			Leaf	Astrin., diru., depurative, aphrodis.
			Bark, seed	In snake bite.
Caesalpinia crista	–	Leguminosae	Seed	Antiper., antipyr., tonic, febge., in ashtma, in
			snake bite.	
			Leaf, bark	Emmen., febge., anthelm.
			Seed oil	Emol.
Calophyllum inophyllum	Alexandrian laurel	Guttiferae	Bark	Astrin. internal haemor.
			Gum	Emetic, purg.
			Juice	Purg.
			Leaf	Fish poison
Calotropis procera	–	Asclepiadaceae	Root bark	Diphor., expect., emetic.
Cassia auriculata	–	Leguminosae	Bark, root	Astrin.
			Leaf, fruit	Anthelm.
Cassia fistula	Purging cassia, Pudding pipe, Indian laburnum	Leguminosae	Root bark, seed, leaf	Laxative
			Fruit	Cath
			Seed	Emeticd
			Root	Astrin., tonic, febge., purg.

Continued...

...Continued

Botanical Name	Common or Trade Name	Family	Parts Used	Complaints Against Which Used
Cassia tora	–	Leguminosae	Leaf decoct.	Laxt.
Ceiba pantandra	Kapok	Bombacaceae	Gum	Tonic, alter, astrin., laxt.
			Young leaf	Emol.
			Root	Diur. in scorpion sting.
			Unripe fruit	Astrin., demulc.
Centratherum anthelminticum (*Veronia anthlmintica*)	Purple fleabane	Compositae	Seed	Anthelm., in skin diseases, tonic, stomch., diur.
Cinnamomum tamala	–	Lauraceae	Bark	Arom., in gonor.
			Leaf	Stim., carmin., used in colic, diar., scorpion sting.
Gissampelos pareira	–	Menispermaceae	Root	Antipe., diur., purg., stomch.
Clerodendrum incerme	–	Verbenaceae	Leaf juice	Alter., febge.
			Root juice	Alter.
Clerodendrum viscosum	–	Verbanaceae	Leaf	Tonic and antiper.
			Fresh leaf juice	Vermifuge, tonic, febge.
			Leaf, flower	In scorpion sting.
			Sprout	In snake bite
Commiphora mukul	Indian bdellium	Burseraceae	Gum resin	Astrin., antispe., expect., aphrodis., enriches the blood, demulc., aper., carmin., alte., antisp., emmen., in snake bite and scorpion sting.

Continued...

...Continued

Botanical Name	Common or Trade Name	Family	Parts Used	Complaints Against Which Used
Mesua fenca	Ironwood tree	Guttiferae	Flowers	Astrin., stomch.
			Unripe fruit	Arom. Sudorific.
			Bark	Astrin., arom.
Michelia champaca	Champak	Magnoliaceae	Bark	febge.,stim., expect., astrin.
			Dried root and root bark	Purg., emmen.
			Flower, fruit	Stim., antisp., tonic, stomch, carmin, bitter and cooling.
Mimosa pudica	Sensitive plant	Leguminoae	Root decoct.	Useful in gravel and other urinary complaints.
			Leaf, root	Used in piles and fistula.
			Leaf	Rubbed into paste and applied to hydrocele
			Leaf, stem	In scorpion sting.
Merinda tinctoria	–	Rubiaceae	Root	Cath.
			Leaf	Tonic, febge.
Murraya koenigii	Curry leaf tree	Rubiaceae	Plant	Tonic, stomch.
			Bark, root	Stim.
Nyctanthes arbor-tristis	–	Oleaceae	Leaves	Used variously
Ocimum sanctum	–	Labiatae	Leaf	Expect.
			Leaf juice	Diaphor., antiper., stimulating expect.
			Leaf infusion	Used as stomch.
			Seed	Demulc.
			Root	given in decoct. as a diaphor.
			Plant	In snake bite and scorpion sting.

Continued...

...Continued

Botanical Name	Common or Trade Name	Family	Parts Used	Complaints Against Which Used
Ficus religiosa	Pipal	Moraceae	Bark	Astrin.
			Fruit	Laxt.
			Seed	Cooling, alter.
			Leaf and young shoot	Purg.
Flacourtia jangomas	–	Flacourtiaceae	Fruit	For biliousness, in liver complaints.
			Leaf	In diar., diaphor.
			Bark decoct.	For biliousness.
Garcinia morella	Gamboge	Guffiferae	Gum resin	Purg., anthelm.
Gmelina arborea	–	Verbenaceae	Leaf juice	Demulc.
Helicteres isora	East India screw tree		Root, bark	Expect., demulc., astrin., antigalactagogue.
Jatropha curcas	Physic nut	Euphorbiaceae	Roasted nut	Purg.
			Seed	Purg.
			Plant	Fish poison
Lannea coromandelica (*L. grandis*)	–	Anacardiaceae	Bark	Astrin.
Lawsonia inermis	Henna	Lythraceae	Flower	Refrig.,soporific.
Melletus philippensis	–	Euphorbiaceae	Gland and hair on fruit	Btter, anthelm., cath., syptic.
Mangifera indica	Mango	Anacardiaceae	Ripe fruit	Laxt., diur., astrin.
			Fruit rind	Astrin., stim., tonic.
			Kernel	Astrin., anthelm.
			Bark	Astrin.

...Continued

Continued...

Botanical Name	Common or Trade Name	Family	Parts Used	Complaints Against Which Used
Melia azedarach	Persian lilac bead tree	Meliaceae	Root, bark and fruit	Deobstruent., resolv., alexipharmic.
			Leaf juice	Used internally as anthelm., anthilic, diur., emmen.
Cardia dichotoma (*C. myxa*)	Sebestens	Boraginaceae	Fruit	Astrin., anthelm., diur., demulc., expect.
Crataeva movala	—	Capparaceae	Bark	Demulc., stomach., laxt., diur., antipyr., alter., tonic.
			Fresh leaf and root bark	Rubft.
Cynodon dactylon	Bermuda grass Brahmas grass	Gramineae	Root decoct.	Diur.
			Plant juice	Astrin., diur., astrin.
Cyperus rotundus	Nut grass	Cyperaceae	Tuber	Diur., emmen., anthelm., diaphor., astrin., stim.
Diospyros peregrina (*D. embryopteris*)	—	Ebenaceae	Fruit and stem bark	Astrin.
Dipterocarpus turbinatus	Gurjan	Dipterocarpaceae	Oleo-resin	Applied to ulcers, ringworm and cutaneous affections, diur., in gonor.
Embelia ribes	—	Myrsinaceae	Dried fruit	Anthelm., astrin., alter., tonic.
Erythrina suberosa	—	Leguminosae	Bark	Used in medicine.
Eurphorbia antiquorum	—	Euphorbiaceae	Plant	Purg., digest., pungent.
			Root bark	Purg.

Continued...

...*Continued*

Botanical Name	Common or Trade Name	Family	Parts Used	Complaints Against Which Used
Euphorbia neriifolia	—	Euphorbiaceae	Milky juice	Used as purg., and expect.
			Root	In scorpion sting and snake bite, antisp., fish poison.
Feronia limonia (*F. elephantum*)	Wood apple Elephant apple	Rutaceae	Fruit	Astrin., stomch., stim.
			Leaf	Arom., carmin.
Ficus benghalensis	Banyan	Moraceae	Bark infusion	Tonic, astrin.
			Seed	Cooling, tonic.
Ficus racemosa (*F. glomerata*)	—	Moraceae	Bark	Astrin.
			Fruit	Astrin., stomch., carmin.
Opuntia dillenii	Prickly pear	Cactaceae	Fruit	Refrig.
			Milky juice	Purg.
			Leaf	Used variously.
			Plant	In snake bite.
Oroxylon indicum	—	Bignoniaceae	Root bark	Astrin., tonic.
			Bark	Used variously.
			Tender fruit	Carmin., stomch.
			Seed	Purg.
			Stem	In scorpion sting.
Salvadora persica	—	Salvadoraceae	Leaves	In rheumatism and scurvy.
			Shoot, leaf	Pungent.
			Fruit	Carmin., diur., deobstruent.
			Stem bark	Stim., tonic.
			Root bark	Acrid.

Continued...

...Continued

Botanical Name	Common or Trade Name	Family	Parts Used	Complaints Against Which Used
Santalum album	Sandalwood	Santalaceae	Wood Heartwood oil	In headache, fevers, local inflam., skin diseases, diaphor. In dysuria, urethritis, cystitis.
Sapindus emarginatus	Soapnut tree	Sapindaceae	Fruit	Tonic, alexipharmic, expect., emetic, purg., nauseant.
Saraca indica	Asoka tree	Leguminosae	Bark	Astrin.
Semecarpus anacardium	Marking nut tree	Anacardiaceae	Nut, nut oil, bark gum and plant ash	Used variously
Seymuda febrifuga	—	Meliaceae	Bark	Astrin., bitter tonic, febge., debility, diar., dysen.
Tamarindus indica	Tamarind Indian date	Leguminosae	Fruit	Refrig., digest., carmin., laxt.
Tamarix troupei (*T. gallica*)	Tamarisk	Tamaricaceae	Gall Manna	Astrin. Laxt., expect., detergent.
Terminalia arjuna	Arjun	Combretaceae	Bark Fruit	Tonic, astrin., febge. Tonic, deobstruent.
Terminalia bellirica	Bahera	Combretaceae	Fruit Kernel	Bitter, astrin., tonic, laxt., antipyr. Narcotic.
Terminalia chebula	Chebulic myrobalans	Combretaceae	Fruit Bark	Astrin., laxt., alter. Diur., cardiotonic.

Continued...

...Continued

Botanical Name	Common or Trade Name	Family	Parts Used	Complaints Against Which Used
Vitex negundo	—	Verbenaceae	Leaf	Arom., tonic, vermifuge, discutient.
			Root	Expect., febge., tonic.
			Dried fruit	Vermifuge
Woodfordia fructicosa	—	Lythraceae	Dried flower	Astrin.

Abbreviations

Abortif.	abortificient	Carmin.	carminative	Febg.	febrifuge
Alter.	alterative	Cath.	cathartic	Haemor.	haemorrhage
Amenor.	amenorrhoea	Chr.	chronic	Inflam.	inflammation
Amorph.	amorphous	Decoct.	decotion	Irrit.	irritant
Anthelm.	anthelmintic	Demulc.	demulcent	Laxt.	laxative
Antid.	antidote	Diaphor.	diaphoretic	Purg.	purgative
Antiper.	antiperiodic	Diar.	diarrhoea	Refrig.	refrigerant
Antipyr.	antipyretic	Digest.	digestive	Resolv.	resolvent
Antisep.	antiseptic	Diur.	diuretic	Restor.	restorative
Antisp.	antispasmodic	Dysmen.	dysmenorrhoea	Rheum.	rheumatic
Aper.	aperient	Dyspep	dyspepsia	Stim.	stimulant
Aphrodis.	aphrodisiac	Emmen.	emmenagogue	Stomch.	stomachic
Arom.	aromatic	Emol.	emollient	Syn.	synonym
Astrin.	astringent	Expect.	expectorant	Tox.	toxic

TABLE 7
Yield and Secondary Plant Products of Some Arnica-Montana Origins (Weyel, 1989)

Origin (Selection)	Flowers		Roots	
	Dry Mass (g/m^2)	Flavonoids (%)	Dry Mass (g/m^2)	Ess. Oil (%)
Marburg (D)	38.5	0.36	42.2	0.91
Vosges (F)	3.7	0.28	7.5	0.66
Bordolone (I)	1.3	0.25	0.3	N.C.
Orocco (I)	1.3	0.19	2.7	0.59

TABLE 8
Number of Recorded Plant Species in India (National Biodiversity)

No.	Taxon	No. of Species	Global
1.	Bacteria	850	3,600
2.	Algae	2,500	3,700
3.	Fungi	23,000	46,983
4.	Lichens	1,600	NA
5.	Bryophytes	2,700	3,900
6.	Pteridophytes	1,022	NA
7.	Gymnosperms	64	750
8.	Angiosperms	17,000	25,000

insects, 40,000 are vertebrates and 360,000 are microbes. Species biodiversity is much higher in the tropics than in the temperate regions. The nodal agency for such studies (Global biodiversity of plants and its conservation) is IPGRI, Rome, Italy.

II. National Biodiversity

Tremendous biodiversity of Indian plants has attracted the attention of many advanced countries. This wealth of plant biodiversity has developed with time due to great variation in climates, altitude and ecological niches. The National Bureau of Plant Genetic Resources (NBPGR), Pusa, New Delhi, has been a pivotal organisation in this field. The biodiversity is reflected in medicinal plants, trees, shrubs and cultivated plants-found in mountains, deserts, forests, grasslands, wetlands, mangroves and water bodies (Table 8).

III. Regional Biodiversity

In a country, plant diversity exists depending upon agro-ecological zones. In India, such a genetic diversity of plant wealth is found from Kashmir to Kanya Kumari due to climatic and edaphic diversity. In the recent past, crop diversification has been recommended. This will further strengthen regional diversity. Occurrence of species of *Ephedra,* a medicinal herb (Gymnosperms group) in high altitude Himalayan cold desert (Gangotri-Gaumukh) and also in hot arid desert (Thar desert of Rajasthan) is an excellent example of regional plant biodiversity. This biodiversity is evident from the pharmaceutical and therapeutic qualities of crude drugs collected from various regions in plants like *Plumbago, Terminalia, Ephedra, Arnica,* etc.

THREATS TO PLANT BIODIVERSITY

The great wealth of phytobiodiversity is under threats of various kinds and orders, both in developed and developing countries as well (Anonymous, 1981; Bunders *et al,* 1996; Kumar and Sharma, 2001; Deb, 2002). These threats originate from various biotic and abiotic factors/pressures. They include:

1. Over Exploitation

Medicinal herbs are being over exploited by pharmaceutical industries. Little efforts have been made to domesticate and bring them under cultivation, especially in India. These little efforts have been found insufficient to meet the growing demands of pharmaceutical industries (Ayurvedic, Homeopathic, Unani and Allopathic drug factories). Example: *Aconitum deinorrhizum, Centenella,* etc.

2. Unscientific Exploitation

Plants are being extracted from Indian forests for various purposes. No studies have been conducted on reproductive biology. Hence, the re-growth, replacement and the realistic substitution are hampered. Medicinal plants like *Atropa acuminata* (Solanaceae), *Balanophora dioica* (Balanophoraceae), *Commiphora wightii* (Burseraceae) and *Withania somnifera* (Solanaceae) are glaring examples being met with such threat (Jain and Sastry, 1980).

3. Environmental Degradation

Natural calamities like floods, cyclones, typhoons, shifting sand dunes, earthquakes and various types of soil erosion adversely affect the natural flora and fauna too. Some of the species are known to vanish due to such threats. Extraction of plants for purposes (other than drug industry) is continuing (*Calligonum polygonoides*–phog = for firewood by local population in Thar desert). Uncontrolled and unscientific grazing (overgrowing) has also led to extinction of some species (Kakralya and Singh, 1995; Chaudhary *et al,* 2000, 2001). Hunting wild animals, intensive cultivation, various types of pollution are other threats to natural flora and fauna.

4. Human Population

Alarmingly increasing human population has caused enormous biotic pressure on natural resources. This is especially factual for plant biodiversity in the fragile desert ecosystem of Thar (Chaudhary *et al,* 2000, 2001). The population pressure has resulted in deforestation and also climatic changes in several parts of the world. Ozone depletion, greenhouse gases, industrial pollution and acid rain are some climatic consequences of human activities. Adverse affects of pesticides used for crop cultivation on natural flora and fauna are evident in several parts of the world. Effect of DDT on fish population and effect of some metal organic pesticides on vulture population have been reported. Such effects on plant biodiversity have also been reported in the recent past (Oag and Rao, 2001).

5. Intensive Cultivation

Intensive cultivation is a natural consequence and compulsion of feeding the increasing human population. But its adverse effects on plant biodiversity are also equally true. Excessive use of fertilisers, pesticides, monocultures have caused ill effects on soil health and later on plant biodiversity (Cassman, 2001). Cassman (2001) therefore, advocated conduction crop science research so as to assure food security keeping in view the sustainability concept.

6. Genetically Modified Organisms

Molecular biology and gene transfer technology has undoubtedly opened new vistas in food security (Transgenic plants like BT cotton, BT corn, BT potato, BT tobacco, BT soybean). However, Janick (2001) and Keller and Carabias (2001) have cautioned about the effects of such efforts on plant biodiversity and sustainable development. The efforts of introduction and cultivation of GMC on natural fauna and flora must, therefore, be carefully investigated.

THREATS TO PLANT BIODIVERSITY IN INDIA

The Botanical Survey of India, Man and Biosphere Programme, Department of Environment and Forests, Department of Science and Technology and some ICAR institutions and universities have joined hands in this regard. In this context the classification given by Jain and Sastry (1980) is important.

1. Endangered Species (E)

Taxa in danger of extinction and whose survival is unlikely if causal factors continue to operate (Table 9).

2. Vulnerable Species (V)

Taxa likely to move into (E) in the near future if the causal factors continue to operate.

3. Rare (R)

Taxa with small population that are not presently vulnerable or endangered but are at risk. Thus, such plants should be domesticated in the near future.

4. Threatened (T)

This word is generally used in the context of conservation of species jointly for all the above three categories of species (Table 10).

5. Out of Danger (O)

Taxa which were formerly included in the above groups but are not considered safe because of effective conservation efforts/measures showing positive results.

TABLE 9
Endangered Medicinal Plants of India

No.	Common Name	Botanical Name
1.	Mitha guggal	*Commiphora wightii (E. stocksiona)*
2.	Cheryata	*Sivertia chirayita*
3.	Maniera	*Coplis teetha*
4.	Hing	*Ferula faeskeona*
5.	Yogespada	*Saussurea sacra*
6.	Indian belladonin	*Atropa acumirata*
7.	Kutaki	*Gentiana kurro*
8.	Kulaki	*Picrorrhiza kurroo*
9.	Jatamonse	*Nardostochys grandiflora*
10.	Aconites	*Aconitum chasmanthum* *E. violaceum, A. hotirophyllum*
11.	Rewad chine	*Rheum austrata*
12.	Kinis	*Dioscorea deltoidea, D. prozeri*
13.	Kiramai	*Aristolochia bracteata*
14.	Bankabri	*Podophylum hexandrum*
15.	Sarpgandha	*Rauwolfia serpentina*
16.	Indian ginseng	*Panoix pseudo-ginseng*
17.	Safed musli	*Chlorophytum arundinaceum*
18.	Somlata	*Ephedra gerardiana*
19.	Salam punja	*Orchis latifolia*
20.	Salib misri	*Eulolphia campestris*
21.	Puskar mool	*Inula racemosa*
22.	–	*Nepenthus khosiana*
23.	–	*Orosma bracteatum*
24.	Kalazeera	*Byunium bulbocastam*
25.	Suranjani-i-talka	*Colchicum luteum*
26.	Kabab chini	*Piper cubaba*
27.	Indian thyme	*Thymus serphyllum*
28.	Jeraka	*Microstylis nucifera*
	Rishavak	*M. wallichic*
29.	–	*Podygonatum cirrhifolium*
30.	Meda	*P. verticillatum*
31.	–	*Roscorea procera, R. alpina*
32.	Shera kankoli	*Lilium polyphyllum*
33.	Resha katuni	*Larateria khashmiriana*
34.	Gaozaban	*Anchusa strigosa*
35.	–	*Coscinium fanostaleim*
36.	Kasturi manzil	*Holostemna annulare*

TABLE 10
Some Threatened Medicinal Plants of Rajasthan

No.	Sanskrit Name	Botanical Name	Depletion Factor
1.	Gunja	*Abrus precatorius* Linn.	Biotic (Exploitation)
2.	Satavari	*Asparagus racemosus* Willd.	Biotic (Over-exploitation)
3.	Sahachara	*Barleria prionitis* Linn.	Natural factors (Drought)
4.	Bilva	*Aegle marmelos* (L.) Corr.	Biotic (Exploitation)
5.	Kunduru	*Boswellia serrata* Roxb.	Biotic
6.	Jyotishmati	*Celastrus paniculatus* Willd.	Biotic and natural (Exploitation)
7.	Mandukaparni	*Centella asiatica* (Linn.) Urban	Natural and biotic (Drought)
8.	Kshavak	*Centipeda minima* (L.) A. Br. & Ascher	Natural and biotic (Drought)
9.	Musli	*Chlorophytum tuberosum* Baker	Biotic and natural (Over exploitation)
10.	Guggulu	*Commiphora wightii* (Arn.) Bhand.	Biotic (Over exploited)
11.	Shankhapuspi	*Convolvulus micophyllous* Steb. ex. Spreng.	Biotic and natural (Over exploited, drought)
12.	Bhringaraja	*Eclipta prostrata* (Linn.)	Biotic and natural (Over exploited and drought)
13.	Langali	*Gloriosa superba* Linn.	Biotic (Exploited)
14.	Gambhari	*Gmelina arborea* Roxb.	Biotic
15.	Gangeru	*Grewia tenax* (Fork.) Fiori	Biotic
16.	Kutaja	*Holarrhena antidysenterica* (Roth.) A.Dc.	Biotic
17.	Kokilash	*Hygrophila auriculata* (Schum.) Heine	Biotic and natural

Continued...

...*Continued*

No.	Sanskrit Name	Botanical Name	Depletion Factor
18.	Changeri	*Oxalis corniculata* Linn.	Natural (Drought)
19.	Chitraka	*Plumbago zeylanica* Linn.	Biotic and natural
20.	Vidari	*Pueraria tuberosa* (Roxb.) DC.	Biotic
21.	Asana	*Pterocarpus marsupium* Roxb.	Biotic
22.	Munditika	*Sphaeranthus indicus* Linn.	Biotic and natural
23.	Rohitaka	*Tecomella undulata* Seem.	Biotic
24.	Bibhitaka	*Terminalia ballerica* (Gaetn.) Roxb.	Biotic
25.	Ashvagandha	*Withania somnifera* Dunal	Biotic and natural

6. Indeterminate (I)

No reliable and scientific information is available.

MEASURES FOR CONSERVATION AND DEVELOPMENT OF BIODIVERSITY IN MEDICINAL PLANTS

Medicinal plants are potential renewable natural resources. Therefore, the conservation and sustainable utilisation of medicinal plants must necessarily involve a long term, integrated and scientifically oriented action programme. This should also involve the pertinent aspects of protection, preservation, maintenance, exploitation, conservation and sustainable utilisation. A holistic system will be a more desirable one. There are two broad lines of biodiversity conservation and development.

(A). *In-Situ* Conservation

It has been well established that the best and cost-effective way of protecting the existing biological and genetic diversity is the '*in-situ*' or on the site conservation wherein a wild species or stock of a biological community is protected and preserved in its natural habitat. The prospect of such an 'ecocentric', rather than a species centred approach is that it should prevent species from becoming endangered by human activities and reduce the need for human intervention to prevent premature extinction. The idea of establishing protected area network has taken a central place in all policy decision processes related to biodiversity conservation at the national, international and global levels (Singh *et al,* 2003). Important *in-situ* conservation methods are as follows:

1. Establishment of National Parks and Gene Banks

Areas of greatest genetic diversity should be demarcated and protected from human interference, so evolutionary potential of the local population of environment would be preserved. It will be preserved so the variability exists and also allow evolution to continue and create new types. At present there are 87 National Parks and 447 Wild Life Sanctuaries extending over an area of about 1.5 lakh sq km, which is more than 4.5 per cent of the geographical area of the country. *In situ* conservation programme for medicinal plants in the national parks and sanctuaries would be taken up through the Chief Wildlife Wardens. The programme needs to be in consonance with the objectives of the national parks and sanctuaries. However, the details of medicinal plants which have been conserved by this approach are not available (Jakhar *et al,* 2003).

2. Preservation of Natural Diversity in Biosphere Reserves

There are areas of high endemism and biological diversity and possess rich genetic wealth of wild relatives of crop plants. The Department of Environment (Man and Biosphere Programme) has identified 12 biosphere reserves. These are reserves located in the:

(i). Humid tropical regions of Western Ghats.

(ii). The hilly tracts of North-East.

(iii). The temperate Himalayas.

3. Controlled Exploitation of Naturally Occurring Medicinal Plants

These are areas which are rich in natural diversity located or dominated by tribals who depend on wild edible forests plants. They not only exploit the curbing the habitats by trampling vegetative cover by cutting off bushes so selective gathering of local produce can be operated by the forest department and BDOs for distribution among the native inhabitants.

4. National Species

Adopting suitable legal measures some plants and animals are allotted national and state plant and animal status based on endevity and nativity. A list of 108 of such species has been prepared (27 each of mammals, birds, wild flowers and trees) allotting, four species to each State.

5. Adopting Extension and Educational Programmes

Socio-economic survey of tribal areas and preparing write-ups (in local dialects) providing information on native types that need to be conserved, preparing inventories of such species with local names and distributing these to villagers through block officers and VLWs, organising educational programmes through block officers/extension workers to generate such awareness among people using audio-visual aids or through other agencies.

6. Sacred Groves

There is no separate scheme for the conservation or restoration of sacred groves under the National Afforestation and Eco-Development Board (NAEB). Documentation of the sacred groves has been carried out by the regional centres of the NAEB under the scheme to "Support to Regional Centres." There are seven regional centres and their activities include helping the State/UT forest departments and Forest Development Corporation in formulation of projects, conduct study research and educational programmes for the protection, development and improvement of forest area and the degraded forest areas (Table 11).

Some regional centres (Table 11) have taken up the study of sacred groves under the forest protection and documentation. Such studies are proposed in the Annual Work Programme to the NAEB. The cost of the documents prepared are fixed on a case-by-case basis. The work done so far is included. Studies have also been conducted by NGOs and research organisations to evaluate the status of sacred groves. The C.P.R. Environmental Education Centre, Chennai, is one of such an autonomous centre of excellence of the Ministry of Environment and Forests. They have published books on the Sacred Trees of Tamilnadu and Ecological Traditions of Tamilnadu. A UNESCO study on the sacred groves of India provides a comprehensive picture of these groves along with their status. Some of the large groves and communities associated with them have been presented as case studies. However, a systematic nation-wide survey of sacred groves has not been undertaken to account for the status of these groves in terms of the conservation of biological diversity by the traditional community. The most important of all is the legal status and ownership of the grove. The changing pattern of lifestyles and religious beliefs are also responsible for the deteriorating conditions of some of the groves. The success of any conservation programme vests solely on the efficient management of protected areas. The involvement of local communities in conservation activities has now been increasingly realised. A people nature-oriented approach thus becomes highly imperative. This will help to generate a sense of responsibility among the local people about the values of biodiversity and the need to use it in a sustainable manner for their own prosperity and the maintenance of ecosystem resilience (Kato, 2002).

TABLE 11
Regional Centres of Sacred Groves

No.	Sacred Grove	Regional Centre	Year
1.	Study of sacred groves in Kurukshetra	AFC, Delhi	1996
2.	Sacred Groves of Rajasthan—relevance to afforestation and eco-development	AFC, Delhi	1997
3.	Study of sacred groves in Varanasi and Mathura districts of U. P.	AFC, Delhi	N.A
4.	Study of sacred groves of Karnataka, Kerala and Tamil Nadu	U. A. S., Bangalore	1997
5.	Sacred groves of Bihar	Jadavpur University, Kolkata	
6.	Sacred groves in Himachal Pradesh	UHF, Solan	N.A.
7.	Sacred groves of eastern M. P.	IIMF, Bhopal	1997
8.	Sacred groves of Meghalaya	NEHU, Shillong	1995
9.	Study on the status and regeneration of forest trees in the sacred groves of Khasi Hills	NEHU, Shillong	1996

In-situ conservation of medicinal plants in India can be accomplished through the active support and participation of the people who dwell in or near and around the protected forest areas. Involving the local mass in all phases of conservation programmes, such as planning, policy-decision process, implementation, etc. will be a significant component in achieving efficient management and utilisation of medicinal plant resources. To enhance *in situ* conservation of medicinal plants, conservation areas must also be set up for repositories of the genetic material and the areas would be demarcated as "no harvest zones." One of the important features is the threat assessment of the medicinal plant species by conducting "Rapid Threat Assessment" using IUCN methodology. The programme comprises of extensive field visits and preparing herbarium sheets. The community programme envisaged under this project would provide an opportunity for interaction and exchange of views among the different communities. Extensive training programme is also envisaged to train different sections of the community, the forest officers and other field staff (Barthiott and Winiger, 1996).

(B). *EX-SITU* CONSERVATION

Conservation of medicinal plants can be accomplished by the *ex-situ,* that is, outside natural habitat by cultivation and maintaining plants in botanical gardens/parks, other suitable sites and though long-term preservation of plant propagules in gene banks (seed bank, pollen bank, DNA libraries, etc.) and in plant tissue culture repositories and by cryopreservation.

1. Role of Botanical Gardens

The importance of these establishments was realised in 1759 when the Royal Botanical Garden, Kew (London) was established. This garden is playing a key role in plant exploration, introduction and phytobiodiversity conservation. At present it has an areas of 225 acres with well-equipped laboratories of all the disciplines of plant sciences. More than 30 such botanical gardens have gained international reputation (Table 12). India has a network of 140 botanical gardens which include 33 botanical gardens attached to 33 universities and their Botany departments. But hardly 30 botanical gardens have any active programme on conservation. Botanical gardens can play a key role in *ex-situ* conservation of plants, especially those facing imminent threat of extinction (Table 12). Several gardens in the world are specialised in cultivation and study of medicinal plants, while some contain a special medicinal plant garden or harbour special collection of medicinal plants (Singh, 2002).

2. Field Gene Bank of Medicinal Plants

The concept of establishing field gene banks of plants provide ample options for long term preservation of the genetic variability (inter-specific) or species. Field gene banks are better established in degraded forests where efforts are made to reforest/restock the missing species complexes, trees, shrubs, herbs, climbers, etc. The field gene bank of the Tropical Botanical Garden and Research Institute (TGBRI), Thiruvananthapuram, has covered 30,000 accessions of 250 medicinal and aromatic plant species which include 100 endemic, rare and endangered medicinal and aromatic plants of the tropical regions of India. A broad spectrum of the genetic diversity of these species was captured and introduced in this gene bank which covered morphotypes, cytotypes and chemotypes and the number of samples from each species varied from 50-100 plants.

3. Role of Seed-Propagule Banking System in Biodiversity Conservation and Development in Medicinal Plants

Seeds and propagules are the basic requirement for plant propagation, production and also for biodiversity conservation and development. It is true for natural (forests, aquatics, ponds, lakes, deserts, etc.) as well as for man-made ecosystems (agro-ecosystem) and all other efforts revolve around this nuclear (central) input (Singh *et al,* 1995; Mc Donald and Copeland, 1997). Seed is basically a mature ovule having potential of giving rise to a normal and healthy seedling. It develops after double fertilisation. However, there are deviations from this conventional definition and several other forms of planting material are grouped as seeds or propagules including corms, bulbs, rhizomes, tubers, cuttings, grafts, buds, layers, synthetic seeds (cultures, excised embryo with calcium alginate layer as protective covering). Modern plant biotechnology also includes some tissue culture regenerate plant segment, embryos, calli, anthers, ovules, cells, protoplast, shoot/root-like pollens, etc. (Kumar and Sharma, 2001).

Sufficient experimental evidences are now, available to indicate that seed and propagule quality has the potential to enhance primary productivity of the ecosystem up to 28-33 per cent (Singh *et al,* 2002). But the seed replacement rate in some developing countries including India is hardly 10-11 per cent. Hence, various methods, techniques have been developed, devised to improve physical, genetic and physiological quality of the seed and propagules including physical purity, genetic purity (genuineness of the variety) and physiological vigour. These goals are achieved through a systematic and well-programmed procedure adopted by national and international organisations concerned with seed science, technology and trade (Mc Donald and Copeland, 1997). Specific procedures, norms and guidelines have been developed for seed crop production, harvest, drying,processing,testing, certification, storage and distribution, details of these procedures and distribution.

TABLE 12

Botanical Gardens for the *ex situ* Conservation of Plant Biodiversity

Botanical Gardens of the World

1. Padua, Italy
2. Pisa, Italy
3. Palermo, Italy
4. Vidlla Taranto, Italy
5. Leyden, The Netherlands
6. Royal Botanical Garden, Edinburgh, Scotland
7. Glasnevin, Ireland
8. Meise, Belgium
9. Munich, Germany
10. Berlin-Dahlem, Germany
11. J. D. Plantes, France
12. Les Cedres, France
13. Oxford Botanical Garden, England
14. Kew Botanical Garden-Royal Botigarden, England
15. Arnoldarboretum, U. S. A.
16. Uppsalla, Scandinavia
17. New York Botanical Garden, U. S. A.
18. Brooklyn Botanical Garden, U. S. A.
19. Long Wood Garden, U. S. A.
20. Missourie Botanical, U. S. A.
21. Huntington, U. S. A.
22. Fairchild, U. S. A.
23. Montreal, Canada
24. Moscow, Russia
25. Yalta, Russia
26. Bogor, Java
27. Peradeniya, Sri Lanka
28. Singapore Botanical Garden, Singapore
29. Melbourne Botanical Garden, Australia
30. Sydney Botanical Garden, Australia
31. Japan Botanical Garden, Tokyo

Important Botanical Gardens in India

1. Indian Botanical Garden, Kolkata
2. National Botanical Garden (N. B. R. I.), Lucknow
3. Lloyd Botanical Garden, Darjeeling
4. Botanical Garden FRI, Dehradun
5. Tropical Botanical Garden, Mysore

(A). ORGANISATIONAL SET UP OF SEED PROPAGULE BANKING SYSTEM

World wide non-formal seed propagule banking system is operative having participatory roles and contributed by many nations, organisations (both governmental as well as NGOs), establishment and academic/research institutions. This is a very large system. This also involves many scientific societies and institutions. Looking at the importance of food security, environmental safety and sustainability of the "development" a great awareness has been generated about such a system in the recent past (Kumar *et al,* 2002). However, more conventionally, this system is termed as gene banking system (Boef *et al,* 1996). Boef *et al* (1996) mentioned that whatever term is used for such widely operative system, its efficacy should be assured and further improved by the participation of local people, farmers both for the purpose of *ex situ* and *in situ* conservation and development of the plant germplasm biodiversity. They also use the term 'local crop development system', which includes the partnership by the farmers and the scientific community concerning plant biodiversity conservation. Boef *et al* (1996) and Heide and Tripp (1996) opined that there is need of realistic integration of two systems (one that constitutes partnership of farmers with scientists—local crop development—and the other with exclusively seed production societies). However, the formal name of seed-propagule banking system was not used by them.

Two complementary approaches have been developed for plant biodiversity conservation and improvement. *Ex-situ* conservation is affected through seed banks (gene banks) which store samples of seeds and propagules under controlled conditions of temperature and humidity. Plant materials are collected through plant exploration and are briefly described (Passport data) before being stored. However, such so called 'gene banks' have their limitations. *In situ* conservation involves living species in their natural resources management to conserve wild, semi wild and cultivated forms of plants in botanical gardens, farmer's fields and wildlife sanctuaries. Biodiversity conservation must also be fortified by plant biodiversity improvement (Development) through selection, hybridisation, mutation researches in close collaboration with farmers. But such genetic diversity conservation and development should also be followed by varietal dissemination. A list of few partners of seed propagule banking system (SPBS) is given in Table 13.

Seeds and propagules are exchanged between countries/organisations for various purposes. Rules framed by I Convention on Conservation of Biodiversity (CCBD) and II Convention on Conservation of Biological Diversity (1995) in collaboration with FAO, CGIAR and CITES (Conservation on International Trade in Endangered Species) are strictly followed. Quarantine rules, seed health and quality rules, seed and seedling vigour rules are taken care of). These are summarised as follows:

1. Involvement of national plant germplasm system is essential.
2. For harmonisation of methods, prescribed methods by applied for collection, characterisation, evaluation, documentation and conservation of germplasm.
3. Germplasm prospecting system be developed.
4. Safeguarding the local and global plant germplasm biodiversity be assured.
5. Better and prioritised use of local and indigenous germplasm be looked into first exchange.

TABLE 13

A Few Organisations Involved in Seed-Propagule Banking Systems for Plant Biodiversity Conservation and Development (Improvement)

No.	Abbreviation	Name and Headquarters
1.	IPGRI	International Plant Genetic Resources Institute, Rome, Italy
2.	IPGRI	Regional Centre for South Asia, Pusa Campus, New Delhi, India
3.	IPGRI	Regional Centre for Asia, the Pacific and Oceania (APO), Singapore
4.	IPGRI	Regional Centre for East Asia, Beijing, China
5.	CPRO-DLO	Centre for Plant Breeding and Reproductive Research, Centre for Genetic Resources, Wageninger, The Netherlands
6.	ODI	Overseas Development Institute, London, U. K.
7.	USDA	United States Department of Agriculture, Dovis, California, U. S. A.
8.	UPOV	Union (for the) Protection (of New) Varieties of Plants
9.	IDRC	International Development Research Centre, Canada
10.	ISTA	International Seed Testing Association, Zurich, Switzerland
11.	SCST	Society of Commercial Seed Technologists, Coffey Road, Columbus, U.S.A.
12.	AOSA	Association of Official Seed Analysts, Coffey, Columbus, U. S. A.
13.	ICAR-CAU-SAU-NARS	New Delhi, India
14.	NBPGR	National Bureau of Plant Genetic Resources, Pusa Campus, New Delhi, India
15.	ICFRE	Indian Council of Forestry Research and Education, Dehradun, India
16.	ISST	Indian Society of Seed Technology, New Delhi, India
17.	SAI	Seed Association of India, New Delhi, India
18.	FA O (UNO)	Rome, Italy
19.	FIS	Federation of International Seed Trade
20.	ISHI	International Seed Health Institute, The Netherlands
21.	OECD	Organisation for Economic Co-operation and Development
22.		International/National seed companies like NSC, Mahyco, Monsanto, Pioneer, PGS, Ciba Geigy
23.	ASTA	American Seed Trade Association, U. S. A.
24.	APAFRI	Asia Pacific Association of Forestry Research Institution, Bangkok, Thailand
25.		PGRFA: FAO Global System for Conservation and Utilisation of PGRs for Food and Agriculture, Rome, Italy
26.	CGIAR	Consultative Group of International Agricultural Research, Washington, U. S. A.
27.	ICRISAT	International Centre for Research in Semi-arid Tropics, Hyderabad, India
28.	CAZRI	Central Arid Zone Research Institute, Jodhpur
29.	ICARDA	International Centre for Research in Semi-arid Tropics, Hyderabad, India
30.	CAIT	Centro International de Agril. Tropical, Cali, Columbia, U. S. A.
31.	CIMMYT	Central International de Majoramiento de Maiz y Trigo, Apdo, Mexico
32.	CIP	International Potato Centre, Lima, Peru
33.	ICRAF	International Council for Research in Agroforestry, Nairobi, Kenya
34.	IITA	International Institute of Tropical Agriculture, Ibadan, Nigeria
35.	IRRI	International Rice Research Institute, Manila, The Philippines
36.	ISNAR	International Service for National Agricultural Research, The Hague, The Netherlands
37.	AVRDC	The Asian Vegetable Research and Development Centre, Shanhua, Taiwan, China

TABLE 14
Selected Medicinal Plants Domesticated Within the Last Decennial

Species	Active Principle
Achillea millefolium	Essential Oils
Arnica montana	Sesquiterpenelactones
Artemisia annua	Sesquiterpenes
Catharanthus roseus	Alkaloids
Cephaelis ipecacuanha	Alkaloids
Chelidonium majus	Alkaloids
Convullaria majalis	Cardenolides
Costus speciosus	Steroids
Dioscorea sp.	Steroids
Dracocephalum moldavica	Essential oils
Duboisia myoporoides	Alkaloids
Echinacea sp.	Immunostimulants
Gentiana lutea	Bitter substances
Pimpinella saxifraga	Essential oils
Rauwolfia sp.	Alkaloids
Silybum marianum	Flavonolignans
Valleriana edulis	Iridoids
Panax ginseng	
Panax guinuifolius	
Hydraceus canadensis	
Hypericum sp.	
Screnoa serrulata	
*Taxus brevifolia**	
*Vinca minor**	
Punus afric	

* Anti-cancer

B. FUNCTION AND ACTIVITIES OF THE SYSTEM

Worldwide seed propagule banking system has specific prescribed and well-documented procedures for performing its functions and activities. These are as below:

For scientific exploitation of plant biodiversity, plant biodiversity, plant taxonomy conduct plant collections, identification and phonological studies, seeds are collected at proper stage. Herbaria are established. These may be new genera of species or may be new/first reports in an area or may be wild relatives already existing taxa (role of taxonomists, ecologists). This is followed by seed studies which includes seed collection, drying, storage, germination studies, dormancy, viability, documentation and other physiological studies.

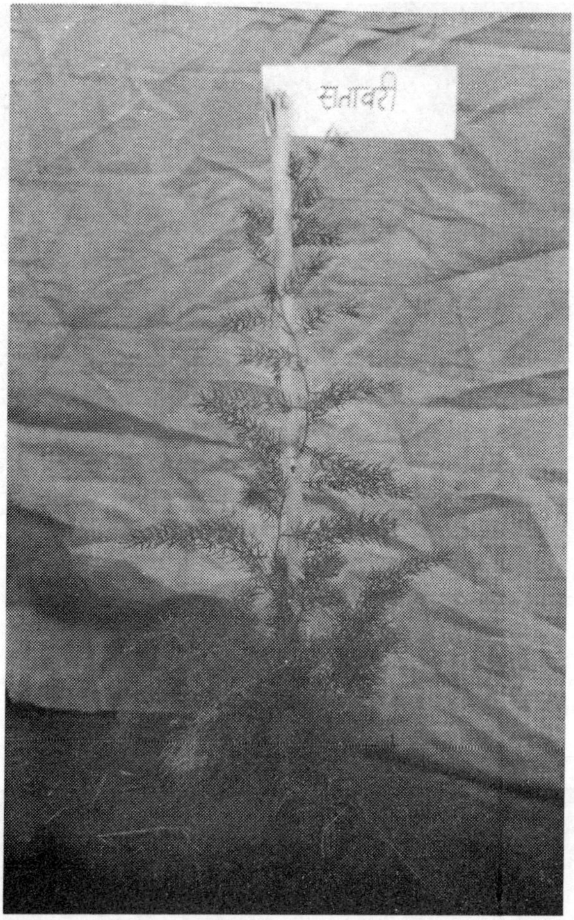

Figure 1. Satawar: *Asparagus racemosus* domesticated and cultivated in Rajasthan, SKNCOA, Jobner.

The collected and documented germplasm is evaluated for its laboratory and field performance.

After primary taxonomic/economical/physiological investigations, wild plants are subjected to domestication efforts. It is realised that since the human utilisation began, very few plant species have been brought under cultivation web. Hence, an extensive work on plant domestication is required. Necessity of such activity was also found by Heide and Trippe (1996), Bunders *et al* (1996), Kumar *et al* (2002) and Kumar and Sharma (2001).

The situation with medicinal plants is more grim. Very limited work has been done on such aspects. Franz (1993) reviewed the world literature on these aspects and detailed strategies for domestication and cultivation of wild medicinal plants, otherwise potentially useful as human and veterinary medicines.

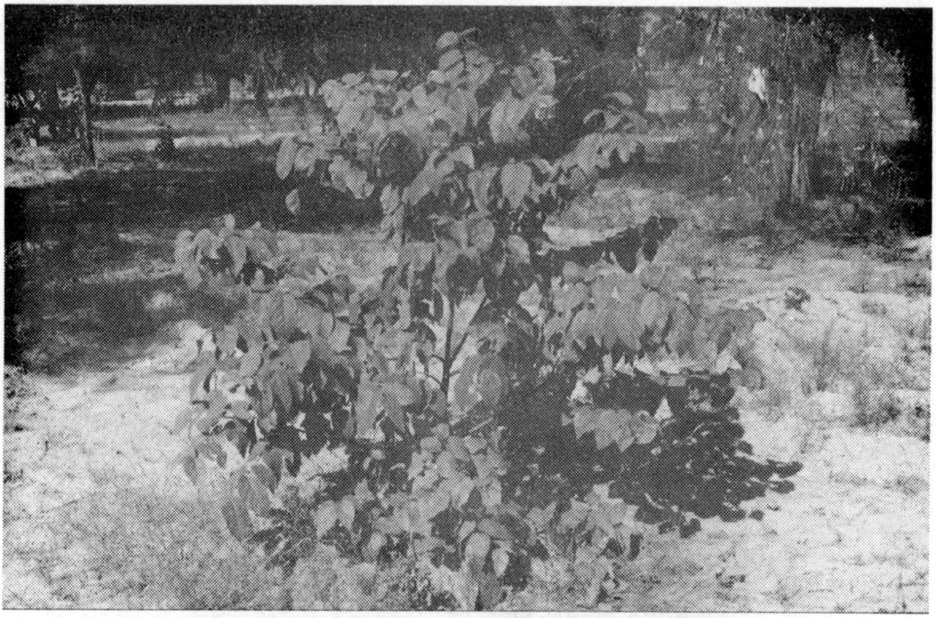

Figure 2. Utrassum bead tree = Rudrak (sh): *Elaeocarpus sphaericus* domesticated and cultivated in Rajasthan, SKNCOA, Jobner.

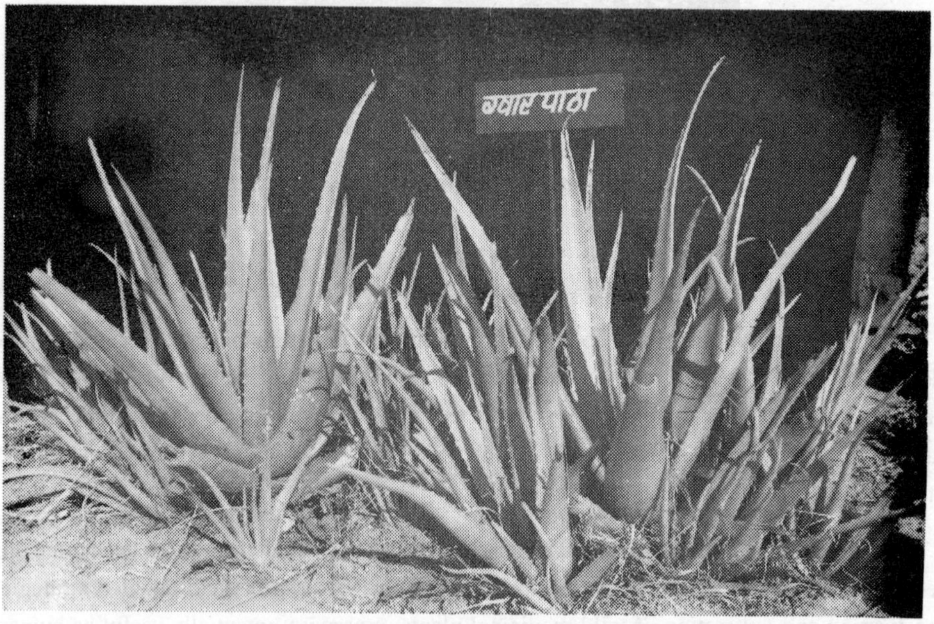

Figure 3. Aloe: *Aloe vera* cultivated at Jobner.

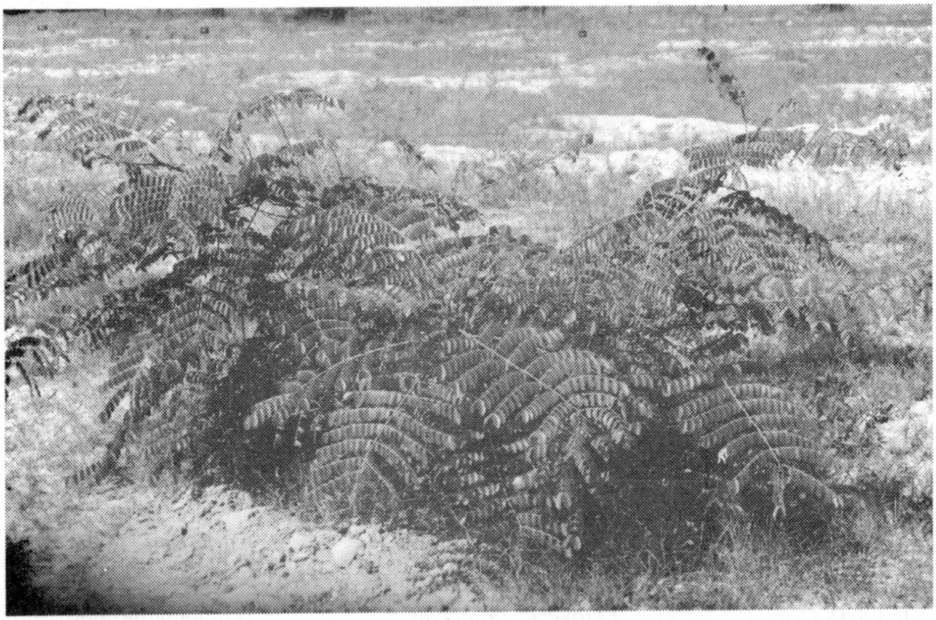

Figure 4. Malluca bean: ***Caesalpinia crista*** **domesticated and cultivated in Rajasthan, SKNCOA, Jobner.**

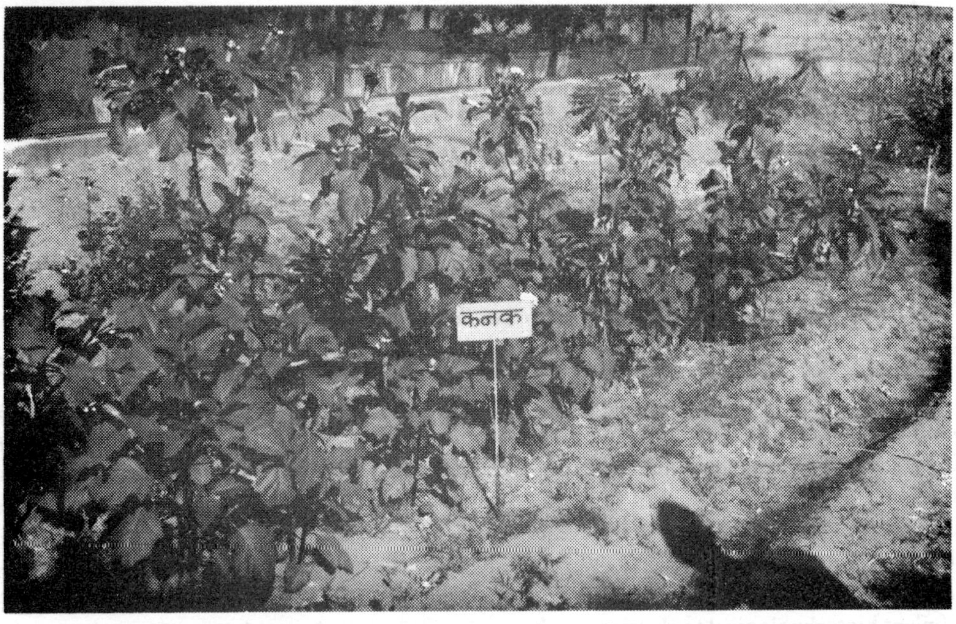

Figure 5. Jimson weed: ***Datura stramonium*** **domesticated and cultivated in Rajasthan, SKNCOA, Jobner.**

TABLE 15
Some Medicinal Plants Collected in the Wild to be Domesticated Within the Near Future

No.	Family	Species	Activity
1.	Acanthaceae	*Adhadota vasica*	Spasmolytic
2.	Apocynaceae	*Aspidosperma quebr.* Blanco	Respirostimulant
3.	Asclepiadaceae	*Marsdenia condurango*	Bitter substances
4.	Asteraceae	*Baccharis* sp.	Anti-inflammatoric
5.	Asteraceae	*Eclipta alba*	Hepatoprotective
6.	Asteraceae	*Gnmaphalium* sp.	Anti-inflammatoric
7.	Asteraceae	*Neurolaena lobata*	Anti-malarial
8.	Asteraceae	*Tagetes lucida*	Spasmolytic
9.	Droseraceae	*Drosera* sp.	Proteolytic
10.	Euphorbiaceae	*Phyllanthus niruri*	Antiseptic
11.	Liliaceae	*Urginea* sp.	Cardioactive
12.	Myrtaceae	*Psidium guajava*	Spasmolytic
13.	Phytolaccaceae	*Petoveria alliaceae*	Immunostimulant
14.	Rutaceae	*Closemma amosata*	Flavouring
15.	Zingiberaceae	*Siphonichilus natalensis*	Anti-malarial
16.	Fabaceae	*Abrus precatorius*	Aphrodisiac
17.	Amaranthaceae	*Achyranthus aspera*	Bronchial infection
18.	Liliaceae	*Aloe barbedensis*	Purgative
19.	Compositae	*Artemisia absinthium*	Vermicide
20.	Nictaginace	*Boerhaavia diffusa*	Diuretic
21.	Mimosaceae	*Caesalpinia crista*	Antipyretic
22.	Asclepiadaceae	*Calotropis procera*	Diaphoretic
23.	Caesalpiniaceae	*Cassia fistula*	Laxative
24.	Apiaceae	*Centella asiatica*	Diuretic
25.	Euphorbiaceae	*Euphorbia antiquorum*	Anthelmintic

In all these efforts, seed propagule banking system plays a key role. For this purpose, conventional methods like selection, hybridisation, mutation and introduction are still prevalent and playing effective and economic roles. After new varieties are developed, their improved seed production strategies are required through seed technology and production sciences. These also include seed testing, certification, processing, storage, treatment invigoration and conditioning coupled with timely distribution to growers and farmers. With biodiversity conservation point of view, the effective participation of local farmers is the need of the day (Kumar *et al,* 2002). Modern methods include the use of plant biotechnological tools (tissue culture, etc.) and applied cryobiology (Figures 1-5)..

Singh (1984), Singh and Kumar (1984), Kumar (1986), Franz (1993) and Padulosi *et al* (2002)

TABLE 16
List of Medicinal Plants Recommended for Cultivation on Priority Basis

No.	Common Name	Scientific Name	Family
1.	Aonla	*Emblica officinalis*	Euphorbiaceae
2.	Aswahagandha	*Withania somnifera*	Solanaceae
3.	Ashoka	*Saraca asoca*	Leguminoseae
4.	Atis	*Aconitum heterophyllum*	Ranunculaceae
5.	Bael	*Aegle marmelos*	Rutaceae
6.	Brahmi	*Bacopa monnieri*	Scrophulariaceae
7.	Baiberang	*Embelia ribes*	Myrtanaceae
8.	Chandan	*Santalum album*	Santalaceae
9.	Giloe	*Tinospora cordifolia*	Meninspermaceae
10.	Guggal	*Commiphora wightii*	Burseraceae
11.	Indian barbery	*Berberis aristata*	Berberidaceae
12.	Isabgol	*Plantago ovata*	Plantaginaceae
13.	Jatamansi	*Nardostachys jatamansi*	Valerianaceae
14.	Kalmegh	*Andrographis paniculata*	Acanthaceae
15.	Katki	*Picrorrhiza kurroa*	Scrophulariaceae
16.	Kokum	*Garcinia indica linnacus*	Clusiaceae
17.	Kur	*Saussurea lappa*	Compositae
18.	Liquorice	*Glycyrrhiza glabra*	Papilionaceae
19.	Long pepper	*Piper longum*	Piperaceae
20.	Madhunashini	*Gymnema sylvestre*	Asclepiadaceae
21.	Satavari	*Asparagus racemosus*	Liliaceae
22.	Shankapushpi	*Convolvulus pluricaulis*	Convolvulaceae
23.	Safed musli	*Chlorophytum borivillanum*	Liliaceae
24.	Senna	*Cassia angustifolia*	Caesalpinaceae

made valuable contributions in enhancing the potential of plant domestication, introduction and cultivation activities relating to medicinal plants. Franze (1993) has given an excellent scheme of domestication and biodiversity development in medicinal plants and also listed recently domesticated medicinal plants in the world (Table 14 and 15). Jakhar *et al* (2003) also made similar efforts in the context of Indian agroclimatic conditions (Tables 15 and 16).

IV. APPLIED CRYOBIOLOGY AND PLANT BIOTECHNOLOGY

Applied aspects of cryobiology and biotechnology have assumed, now, a very important status in biodiversity conversation and development. These scientific technologies have become part and parcel of seed and propagule banking system. Cryopreservation of seeds and propagules is the storage at ultra low temperature in cryogenic medium such as liquid nitrogen. This technique has been developed as modification of classic procedures such as chemical cryoprotection, slow dehydration, cooling, storage in liquid nitrogen, rapid thawing, washing and recovery (Kumar and Sharma, 2001). Cryostorage or long-term storage at –196°C in liquid nitrogen is potent in reducing the metabolism of seeds, propagules, tissues, cells and even protoplasts. Chin (1993) reviewed the literature and compared the relative merits and demerits and limitations of conventional propagule storage practice and modern techniques (cryopreservation). These techniques are integral parts of seed propagule banking system for biodiversity conservation purpose. Vitrification is a new addition to the technology of cryopresentation. Vitrification is the process of transition of water directly from liquid phase into an amorphous phase or glass, thus avoiding the formation of ice crystals in cells of seeds-propagules and tissue culture regenerates. This technique has been found still more successful in the cryopreservation of somatic embryos and synthetic seeds (Table 17).

Ways to conserve plant biodiversity through tissue biotechnology have been comprehensively reviewed by Kumar and Sharma (2001) taking the example of several rare and threatened plant species.

FUTURE PROSPECTS AND LINE OF ACTION

For sustainable and equitable development of medicinal plants, various departments (both public sector and NGOs as well) may adopt the following approaches:

1. The institutes of ICFRE should concentrate on collection of germplasm of the 25 plant species identified by the Task Force on Medicinal Plants constituted by the Government of India (Table 16). With well-developed infrastructure these institutes should try to develop agrotechnique and protocols for mass multiplication to provide quality planting material to the cultivators and foresters. It should also collect information on inter cropping, rotational-cropping use of biofertilisers and organic farming for providing know-how to the farmers and Forest Department for developing "Vanaspati Van' and cultivation of medicinal plants. The Council should attempt to make available high quality planting material by developing a network of nurseries of medicinal plants. Attempts should also be made for human resource development by organising training programmes on agro-practices, post-harvest technology and quality control techniques.
2. For conservation of medicinal plants, the Wildlife Wing of the Forest Departments may consider establishment of Medicinal Plant Conservation Area (MPCA) covering all ecosystems, forest types and sub types in the country.
3. The main problems which the Forest Departments are facing is continuing degradation of India's forest cover, which is a source of most of the medicinal plants; and it is in this extremely difficult situation that the country has to implement its commitment to the conservation of biodiversity and its sustainable use. Considering that at present 90 per cent collection of medicinal plants is from the wild, generation of about 40 million man-days employment, current practices of harvesting are unsustainable and responsible for depletion of resource base. To reverse this process, Forest Department has to initiate the following actions:

   (i). Identify forest areas rich in medicinal plants, formulate a management

TABLE 17
Medicinal Plant Biodiversity Conservation Through Tissue Culture Biotechnology

No.	Plant	Explant Used	Medium	Mode of Regeneration	Reference
1.	*Caralluma edulis*	Shoot segments	MS	Clonal multiplication	Hatanco *et al,* 1987
2.	*Commiphora wightii*	Shoot segments	MS	Axillary shoot proliferation	Barve & Mehta, 1993
3.	*Coptis teeta*	Hypocotyl segment	MS	Callus culture	Tandon & Rathore, 1991
4.	*Gerbera qurantiaca*	Axillary bud	MS	Axillary shoot proliferation	Mayer Vanstaden, 1998
5.	*Nepenthes khasiana*	Mature nodal segment	MS or Wood Pt. medium	Axillary bud	Latha & Seeni, 1994
6.	*Ocolea cathannensis*	Zygotic	MS	Somatic embryogenesis	Casta *et al,* 1993
7.	*Opcidium varicosum*	Seeding	Knudson medium	Root tip culture	Kerbeay, 1993
8.	*Prorhiza kumba*	Axillary bud	MS	Axillary shoot proliferation	Upadhyay *et al,* 1989
9.	*Podophyllum haxandrum*	Zygotic embryo	MS	Somatic embryogenesis	Arumugan & Bhojwani, 1989
10.	*Rauwolfia serpentina*	Low temperature	MS	Storage	Sharma & Chandel, 1982

plan for intensive management and sustainable harvesting of herbal products.

(ii). Establishment of 'Vanaspati Van' in degraded forest areas where medicinal plants exist or existed. Each 'Vanaspati Van' should have an area of 3,000-5,000 hectares, with irrigation facility and managed by a registered society headed by Divisional Forest Officer.

(iii). It should effectively regulate extraction and transport of medicinal plants from the wild. The Department should maintain a list of petty traders, private agents, wholesale dealers and final consumers of medicinal plants. It should organise training and awareness camps on various aspects of medicinal plant development.

(iv). Creation of awareness among rural folk of medicinal plants around them and also encourage them for cultivation of these plants for health care and as alternative crops.

4. The role of organisations like National Medicinal Plant Board, Rajasthan State Medicinal Plant Board, Multifaculty Universities, State Agricultural Universities, etc. is also valuable. The effective and realising coordination/cooperation/interdisciplinary/integrated/inter-institutional approach is unavoidable. Farmers participation/extension education/training/workshops/marketing procedure/remunerative price motivation/exporter, scientific information on domesticational and cultivational aspects of medicinal plants other than flowering plants is very meagre. Therefore, we must also give due and prioritised attention to therapeutically useful bacteria, fungi, lichens, algae, bryophytes, pteridophytes and gymnosperms. Medicinal and export potential of these groups of plants is reflected in the literature but systematic initiation is immediately required.

REFERENCES

Anonymous. IPGRI, Rome, Italy Newsletter No. 32 (August 2000), pp. 22-23, 2000.

Anonymous. Task Force Report, 2000.

Anonymous. *Tropical legumes: Resources for Future.* Washington, DC. USA: National Academy of Sciences, 1981.

Boef, W. S., Berg, T. and Hawerkort, B. 'Crop genetic resources'. In *Biotechnology-Building on Farmer's Knowledge.* (Eds.). Bunders, J., Hawerkort, B. and Hiemsira, W. London: MacMillan, pp. 103-128,1996.

Borthiott, W. and Winiger, M. *Biodiversity A Challenge for Development Research and Policy.* Springer For Science, Ij muiden The Netherlands, 1998.

Cassman, K. G. 'Crop science research to assure food security'. In: *Crop Science: Progress and Prospects.* (Eds.). Nosberger, J., Geiger, H. H. and Struik, P. C. Wallingford, UK: CABI Publishing, pp. 33-52, 2001.

Chaudhary, V., Singh, Karan and Kakralya, B. L. (Eds.). *Environmental Protection.* Jaipur: Pointer Publishers, pp. 231-240, 2000.

Chaudhary, V., Singh, Karan; Kumar, A. and Bora, K. K. 'Environmentalists, agrihorticulturists, foresters, industrialists and exporters expectations from phytophysiologists'. In: *Production and Developmental Plant Physiology.* (Eds.). Bora, K. K., Singh, Karan and Kumar, Arvind. Jaipur: Pointer Publishers, pp. 5-39, 2001.

Chin, H. F. 'Germplasm conservation in year 2000'. *Seed Res. Special,* vol. No. 1, pp. 207-216, 1993.

Connor, D. J. 'Optimising crop diversification'. In: *Crop Science: Progress and Prospects.* (Eds.). Nosberger, J., Geiger, H. H. and Stuirik, P. C. Wallingford, UK: CABI Publishing, pp. 5-39, 2001.

Deb, C. R. 'Cryopreservation of somatic embryos and artificial seeds of *Melia azedarch* by vitrification'. *J. Plant Biol.* 29: 71-76, 2002.

Edwards, P. J. and Hitlbeck, J. *Biodiversity of agroecosystems.* (Eds.). Nosberger, J., Geiger, H. H. and Struik. P. C.. Wallingford, UK: CABI Publishing, pp. 213-230, 2001.

Franz, C. 'Domestication of wild growing medicinal plants'. *Plant Res. and Development* 37: 101-111, 1993.

Govil, J. N., Pandey, J., Shivakumar, B. G. and Singh, V. K. 'Recent process in medicinal plants. V. Crop improvement, production technology, trade and commerce'. H. 1-42 Sci. Tech. Publ. Co. LLC. Texas, USA, 2002.

Heide, W. M. and Tripp, R. *Local Crop Development.* Rome, Italy, 1996.

Jain, S. K. and Sastry, A. R. K. *Threatened Plants of India.* New Delhi: Department of Science and Technology, 1980.

Jakhar, M. L., Singh, Karan and Kakralya, B. L. 'Prospective strategy for biodiversity conservation and development in medicinal and aromatic plants'. In: *Environmental Conservation: Depleting Resources and Sustainable Development.* Jaipur: Aavishkar Publishers Distributors, pp. 145-156, 2003.

Janick, J. 'New crops for 21st century'. In: *Crop Science: Progress and Prospects.* (Eds.) Mosberger, J., Geiger, H. H. and Struik, P. C. Wallingford, UK: CABI Publishing, pp. 307-328, 2001.

Kakraliya, B. L. Zoogenic factors in desertification in Thar Desert of Raj. Ph.D. Thesis. University of Rajasthan, Jaipur, 1989.

Kakraliya, B. L. and Singh, Karan. 'Ecophysiological factors in desertification'. In: *Plant Productivity Under Environmental Stress.* (Eds.). Singh, Karan and Purohit, S. S. Bikaner: RAU and *Agros*, pp. 35-44, 1995.

Kakraliya, B. L. and Singh, Karan. 'Seed quality of Indian mustard'. In: *Seeds Bioregulants and Applied Plant Biotechnology.* (Eds.). Bora, K. K. and Singh, Karan and Kumar, Arvind. Jaipur: Pointer Publishers, pp. 146-155, 2002.

Kato M. *The Biology of Biodiversity.* Springer for Science, Ij muiden, The Netherlands, 2002.

Kumar, A., Singh, Karan; Kakralya, B. L. and Manohar, S. S. 'Traditional ecophysiological knowledge (TEK) in sustainable agriculture'. In: *Seeds, Bioregulants and Applied Plant Biotechnology.* (Eds.). Bora, K. K., Singh, Karan and Kumar, Arvind. Jaipur: Pointer Publishers, pp. 51-57, 2002.

Kumar, S. Ecophysiological studies on Indian medicinal plants. Ph.D. Thesis. Meerut University, Meerut, 1986.

Kumar, U. and Sharma, A. *Plant Biotechnology and Biodiversity Conservation*. Jodhpur: *Agro-Bios*, 2001.

Mc Donald, M. B. and Copeland, L. *Seed Production—Principles and Practices*. New York and London: Chapman and Hall, 1997.

Nosberger, J., Geiger, H. H. and Struik, P. C. *Crop Science—Progress and Prospects*. Wallingford, UK: CABI Publishing, 2001.

Oago, C. K. and Rao, M. R. 'Management of complex interactions for growth resources and of biotic stresses in agroforestry' In: *Crop Science—Progress and Prospects*. (Eds.). Nosberg, J., Geiger, H. H. and Struik, P. C. Wallingford, UK: CABI Publishing, 2001.

Podulosi, D., Leaman, D. and Quick, F. D. 'Challenges and opportunities in enhancing the biodiversity conservation and uses of medicinal plants'. *Herbs, Spices and Medicinal Plants* 9: 243-279, 2002.

Sankhla. N. 'Facing the flash flood of new knowledge and innovation: a plant physiologist in biotechnological wonderland'. In: *Seed Bioregulants and Applied Plant Biotechnology*. (Eds.). Bora, K. K., Singh, Karan and Kumar, A. Jaipur: Pointer Publishers, pp. 94-101, 2002.

Singh, K. B. 'Exploitation and evaluation of chickpea genetic resources'. In: *Genetic Resources and Their Exploitation*. (Eds.). Witcombe, J. R. and Erstkine, W. The Hague: Martinus Nishoff/Dr. W. Junk Publishers, pp. 105-130,1984.

Singh, Karan and Kumar, S. 'Ecophysiological observations on Indian medicinal plants'. *Acto Bot. Indica* 12: 216-219, 1984.

Singh, Karan; Kakralya, B. L. and Singh, B. 'Production physiology of Indian medicinal plants under abiotic stress'. In: *Plant Productivity Under Environmental Stress*. (Eds.), Singh, Karan and Purohit, S. S. Bikaner: RAU & *Agros*, pp. 55-66, 1995.

Singh, Karan; Singh, K. P. and Kumar, S. 'Seedling growth responses of medicinal plants to certain physical and chemical treatments'. *Indian J. Plant Physiol* 27(3): 295-299, 1984.

Singh, S. J., Singh Karan; Gupta, S. C. and Kakralya, B. L. 'Seed propagule banking system and applied cryobiology: Potential tools for plant biodiversity conservation and sustainable development'. In *Environmental Conservation Depleting Resources and Sustainable Development*. Jaipur: Aavishkar Publishers Distributors, pp. 55-66, 2003.

Singh, V. *Taxibint of Angiospersus*. Meerut: Rastogi Publications, 2002.

Wilkings, R. J. 'Facng the growing needs of mankind: grasslands and rangelands'. In: *Crop Science: Progress and Prospects*. (Eds.). Nosberger, J., Geiger, H. H. and Struik, P. C. Wallingford, UK: CABI Publishing, pp. 65-80, 2001.

—oo(O)oo—

4

Medicinal Plants: Biodiversity Conservation, Export Potential and Intellectual Property Rights

M. M. Bhandari

FROM earliest times, herbs have been used for pain-relieving and health care needs. They have provided all the medicament to man and his domestic animals for a wide spectrum of ailments and to soothe his aches and pains. Until comparatively recent times they remained mankind's chief method of healing. Even now in an age dominated by scientific and technological marvels, by miracle drugs and miracle cures, botanicals or their synthetically derived equivalents account for a majority of prescriptions or even non-prescription medicines. Over the ages the magical and mystical powers were ascribed to plants. Occasionally these beliefs were mere superstitions; more commonly they were based on keen observations. At that time although people knew that certain plants had indispensable healing powers, they could not explain how the medicinal powers of plants worked. Therefore these were attributed to supernatural forces.

Initially, the plants were part of folk-medicine practised by ancient man in different parts of the world, which include India, China, the Middle East, Africa and South America. The same herbs, trees and shrubs employed by ancient people have continued to be valued through the ages-by Egyptians, Greeks, Romans and Indians. In the long struggle to achieve mastery over the powerful forces of nature man, has always turned to plants for help. Plants provide vital energy in their growth and seasonal rebirth. When pain, injury or disease struck early man, he had little choice but to turn to plants. Developed empirically by trial and error, many herbal treatments were remarkably effective. But the herbal treatments fell out of favour and branded as ignorant superstition. Now the new medical science is affirming much of the old herbal lore and extending its horizons to botanical medicines.

Long before the earliest record that is available today, it seems many different people and cultures discovered that some plants are not only good to eat, but many plants have healing properties. Slowly by trial and error, some tried and trusted herbal remedies were amassed resulting in a corpus of information about the medicinal herbs. A fund of information developed by word-of-mouth and by inspection ad direct appreciation and experiences handed down from one generation to the next. Those who took special interest in the healing qualities of plants became especially skilled in the application of plants for this purpose, gradually gained an honoured place in society. Fortunately for us today, however, this accumulated traditional knowledge of the early past has been preserved in the writings and practice of herbalists. As civilisation grew from 3000 BC onwards, that is, in Egypt, India, China and the Middle East, the use of herbs became more sophisticated and gradually the first written account of plants of medicinal value were made. Nearly half or more of all medicines currently prescribed are derived from members of the plant kingdom. Ancient Egypt was not alone in recording the healing power of plants and gave the world the famous *Eberus papyrus* of *circa* 1500 BC.

At least 2,000 years ago, the earliest known Chinese Pharmacopoeia *Pen Taso*, mentions choolmugra oil obtained from *Hydnocarpus* to treat leprosy. The ancient Chinese also first recorded the use of desert the shrub *Ephedra* from China to improve the circulation of blood, reduce fever, help urinary function and suppress lung and bronchial disorders. We also have desert *Ephedra—Ephedra foliata*. Although the preliminary survey made by the Forest Department some 50 years ago mentions that the ephedrine contents of our *Ephedra* is much less than is found in *Ephedra narbadensis*, a Himalayan species, but in view of the fact that the Ephedrine contents decreases with the increase in rainfall (as mentioned by Chopra), it is worth fresh analysing by modern methods of chemical analysis.

Thousands of years ago, India's greatest sages established the Ayurveda or the knowledge of life, the main goal of which was alleviation of human suffering. The sages of Ayurveda saw all illnesses and all health as part of an interlocking whole—mind, body and spirit–that they thought should be treated as one. For medicines and treatments, they looked to the natural world around them, to the plants used by forest tribes since the beginning of history.

The traditional system of medicine in India prescribing plant extractives in therapy dates back to the early age of the *Rig Veda* (4500 to 1600 BC). The therapeutic efficacy of herbal medicines led to the evolution (2500 to 600 BC) of Ayurveda which literally means "science of life." All the Vedas—*Rig, Yajur, Sama* and *Atharva* have contributed to the development of Ayurveda. The *Rig Veda* mentions 67 herbal drugs, the *Yajur Veda* 81 and the *Atharva Veda* about 290.

The sages of Ayurveda were aware of the medicinal plants known and used by the so called aboriginal Indian tribes that had inhabited India's forests from the beginning of history. So the second task they set themselves was the collation and examination of medical information into what we would call today the first Indian medical and botanical encyclopaedia. The growing mass of knowledge, constantly expanded by successive Ayurvedic physicians, was committed to memory and handed down orally from teachers to students for over thousands of years before it was finally written down in the first century AD by Ayurveda's third legendary physician, Charaka. Charaka provided Indian medicine with its first written text in the *Charaka Samhita* or treatise of Charaka, which describes 1,500 plants and identifies 350 of them being valuable for medicinal purposes.

Charaka Samhita (700 BC), the first recorded treatise on Ayurveda, was followed by *Sushruta Samhita* (600 BC) both compiled a century apart, believed to be not later than 900 BC. *Charaka Samhita* and *Sushruta Samhita* are the beacon lights of Ayurveda even to the present day. *Charaka Samhita* gives the properties of drugs prepared from indigenous plants and their uses and the methods of their administration as in the present day practice clearly showed the extent of advancement of the indigenous system of medicine as well as the depth of knowledge of the then practitioners with regard to drug therapy and toxicology.

The fifteenth century saw expelling the Arabs from Spain. The European powers sought to break the Arab monopoly on the trade of Indian spices and medicines and find their own routes to India. At this moment of History, India's vast knowledge of plant pharmacopoeia led to launching fleet after fleet of Europeans, British, French, Dutch, Spanish and Portuguese. The rulers of Spain financed and expedition by Columbus and it can be said that Ayurveda led to the discovery of America since Columbus' mission was to find new access to the spices of India. While Europe was searching for means to acquire India's spices and plants, Ayurvedic medicine was flourishing in India. At the beginning of the Mughal empire, the Ayurvedic knowledge was at its zenith in India. With the fragmentation and decay of the Mughal empire at the end of the 17th century, as India disintegrated into civil wars, the great centres of India's learning fell apart and scholarship was dispersed by two centuries of political unrest. Ayurvedic knowledge retreated into the villages, temples and small princely courts of India. For the whole century, British rule despised Indian scientific learning. Fired by new nationalism, patriotic Indian physicians began to examine the claims made by Ayurvedic medicines. Small Ayurvedic centres began to flourish again. New ones were established. But it was not until India became independent that Ayurveda began to regain as a valid school of medicine.

It has been suggested that the ancient Greek School of Medicine was indebted to the Hindu System since reference to indigenous Indian drugs are found in the works of Hippocrates as *kardamoman* from the Sanskrit *kardama* (cardamom). Hindu thoughts influenced the Greek medical literature in the fifth and sixth centuries BC. About 400 BC, a Greek named Hippocrates asserted that medicine was a science and art rather than a religious ritual full of incantation and mystery. Hippocrates believed that the four elements of fire, water, earth and air were represented in the human body by yellow bile, phlegm, black bile and blood. The picture at the beginning of first century AD is one of increasing experimentation and knowledge.

Before Dioscorides, to the west, Rome had begun its rise to power in Europe and the lands around the Mediterranean sea. Pliny was the most important writer on plants in ancient Rome. Seven out of his 37 volumes of his *Historia Naturale* composed in 77 AD, were devoted to the medicinal uses of plants. However, Pliny's writing being uncritical and his information remained unverified, this work later on become of little value. The Arabs also gave the peculiar mixture of philosophy and chemistry known as alchemy.

The Vedas originally written down in Sanskrit made many references to the healing plants, including the snake-root plant *Rauvolfia serpentina*, used in India to treat snake bite and mental disorders. Known from very early times in Bihar as 'Pagal-ki-dava', *Rauvolfia serpentina* is a modern source of reserpine—a modern source of tranquilliser and hypertensive agent. Its active ingredient reserpine is the basic ingredient of a variety of tranquillisers first used in the 1950s to treat certain types of emotional and mental problems. Though reserpine is seldom used today for this purpose, its discovery was a breakthrough in the treatment of mental illness. Other important constituents of *Rauvolfia* are serpentine and ajmantine. The German pharmaceutical company Hoechst capitalised on it. I had an opportunity to visit Hoechst's establishment at Mumbai in 1990 and I was told that the entire Hoechst Co. was based basically on *Rauvolfia serpentina*.

A very important medicinal plant mentioned in our ancient Ayurvedic literature is *Commiphora wightii*, formerly known as *Balsemodendron mukul* or, the guggal plant. This is the only medicinal plant of Rajasthan now included in our Red Data Book of rare and threatened medicinal plants. Many preparations like Yograj Guggal, Mahayograj Guggal, Triphala Guggal, Kishore Guggal, Kachnar Guggal, etc have been made from the pale-yellow oleo-gum-resin of this species with the mixture of different plants. Guggal is used in arthritis, water retention, rheumatism and glandular and neurological disorders. Contemporary clinical tests have located a steroid fraction in the resin which had proved effective in the treatment of secondary arthritis. Recently, CDRI, Lucknow, has prepared Gugulip from this species which has now been taken up by many other pharmaceutical companies. The importance of guggal has reached far and wide. In 1991, while I was attending a conference organised by the Open University of Complementary Medicines, Srilanka, while we were going through the book exhibition there, a Swedish professor met me. He was fantastically searching for literature on the guggal plant, his wife being seriously suffering from arthritis. When I told him that you have met the right person since my name is permanently associated with guggal plant, *Commiphora wightii* (Arnott) Bhandari formerly based on *Balsamea wightii*. Not only I showed him the description and photograph of this plant from my flora, I also sent him one kg of real guggal on my return to Jodhpur. Nearly two years latter, he confirmed that his wife was greatly relieved from arthritis by guggal treatment.

This guggal plant though widely available in drier parts of Rajasthan and Gujarat, but today, hardly one can find new seedlings of this plant anywhere in its range of distribution. We, therefore, had the opportunity to study the ecology of this plant particularly from the point of view of conservation of this species. We found that this plant produces flowers twice in the year, once in September-October and then again in March after winter rains. The seeds produced in March are viable and on germination produced plants but no seeds germinated from rainy season flowers. We raised nearly 700 plants of guggal both by seed germination as well as by cuttings and distributed to numerous botanical gardens and institutions.

While examining the guggal plant from its range of occurrence, we found that there is diversity in the production of oleo-gum resin from the plant. The plants collected from Mevanagar near Balotra had a thinner consistency of resin than the one found at Jodhpur and Barmer. The samples of guggal collected from a grocer's shop examined by us revealed that the guggal samples very often were a mixture of salai and other cheaper gums. It is this type of substitute medicines available with grocers that has led to undermining the importance of Ayurvedic treatments.

Genetic diversity refers to the heritable variation within and between populations and organisms. Each variety within a species contains unique genes, and the diversity of genes within species increases its ability to adapt to pollution, disease and other changes in the environment.

The pool of genetic variation thus enables both natural evolutionary change and artificial selective breeding to occur. When these varieties or populations of these species are destroyed, the genetic diversity within the species is diminished. The planet's natural wealth lies not just in its species, but in the genetic variation within them. Until recently, measurements of genetic diversity were applied mainly to domesticated species and population. With modern biotechnological tools, where genes of wild relatives of cultivated plants are introduced in domesticated plants, this technique is proving to be of immense potentiality. Genetic engineers can use these genes to develop medicines and foods. In the Indian desert, there are numerous populations of a number of genera such as *Tephrosia, Citrullus, Cucumis, Tribulus, Convolvulus, Lasiurus,* etc. and the genetic diversity present in them could be made use of in the improvement of useful traits of these species for their better utilisation. To give one example, there is a large number of strains of *Citrullus colocynthis*, the tumba plant, which is an important sand-dune stabiliser, found throughout the desert spreading on the loose sand. However, in the last nearly 15 years ever since its seeds have been collected for oil, it has become a threatened plant in the desert. Moreover, a natural hybrid between *Citrullus colocynthis* and *C. lanatus*, the water melon, has been found in the Indian desert. Therefore, there is a possibility of transferring the genes responsible for disease resistance, drought hardy and perennial nature of *Citrullus colocynthis* into the water melon. This will open new vistas for improving our water melon.

In this connection let me tell you the story of genetically improved corn—the *Zea mays* plant. Prof. Hugh H. Iltis of Wisconsin University is a taxonomist turned evolutionary conservationist. He led a number of botanical exploration tours in Mexico, Peru and Costa Rica. In one of the collection trips to Mexico he collected a diploid strain of this plant, and named it as *Zea diplensis*. Unfortunately he lost all the seeds of this strain. Few years latter he issued a New Year card to all his geneticist and taxonomic friends throughout the world. In response to his appeal, soon came a reply from Canadian geneticist, informing him that he has a Mexican student who knows where this diploid maize grows in Mexico. Soon funds were collected and a trip was organised for Mexico. Instead of that diploid strain, Dr. Iltis collected a perennial diploid strain of maize, which he latter named as *Zea diploperennis*. The latter was hybridised with normal *Zea mays*, since both of them had the same basic chromosome numbers to produce a perennial maize which resulted in America earning a profit of nearly 3 billion dollars per year.

ECOSYSTEM DIVERSITY

The quantitative assessment of biodiversity at the ecosystem, habitat or community level is known as ecosystem diversity.

Ecosystem diversity could best be understood if we study the communities in various ecological niches within each ecosystem, each associated with definite species complexes. Each community has its own relative abundance of species and population complex. These complexes are all related to composition and structure of the biodiversity. Habitat destruction has dangerously narrowed the genetic variability of many species cutting their ability to adapt to number of adversities, which they can possess, if allowed to grow in different habitats. This may result from the habitat being made unsuitable for the species (for example, clear-felling of forests, severe pollution of rivers or through the habitat becoming fragmented. The maintenance of biological diversity at all levels is fundamentally the maintenance of viable populations of species or identifiable populations.

Thus the diverse array of genes, species and ecosystem is a resource which can be tapped as human needs and demand change since biodiversity is so closely intertwined with human needs. Therefore, conservation of biodiversity at all costs should rightfully be considered as an element of national security. National security will be strongest in countries that care for their biodiversity. Indiscriminate collection and extraction of biodiversity resources, without an opportunity for them to resurge and rejuvenate, conversion of land use for development and other purposes, destruction of forests have raised questions about the conservation and sustainable use of biodiversity in the interest of the survival of the planet. These concerns got articulated in an international treaty called the Convention on Biological Diversity, which was signed at the Rio Summit in 1992 and entered into force in December 1993.

BIODIVERSITY IN RELATION WITH HUMAN HEALTH

As mentioned earlier, all medicines once used to come from plants and animal resources. Even today medicinal drugs derived from natural sources make an important global contribution to health care. An estimated 80 per cent of people in less-developed countries rely on traditional medicines for primary health care; this shows no signs of decline despite availability of Western medicine.

Even now 80 per cent people in the developing countries depend upon traditional medicines. Penicillin and tetracycline are amongst the 3,000 antibiotics from micro-organisms and the recent discovery of cyclosporin from soil fungus has revolutionised the heart and kidney transplant surgery.

There are as many as 200 species of desert plants of minor medicinal uses such as *Phyllanthus amarus*, *Balanites aegyptiaca, Boerhaavia elegans* and *Vicoa indica* which have proved to be of great use in the desert.

Catharanthus roseus, a pretty pink-flowered plant of Madagascar is a wonderful plant, since the extract from these flowers can stop childhood leukaemia. It has many different stains. This herb contains more than 100 alkaloids. More important ones are *vincristine* and *vinblastine*, both of which are prescribed by physicians to fight certain types of cancer. Synthetic *vincristine*, used to treat childhood leukaemia is only 20 per cent as efficacious as the natural product derived from *Catharanthus roseus* (Rosy Periwinkle). In Tamil Nadu and Kerala there are firms which are exporting the roots of this plant. They supply the seeds of the selected strains of this species and collect the root crops themselves, thus solving the buy-back problem—one of the greatest hurdles in the cultivation of medicinal plants.

The Indian Desert contains a large number of biodivertic entities such as *Commiphora wightii, Withania somnifera, Urginea indica, Solanum surattense,* etc., which are all of immense medicinal value having enormous export potential. The bulbs of *Urginea indica* of the Indian Desert, though have a smaller tuber size in comparison to more humid samples, yet are richer in total glycoside contents (Gupta, 1988). As mentioned earlier, *Commiphora wightii*, the guggal plant, is an important medicinal plant endemic to N. W. Rajasthan and Gujarat of the desert, which apparently has become a threatened plant in the desert due to over exploitation as a result of ignorance and greed of the people particularly during famines. This plant faces serious threats due to its medicinally valuable gun resin. The demand for the guggal gum is estimated to be 300-500 tonnes per annum and in 1986 we had to import 50 tonnes of this gum from Pakistan (Gupta, 1988). We have therefore started Guggal Farm as in Mangaliawas near Ajmer. The demand of guggal, an oleo-gum resin, which has long been used n Ayurvedic medicines, has of late attracted the attention for its anti-inflammatory, anti-rheumatic, hypocholesterolemic and hypolipaemic activity. The Anand Centre has collected 55 populations and the Agriculture College at Jobner collected 58 samples of this plant from 11 districts of Rajasthan. Proper evaluation from the point of view of productivity will enable to choose the best available strain for commercial cultivation.

Similarly, the estimated demand of 500 tonnes of Nagori Ashgandh (*Withania somnifera*) roots has been mentioned to be of high value in comparison of other samples. *Nagori Ashagand*, which is proving to be Indian Ginseng, is now no longer available in Nagaur.

Solanum surattense (*Solanum xanthocarpum*), a ruderal weed of arid zone, demonstrated in Indian Parliament when Pandit Nehru was Prime Minister, can open up new vistas for economic development in this region (Gupta, 1988). The crude drug market plants and their parts are not kept in proper conditions and many of them are adulterated and substituted with genuine drugs. There is a need to discuss this problem and evolve its solution so that standard and quality medicines are produced.

EDIBLE PLANTS

Man has been in search of useful edible plants from amongst the wild flora from time immemorial. It was his trial and error method, which resulted in selection of some of the more useful edible plants for purposes of his needs. Species growing in nature are never cultivated but local people display a remarkable knowledge of their food value, which is mostly undocumented. These have so profusely been adapted by the local population that they have come to stay as permanent food articles in their diet in the desert areas.

In course of time, these plants were used during famines and other scarcity conditions. However, not all plants which were found edible and useful could be cultivated on a large scale. Some of these wild edible plants started as emergency foods. Their adjustment of these foods is a result of long-standing struggle against nature and acts as a palliative and modifies or almost nullifies the effects of deficiency or failure of rains which in other regions would have resulted in serious and widespread distress. Over the centuries of use of these plants, when their seeds and fruits are collected and stored for future use, their regenerative power has decreased considerably.

These dry vegetable fruits are being exported out of the desert and their cost has also increased enormously due to paucity of their availability. The intensity with which this seed collection is made, and in particular the seeds of *Capparis* and *sangari* fruits are collected when they are not fully mature, has seriously affected the natural process of regeneration of these desirable species in this difficult terrain. Proper and judicious uses of these foods, propagating them from their high-yielding strains, and educating people for their proper utilisation are some of the methods of improvement in this regard. Export and price rise over the last two decades of *sangari* (young pods of *Prosopis cineraria*), kair (young fruits of *Capparis decidua*), kumbat (seeds of *Acacia senegal*), gawar (immature dried fruits of *Cyamopsis tetragonoloba*), etc. have skyrocketed. As a result, on the one hand due to over exploitation their market value has increased enormously, on the other hand it has gradually resulted in the depletion of these resources. This diversity preserved and maintained by them over the centuries has become a source of deprivation for them since the material they have preserved through centuries of sustenance, has gone in the hands of the elite.

TRADITIONAL MEDICINES AND INTELLECTUAL PROPERTY RIGHTS

Intellectual property is the term used to describe the branch of law which protects the application of thoughts, ideas and information which are of commercial value. It thus covers the law relating to patents, copyrights, trademarks, trade secrets and other similar rights.

The development of the genetic resources of biodiversity is known as biotechnology. Broadly defined, biotechnology includes any technique that uses living organisms or part of organisms to make or modify the products, to improve plants or animals or develop micro-organisms for specific uses. It has been the recent development of new biological techniques (for example, recombinant

DNA, cell fusion and monoclonal antibody technology) which has raised fundamental social and moral questions and created problems in intellectual property rights.

The idea of using patents to protect the rights of the inventor is not new. Ever since commercialisation started, the use of patent and copyrights also began throughout the world. In the beginning it was more an issue of trust and respect but gradually it became the matter of law, firstly within the countries and lately internationally. In the present times, the patent system is an extremely aggressive legal order and the growing trade and commercial temper has created a patent culture in Western countries with aggressive tone. The debate on the comparative benefits of the patent regime to developed and developing countries has still not concluded. The developed countries argue that the patent will help the developing countries for their economic growth while on the other hand other people believe that the patent regime will help more to the developed countries like the U. S. A. and will help them to monopolise world trade and economy. However, the patent regime should be considered in the present context in the totality of the Indian Patent Act, GATT, TRIPS and issues of intellectual property rights.

The Convention on Biological Diversity held at Rio and subsequent national level meetings organised in India recognised the sovereign rights of the countries over their biodiversity. Till the end of the 20th century the biotechnological-rich developed countries continued to exploit the bio-resources of biodiversity-rich developing countries through their gene technology leading to a situation of 'Biopiracy' or 'gene robbing'.

It is high time that the Indian botanists, specially the plant taxonomists, begin to play a key role in the protection of the sovereign rights of our country over their resources through chemical and gene prospecting. Taxonomists should not only collect and identify the plants but they also have to play a key role in bioprospecting the plants resource for their different medicinal properties and in the discovery of newer drug plants and in the development of databases for national and international bio-information sectors.

Ayurvedic medicines and Indian herbs form one of the most vulnerable sectors in the context of patent regimes. A number of known herbs and plant drugs of India have been patented by outsiders on the basis of secondary research. Neem, haldi and aswagandha are a few among many examples. Because of the lack of awareness and fallacies in law, patents are being granted to individuals on the basis of minor secondary research ignoring the obvious traditional knowledge. In order to promote traditional medicine in any country, there is an urgent need to change the patent laws designed to protect the national heritage of a country which should be considered its intellectual property and should not be allowed to be patented in the name of any individual, national or foreigner. An ancient traditional knowledge claimed to have originated in any country should be treated as the National Intellectual Property of that country. There is need for making necessary legal provisions for National Heritage Patent. For this, there is a need for nation-wide awareness and national debate.

The first task is to precisely define and describe the National Heritage Intellectual Property of the country with substantial proof and textual records. It would be necessary to enlist and to officially register the ancient classical texts and the oral traditions historicity-wise which may be projected as 'National Heritage Record' to be used as a document in support of a national claim. Such homework and suitable law reform will go a long way in protecting the ancient heritage knowledge of a country from being patented by foreign agencies. The interim strategy should be titled 'Protection' rather than 'Patents' to prevent any kind of piracy or infringement. Certain corners in India have been raising the slogan of "to combat the negative impact of globalisation." But in spite of being a solid reality, 'Swadeshi' has so far been used only as a slogan, and not as realistic work strategy. As such, the developing countries like ours are carrying a big risk which can be overcome only by reasonable defensive strategies and by generating the sense of activism and work culture among our people.

CONCLUSION

Of late there has been a growing awareness for conservation of genetic resources of our medicinal plants. In fact, the role of these in health care programmes is much appreciated in most south and south-Asian countries which led to the establishment of national research institutes in these countries to work on cultivation, chemistry and clinical screening of traditional medicinal plants. There is need for developing a code of practices for growing, harvesting, collecting, handling, packaging, storing and exporting these plant materials. All this will have a multifold effect in developing superior varieties and better cultivation practices for these life support species.

—oo(O)oo—

5

Evaluation of Cultivation and Extraction Practices of Guggulu [*Commiphora wightii* (Arn) (Bhand)] at Guggul Herbal Farm, Mangliawas

K. C. Audichya

THE Guggul Herbal Farm, Mangliawas, was established by the Government of Rajasthan in the year 1969 and was handed over to the Institute (under CCRAS) in the year 1972 and presently under the control of the Central Research Institute (Ay.), Jaipur. The farm is spread over 142 acres of forest land and maintains extensive cultivation of Guggulu. At present, +15,000 mature guggulu plants are growing in the farm. Severe drought conditions prevailed for the last several years in the guggulu growing area of Rajasthan and Gujarat States and its over exploitation in nature has resulted in depletion of this species to the status of endangered species. The cultivation and conservation of guggulu at the Herbal Farm has saved the species from extinction.

CULTIVATION AT GUGGUL HERBAL FARM, MANGALIAWAS

Guggul Herbal Farm, Mangliawas, is situated at village Mangliawas about 26 km from Ajmer along with the main chain of Aravalli range. The topography of the farm is undulating marked by the slopes of the hills and hillocks including plain area. The bulk of the plantation is on the foothills and along plain areas covering about one-third of the total area. The farm is protected by random stone boundary wall on all sides. Motorable, katcha roads and pathways traverse the whole area of the farm. Irrigation is managed by a tubewell, one overhead reservoir and pipe line connection to the different areas of the farm.

At present, there are about 15,000 mature guggul plants 10-12 years old. The natural vegetation and flora of the farm typical of the Aravallis is not distributed. The dominant species comprises *Grewia flavescens, Grewia tenax, Acacia senegal, Acacia leucophloea, Acacia nilotica, Rhus mysurensis, Asparagus racemosus* and *Anogeissus pendula*. Ground flora is mostly covered by *Barleria prionitis, Tephrosia purpurea* mostly on the plains along with grasses like *Apluda mutica, Heteropogon contortus, Cenchrus* sp., etc.

Besides guggulu plants, *Caesalpinia bonduc* (Kuberaksh), *Aloe vera* (Ghrit-Kumari), *Gloriosa superba* (Langli), *Tinospora cordifolia* (Amrita), etc. are also growing in the farm.

Propagation of guggul is done by the following methods:

1. Through seeds
2. Stem cuttings
3. Air layering method

Through Seeds

As undergrowth of many species of plant seedlings are often found under thicket *Euphorbia caducifolia* or bushes of *Grewia* sp., *Rhus*, sp., etc. indicating propagation of guggul through seeds in nature regeneration through seeds is very poor due to low percentage of viable seeds.

Vegetative Propagation (Through Stem Cuttings)

Guggul can be successfully propagated through stem cuttings. The sprouting and establishment of cutting varies between 60-100 per cent.

(i). Time of Planting

The cuttings are planted during late summer, that is, June, when the plant is almost leafless. With the onset of monsoon the plant becomes physiologically active and shows signs of sprouting within 25-50 days.

The cuttings established in nursery beds are transferred into polyphone bags after one year and then planted in the field during rainy season.

The experimental studies conducted in farm showed maximum sprouting 94.5 per cent in the third week of June.

(ii). Preparation of Bed

Soil must be pulverised and thoroughly mixed with farmyard manure and a small quantity of BHC or Aldrin to prevent termite infestation. Beds are prepared in various sizes such as 6' × 3' or 10' × 4'.

(iii). Preparation of Planting Stock

Stem cuttings are selected from a healthy plant. Experimental observations at G. H. F., Mangliawas, has shown that 25-30 cm long and 6-10 mm diameter are most suitable for planting. The cuttings are planted at a distance of 25-30 cm and at a depth of 15 cm in soil to avoid drying in severe drought condition in Rajasthan.

Sprouting of Cuttings

The cuttings usually sprout within 8-15 days after planting during monsoon. However, rooting starts 20-25 days of sprouting. Cuttings treated with NAA (500 mg/l) (Naphthalene acetic acid) and IBA (100 mg/l), (Indole-3-butyric acid) increased percentage of sprouting to 87.5.

Experiments at Guggul Herbal Farm, Mangliawas, using Ceredik-1, ceredik-2 and Ceredik-3 on the stem cuttings increased the sprouting percentage.

Air Layering

Air-layering is practised in India and China from early times in pomes and other plants. Air layering has been successfully developed at Guggul Herbal Farm, Mangliawas, as propagation method. A 5-cm long bark is removed from the stem or branch. The exposed portion is covered by applying a ball of adhesive soil holding it securely together with coir fibre and bandaging around the branch. The bandaged portion is supplied with drip irrigation drop by drop system so that the portion gets enough moisture. The portion is severed from the parent after development of root system.

Experiments conducted at Guggul Herbal Farm, Mangliawas, showed July to September as the most suitable period for air layering. Air layering is successful and quick method for propagation of guggul.

EXTRACTION OF GUGGUL

"Guggul-gum" oleo-resin is the exudate of *Commiphora wighti*. It oozes out sometimes naturally as well as on injury. The gum-oleo-resin is located in the gum-oleo-resin ducts scattered throughout the bark. The flow of gum is more during winter, that is, December to February (Shah, 1983; Yadava *et al*, 1999).

Extraction in Rajasthan

In Rajasthan, the extraction of the gum previously was done by the agency of contractors who engaged local people belonging to the Bhil, Meena, Rawat and other tribes. The payment of the labour was made on the quantity of the gum collected. The contractors used chemicals, etc. to extract maximum yield of gum and as a result large-scale destruction of guggulu was brought about.

Extraction in Gujarat

Guggul gum is collected in the whole of Kutch Division. The tapping is done by "Samma" (Sindhi Mohamedans) and "Kanbi" tribes in Kutch (Atal *et al*, 1975). Gum is also collected from Mahi ravines and surrounding areas of Borsad Taluka. Along the border of Gir forests there is a community known as "Gugali Brahmin" whose main profession is tapping and collection of guggulu. In order to increase yield after 2-3 collections, a paste consisting of horse/wild ass urine, guggul gum and copper sulphate is applied (Atal *et al,* 1975).

Tapping Method

Well-grown plants of Guggul 10-20 years old are suitable for tapping. Tapping is done usually by giving an incision 3-4 cm long on the main trunk of the plant with a sharp knife. The knife is dipped in an activator like guggul gum paste. The guggle gum paste is prepared with 100 gm of gum with 200 cc fresh water in an earthen pot stirred with a guggul stick till a fine paste is prepared.

The knife is dipped in the guggul paste and incision is given in such a way that guggul solution on the edge of the knife enters the incised portion of the branch.

Yellow latex oozes out through the wounds and slowly solidifies forming big lumps, which are collected after 15-20 days of incision. Subsequent collection is made at intervals of 10-15 days.

Some of the general observations are given below:

1. Tapping time	January and February
2. Age of tapping	10-20 years old plant
3. Tapping instrument	Knife (Choori) 9" 1'
4. Incision on plant part	Main trunk and main branches
5. No of incisions per plant	2-4
6. Type of incision	Horizontal usually at an angle of 60°
7. Distance between two incisions	30 to 40 cm
8. Interval between tapping and gum collection	15-20 days
9. Interval between two collections	10-15 days
10. No. of collections	3-6 times
11. Period of collection	January to May
12. Depth of incision	Thickness of bark (5 cm to 1 cm)
13. Tribals involved in tapping	Bhil, Mehrat, Banjara, Meena, Rawat and Samara

The above data is based on our observations and experience. Time of collection and intervals between two collection may vary depending upon the prevailing weather conditions.

It is observed that usually the exudation increases as the heat of the summer increases. The tapped plants, which yield gum dried up gradually. So far there is no method/technique known by which guggulu can be extracted without mortality of the plant.

Tapping with Ethephon

Experiments by Bhatt *et al* (1989) on guggul plants growing in ravines near Vasad area of Gujarat for 3 years in 27 plants using 3 methods and 3 concentrations (100, 200, 400 mg) showed an increase in gum by about 22 times over control

Tapping Trials at G. H. F., Mangliawas

Tapping trials using Ethephon was carried out at G. H. F., Mangliawas and Dadupalki forest near S. K. N. College of Agriculture, Jobner. The plants selected at Dadupalki forest area are naturally growing ones. In both the locations enhancement of exudation in a short duration was observed.

Observation at Dadupalki are as follows:

TABLE 1
Ethephon Treatment at Different Concentrations

	Method of Treatment	Concentration of Ethephon						Remarks No. of Plants
		150	300	450	600	800	Control	
1.	Making hole (Average yield per plant in gm)	91	97	138	89	—	59	14
2.	By stem soaking	73	184	127	155	—	60	14
3.	By root feeding	153	323	389	334	126	167	17

Location	Dadupalki (near Jobner) Jaipur District
Number of plants	24
Ethephon concentration	Average yield
300 mg	180 gms
400 mg	135 gsm
500 mg	200 gms
Control	40 gms

STUDIES AT G. H. F., MANGALIAWAS

Forty five plants were selected more or less of the same age group at G. H. F., Mangliawas. Solution of Ethephon was selected in concentrations of 150, 300, 450, 600 and 800 mg of active substance (Table 1).

OBSERVATIONS

1. Ethephon treated plants started exuding gum within 5-7 days after incision compared to 10-12 days of control group.
2. Exudation at faster rate.
3. Plants treated with Ethephon through root are better method as compared to other two methods.
4. Yield was highest in 450 mg. Concentration of Ethephon is suitable for optimum yield.
5. 40 plants which yielded gum dried up out of 45 plants.

EXPERIMENTS TO FIND OUT IDEAL PERIOD OF TAPPING

Guggul gum is tapped during December to March in 1989, 1991 and 1992 and 162 guggul plants were tapped from January to May using guggul gum and Ethephon.

INFERENCES

1. Plants tapped in February and March yielded maximum in 1989 while May to December yielded nil.
2. Plants tapped from January to April, February and March yielded more in 1991.
3. Period showing increase in temperature and decrease in humidity coincides with maximum yielding period.

CONCLUSION

1. Guggul cultivation can be spread to other neighbouring States like Uttar Pradesh and Madhya Pradesh as it is successfully growing in areas like Jhansi.
2. Guggul distribution in Chambal area and Chambal ravines prove that it can be cultivated in similar habitat where the soil is more or less sandy.
3. Existence of *Commiphora agallocha* in Sambalpur areas showing luxurious growth as a hedge plant around fields and house boundaries prove that guggul can be grown in variable weather conditions. Shepherds from Rajasthan originally planted the plant in Orissa State.
4. Likewise, chance of *Commiphora wightiii* being successful in other climates in India cannot be ruled out.
5. Solution to save *Commiphora wightii* from extinction is spreading of extensive cultivation to more areas in Rajasthan and Gujarat.
6. Extension of cultivation of guggul to neighbouring States like Uttar Pradesh and Madhya Pradesh in semi-arid areas.
7. Since yield of gum causes death of the plant tapping should be done only after planting at least two plants in lieu of one plant tapped.
8. To maintain total number of guggul plants in G. H. F., Mangliawas, particular area was chosen for tapping and re-plantation was planned for the areas where plants were tapped within one year of drying up of plants.
9. To continue tapping experiments for further modifications of the existing methods to increase quantity of gum and to save plant from drying up.
10. The cost of chemical for tapping is between one to two rupees only and does not affect much on the overall expenditure or quality of gum.

REFERENCES

Anonymous. 'Guggulu and its cultivation'. *Newsletter*, CCRAS, New Delhi 4 (4): 1-8, 1982.

Anonymous. Monograph on cultivation of guggulu. New Delhi: CCRAS Publication, 2000.

Bhatt. J. R., Nair, M. N. B. and Mohan Ram, H. Y 'Enhancement of oleoresin production in *Commiphora wightii* by improved technique'. *Current Science* 58(7): 318-357, 1989.

Billore, K. V., Audichya, K. C. and Dhar, Bishnupriya. 'Conservation of medicinal plants in Rajasthan with special reference to conservation and propagation of guggulu'. *Bull. Med. Ethn. Bot. Res.* 8 (1-2): 118-127, 1987.

Billore, K. V. 'Note on the confused identity and nomenclature of *Commiphora* species'. *Bull. Med. Ethno Bot. Res.* 12(1-2): 87-90, 1991.

Chaturvedi, D. D., Yadav, B. B. L. and Mishra, K. P. 'Cultivation/extraction of gum oleo-resin of *Commiphora wightii* (Arn.) Bhand. at Guggul Herbal Farm, Mangliawas—Problems & prospects'. *Bull. Med. Ethno. Bot. Res.* 8 (3-4): 166-170, 1987.

Chhipa, R. P., Billore, K. V., Yadav, B. B. L. Mishra, Ratan and Mishra, K. P. 'Some indigenous method for tapping of gum guggulu—a pilot study'. *Bull. Med. Ethno. Bot. Res.* 3(i): 68-73, 1982.

Yadav, B. B. L., Joseph, T. G., Billore, K. V. and Chatuvedi, D. D. 'Some observations on the tapping trials on *Commiphora wightii* (Arn.) Bhand. using Ethephon'. Seminar of Silver Jubilee Celebration, Tarikhet, 1993.

Yadav, B. B. L., Billore, K. V., Joseph, T. G., Mishra, K. P. and Chaturvedi, D. D. ' Ideal period for extraction of gum oleo-resin in *Commiphora wightii* (Arn). Bhand'. Seminar of Silver Jubilee Celebration, CCRAS, New Delhi, 1995.

Yadav, B. B. L. 'A successful method of propagation through air layering in *Commiphora wightii* (Arn.) Bhand'. Seminar of Silver Jubilee Celebration, CCRAS, New Delhi, 1995.

—oo(O)oo—

6

'GREEN HEALERS': A REVIEW

PADMA KUMAR

"WE come on this earth as guests of plants" is a monumental ancient aphorism. Since time immemorial, nature's own supreme creation, man, has completely been dependent on plants and as civilisation developed, he has learnt to exploit natural resources and to make use of every bit of it. In fact from the start of life to the last breath, almost every aspect of human life is deeply associated with plants. Primitive man tried to cure diseases from plants growing abundantly around him. His experience through trial and error taught him a lot about the medicinal properties of different plants.

In India, the names of Charaka and Sushruta are well known even today. Since their time, the collection and identification of medicinally important plants led to the development of the branch of pharmcognosy to the present state in which pharmaceutically important plant products are studied.

There are hundreds of medicinal plants that have a long history of curative properties against various diseases and ailments. However, screening of plants for their activity is very essential and needs urgent attention in order to know the real value of plant genetic resources, which is eroding fast. The screening of plants for their biologically active principles is done on the basis of either their chemo-taxonomic investigations or ethno-botanical knowledge for a particular disease. Chemotaxonomic investigations involve the use of biomolecules. Identification of action of a particular compound against a specific disease is a challenging and long process. The importance of medicinal plants lies in their biological active principles, which are the real healers in the process of medication. There are two types of plant chemicals: Primary metabolites such as common sugars, carbohydrates, proteins, amino acids and chlorophyll. These are universally present in all kinds of plants whether medicinal or non-medicinal. The other types of chemicals called secondary metabolites include alkaloids, terpenoids, phenolics, etc. which do not have an essential role in plant metabolism and vary in their distribution from plant to plant. Secondary metabolites are mostly accumulated by plant cells in smaller quantities than primary metabolites. They are synthesised in specialised cells at particular development stages, making their extraction and purification difficult. These secondary metabolites exert a profound physiological effect on the mammalian system and thus are known as the active principles of that plant. The physiological effect of these active principles is used for curing ailments. The use of crude drugs of plant origin is used in the Indian system of medicine (Ayurveda) and large number of drugs of plant origin are used in Western medicine. Given below is a brief account of important commercial medicinal plants:

1. *Aegle marmelos* (Rutaceae)

Commonly known as 'beal', is a well-recognised medicinal plant in the Indian system of medicine and has been used for centuries. Ripe fruits are used in constipation, chronic dysentery. Roots and stems are used as antipyretic. It contains alkaloids, coumarins, flavonoids and sterols (Waterman and Grundon, 1983). Umbelliferone, marmesin, skimmin, marmeline, aegelin, imperatorin, alloimperatorin, xanthotoxtol, scoparone, scopoletin and β-sitosterol, β-D-glucoside have been isolated from fruits, rutin marmesinin aegeline and lupeol from leaves, marmin, umbelliferone, skimmianine, lupeol and aurapten isolated from bark.

Aqueous and alcoholic extracts showed cardiac stimulant, smooth muscle relaxant and uterine stimulant activities. Skimmiane showed sedative bypnotic, analgesic, anti-convulsion and anti-pyretic activities in various experimental animals. Leaves, fruits and bark are used for the treatment of intestinal diseases. Essential oil from leaves has a broad spectrum anti-fungal activity. Extracts of fruits lowered blood sugar level in normal rabbits significantly but in diabetic rabbits reduction level was insignificant. Aegeline, an alkaloid isolated from leaves, is used as an active principle in allopathic medicines. Bhardwaj and co-workers obtained different cell lines grown on hormone supplemented and hormone-free medium or hormone-free but inhibitor containing medium.

2. *Aconitum heterophyllum* Wall. (Ranunculaceae)

Extracts from these plants are used in stomach ache and as an aphrodisiac. The roots contain alkaloids and have found use in the treatment of hysteria and throat diseases. They are considered astringent and are prescribed in diarrhoea, vomiting and cough. The root is also considered anti-diabetic and very efficacious for irritability of stomach and in abdominal pains.

3. *Allium* sp. (Alliaceae)

Garlic (*Allium cepa.* L.) and onion (*Allium sativum* L.) of this group are used to treat various kinds of ailments like abdominal pain, hypertension, heart disease, rheumatism, stomach disorders, etc. The medicinal properties of these plants are usually attributed to sulphur containing compounds. The ability of garlic to decrease the concentration of serum lipids and serum fibrinogen has been attributed to ajoene. The flavonoids which occur in low concentrations are thought to add to the anti-oxidant properties of *Allium* sp. Clinical studies have shown that extracts of garlic can decrease serum levels of cholesterol and triglycerides. Fresh garlic extracts have been found to inhibit many fungal species, bacteria and parasites. Garlic also possesses anti-cancer activity. Garlic reduces platelet aggregation and blood glucose level and increases blood insulin levels.

4. *Aloe barbadensis* Mill. (Liliaceae)

The plant was used in skin infections and wound healing. The leaf contains three medicinally important and distinct parts: the leaf exudates, the leaf epidermis and the leaf pulp. The leaf exudates a bitter yellow liquid can be heated, concentrated and dried to a black powder which is used as purgative. The whole leaf of *Aloe vera* or its products have been used directly on radiation burns, thermal burns, wounds, ulcers. The whole drug is stomachic, tonic in small doses and purgative in large doses.

5. *Artemisia annua* L. (Asteraceae)

The anti-malarial compound artemisinin was first isolated by Chinese scientists in 1972. Other properties of the plant include anti-periodic, tonic, cardiac stimulant and expectorant. In an attempt to produce artemisin through *in vitro* methods, Fulzele *et al* (1975) established cultures of *Artemisia annua.* Shoot cultures from the bioreactor produced 1.08 mg per cent camphor on fresh weight basis. A protocol for quick regeneration of large number of plants was developed. Hairy root cultures have been obtained through genetic transformation by *Agrobacterium rhizogenes.*

6. *Asparagus* species (Liliaceae)

Common name shatawar is a xerophytic climber. Roots are known to contain a number of pharmacologically active saponins. Asparagine shataverin I to IV are the principal steroidal saponins. The alcoholic extracts of roots of *Asparagus racemosus* exhibit anti-cancer and cardiac stimulant activities.

Protoplast isolation, somatic embryogenesis and organogenesis have been achieved in *Asparagus officinalis*, an economically important species (May and Sink, 1995). Callus cultures of *Asparagus racemosum* produce sterols (Kar and Sen, 1985).

7. *Atropa belladonna* (Solanaceae)

Roots and leaves are known to contain hyoscymine and some other compounds. These are northyoscyamine, hygrine, hygroline, atropine, scopolamine. The drug obtained from roots and leaves is considered to be anti-asthmatic, sedative. It is used to check secretion in the throat and respiratory passages. Belladona preparations are used for asthma, bladder stones, convulsions, gastric ulcers, kidney stones, Parkinson's disease and whooping cough. Efforts are being made by many workers to raise cultures differentiated or undifferentiated in a synthetic culture medium to develop methods for high alkaloid yield. *In vitro* multiple shoot formation from stem explants and root cultures of *Atropa belladona* has been achieved. Hairy root cultures were developed for alkaloid production (Kamada *et al,* 1986). Cultures have been used to study the effect of amino acid precursors on alkaloid production *in vitro.* Incorporation of 50 mg tyrosine per 100 ml medium resulted in 0.98 per cent alkaloid production.

8. *Azadirachta indica* (Meliaceae)

Azadirachtin, a triterpenoid, is an important active principle isolated from fruits in addition to several other constituents. Azadirachtin proved to be a natural insecticide. The plant also shows activities like anti-microbial, hypoglycaemic, anti-inflammatory. Micropropagation through somatic embryogenesis (Muralidharan and Mascarenhas, 1989) and through axillary bud has been reported.

9. *Camellia sinensis* (Theaceae)

Commonly known 'Tea' is an important medicinal plant. The active principle obtained from tea waste or from the dried leaves is caffeine, which provides a condition of wakefulness and increases mental activity. Caffeine is included in analgesic preparations with aspirin or codeine.

10. *Cannabis indica* (Cannabinaceae)

Cannabis-based drugs are used for treatment of pain, asthma, etc. The chief active principles of the plant are cannabinoids which have hallucinogenic properties. Other therapeutic properties are stomachic, anti-spasmodic, analgesic stimulant, aphrodisiac and sedative. Callus cultures were raised from leaves and seeds on hormone-free MS medium. It has been reported that the cultures lost their ability to organise and synthesise cannabinoides. However, some workers have achieved by medium modifications (Petri, 1988).

11. *Catharanthus roseus* (Apocyaceae)

The plant contains more than 100 alkaloids, two of which, vinblastine and vincristine, have potent activity in the treatment of different forms of cancer. Vinblastine is used for the treatment of Hodgkin's disease whereas vincristine is used for the treatment of paediatric leukaemia. They are also used in the treatment of breast, ovarian and renal cancer.

12. *Cephaelis ipecacuanha* (Rubiaceae)

Roots of the plant contain 2 per cent alkaloids. Main active alkaloids are emetine and cephaeline. It is a source of the well-known drug ipecacuanha. The drug consists of bark and root and is used in amoebic dysentery. Jha and Jha (1989) developed a micropropagation method using tips obtained from aseptically grown seedlings. The alkaloid content of regenerated plants was comparable to that of the mother plant.

13. *Chlorophytum borivilianum* (Liliaceae)

Commonly known as 'safed musli'. Tuberous roots of *Chlorophytum arvndinaceum* contain steroidal saponins. Dried tuberous roots of the plant are the products of commerce. Roots or its extracts are widely used in several herbal tonics. The plant is known for its vitaliser activities and used along with extracts of *Withania somnifera* and *Asparagus racemosus* in fatigue and general weakness.

Tissue cultures were initiated from underground modified stem explants and seedlings to develop technology for mass propagation. (Ramawat *et al*, 1998).

14. *Commiphora wightii* (Burseraceae)

Commonly known as 'guggul'. This is one of the most important medicinal plants used in the herbal system of medicine (Dalal and Patel, 1995). Important compounds of pharmacological interest isolated from resin fractions of guggal are guggulsterone z and E. The resin is a mixture of terpenoides, volatile oils, gum and minerals. The drug possesses potent anti-flammatory, anti-arthritic and hypocholesterolemic activities. Guggul is also used as an antiseptic, astringent and lotion for ulcers and improves digestion.

A technique for rapid multiplication of *Commiphora wightii* through direct somatic embryogenesis has been developed (Singh *et al,* 1997). Guggulsterone production is very low in undifferentiated callus cultures, cell suspension cultures and immobilised cells.

15. *Datura innoxia* (Solanaceae)

Datura species are the source of hyoscyamine and scopolamine. Hyoscyamine, hyoscine and metaloidine were isolated from roots and leaves, tropine, pseudotropine from roots, scopolamine from aerial parts of the plant. It is reported to be analgesic, anaesthetic, expectorant, narcotic, sedative and a folk remedy for asthma, boils, bronchitis, cough, dandruff, earache, Parkinsonia, piles and tumours.

The plant has been extensively used for developing plant tissue culture techniques. Alkaloid production and plantlet regeneration were used to develop various models of secondary metabolite production (Petri, 1988).

16. *Digitalis lanata* (Scrophulariaceae)

The plant contains a number of therapeutically active groups of compounds such as flavanoids and chalcones. Digoxin, digitalin and digitoxin, the main cardioactive glycosides isolated from the leaves of *Digitalis lanata,* are being used in the allopathic system of medicines as a cardio-tonic. *Digitalis* species have been extensively studied in tissue culture for the production of lanatosides. Biotransformation of digitoxin to digoxin by *Digitalis purpurea* cell cultures has become an example of application of plant tissue culture for the production of secondary metabolites at an industrial level.

17. *Ephedra gerardiana* (Ephedraceae)

Ephedra species is said to improve the lung condition and control wheezing. It also promotes sweating and urination. The multifarious effects of this plant are related to stimulation of the sympathetic nervous system. The whole plant possesses oxytoxic, divertic and anti-fertility properties.

18. *Ginkgo biloba* (Ginkgoaceae)

This plant contains terpenes, steroids and flavonoid derivatives (Kleijnen and Knipschild, 1992). The extract is prepared in a defined way and sold in the market under the trade name EGB-761. It is mainly used as an anti-fatigue and anti-ageing agent which enhances mental alertness. Ginkgolide production in cell and callus grown in shake flasks and 2-6 litres bioreactors was attempted (Carrier *et al*, 1991). The production of ginkgalido in gametophyte derived cell cultures varied from 0.065–0.087 per cent dry weight basis (Laurain *et al,* 1997).

19. *Gloriosa superba* (Liliaceae)

The main active principle of the plant is colchicines which is effective in treatment of gouty arthritis. The whole rhizome is oxytoxic and antibiotic but poisonous in large doses. Fresh juice of plant is uterine stimulant.

20. *Gossypium herbaceum* (Malvaceae)

The cotton seed oil contains a phenolic compound known as gossypol. Gossypol has been shown to be an effective anti-fertility agent in humans with an efficacy of 99 per cent. The aerial part of the plant shows diuretic and oxytoxic activities while the leaf is anti-bacterial. Other properties are laxative expectorant, aphrodisiac.

21. *Hyoscyamus* Species (Solanaceae)

Active principles of the plant are atropine, hyoscyamine, scopolamine. Hyoscyamine is used as a mydriatic sedative, pain killer. The herb is used for treatment of cough, asthma, bronchitis, hydrophobia.

The plant has been investigated for tropane alkaloid production in cell cultures. Other species investigated for alkaloid production in callus, cell and root cultures are *Hyoscyamus albus, Hyoscyamus pusillus, Hyoscyamus aureus* (Strauss, 1989).

22. *Panax ginseng* (Araliaceae)

The dried roots of ginseng species contain complex mixture of saponin glycosides termed as ginsenosides. Other important compounds include panaquilon, resin, tannin, choline, etc. Ginseng has a wide range of pharmaceutical activities like enhancing natural resistance. It has both stimulant and sedative activity with a low level of toxicity. It has the capacity of reducing high blood pressure and raising low blood pressure to the normal level. Complete work regarding production of saponins in cells and root culture in flasks, jar fermenters and industrial fermenters was carried out by Furuya *et al,* 1988. Details of cultivation and *in vitro* production of genosides are presented by Choi (1988, 1995).

23. *Papavar somniferum* (Papavaraceae)

The plant is the source of opium. Morphine, codeine, narcotine, laudanine, papavarine and thebaine are principal alkaloids. The cultures produced several alkaloids but the production of morphine and related alkaloids was always low. The benzophenanthridine alkaloids found in callus cells are not present in the original plant (Roberts, 1988).

24. *Phyllanthus fraternus* (Euphorbiaceae)

Phytochemical occurrence of lignans phyllanthin and hypophyllanthin have been reported. Plant is used as diuretic, for infection of the urinary tract and for jaundice. The plant gained importance after discovery of anti-AIDS compounds (Phyllanthosides) in *Phyllanthus niruri.*

25. *Rauvolfia serpentina* (Apocyaceae)

Of the 30 important alkaloids, reserpine found in the root is the most important. Other alkaloids are ajmaline, ajmalicine, papavarine, serpentine, etc. Alkaloids are mostly used in treating high blood pressure, insomnia, hyperglycaemia.

26. *Taxus baccata* (Gymnosporium)

The chief active principle of various *Taxus* species is paclitaxel, an anti-cancer compound. A commercial drug taxol is isolated from the bark of this plant. The other pharmacological actions of the plant are carminative, expectorant, stomachic, tonic, sedative and anti-spasmodic.

27. *Withania somnifera* (Solanaceae)

The active compounds of the plant comprise mainly alkaloids and withanolides. The whole plant, especially the leaves and the root bark, are enriched with medicinal properties. Mainly acting on the reproductive and nervous systems, it has strong tranquillising effects as well. It also stimulates the immune system, inhibits inflammation, improves memory while counteracting the effects of stress.

The importance of plant-derived drugs in modern medicine is usually not fully recognised. Plants are not only the source of pharmaceuticals, they also provide structures. These compounds provide new pharmacological properties and may serve as a starting material for more complex biologically active compounds. But all the plants present on the earth are still not known. Many more plants have yet to be evaluated chemically and pharmacologically.

A large majority of these medicinal plant raw materials are still collected from forest areas. Pharmaceutical industries throughout the world have been making consistent endeavours to discover newer, more potent and cheaper sources of raw materials and their derived chemicals to broaden the product range in the trade. Plant cells are highly sophisticated chemical factories in which a large variety of chemical compounds are manufactured with great precision from simple raw materials. Plants are thus a very important renewable source of raw materials for the production of a variety of chemicals and drugs. India being a tropical country and rich in biodiversity, produces and exports raw medicinal plants and their extracts. A number of plants are cultivated for the purpose. These plants require biotechnological inputs to maintain their quality. According to one estimate, the present world trade in plant-based dry raw materials and phytochemicals is around US $ 33,000 million. Cell culture technology has been applied to a number of medicinal plants to obtain pharmaceutically important drugs but the results have not been encouraging as the yield is too low to be commercially feasible. Only a few products such as shikonin and ginseng biomass are manufactured on a large scale. However, the techniques such as biotransformation, cell permeabilisation, immobilisation, elicitation and hairy root culture indicate the likelihood of many products to reach commercial level.

Screening of medicinal plants in India is going on at a very slow pace as compared to other countries, in spite of the fact that India possesses a major chunk of the medicinal plant pool of the world. Except for few individual research organisations working on individual plants, India has no systemic plan to screen all the medicinal plans available in the country. However, this precious material is finding its way out to foreign shores where research is being carried out followed by patenting.

REFERENCES

Carrier, D. J., Chauret, N., Mancine, M., Coulombe, P., Neufeld, R., Weber, M. and Archambault, J. 'Detection of ginkgolide–A in *Ginkgo biloba* cell cultures'. *Plant Cell Rep.*, 10:256-259, 1991.

Choi, K. T. '*Panax ginseng* CA Meyer: Micro-propagation and the *in vitro* production of saponins'. In: *Biotechnology in Agriculture and Forestry.* vol. 4. *Medicinal and Aromatic Plants*, I. (Ed.). Bajaj, Y. P. S. Berlin-Heidelberg: Springer-Verlag, pp. 484-500, 1988.

Choi, K. T., Lee, H. C., Ahn, I. O., Lee, J. H. and Park, J. C. 'Characteristics of the growth and ginsenosides in the suspension cultured cells of Korean ginseng (*Panax ginseng* CA Meyer)'. In: *Proc. Int. Ginseng Conf.* 1994, (Eds.). Bailey, E. G., Whitehead, C., Proctor, J. T. C. and Kyle, J. T. Vancouver, Canada, pp. 259-268, 1955.

Dalal, K. C. and Patel, M. A. 'Guggul'. In: *Advances in Horticulture*, vol. 11. *Medicinal and Aromatic Plants.* (Eds.). Chadha. K. L. and Gupta, R. New Delhi: Malhotra Publ. House, pp. 491-501, 1995.

Fulzele, D. P., Heble, M. R. and Rao, P. S 'Production of terpenoids from *Artemisia annua* L. Plantlets culture in bioreactor'. *J. Biotech.* 40: 139-143, 1995.

Furuya, T. 'Saponins (Ginseng saponins)'. In: *Cell Culture and Somatic Cell Genetics of Plants*, vol. 5. (Eds.). Constabel, F. and Vasil, I. K. San Diego, Cal, U. S. A.: Acad. Press, pp. 213-234, 1998.

Jha, S. and Jha, T. B. 'Micropropagation of *Cephalis ipecacuanha* Rich.' *Plant Cell Rep.*, 8: 437-439, 1989.

Kamada, H., Okamura, N., Satake, N., Harade, H. and Shimomura, K. 'Alkaloid production by hairy root cultures in *Atropa belladonna*'. *Plant Cell Rep.* 5: 239-242, 1986.

Kar, D. K. and Send, S. 'Propagation of *Asparagus racemosus* through tissue culture'. *Plant Cell Tiss. Org. Cult.* 14: 89-95, 1985.

Kleijnen, J. and Knipschild, P. '*Ginkgo biloba*'. *Lancet* 340: 1136-1139, 1992.

Laurain, D., Tremonillaux–Guiller, J., Chenieux, J. C. and Beek, T. A. 'Production of ginkgolede and bilobalidein transformed and gametophyte derived cell cultures of *Ginkgo biloba*'. *Phytochem.* 46: 127-130, 1997.

May, R. A. and Sink, K. C. 'Genotype and auxin influence direct somatic embryogenesis in protoplasts derived from embryogenic cell suspension of *Asparagus officinalis* L.' *Plant Sci.* 108: 71-84, 1995.

Muralidharan, E. M. and Mascarenhas, A. F. '*In vitro* morphogenesis in *Azadirachta indica*. A Juss and *Eucalyptus citriodora* Hook F.' In: *Tissue Culture and Biotechnology of Medicinal and Aromatic Plants.* (Eds.). Kukreja, A. K., Mathur, A. K., Ahuja, P. S. and Thakur, K. S. Lucknow: Central Institute of Medicinal and Aromatic Plants, pp. 49-55, 1989.

Petri, G. '*Cannabis sativa*: *In vitro* production of cannabinoids' In: *Biotechnology in Agriculture and Forestry*, vol. 4. *Medicinal and Aromatic Plants.* (Ed). Bajaj, Y. P. S. Berlin-Heidelberg, Springer-Verlag, pp. 333-349, 1988a.

Petri, G. 'Tropanes'. In: *Cell Culture and Somatic Cell Genetics of Plants*, vol. 5, *Phytochemicals in Plant Cell Cultures*, (Eds.). Constable, F. and Vasil. I. K. San Diego, Cal., U. S. A.: Acad. Press, pp. 263-275, 1988b.

Ramawat, K. G., Jain, S., Suri, S. S. and Arora, D. K. 'Aphrodisiac plants of Aravalli Hills with special reference to safed musli'. In: *Role of Biotechnology in Medicinal and Aromatic Plants.* (Eds.). Khan, A. and Khanum, A. Hyderabad: UK92 Pub., 1998.

Roberts, M. F. 'Isoquinolines (Papavar alkaloids)'. In: *Cell Culture and Somatic Cell Genetics of Plants*, vol. 5. (Eds.). Constable, F. and Vasil, I. K. San Diego, Cal, U. S. A.: Acad. Press, pp. 315-334, 1988.

Singh, A. K., Suri, S. S., Ramawat, K. G. and Sonie, K. C. 'Somaticembryogenesis from immature zygotic embryos of *Commiphora wightii*, a woody medicinal plant'. Gartenbauwissenschaft. 62: 44-48, 1997.

Strauss, A. C. '*Hyoscyamus* spp. *in vitro* culture and the production of tropane alkaloids'. In: *Biotechnology in Agriculture and Forestry*, vol. 7, *Medicinal and Aromatic Plants, II.* (Ed.). Bajaj, Y. P. S. Berlin-Heidelberg: Springer-Verlag, pp. 286-314, 1989.

Waterman, P. G. and Grundon, M. F. *Chemistry and Chemical Taxonomy of the Rutales*. New York: U. S. A: Acad. Press, 1983.

—oo(O)oo—

7

Rajasthan Bhils Conserve Biodiversity Especially Medicinal Plants

V. S. Saxena

THE linkage between the tribals and the forest is traditional. Tribals are economically and ecologically inseparable from forests. Be it food, fodder or fuel needs, the tribal inescapably and assuredly depended on his surrounding forests for sustenance every during troubled drought.

TRIBAL—A COMPONENT OF FOREST ECOSYSTEM

Their dependence on forests is so much so that they constitute one of the integral components of forest ecosystem. Forests have been the base on which tribal habitat and life has revolved and evolved so far; their religio-cultural artefacts, beliefs and practices, technologies and tools have been nurtured and cultivated under perennial plant associations and benign environment. The Bhil totem is reflected through worship of certain trees. Some Bhils have their 'gotras' (surnames) after the trees they worship. The tribals and forests live in a symbiotic and mutually reinforcing relationship.

The Dhebar Commission emphasised the need to provide employment by the Forest Department to the tribals living in and around the forests. It also strongly suggested that collection of minor forest produce did not hinder the forest either in its growth or its preservation and that, therefore, there was no justification for auctioning out the right to collect the minor forest produce or to have a contractor or a middleman to exploit it. The vital place the forests have in tribal economy has been recognised in the National Forest Policy of India 1952. The National Commission on Agriculture has also attached considerable importance to forestry vis-à-vis tribal economy and has reiterated the earlier findings by stating that almost all tribes depend upon dual economy based on crop production and collection from forests and stressed the need for developing a mutually beneficial relationship between the forests and tribals.

POVERTY, THE BANE OF TRIBALS

It is however a sad fact that forests have been destroyed, denuded and degraded at an alarming rate and has thus undermined the economic base of the tribal. It has become rather a fashion to blame the tribal for forest devastation. But if we critically analyse the position, it will sound irrational, illogical and even untrue to raise an accusing finger today at the exploited and helpless tribal for destroying forests on which his generations have lived securely and safely since historic times. Tribals looked upon the forests as Nature's gift, as their own property and they had unfettered freedom to do as they pleased and the way they pleased. But the situation continued to change after the enactment of the Indian Forest Act 1937. The master of the forest, the tribal, is now no more than a wage earner. He has been gradually alienated from forest management. He no more shares the profit received from the forests. The tribal today lives below the poverty line. He is in knee-deep poverty on account of exploitation by unsocial elements like money lenders, petty shopkeepers and even pseudo social workers staying in and around the forests. These tribals today, in many cases, are just a tool in the hands of these elements who are largely responsible for the destruction of forests. Bhils are, in fact, the weakest of the weak who are unable to eke out even a miserable existence. The tribal is driven to cut the same branch on which he is sitting. Land hunger is an eternal characteristic of human beings. In the process of owning or usurping more land, the economically well-off people, traders, industrialists, social workers and leaders have occupied tribal lands turning these people landless. In many cases, the tribal roots have thus shaken. Today, the landless tribal only either looks after his new master's interest in the forest or goes to work for earning a livelihood on it. Large number of 'bidas' (individually owned forest pockets) owned by urban people in the tribal periphery is symptomatic of the scenario.

BIOLOGICAL ILLITERACY

The open book of Nature was written in millions of years. We have not understood it properly. We are not yet aware that there are friendly plants, enemy plants and neutral plants to serve as the bio-indicators for the growth of specific plants. Among the friendly plants we might refer to the presence of *Opliomanus* grass as an indicator for successful regeneration of *dhok—Anogeissus pendula* whose propagation is difficult in Rajasthan. A very distinct example of enemy plants is *vilayti babool* (*Prosopis chilensis = Prosopis juliflora*), *khejadi* (*shami*) (*Prosopis cineraria),* the State tree of Rajasthan. The carrot grass or Congress weed, *Parthenium hysterophorus* (invaded with wheat under PL 480 from the U. S. A. in the 1950s) avoids patches covered by *punwad* (*Cassia tora*). Plants like *sirio* (*Albizia lebbeck*) and *shisham* or *tali* (*Dalbergia sisoo*) are considered neutral as their occurrence in an area is neither inimical nor favourable to other plants. There is, however, a silver lining—the forest dwellers like Bhils in Rajasthan have lived for generations in harmony with plant-kingdom possess a treasure of knowledge and practical approach to maintain them. As a matter of fact, trees and tribals go together. It is heartening that the latest Forest Policy of India continues to lay emphasis on making use of this wisdom.

Biodiversity, the library of life, is on fire. Biological hazards take place when we make our surroundings simpler, less variable and homogenous. Presently, man-made order of oversimplification as against the natural order, which sustains polyculture and diversity, is presiding over the holocaust of disappearance of a million species permanently and many others, which we have not identified yet.

Diversity is a valuable resource, which promotes stability. Monoculture gives rise to increased prospective instability. Our consumerist approach to exploit nature and its bountiful resources without replenishing it is responsible for the current environmental degradation. We appear to have forgotten (under the impact of materialist glamour of Western culture) our conservation concepts as enshrined in the *Atharva Veda*: "Mata bhumi: Putroaham prithiviya." (the earth is my mother and I am the son of the soil). We take pride in calling ourselves as the master of nature. It is this disruption of family bond with benevolent nature that environmental crisis has taken place. We have already committed ecocide and are hastening to bring about a tree-less moonscape to appear on earth. We conveniently tend to ignore that plants can live without us, but our survival will be threatened without them.

The natural resource management and conservation efforts are at the crossroads today. Fortunately, it is gaining ground that biological inputs combined with societal contributions can abate depletive forces that lead to biodiversity impoverishment and collapse of ecological processes and life support systems.

THE BHILS

The Aravallis, the oldest mountain chain of India, harbour most of the forests in Rajasthan and within and around them, especially in the southern region, the major tribes, namely Bhils, Garassias, Damors and Kathodias.

The Bhils are the aboriginal inhabitants of Rajasthan dwelling in the Aravallis. They are a hill tribe adapted to a style of living which their territory demands. They are known for their bravery, carefree disposition and excellence at archery. In our Sanskrit texts, they have been called as *van putras* (sons of the forest) and *nishads* (Joshi, 1995). They are concentrated in Udaipur, Dungarpur, Banswara, Sirohi and Chittorgarh districts. Sage Valmiki, who wrote the monumental epic, the *Ramayana*, is said to be a notorious, ruthless dacoit, Valia Bhil.

Bhils live in a scattered hamlet pattern where the huts are on hillocks or hill slopes. Every village, called as *phalan* has a headman honoured as *gameti* or *mukhi*, a position that is hereditary. The *bhopa* is the village *vaidya* or medicine man who is next to the *gameti* in the social hierarchy. He is also the religious leader, commanding respect and awe. The *bhopa* looks after the spiritual needs of the tribals and also serves as a village healer. The Bhils have an animistic faith and are deeply steeped in superstition. The *Bhagat* cult started in the 19th century, which inspired the Bhils to lead a life of righteousness and devotion, deterring them from partaking liquor and meat, committing crimes and craving for material desires. *Bhagats* wear white apparel and fly a white flag on their huts. Today, one can see Bhils in various stages of advancement from the primitive Bhils in remote areas to semi-acculturised ones near towns and large non-tribal villages.

PLANT CONSERVING TRADITIONS IN BHILS

The Bhils, like other tribes, have traditional dependence on forests and trees. Some of the plant conserving practices include

1. *Kesarchhanta;*
2. *Deobans* or sacred groves;
3. Clan nomenclature—*gotra* naming;

4. Naming villages after tree names;
5. Marriage customs—*mahuwa* hugging;
6. Using *salas* branches in *mandaps* and *sandeshada* branches in fences;
7. Using biodegradable material like leaf plates and leaf cups, earthen containers (*shakora*) in their ceremonial functions;
8. Saving fuelwood trees; and
9. Reverence to trees including *kalpataru*.

Let us briefly describe these tree-friendly practices in the tribals of Rajasthan with special reference to the Bhils.

Kesar-Chhanta

In southern Rajasthan, when villagers decide to provide protection to a certain patch of forest, they collect kesar (*Crocus sativus*) from a temple (generally Kesariaji) and on a pre-fixed date, the village community announces with drum beat that they gather at a definite point and then proceed to the forest area proposed to be so safeguarded against felling and other adverse biotic factors inimical to the perpetuation of the forest vegetation. After reaching the predetermined spot, they sprinkle the kesar on the trees standing on the outer periphery of the desired forest land. They thus, collectively, impose a self-restraining ban on cutting of trees, grazing, etc. In some cases, they appoint a watchman also to ensure complete protection to this forest almost like a sanctuary. This watchman also collects dry, fallen and waif wood to be distributed among the village community. The grass and non-timber forest products (NTFP) are also collected for equal distribution among the people. The vandals who flout these social dictates are condemned publicly and fined by the elders of the village. This is a kind of 'social fencing'. According to Deep Narain Pandey (1996), an area of 12,000 hectares is getting protected in Udaipur forest division like Vijai-talai (Salumbar), Madri (Jhadol), Nayanwada (Kherwada) Alsigarh, Madonpur, etc.

Deobans (Pavitra Kunjs/Sacred Groves)

These *kunjs* (tree groves) are observed practically over the whole of Rajasthan and there is a preponderance of these in the Aravallis. In *Beyond the Vanishing Woods*, D. N. Pandey (1996) has devoted a chapter on sacred groves particularly existing in Udaipur forest division of southern Rajasthan. He has classified these into three groups.

In the first category are those sacred groves, which are in the tribal villages, often near the water source. These forest-like areas are often preserved on hill tops or hillocks and are devoted to a local deity, for example, Bherunji, Khanpa Bherunji, Kukawas Bherunji, Bhakar Bawasi, Magra Bawasi, Mataji, Badi Rupan Mata, etc. They are for maintaining congenial environments and at the same time to check water erosion.

The second category of these sacred groves comprises those which are dedicated to Lord Mahadev or Shiva. These aim at the protection of watershed areas. Sometimes stepped wells (*baori*) are made in these. Few instances are Ubeshwarji, Gautemeshwarji, Taneswarji, Jhameswarji and Kamaloath in Udaipur. Gangeshwar Mahadev forest in Dungarpur is protected similarly.

In the third category fall such groves in which only one species constitutes the grove. In Kotra range of Udaipur division, there are many *bargad* (*vat vriksha*) trees with their aerial roots forming props at the ground and looking like big groves. In Jhed and Devala there are sacred groves of *khajur* (palm) only while in Malpur, Rama Rathod, Baliakheda and Daikheda, the trees of *sagwan* (teak) make up these groves. In Amarakji, there are large dimensioned trees of only *papdi* or *chudel*; one such tree in 1995 measured about 33 metres in height and 6.91 metres in girth. It may be easily one of the largest trees of this species in India. In Dungarpur district also, there is an even-aged grove of *kalam* or *phaldu* trees. In Madar village of Udaipur district, a grove has big-sized *haldu* trees. The folklore prevalent here is that once a person in Ekpania *devban* of Madar village started to cut one such tree and when he aimed the first axe at the base of the tree, there oozed milk-like white fluid, and on the second cut came out water like liquid. Strangely, at the third stroke of the axe, a blood-red sap started flowing and the person lost his eyesight at this stroke and became permanently blind. This is termed as *dev prakop* or the 'wrath of the god or deity'. In some of these groves, the wood is taken out only for repairs of religious buildings. In the famous Shri Nath temple of Nathdwara, there is a forest block named as Ghasiara from where firewood is cut to prepare the dishes for the grand ceremony of *annakoot*, following Diwali.

Such sacred groves while providing the welcome greenery and comfortable climate, also serve as shelter to wildlife and birds. In one of the *khajur* tree groves in Udaipur were enumerated 23 avian species of which three species of parakeets (*tota*), five species of woodpeckers (*khatichida*), seven species of owls (*ulloo*), two species of myna, two species of grey tit (*ramgangra*), one species each of kingfisher (*kilkila*), blue jay (*nilkanth* or Indian roller), hoopooe (*hudhud*) and tree creeper. The Dadalia Mahadev in Raoli range of Ajmer division has a hot spring and lush green and luxuriant vegetation which provides refuge to uncommon birds like paradise flycatchers (*dudhraj*), hornbill (*dhanesh*), white cheeked bulbul (*bulbul*), etc. besides water point for *sambar, nilgai* and even panthers. In brief, these groves are a treasure house of genepool and indicators of climatic climax of the forests of the site like preservation plots.

In these *deobans* one can see the offerings of coconuts, camphor, clay terracotta and *sindoor* (vermilion) on the deity. There is always a flag hoisted on a bamboo staff. The shrine is also adorned with fresh leaves of mango and *jamun*.

The Forest Department of Rajasthan launched 'Aravalli Deoban Conservation Programme' in 1992 with the objectives of protection of groves, soil and water conservation, plantation of indigenous species and participative approach for the restoration of these groves.

A few more groves in existence are listed below:

Dungarpur District
1. Paoti Koda
2. Boreshwar
3. Rangela
4. Charwara

Sirohi District
5. Bosa
6. Jamburi

Udaipur District
7. Ram Kunda

In addition to these, Peepasar and Mukam of Nagaur district, Kiradu and Safed Oakda of Barmer district, Khejadali, Golinga Magra and Samrathal Dhora of Jodhpur district are also important besides Talvriksha of Alwar and Sita Badi of Baran district.

Gotra Namkaran (Clan Nomenclature)

Some Adivasis (tribal people), particularly Bhils, feel honoured in getting themselves named after a particular tree. Some of the surnames are salaria (after *salar),* semalia (after *semal*), palasia (after *palas*), jamania (after *jamun*), anwalia (after *aonla*), etc.

Khandelwal and Shrivastva (1999) made extensive studies on tribal clans and their totemic deity (plant). They neither cut the totemic tree (or its branches) nor burn its wood. Some important instances are:

1. Amaliyan (*Papavar somniferum*)
2. Bhagora (*Butea monosperma*)
3. Bilwal (*Aegle marmelos*)
4. Dangi (*Dendrocalamus strictus*)
5. Gamar (*Gmelina arborea*)
6. Ganawa (*Cochlospermum religiosum*)
7. Gundia (*Cordia gharal*)
8. Hingoda (*Trapa natans*)
9. Kanwi (*Mitragyna parvifolia*)
10. Maina (*Sterculia urens*)
11. Maira (*Carissa congesta*)
12. Meheda (*Terminalia bellerica*)
13. Ninama (*Ficus religiosa*)
14. Rana (*Ficus benghalensis*)
15. Rohini (*Soymida febrifuga*)
16. Tad (*Borassus flabellifer*)

Gram Namkaran (Naming the Village After a Tree)

Some places are named after the preponderance of a particular tree or some incident related with a tree. In Rajasthan, instances are Banswara (after *bans*), Kherwada (after *khair*), Sagwada (after *sag* or *sagwan*), Semalwada (after *semal*), Sariska (after *siris*), Neemada (after *neem*) and Peepalu (after *peepul*), etc. although the trees do not exist in abundance now there. The Bhils are not harbouring Bhilwara as they might have been centuries ago.

Marriage With Plants

A girl whose *mangal* (Mars) is too strong is likely to become a widow soon. In such Mars-strong virgins, the pandits first perform wedding rituals with a living *peepal* tree so that the death of the husband is avoided, for the first husband, that is, the *peepal* tree, bears the brunt of the wrath of *mangal* or Mars. In Nepal also, the virgin is first married to a *bilva* tree to ward off the evil effect of bad stars. In the Bangad area of Rajasthan (Banswara, Dungarpur, etc), the Bhils have the practice of asking the bridegroom to go below a *mahuwa* tree and then lovingly hug the tree and put *sindoor* (vermilion) on it before going to marry the bride.

Salar (Putting Branch Cutting, Sprouting Trees in Rituals) and *Sandeshada* (Fences)

Our tribals are excellent ethno-botanists. The Bhils put hand-thick tall branches of *salar* in *mandap* (posts put in marriage customs). This *salar* post has the inherent capacity to sprout and assumes a tree form in due course of time and thus not only becomes a commemoration plant of marriage but also provides its products including oxygen and, as a matter of fact, it acts as a fixed deposit which can provide finances in unforeseen circumstances. These people prefer to make their *taparies* (huts) on hillocks and to protect their huts, put fences around them so that unwanted cattle, wild animals and vandals do not get an easy access to their campus. They often put thick branches of an indigenous plant *sandeshada* (*Delonix alata*) along the fence in close proximity so that these make rather impenetrable physical barrier for intruders. These branches, in a few months, strike roots in the ground and become trees which besides keeping the atmosphere and environment nice, serve as a source of firewood and leaf-fodder for the inhabitants and animals. These plants also serve as support for the climbers grown by them for beans and vegetables.

Using Biodegradable Products in Functions

In our social functions like marriages, *goths* (community feasts/picnics) and other large-scale party-gatherings, they use leaf-plates and cups (*pattal dauna*) and earthen pots (*shakora* or *kulhads* for water) instead of plastic articles, which cannot decompose. The leaf products and earthen utensils soon get degraded biologically and provide nutrients to the soil. The sacred tank of Pushkar and other places are gradually getting polluted because of throwing of used plastic and glass bottles by foreigners and even local and domestic visitors to this holy lake of Pushkar, where persons in lakhs gather together in the annual fair held in *Kartik* (October-November) besides every day pilgrims in this holy place.

Saving Fuelwood

Fuelwood saved is forest saved. Efficient use of firewood is followed by tribals even today. Whenever a death occurs, each of them brings a piece of dry wood log and thus green trees have not be felled for this necessary ritual. Bhils realise the worth of a green forest.

REVERENCE TO TREES INCLUDING *KALPATARU*

Plants too are held sacred and worshipped as deities. Some important examples will elucidate:

Adansonia digitata Linn. (Kalpa dev)

This tree is acclaimed universally as a wish-fulfilling deity. Two trees are existing near Banswara on the banks of the river Mahi. Tribal people desirous of getting married or getting a child, for fulfilment of wishes or with newly-born babies in anticipation of getting long life conferred on them, circle around the tree tying thread on the trunk and pouring offerings. Vows taken are also kept this way.

Ficus benghalensis Linn. (Vadla)

As in Hindu society, this tree is worshipped by the tribals also.

Ficus religiosa **Linn. (Pipali, Pipli Mata)**

The tree is taken as a female deity unlike Hindus who take it as a male one. If growing near the hut, it may be transplanted elsewhere but destroying it is considered a sin. During the day of 'Dasha Mata' celebration (in the month of March) womenfolk move around the tree five times and tie a thread around its trunk. A story (katha) is used by the priest to narrate while a drummer drums nearby. A thread given by the priest is worn as a 'dora'.

Mangifera indica **Linn. (Amba)**

At Ghotia Amba, (a pilgrim spot) in Banswara district, tribals worship this mango tree believed to have been planted by Bhim of the Pandavas during their exile period to please Inder Dev, the god of rain. A two-day fair is held in March when tribals congregate at this spot, bathe the trunks of the ancient mango trees, apply turmeric (*Curcuma domestica* Linn.) paste and offer coconuts (*Cocos nucifera* Linn.), incense sticks and coins.

Musa paradisiaca **Linn. (Keli, Kela)**

This plant is associated with Aryan rituals too. The plant is believed to prosper only under strict taboos and codes of worship. Persons with a form of pollution, for example, in a drunken state, women with menses, etc. are forbidden to go in its proximity.

Phyllanthus emblica **Linn. (Amli, Anwla)**

Valia Bhil, later known as the great celebrated saint, Valmiki, used to loot and murder travellers and took a piece of their flesh which he stored in bins. When his crimes amounted to a big magnitude, that seven earthen bins were filled with pieces of human flesh, God came to intervene. On asking how he could achieve salvation, he was told to take seven circles around the emblica tree. Even today, Bhils seeking absolution do the same.

Tamarindus indica **Linn. (Amli, Imli)**

Singh and Pandey (1982) report the worship of the tamarind tree on the day of 'Amil gyaras'. Young boys and girls take seven rounds of a twig of this tree planted on the ground, offering maize and millet grains to it. They collect some of the latter storing them in granary in their homes under the belief that the bins will never be empty.

Vetiveria zizanioides **(Linn.) Nash (Kator Mata)**

This perennial grass grows in marshy and wet habitats and is believed to be the abode of Kator goddess, responsible for the safety and welfare of children. On a day in the month of September, the weeds are worshipped and food cooked a day earlier is eaten.

Place of Worship and Allied Functionaries

The most important place associated with sacred nature in the tribal villages is the *devra* where the deity is housed. There may be more than one deity at a *devra*. It may be an elaborate construction or a raised square platform often below an auspicious tree like *Azadirachta indica* A.

Juss, *Ficus benghalensis* Linn., *Ficus religiosa* Linn., etc. Generally, the land left aside for the deity and *devra* supports a grove of old, large and well-preserved trees where cutting of trees, even plucking a twig is considered a blasphemy. This stand or sacred grove is known as a *maalvan* and may comprise a single or many plant species. The most common ones are *Butea monosperma* (Lam.) Taub, *Ficus* species, *Diospyros melanoxylon* Roxb, *Boswellia serrata* Roxb. ex Colebr, *Mangifera indica* Linn., *Musa paradisiaca* Linn., *Jasminum sambac* (Linn.) Ait and *Tectona grandis* Linn. f.

PLANTS USED FOR MEDICINAL PURPOSES

Bhils still use their readymade pharmacopoeia, the vegetation around them, through their magico-medicine person, the *bhopa*. Many workers have done research on this aspect in various tribes of the country.

Prabhakar Joshi in *Ethnobotany of Primitive Tribes of Rajasthan* (1995) listed 100 local plants of which different parts are used as drugs (Roots 22, rhizomes 2, root bark 6, stem 11, stem bark 19, exudates 10, leaves 39, flowers 5, fruits 10, seeds 15, seed oil 2 and whole plant 15..

Joshi (1995) has further classified these plants on the basis of diseases in which these 100 plants are used. These diseases are abdominal pains, abortion, acne, anaemia, appetite (loss of), asthma, backache, bitter mouth, bleeding, burns and scalds, carbuncles, centipede bite, child birth (difficulty), constipation, coughs and colds, cracked skin, cramps, cuts, diabetes, diarrhoea, dandruff, dropsy, dysentery, eye inflammations, facial swelling, fever, fontanel (infants), gangrene, gastric disorders, guineaworm, haemorrhage, headache, heartburn, hoarse voice, inflammation of teats (milch cattle), ingestion of iron pieces (cattle), intestinal obstruction, itching, jaundice, lactation (painful), malaria, malnutrition (cattle), migraine, mumps, myotic wounds, night blindness, parasites (external), pimples and boils, poisoning, post parturition (weakness), proper foetal development, pulmonary inflammation, pustular skin eruptions, (rainy season), ringworm, scabies, scorpion sting, snakebite, sore throat, sore sprains and fractures, sunstroke, teeth and jaw diseases, tonsillitis, typhoid, urinary tract problems, urine (retention of) uterus protrusion, virility (lack of), vomiting, worms, wounds, etc.

Plants Found Effective in Cuts and Wounds

Plants, besides providing shelter, are of utility for treatment of ailments and mundane necessities of life. The paper deals with healing of cuts and wounds through indigenous plants. These plants are:

Bleeding

Tridax procumbens.

Burns

Chretia laevis, *Capidagethia cristata*, *Marsilea* sp. *Sesbania bispinosa*, *Sida orientalis.*

Cracked skin

Crataeva nurvula, *Ficus racemosa*, Schreber's swietenioides, *Sterculia urens.*

TABLE 1
Indigenous Plants Used for Cuts and Wounds by Bhils

Latin Name	Family Name	Local Name	Habit	Parts Used	Mode of Use	Preparation of Drug
Bleeding						
1. *Tridax procumens*	Asteraceae	Kalal, Pabula ka mocha	Tall herb, hairy	Whole plant	Dripped over injured spot	Crush the plant to get juice
Burns						
2. *Ehretia laevis*	Ehretiaceae	Luni, Tambolia	Tree, leaves with foul smell	Stem, bark	Like ointment	Crushing bark, paste made
3. *Lepidagathis cristata*	Acanthaceae	Jamunghota, phootaliya	Perennial, spiny herb	Stem	Like ointment	Globose aerial parts lifted, burnt, powdered and paste made
4. *Marselia* species	Pteridophyte	—	Aquatic herb	Leaves	Like ointment	Leaves crushed as paste
5. *Sesbania bispinosa*	Papilionaceae	Daden, dadon	Shrub, weak stem	Seeds	Like ointment	Seeds crushed as paste
6. *Sida orientalis* = *S. rhombifolia*	Malvaceae	Bagulia, kharaiti	Under-shrub, hairy stem	Leaves	Like ointment	Paste made of fresh leaves
Cracked Skin						
7. *Crataeva nurvula*	Capparaceae	Valvarna, vanno, vanni, varno	Deciduous, small tree	Stem bark	Locally	Paste made along with bark of *mokha*

Continued...

...*Continued*

Latin Name	Family Name	Local Name	Habit	Parts Used	Mode of Use	Preparation of Drug
8. *Ficus racemosa*	Moraceae	Umar, umba	Evergreen tree	Latex	Locally	Fresh latex
9. *Sehrebera swietenoides*	Oleaceae	Mokha, mokhdi	Tall tree	Stem, bark, leaves	As ointment	Paste along with bark of *varno*. Crushed along with leaves of *varno* as paste
10. *Sterculia urens*	Sterculiaceae	Kadaya	Tree, smooth white bark	Leaves	As ointment	Fresh crushed to make paste
Cuts						
11. *Adiantum caudatum*	Pteridophyte	Aadisha	Fern-herb	Whole plant	As ointment	Crushed into paste
12. *Cocculus hirsutus*	Menispermaceae	Vev-no-vela	Scandent shrub, villose branch	Leaves	Dripped over affected spot	Crushed and juice taken out
13. *Grewia flavescenes*	Tiliaceae	Gangeshri, kharbata	Large shrub	Leaves	Ointment	Crushed and juice taken out
14. *Gymnema sylvestre*	Asclepiadaceae	Gurmar, jungli urad	Twining shrub	Leaves	Locally	Paste of crushed leaves
15. *Marsilea* species	Pteridophyte	—	Aquatic herb	Leaves	Locally	Paste of crushed juices

Continued...

...Continued

Latin Name	Family Name	Local Name	Habit	Parts Used	Mode of Use	Preparation of Drug
16. *Sesbania bispinosa*	Papilionaceae	Daden, dadon	Shrub	Seeds	As ointment	Paste of seeds + white stone powder
17. *Sida orientalis*	Malvaceae	Bagulia, kharaiti	Under-shrub	Leaves, roots	Locally Locally	Paste made Paste made
Wounds						
18. *Abrus precatorius*	Papilionaceae	Charmdi, chanbol	Slender twiner	Leaves (for cattle neck)	Rubbed locally	Paste of leaves
19. *Cocculus hirsutus*	Menispermaceae	Vev-no-velo	Shrub	Leaves	Dripped over wound	Juice of fresh leaves
20. *Derris indica* = *Pongamia pinnata*	Papilionaceae	Karanji, kannaji	Tree, big crown	Seed oil	Locally	Seeds to yield oil
21. *Grewia flavescens*	Tiliaceae	Gangeshri, kharbata	Large shrub	Roots	Locally	Crushed to make paste
22. *Gymnema sylvestre*	Asclepadaceae	Gurmar, jungli urad	Twining shrub	Seed, Stem bark	Ointment Ointment	Paste made by crushing seeds Paste made of bark
23. *Haldina cordifolia*	Naucleaceae	Haldu, halda	Large tree, crown big	Stem bark, leaves	Poultice Poultice	Bark paste Leaves boiled
24. *Marsilea* species	Pteridophyte	—	Aquatic herb	Leaves	Locally	Paste made

Continued...

...Continued

Latin Name	Family Name	Local Name	Habit	Parts Used	Mode of Use	Preparation of Drug
25. *Sesbania bispinosa*	Papilionaceae	Daden, dadon	Shrub	Seeds	As ointment	Paste of seeds + white stone powder
26. *Sida orientalis*	Malvaceae	Bagulia, kharaiti	Under-shrub	Root, leaves	Locally Locally	Paste by crushing Paste by crushing
27. *Typha angustata*	Typhaceae	Patar, pata, era	Perennial, tall herb, scapigerous	Inflorescence	Tied as dressing	Split in 2 halves, half taken to tie

TABLE 2
Hindi Names of Plants Used in the Article With Their Latin Equivalents

Hindi	English	Latin
Am	Mango	*Mangifera indica*
Anwala		*Emblica officinalis*
Arjun		*Terminalia arjuna*
Bans	Bamboo	*Dendrocalamus strictus*
Bargad	Banyan	*Ficus benghalensis*
Churel		*Holoptelia integrifolia*
Dhak		*Butea monosperma*
Dhok		*Anogeissus pendula*
Gular, umbar		*Ficus racemosa* f. *glomerata*
Haldu		*Haldina cordifolia*
Imli, Amli	Tamarind	*Tamarindus indicus*
Kalam		*Mitragyna parvifolia*
Kalpavriksha	Baobab	*Adansonia digitata*
Karpoor	Camphor	*Cinnamomum camphora*
Kesar		*Crocus sativa*
Khair	Catechu	*Acacia catechu*
Khajur		*Phoenix sylvestre*
Mahuwa		*Madhuca indica* = *Bassia latifolia*
Nariyal	Coconut	*Cocos nucifera*
Neem/neemada	Margosa	*Azadirachta indica*
Palas		*Butea monosperma*
Papadi		*Holoptelia integrifolia*
Peepal		*Ficus religiosa*
Sagwan	Teak	*Tectona grandis*
Salar		*Boswellia serrata*
Shami (Khejadi)		*Prosopis cineraria* = *P. spicigera*
Sandeshada		*Delonix alata*
Siria	Indian laburnum	*Albizzia lebbeck*
Simal	Semal	*Bombax ceiba* = *B. malabaricum*
Talvriksha		*Terminalia arjuna*
Tulsi	Basil	*Ocimum sanctum*
Vetvriksha	Banyan	*Ficus benghalensis*
Vilva (Belpatra)		*Aegle marmelos*

Cuts

Adiantum caudatum, Cocculus hirsutus, Grewia flavescens, Gymnema sylvestre, Marsilea species, *Sesbania bispinosa, Sida orientalis.*

Wounds

Abrus precatorius, Derris indica, Haldine cordifolia, Typha angustata, Marsilea sp., *Sesbania bispinosa, Sida orientalis, Cocculus hirsutus, Grewia flavescens, Gymnema sylvestre.*

The botanical description, local names, parts and their modes of preparation are indicated in Table 1.

CONCLUSION

Indigenous cultures are under assault everywhere in the world under the impact of urbanisation and industrialisation. The tribals and Bhils are also dwindling in Rajasthan due to modernisation. The tribals are vanishing relics of primitive human societies. The hill supporting forest cover from where they came and brought down the knowledge of biodiversity and its significance are fast disappearing and have become ecological disasters. These Bhils and tribals are also getting acculturated and losing their well-preserved repository of nature's benevolent and beneficial attributes. It is a challenge for us today to salvage the valuable legacies of the tribals before they get entombed for ever along with culture that gave them birth. We must ensure preservation of species, which we are not promoting today as enshrined in Agenda 21 of the Rio Earth Summit 1992.

REFERENCES

Billore, K. V. *et al.* 'Conservation of medicinal plants in Rajasthan'. *Bull. Medico-Ethnobotanical Research,* C. C. R. in Ayur. and Siddha, New Delhi. 8(1 & 2): 118-127, 1986.

Botanical Survey of India. *Ethnobotany in India.* Howrah: Botanical Survey of India, 1983.

Desai, B. L. 'Tree worship in Gujarat'. *Folklore* pp. 183-186, May 1964.

Doshi, S. L. *Bhils: Between Social Self-Awareness and Culture Synthesis.* New Delhi: Sterling Publishers, 1971.

Jain S. K. and Rao, R. R. 'Ethnobotany in India: An overview'. *Bot. Surv. India,*. Howrah, 1983.

Joshi, P. 'The forest herbal resources and Bhil medicine'. *Tribe* (Udaipur) (Spl. No.). 13(2-4): 129-136, 1981.

Joshi, P., Khandelwal, S. and Shrivastva, Y. 'Drops of nature: Conservation in Rajasthan sacred groves'. Proc. Sem on *Eco-Dev. Habitat and Wildlife Cons. in Rajasthan and Adjacent Areas'.* Hadoti Naturalists Soc. Kota, pp. 40-43, 1994.

Joshi, Prabhakar. *Ethnobotany of the Primitive Tribes in Rajasthan.* Jaipur: Printwell, 1995.

Khandelwal, Sita Ram and Shrivastava, Yogesh. 'Folk beliefs and practices related to plants conservation'. *Ind. Jour. Env. Sciences,* Green Earth Foundation, Jaipur. 3(2): 165-170,1989.

Krishnamurthy, A. V. R. G. 'Management of forest eco-systems for tribal development'. *Tribe* (Udaipur) 13:2-4, 1981.

Mann, R. S. 'Religious attributes of Bhils'. *Tribe* (Udaipur) (Spl, No.). 10:109-122, 1978.

Palat, R. 'Rajasthan ki adam jatiyon mein vaivahik prakriyayen aur sanskarik geet'. *Vanyajati* 33(1)16-26, 1984.

Pandey, Deep Narain and Singh, Samar. 'Aravali ke dev van'. *Rajasthan Patrika, Ravivariya Parishist,* Jaipur, 21.5.1995.

Pandey, Deep Narain and Singh, Samar. *Beyond Vanishing Woods*. Udaipur: Himanshu Publications, 1996.

Saxena, V. S. 'Etho-environmental considerations in traditions and rituals of Rajasthan'. In: *Encyclopaedia Botanica*. (Ed.). Trivedi, P. C., Jaipur: Pointer Publishers, pp 284-304, 2000.

Saxena, V. S. 'Kalpa vrikshon ka aradhan'. *Rajasthan Patrika, Ravivariya Parishist*, Jaipur, 14.8.1996.

Saxena, V. S. 'Parampara khejadi poojan ki'. *Rajasthan Patrika, Ravivariya Parishist*, Jaipur, 20.10.1996.

Saxena, V. S. 'Prachin paramparaon mein paryavaran parirakshan bodh'. *Rajasthan Patrika, Ravivariya Parishist*, Jaipur, 30.7.1995.

Saxena, V. S. 'Rural social forestry in Rajasthan'. *Rur. Soc. For.*, N. I. R. D., Hyderabad, 1983.

Saxena, V. S. 'Tribals and forest policy'. *Tribe* (Udaipur) 13(2-4): 15-22, 1981.

Saxena, V. S. 'Virkshon par palti sanskritika asthayen'. *Dainik Bhaskar*, Jaipur, 14.4.1998.

Saxena, V. S. 'Vrikshon ka dharmik mahatwa'. *Ped Podha Samachar,* Allahabad, 1.3.1998.

Shah, S. A. 'Tribals and social forestry'. *Tribe* (Udaipur) 13 (Spl. No. 2-4), 1981.

Trivedi, P. C. and Jyoti, Nargas. 'Ethnobotanical Studies: Aspects and Prospects'. In: *Encyclopaedia Botanica*. (Ed.). Trivedi, P. C. pp. 305-340, 2000.

—oo(O)oo—

8

Psyllium (*Plantago ovata* F), its Conservation and Utilisation

R. K. Lal, S. P. S. Khanuja and A. K. Agnihotri

The genus *Plantago* comprises 200 species, of which 10 occur in India (Anonymous, 1967). Among the latter are many that are used in indigenous medicine in India and in many countries all over the world. It is a plant of west-Asian origin and was introduced into India during Muslim settlement in the Middle Ages. Another but minor source of seed and seed husk is *Plantago psyllium*, which was earlier cultivated in France. Other species of the genus including *Plantago major*, *Plantago lanceolata, Plantago pumilla, Plantago coronopus, Plantago argentia* and *Plantago lagopus* produce small quantities of mucilage around their seeds. Therefore, none of them find use in the pharmaceutical industry.

The seeds and husk of *Plantago ovata* are used in 60 traditional and modern systems of medicine. Seeds are cooling, demulcent, useful in inflammatory and bilious derangement of the digestive organs, applied as poultice to rheumatic and gouty swelling, good in dysentery and irritation of the intestinal tract, decoction is useful in cough and chronic diarrhoea. The husk from the seeds has the property of absorbing and retaining water and hence, it works as an anti-diarrhoea drug (Luthra, 1950).

At present, Gujarat, Madhya Pradesh and parts of Rajasthan, especially, the Malwa tract and northern belt are the major isabgol (*Plantago ovata*) growing areas in India. India continues to hold monopoly in its production and trade in the world market (Anonymous, 1976). The export of husk and seed was of Rs. 19,993.8 lakh and Rs. 746.8 lakh, respectively, during 2000-2001.

Countries to which the husk is exported are Afghanistan, Bahrain, Canada, Sri Lanka, Dubai, Fiji, France, Germany, Kenya, Kuwait, Oman, Nepal, New Zealand, Saudi Arabia, the U. K., the U. S. A., Somalia and Zambia. Countries to which seeds are exported are: Afghanistan, Belgium, Canada, Ethiopia, France, Germany, Kuwait, Saudi Arabia, the U. K. and the U. S. A.

Though India enjoys monopoly in production of and export of isabgol but hardly 50 per cent requirement of the U. S. A. could be met. In view of its substantial demand, there is scope to increase the area and to intensify its cultivation. There is also an urgent need to evolve high-yielding strains and to examine suitable locations for growing this crop in other States of the country.

BOTANY

Plantago ovata (2n = 8) is a stem-less or short-stemmed annual herb which attains a height of 30-40 cm, has leaves in a rosette or alternate, clasping the stem, strap-like recurved, 7.5 to 25.0 cm long, narrow, varying from less than 6.0 mm to 12.5 mm in width, tapering to a point, three nerved, entire, coated with fine hairs. Flowers white, minute, four parted, erect, ovoid or cylindrical spike 12.5 to 37.5 mm in length. Capsule ovate, 8.0 mm long, 2-celled, the top half lifting up, when ripe releasing the smooth, dull, ovate seeds 1.8 to 3.8 mm long pinkish-grey brown or pinkish-white with a brown about 1.5 gm. Each seed is enclosed in a thin, white, translucent membrane, known as husk, which is odourless and tasteless (Morton, 1977). When soaked in water, the whole seed appears much swollen because of the expansion of the mucilage in the husk (Hyde, 1970). The husked seeds are dark-red and hard (Wren, 1930).

FLORAL BIOLOGY

Flowers small, greenish, spicate, often dimorphic, bracteate, sepals four, imbricate in bud, persistent. Corolla scarious, hypogynous; lobes four, short, imbricate in bud; stamens four, inserted on the corolla-tube; filament filiform, persistent; anthers large, pendulous, versatile, ovary superior, 1-4 celled; ovules 1-8 in each cell. Capsule 1-4-celled, circumscissilely dehiscent, membranous, one or more seeded.

CULTIVATION

Plantago is an irrigated *rabi* crop, which remains in the field for about four months. The crop is grown in marginal, light, well drained sandy-loam to loamy soils having pH between 7 and 8. It requires a climate and dry sunny weather during maturity; even mild dew, cloudy weather or light showers cause seed shedding.

The optimum sowing time is early November; sowing however is extended till the end of December, but the delayed sowing decreases the yield. The seed rate is 7-8 kg/hectare. Sowing is done through broadcasting or line sowing. They are covered thinly by raking the soil. A light irrigation is given immediately.

Germination starts in 6 to 10 days and the crop is given second irrigation after three weeks and a third one at the time of the formation of the spikes; thus the crop needs 6 to 7 irrigations.

Plantago makes a moderate demand for nutrients. Usually 25 kg each of N and P per hectare is given at planting and another 25 kg of N is applied with the third irrigation. Crop is given one to two hand weedings.

The plant bears the flowering spikes in about 60 days after sowing and matures in the next two months. The yellowing of the lower leaves is an indication of maturity, confirmed by pressing a spike between two fingers, when the mature seeds come out. Crop is harvested close to the ground in the early morning hours to avoid losses owing to seed shedding. The average seed yield is one tonne per hectare and after processing about 30 per cent husk by weight is recovered (Handbook of Agriculture, ICAR).

UTILISATION

Plantago seeds are mostly used in medicine because of its mucilage that is colloidal in nature, and serve as a safe bulk-laxative which promotes regular bowel movement, for chronic dysentery of amoebic and basillary origin. This is administered. The seeds and husk are used to cure inflammation of the mucous membrane of gastrointestinal and genito-urinary tracts, duodenal ulcer, gonorrhoea and piles. It can also be used as cervical dilator for termination of pregnancy. Besides its use in medicine, mucilage is also used in various industries like food processing, sizing of textile, paper and in cosmetics as a base. The embryo oil of seeds has 50 per cent linoleic acid, which prevents arteriosclerosis (Kirtikar).

CHEMICAL COMPOSITION

The seeds contain a fatty oil, albuminous matter and mucilage in such large quantities that one part of the seeds with 20 parts of water forms a tasteless jelly within a short time. On addition of a large quantity of water and filtering, little mucilage passes, but the major part of it remains adherent to the seeds. The mucilage can be separated through straining with pressure. It is neutral in reaction, is not altered by adding or precipitated by boiling with alcohol or changed by iodine, borax or perchloride of iron. It is only sparingly soluble in water. A glycoside named aucubin $C_{13}H_{19}O_8H_{20}$ has been isolated from the seeds, leaves, roots and flowering stems. It crystallises in the form of colourless bush-forming needles, which have a melting point of 181°C and a rotation in aqueous solution of –164.9°C. Fatty acid contents of the oils is as follows: linoleinic acid 0.2 per cent, linoleic acid 47.9 per cent, oleic acid 36.7 per cent, palmitic acid 3-7 per cent, stearic acid 6.9 per cent and liguoceric acid 0.8 per cent.

PHARMACOPOEIAL STANDARDS

In the Indian Pharmacopoeia it is specified that the husk should contain not more than 2 per cent foreign organic matter, 2.9 per cent ash and 0.45 per cent acid insoluble ash. Swelling factor of the husk is 40 to 90 per cent compared with 10.25 to 13.50 per cent for seed (Trease *et al*, 1972). However Atal and Kapoor (1963) pointed out the inadequacy in the existing standards and proposed new standards as given below:

1. Foreign organic matter	—	2 per cent
2. Ash	—	2 per cent
3. Acid insoluble ash	—	0.2 per cent
4. Swelling factor	—	55
5. Non-mobile gel volume	—	40 ml

The gel compared with those of sodium alginate, methylcellulose, sodium carboxymethyl cellulose and starch appears to be superior in spreadability, penetration, washability, etc.

THERAPEUTIC USES

These are very useful in all inflammatory affections of the mucous membrane of the alimentary canal on account of their emollient, demulcent and laxative properties. The seeds of *Plantago ovata* in the following conditions give good results (Chopra; Kirtikar).

(a). Chronic Bacillary Dysentery

This condition is invariably associated with the presence of mucus in the stools. The bowels in these conditions are generally ulcerated and the toxins absorbed from the ulcerated surface produce a diminution of tone of involuntary muscle of the gut wall producing intestinal stasis, viscroptosis and a general toxaemic condition in the individual. Chronic diarrhoea with painful peristalsis persists for prolonged periods and may alternate with periods of constipation. The condition is intractable and may persist for years.

(b). Chronic Amoebic Dysentery

These patients may have constipation or irregularity of bowels and the majority shows mucus in their stools. The degree of ulceration varies greatly according to the intensity of the intestinal symptoms. In the above two conditions the administration of the seeds gives a considerable relief to the patient. In chronic amoebic dysentery where constipation is one of the main symptoms, the mucilage covers the faeces, as they become solid in the large intestine and thus facilitates their passage through the large gut by acting as a lubricant. In this condition, as well as in chronic spastic constipation, its action may be aided by giving small doses of saline purgatives.

(c). Hill Diarrhoea

This condition is more common in Europeans. The patient usually passes several stools in the morning and the condition is accompanied by catarrh of the intestines. *Plantago ovata* seeds are useful in the early stages. Not only in the irritated mucous membrane soothed and protected by the mucilage but the fermentation is also inhibited and the stools assume a solid form.

(d). Chronic Diarrhoea

Chronic diarrhoea in children, which is due to the irritation of the gut with bacterial toxins and the mucilage, acts by removing this irritation. Roasted seeds are given to the children.

(e). Inflammation

In Argentina, psyllium seeds are boiled in water for 15 minutes, the liquid strained, chilled and used as eye drops to dispel inflammation. The decoction is taken with honey as a remedy for sore throat and bronchitis.

(f). Cancer

Seeds of *Plantago ovata* soaked in water are recommended for treatment of cancer (Goswami, 1988; Hartwell, 1970).

(g). Serum-Cholesterol Level

The seed husk is effective in reducing serum-cholesterol level. The oil contained in isabgol embryo is rich in linoleic acid and has potential as dietary hypocholesterolemic agent. Isabgol oil is more potent than safflower oil for reducing serum-cholesterol level (Siddiqui *et al*, 1964). The efficacy is increased when the husk is consumed with metronidazole (Imran, 1984). Ingestion of 10 gm isabgol a day for a month reduces serum cholesterol level by 9.6 and triglyceride by 8.6 per cent (Goswami, 1988).

(h). Pimples and Hair Fall

It also controls pimples and hair fall.

(i). Bronchitis

Tribals use isabgol for several purposes. The Santhals use it to relieve pain and treat bronchitis (Jain *et al*, 1970). The tribal inhabitants of North Gujarat consume seeds of psyllium as a cooling demulcent to cure diarrhoea and dysentery.

OTHER USES

(a). They are common ingredients in laxative products of various manufacturers (Claus *et al*, 1980).

(b). The mucilage is sometimes employed as a substitute for agar-agar.

(c). It may serve as a stabiliser in ice cream, filler for wheat starch, an ingredient in chocolate, a sizing for textiles and in the formation of pharmaceutical tablets (Mithal et al, 1971; Patel *et al*, 1966) and in cosmetics.

(d). The CDRI, Lucknow, has developed sweet palatable variously flavoured granules (marketed under the trade name 'Ligafin'), and fine powder for more popular use of isabgol.

(e). Development of 'Isaptent' sticks from isabgol husk for medical termination of pregnancy (MTP). Isaptent is poised to replace the expensive imported 'Laminaria-tent' which takes larger time to dilate the cervix.

(f). As the seeds of isabgol are rich in protein, they are mixed with guar (*Cyamopsis tetragonoloba* Tab) for feeding cattle (Anonymous, 1969; Desai *et al*, 1980; Williams, 1960).

TOXICITY

Use of psyllium as laxative does not induce any side effects. However, the plant causes allergy in work environment (Hussain, 1977). Occasional asthma is reported among people who work with psyllium (Benton, 1969; Basse *et al*, 1975). Unsoaked seeds may cause gastrointestinal irritation, inflammation, mechanical obstruction and constipation whereas powdered or chewed seeds release a pigment which is injurious to the kidneys (Patel *et al*, 1966), psyllium seed cookies, consumed by the unwary, have produced profuse diarrhoea (Morton, 1977).

ADULTERANTS

Psyllium seeds are frequently mixed with the seeds of *Salvia aegyptica* L. which also yield copious mucilage. Commercial samples of isabgol are sometimes adulterated with the seeds of *Plantago lancealato* L., *Plantago arenaria* Waldet and *Plantago major* L. besides *Plantago ovata* Forsk and *Plantago psyllium* L. which can be identified by their external colour, shape and outline.

CONSERVATION

There is an urgent need to collect more variability from wild and cultivated populations of *Plantago ovata.* Collection of genetic diversity requires an understanding of what is a character and how does it vary in a population. Genetic diversity is defined as the heritable variability of plants, animals and micro-organisms of actual or potential value. In a broader perspective it includes diversity within species, between species and of ecosystems of which those are components. In the context of crop improvement, diverse genotypes of specific taxon need to be collected, evaluated and utilised as direct introduction or as parent in the crop improvement programme and conserved. It should be emphasised that the rapid replacement of land races and locally adopted varieties by highly uniform varieties is likely to occur in this crop in the near future, leading to the elimination of these vital resources created by nature over hundreds of years. Thus, there is an urgent need to conserve the existing variability in this species. Further, it is important to formulate procedures, both for regeneration and conservation of germplasm collections in long-term storage with little loss of aggregated diversity within each stock when grown simultaneously. In cross-pollinated species like *Plantago ovata*, if the seeds so formed will be of unknown male parentage it will thus not be the true representative of the type multiplied. Therefore, hand pollination using mixture of pollen collected from a large number of plants in each accession may be done to have enough diversity in the sample. The seeds from these hand-pollinated plants in each accession have to be bulked to reconstitute the stock, which is conserved.

CENTRES FOR CONSERVATION

(a). Proposed Storage Centres

Banaskantha and Mehsana districts of Gujarat in India and Sindh in Pakistan are the most suitable locations for storing the germplasm collections of *Plantago ovata.*

(b). Medicinal Plant Gardens

Counterparts of the main germplasm collection can be conserved in the medicinal plant gardens situated in Gujarat, Rajasthan, Haryana, Uttar Pradesh, Bengal and Mysore States of India and in West Pakistan.

(c). National Reserves

Because of its sporadic distribution in its natural habitat, it would not be possible to locate areas, which can be made national reserves for conserving the genetic diversity in a wild state.

The germplasm collection from different areas of India and Pakistan should be evaluated as under for various characters of economic importance and to classify the stocks and prepare a documented information on their characters.

Genetic resources are supplied by gene banks to individual plant breeders who undertake detailed evaluation of morphological, physiological and biochemical characters, including tolerance to disease and best adaptation to adverse soil and climatic conditions. Breeders should provide data on detailed evaluation to gene banks for incorporating the information in detailed catalogues and in the national database.

The Institute maintains the germplasm of the following categories (*Plant Genetic Resources*):

(a). Land Races

The traditional *Plantago* cultivars collected from the farmers.

Elite Cultivars/Varieties: High-yielding varieties released by the CIMAP, Lucknow (Institute) State and Central variety release committees. This also includes the pure line selections from the land races recommended for general cultivation before the release of high yielding varieties, for example, Niharika, Mayuri, Gujarat Isabgol-1, G.I.-2, HI-5, etc. and Italian strain EC42706.

(b). Donors

Important breeding lines or land races identified as resistant to abiotic and biotic stress situations, superior in quality characters, etc.

(c). Genetic Markers

Genotypes that possess some specific characters useful in the genetic studies branched, feathery, club and long inflorescence mutants (Lal *et al,* 2000; Lal *et al*, 2002). Aberrant cytological types (haploids, triploids, tetraploids, trisomics), CMS lines, etc. belong to this group.

(d). Wild Species

Species of *Plantago* and related genotypes, their ecotypes, inter-specific hybrids, etc. *Plantago exigua, Plantago indica, Plantago himalaica, Plantago lagopus*, etc. with the advancement in plant breeding techniques and development of high yielding varieties, the land races and primitive cultivars are fast being replaced. It is very necessary to conserve the valuable gene pool of the cultivated plants for posterity. To avoid frequent regeneration and to check genetic drift, facilities have been developed for long-term storage of germplasm in the National Gene Bank at NBPGR, New Delhi.

There is an urgent need to pool the entire genetic wealth available in the country at one or two locations and systematically evaluate in phases to check or eliminate duplicates, using biochemical and molecular techniques.

SUMMARY

The seeds of *Plantago ovata* are very beneficial in chronic dysentery of amoebic origin and chronic diarrhoea due to irritative conditions of the gastrointestinal tract. A glycoside named aucubin has been found in the seeds but it is physiologically inactive. The tannins, which are present in appreciable quantity, have little action on the entamoebae or bacteria. The action of the drug would appear to be purely mechanical; being due to the large amount of mucilage, which is contained in the superficial layers of the seeds. This mucilage is shown, not to be acted on by the digestive enzyme and passes through the small intestine uncharged. It lines the mucous membrane of this part of the gut and its demulcent properties give it a protective and sedative action. The toxins present in the gut are absorbed by the gel and their absorption into the system is prevented. Seeds swell up on contact with water, they increase the bulk of the intestinal contents stimulating the intestinal peristalsis. The mucilage of *Plantago ovata* seeds acts in very much the same way as liquid paraffin. It is very much cheaper and is further free from injurious effects

Produced by the habitual use of the latter drug, that is, malignant disease of the colon, eczema, ani, paraffin pains, etc.

For conservation the genetic diversity of the cultivated *Plantago* is quite impressive in India. Collection and conservation of this genetic wealth is in the national interest. Evaluation and documentation of its variability will help the improvement of *Plantago* cultivars of the country.

REFERENCES

Ahmad, J., Farooqui, A. H. and Siddiqui, T. O. 'Zabariyaal-Razi's treatise on botanical, animal and mineral drugs for cancer'. *Hamdard* 28(3): 76-93, 1985.

Anonymous. 'Isaptent, a new cervical dilator'. CDRI Annual Report, p. 12, 1979.

Anonymous. 'Palatable isabgol granules'. *CSIR News* 29(24): 184, 1979.

Anonymous. *Commodity Study of Crude Drugs and Herbs*. New Delhi: Indian Institute of Foreign Trade, pp. 55-99, 1976.

Anonymous. *The Wealth of India: Raw Materials*. vol. VIII: Ph-Rc. New Delhi: Publication and Information Directorate, CSIR, pp. 146-154, 1969.

Atal, C. K. and Kapur, K. K. 'Evaluation of ispaghula husk'. *Indian J. Pharm.* 25(11): 376-378, 1963.

Bernton, S. H. 'The allergenicity of psyllium seed'. *Med. An. d.c.* 39: 313-317, 1969.

Bhattacharya. P. and Dey. S. 'Use of low cost gelling agents and support matrices for industrial scale plant tissue culture'. *Plant Cell Tissue and Organ Culture,* vol. 37: 1, 15-23, 1994.

Bhattacherjee, S. K. *Handbook of Medicinal Plants*. 4th rev. edn. Jaipur: Pointer Publishers, 2004

Bhunvaro, N. B. and Khorana, M. L. 'Plantago mucilage'. *Ind. Jour. Pharm.* 12(3): 68, 1950.

Busse, W. W. and Schoenwetter, W. F. 'Asthma from Psyllium in laxative manufacture'. *Ann. Intern. Med.* 83: 361-362, 1975.

Chandra, V. 'Studies on cultivation of *P. ovata* Forsk'. *Ind. Jour. Pharm.* 29(12): 331-332, 1967.

Chopra, R. N. '*Plantago ovata* in chronic diarrhoeas and dysentery'. *Ind. Med. Gaz.* 65: 428-433, 1930.

Chopra, U. N. *Indigenous Drugs of India.* Dhur & Sons Private Ltd., pp. 379-385.

Claus, E. P., Tyler, V. E. and Brady, L. R. *Pharmacognosy.* 6th edn. Philadelphia, U. S. A.: Lea and Fabiger, 1970.

Desai, M. C., Desai, H. B., Patel, B. M. and Shukla, P. C. 'A note on nutritive value of isabgol byproducts'. *Ind. Jour. Anim. Sci.* 50(10): 890-981, 1980.

Goswami, S. 'Effect of isabgul on serum lipids'. *Ancient Sc. of Life* 7(324): 164-165, 1988.

Hartwell, J. L. 'Plants used against cancer. A. survey'. *Lloydia* 33(3): 288-292, 1970.

Husain, A. 'Achievement in the research of medicinal plants, their present and future value in India'. Proc. 4th Symp. Pharmacognosy and chemistry of natural products of development co-operation in the discovery and use of natural resources for drugs in the Third World, pp. 12-36, 1977.

Hyde, B. B. 'Mucilage producing cells in the seed coat of *Plantago ovata*: Developmental fine structure'. *Amer. J. Bot.*, 57(10): 1197-1206, 1970.

ICAR. *Hand Book of Agriculture.* New Delhi: ICAR, 1997.

Ikram, M. 'Biologically active medicinal plants'. *Hamdard* 27(3): 73-85, 1984.

Jain, S. K. *Medicinal Plants.* New Delhi: National Book Trust, 1968.

Jain, S. K. and Tarafder, C. R. 'Medicinal plant lore of the Santhals'. *Econ. Bot.* 24(3): 241-278, 1970.

Jamal, S., Ahmad, I., Agrawal, R., Ahmad, M. and Osman, S. M. 'Novel oxo fatty acid in *P. ovata* seed oil'. *Phytochemistry* 26(11): 3067-3069, 1987.

Khanna, N. M., Sarin, J. P. S., Nandi, R. C. and Engineer, A. D. 'Isaptent: A new cervical dilator'. *Contraception* 21(1): 29-40, 1980.

Khasgiwal, P. C. and Mithan, B. M. 'Derivatives of *Plantago ovata* seeds husk gum. Part I. Carboxyl derivatives'. *Ind. Jour. Pharm.* 37(2): 53-55, 1975.

Kirtikar, K. R. *Indian Medicinal Plants.* vol. 3. Lalit Mohan Bose, Publisher, pp. 2033-2044.

Laidlaw, R. A. and Percival, E. G. V. 'Studies on polysaccharide extracted from the seeds of *Plantago ovata* Forsk'. *Jour. Chem. Soc.* (London) 6: 1600-1607, 1949.

Lal, R. K. and Sharma, J. R. 'Effects of gamma irradiation (^{60}Co) on economic traits in isabgol'. *J. Med. Aromat. Plant. Sci.* 22: 251-255, 2000.

Lal, R. K. and Sharma, J. R. 'Induction by gamma irradiation (^{60}Co), characterisation and utilisation of mutants for economic traits in isabgol'. *J. Med. Aromat. Plant. Sci.* 24: 689-695, 2002.

Lal, R. K., Sharma, J. R. and Misra, H. O. 'Development of new variety "Niharika" of isabgol. Register of new genotypes of cultivars'. *J. Med. Aromat. Plant Sci.* 20(2): 421-422, 1998.

Lal, R. K., Sharma, J. R. and Misra, H. O. 'Induced changes in the genetic architecture of plants in isabgol'. National Conference on Plant Biotechnology: Towards Strategic Agriculture and Drug Development and one day wet workshop on Recent Approaches in DNA Analysis, March 15-18 at CIMAP, Lucknow. *Souvenir,* p. 96, 1999.

Lal, R. K., Sharma, J. R., Kumar, S., Sharma, S., Misra, H. O. and Neelakshi Singh. 'Stability for economic traits in isabgol'. *J. Med. Aromat. Plant Sci.* 21(4): 1064-1068, 1999.

Lal, R. K., Sharma, J. R., Misra, H. O., Kumar, S., Shukla, N. and Sharma, S. 'Influence of variability and associations on economic traits in isabgol'. *J. Med. Aroma. Plant. Sci.* 21(2): 367-372, 1999.

Luthra, J. C. 'Some important economic plants and their cultivation'. *Indian Farming* 11(1): 10-14, 1950.

Machado, L., Ztterstom, O. and Fagerberg, E. 'Occupational allergy in nurses to a bulk laxative'. *Allergy* 34(1): 51-66, 1979.

Mital, S. P. and Bhagat. 'Studies on the floral biology in *Plantago ovata* Forsk'. *Curr. Sci.* 48(6): 261-263, 1979.

Mithal, B. M. and Bhutiani, B. R. 'Disintegrant properties of *Plantago* seed husk'. *Ind. J. Pharm.* 29(12): 329-31, 1967.

Mithal, B. M. and Zacharias, G. 'Gel-forming properties of *P. ovata* seed husk'. *Indian. J. Pharm.* 33(2): 32-34, 1971.

Mithal., B. M. and Kasid, J. L. 'Evaluation of the emulsifying properties of *P. ovata* seed husk'. *Ind. Jour. Pharm.* 26(12): 316-319, 1964.

Morton, F. Julia. 'Major medicinal plants: botany, culture and uses'. *Illinois*, pp. 325-328, 1977.

Patel, R. P. and Alex, R. M. 'Powdered isabgol husk as a binder for compressed tablets'. *The Pharmaceutist* 12(6): 13-17, 1966.

Plant Genetic Resources. New Delhi: National Bureau of Plant Genetic Resources, 1944.

Roia, F. C. Jr. 'The use of plants in hair and scalp preparations'. *Econ. Bot.* 20(1): 17-30, 1966.

Schwarez, H. 'Plant mucilages in cosmetics'. *Scifensiderztg.* 68: 411-422, 1941.

Shah, N. C. 'Need of systematic cultivation and collection of medicinal herbs used in indigenous systems and traditional medicine'. *Ind. Drugs* 18(6): 210-217, 1981.

Sharma, P. K. and Koul, A. K. 'Mucilage in seeds of *P. ovata* and its wild allies'. *Jour. Ethnopharm.* 17: 289-295, 1986.

Shukla, P. C., Desai, M. C., Purohit, L. P., Desai, H. B. and Patel, B. H. 'Use of isabgol in the concentrate mixture of milch cows'. *Guj. Agric. Univ. Res. Jour.* 9(1): 33-36, 1983.

Siddiqui, H. H., Kapur, K. K. and Atal, C. K. 'Studies on Indian seed oils. Part II. Effect of *P. ovata* embryo oil on serum cholesterol levels in rabbits'. *Ind. Jour. Pharm.* 26: 1964.

Singh, A. K. and Virmani, O. P. 'Cultivation and utilisation of isabgol. A review'. *CROMAP* 4(2): 109-120, 1982.

Trease, G. E. and Evans, W. C. *Pharmacognosy*. Baltimore, U. S. A.: Williams and Wilkins Co., 1972.

Upadhyah, K. G., Patel, Patel and Vyas, S. H. 'Evaluation of isabgol husk and gum acacia as ice cream stabilisers'. *Guj. Agri. Univ. Res. Jour.* 4(1): 45-50, 1978.

Williams, L. O. *Drug and Condiment Plants*. Washington DC, U. S. A.: Agr. Handbook 172, USDA-ARS, 1960.

Wren, R. W. *Potters New Encyclopaedia of Botanical Drugs and Preparations*, VII edn. Rustington, England: Health Science Press, 1920.

—oo(O)oo—

9

Conservation and Cultivation of Ethno-Medicinal Plants in Jharkhand

Narsinha Dayal

JHARKHAND is one of the oldest names of the Chotanagpur and Santhal Parganas plateau, which has been carved out as a new State from Bihar State on November 15, 2000. It has distinct agro-climatic and socio-economic features with geographical areas of about 80 lakh hectares and population of nearly 30 million. The recorded forest area occupies 29.23 per cent of the geographical area of the State. It is generally said that Jharkhand is a rich State where poor people live, which is true in the sense that approximately 40 per cent of all the minerals of the country is stored here and about 85 per cent of the population is rural whose livelihood depends upon poorly developed farming systems. Due to poor productivity and profitability in farm enterprises, there is the problem of food and economic security. Apart from this, there are also threads of environmental degradation, instability in productivity and non-sustainability of natural resources and inequitability. However, the State has immense potential to create a better living for the people due to its vast natural resources and potential in the fields of crop production and forest based enterprises.

Jharkhand enjoys a rich heritage of flora and fauna because of its typical climatic and strategic geographical location. The hilly terrain, the climate, the network of rivers such as Subarnrekha, Kharkai, Damodar, etc., hilly *nalas* and the presence of a wide spectrum of mineral deposits including the radioactive minerals in the soil, make this region a centre of biodiversity witnessed by a number of endemic plants which still remain to be properly investigated.

The tribal dominated tract of Jharkhand and adjoining regions of Orissa and Chhattisgarh constitute one of the major regions of rich crop and other plant diversity. It is an important abode of many plants of ethnobotanical, medicinal and agro-industrial importance. The tribal populations of this State use many plants for various purposes: medicine, food, fodder, etc. The knowledge about various uses of plants should be collected and systematised for they are linked to their cultural heritage.

Unfortunately, the plant biodiversity in this region has been continuously changing over the last 50 years. The rapid growth of industrialisation and mining, indiscriminate exploitation of resources, ecological imbalance due to pollution, forest fire, depletion of soil due to poor agricultural practices, erosion of soil due to deforestation and poor water holding capacity of soil, etc. are the causes which have adversely affected the biodiversity of the region. Consequently, many plant species have become extinct from the area or are on the verge of extinction. Such loss of species is never healthy for the environment and the consequences are grave.

The tribal medicine men, who are trying hard to keep the tribal indigenous healing system alive, have the knowledge about the herbs that heal but are finding it difficult to maintain their source of supply because of large scale destruction of forests. With the extinction of sources of indigenous supply, it is apprehended that the knowledge about these herbs would also dry up.

WHY CONSERVATION

Although interest in environment assets began with the very beginning of human civilisation, the conservation of biodiversity, as we understand it now, is a new venture. Interest in the conservation of ethnomedicinal plants has grown enormously in recent years. In the last two decades or so the need for a clear national and international policy on crop and other plant diversity has been stressed at numerous symposia, seminars, conferences and congresses (Swaminathan, 1983, 1988). The famous "Earth Summit" at Rio de Janeiro in Brazil in 1992 speaks loudly about the significance of biodiversity conservation. Frankel (1974) has described conservation of biodiversity as the 'evolutionary responsibility' of man. This 'responsibility' can be discharged at three levels: political, professional and public. The professional responsibility has to be discharged by plant scientists, ecologists, conservationists and a whole series of scientists and technologies connected with the identification, collection, conservation and utilisation of biodiversity. The political aspect of the problem relates to the development of national policies which will help to accord priority to the protection of the environment, conservation of biodiversity and appreciation of the dangers arising from genetic erosion and vulnerability and the consequent need to provide enough financial and technical resources to all works related to the conservation of biodiversity. Above all, the political leaders must be committed to the cause of considering biodiversity as a common human heritage and hence should promote free exchange of material and co-ordinated action at the regional, national and global levels on the utilisation of biodiversity for the common good. Even if the necessary professional skills and political will are available, the cause of conservation will go by default if there is no widespread awareness among the general public on the need to promote development without destruction and of the pivotal role the people themselves can play in biodiversity conservation. Public awareness can be generated by mass media and through schools and colleges all over the country. We must understand that the ecosystem can be compared with that of a spider's cobweb in the centre of which is man himself. So, if he harms any string of the cobweb, he will ultimately harm himself. It should not be forgotten that the earth does not belong to man; man belongs to the earth, which he has inherited for his children.

According to a recent World Bank report, a large number of medicinal plants are being over-harvested and could become extinct unless stringent conservation measures are introduced by developing countries. Many of these plants have been used since ancient time to treat a variety of ailments, but during the past 10 years there has developed a booming world trade in plant remedies, leading to over-harvesting. Unless swift action is taken, more plants will be gone forever. Given that more than four billion people depend heavily on natural medicines for their daily health, the need for better conservation is beyond question. With the exception of India and China, which are the biggest suppliers of herbal medicines, most developing countries in the West have done little or nothing in conservation, cultivation and use of their medicinal plants.

In order to avoid such losses in the future, the World Bank report suggests that the developing countries should

- organise better co-ordination among government agencies, pharmaceutical companies and departments dealing with environment, natural resources and agriculture;
- arrange for more trade information at the national and the village level;
- get women involved in conservation efforts since mothers and grandmothers use plant remedies in their homes and are generally considered founts of herbal wisdom in villages;
- establish organised cultivation. Most medicinal plants are found in the wild and are at the mercy of the weather, pests and shortage of water.

Fortunately, in recent years, there has been a revival of interest in tribal medicine partly on account of efforts of anthropologists and social activists interested in the study of tribal ways and preservation of its values and partly because of the interest of some Christian missionary groups in the revival of herbal medicine as a part of their efforts towards developing a less costly but effective medicine system for poor tribal groups living in remote rural areas. In some cases, study and practice of herbal medicine has been made a part of the syllabi for training of not only of their rural health workers but also of their religious orders. This has promoted vigorous efforts towards collection of information from various sources and their compilation for training and research purposes.

ETHNOMEDICINE OF JHARKHAND

Ethnomedicine has been defined as indigenous beliefs, concepts, knowledge and practice among ethnic groups; folks, people or races for preventing, lessening and curing diseases and pain. It is a branch of ethnobotany which is also known as tribal medicine, *adivasi aushadhi* or *lok aushadhi;* plant-derived medicines are in vogue in all world cultures and have always played a key role in world health. The WHO has estimated that 80 per cent of the world population rely on traditional medicine for primary health care needs. The ethnomedicine, ethnopharmacology and ethnobotanical disciplines, recognised by the Western research institutions and researchers as a basis to study medicinal plants, represent the inevitable step towards the goal of universal health (Sinha, 1991a, 1991b, 1996; Swaminathan, 1994; Chopra *et al* 1969, 1956-58; Basu & Kirtikar, 1945).

In India, there are about 45,000 plant species of which about 15,000 plant species belong to the higher group. According to All India Coordinate Research Project on Ethnobotany (AICRPE) 1982-93, about 9,500 wild plant species are being used by Indian tribals for meeting their varied requirements of which about 7,500 species are used for medicinal purposes. It is interesting to note that out of this, about 950 species are found to have new claims worthy of scientific enquiry. In Jharkhand about 2,000 wild plant species of great medicinal importance have been recorded so far in different books and literature (Bodding, 1925; Hoffmann, 1987, 1994, 1996; Jain, 1966, 1991).

Forests are a part of tribal life in Jharkhand. It is also a storehouse for them. The tribal people understand this and live a harmonious and symbiotic life with forests. In the ages past, they had surplus forests but in spite of their denudation due to overexploitation by the more 'civilised' man they had been managing their *khutkhati* or village forests in a sustained manner. They are also planting trees around villages for fruits, medicine and timber. Based on their beliefs and experiences, they have framed certain rules for the exploitation of ethnomedicinal plants and the efficacy of the recipe (Hembrom, 1995). Some of the methods practised by them for the conservation of ethno-medicinal plants are as follows:

(i). No exploitation should be carried out during night as plants are believed to be sleeping.

(ii). Tree bark should be chopped from the bottom to the top in one action.

(iii). Exposed roots taken from *nala* banks are supposed to be more effective if taken in one action without being noticed by any one.

(iv). Roots should be dug from one side only so that the shadow may not fall on the plant and the pit should be filled up again.

(v). Rare drugs should be prepared early in the morning without being noticed by any one and without attending the call of nature call. This helps lateral roots to remain intact for further regeneration.

(vi). Taking out the tubers after digging, the pit should be filled back and the head of the tuber should be planted back for regeneration.

(vii). Some roots may be pulled out in one action. This helps lateral roots to remain intact for further growth.

PEOPLE'S PARTICIPATION IN ETHNOMEDICINAL PLANT BIODIVERSITY CONSERVATION

It has already been pointed out earlier that all polices, professional skills and measures of conservation of ethnomedicinal plant biodiversity will go in vain unless the rural people and forest dwellers who have been using biological resources as an assurance for their food, medicine, shelter and other subsistence needs are involved. Today, people's participation (PP) in biodiversity conservation is viewed as a dynamic group process in which all members of a group contribute to the attainment of common objectives, exchange information and experiences of common interest and follow the rules, regulations and other decision-making by the group. In other words, the core concept of PP is sustainable development. Therefore, there is an urgent need for PP in biodiversity conservation because of its

(a). efficiency and/or cost effectiveness;

(b). equity in distribution of benefits,

(c). cheap access to innovative technologies;

(d). sustainability of efforts; and

(e). empowerment of people.

Fortunately, a national programme called the National Biodiversity Strategy and Action Plan (NBSAP) has come up with a new vision and strategy related to environment and development.

The NBSAP process stands in contrast to the general trends of planning and attempts towards truly operationalising people's participation. Previous national policies and plans on environment involved only a handful of bureaucrats and 'experts', usually the urban elite sitting in New Delhi or State capitals who are far removed from the natural environment.

In NBSAP, people from all walks of life such as policy makers, experts, environmental scientists, social workers, industrialists, farmers, forest dwellers, etc. are involved. Some States have already taken the initiative in this direction. In the new State of Jharkhand, the Ministry of Science and Technology should give immediate attention for the creation of a Biodiversity Board consisting of scientists, policy makers and social workers which would be responsible for the implementation of State Biodiversity Strategy and Action Plan (SBSAP) processes and programmes. There is also an urgent need of a Biodiversity Bill in this State in order to put a thorough check on the overexploitation of its forest resources.

POTENTIALITY OF CULTIVATION OF ETHNOMEDICINAL PLANTS IN JHARKHAND

The forests of Jharkhand, which are rich in biodiversity of ethnomedicinal plants, have been overexploited by the growing population and some pharmaceutical companies. This has led to their habitat loss, which may in turn lead to their extinction in course of time. Many of them are endemic and are under constant threat of danger. Therefore, they need our utmost attention. They can be grown commercially to meet the requirements of the drug industry.

There is a great potential of cultivation of medicinal plants as well as plants of ethnobotanical and agro-industrial importance in this area. Special emphasis should be given to the protection of naturally growing plants in the forests of Jharkhand. Legislation should be made for the protection of areas rich in such plants. Besides, public awareness should be created so that these protected areas are given the status of 'sacred groves' as has been done in some parts of Maharashtra and Karnataka. The organised cultivation of medicinal plants in this area will not only meet the requirements of the drug industry but will also go a long way towards the upliftment of the socio-economic condition of the tribal population in the plateau. Many of the tribes inhabiting these forests have the ancient knowledge and wisdom of curing various ailments which has been carried down to them through generations and has become part of their culture and heritage. This must be preserved at any cost. For this, their involvement in mass cultivation of medicinal plants, which they know, should be given top priority.

Some of the medicinal plants can be conserved by people related with social and agro-forestry. Such plants can be planted as avenue trees along the roadside and along with agricultural lands. Some of such plants may be: *Adansonia digitata* L., *Adenanthera pavonina* L., *Ailanthus excelsa* R., *Alstonia scholaris* R. Br., *Artocarpus heterophyllus* L., *Cedrela toona* R., *Lagerstroemia speciosa* L., *Pterospermum acerifolium*, *Thespesia populnea*, *Trewia nudiflora,* etc. Similarly, many medicinal plants may be grown in our gardens or as hedges. Chief among them are: *Adhatoda vasica*, *Argyreia speciosa*, *Anacardium occidentale* L., *Datura metel* L., *Euphorbia antiquorum* L., *Euphorbia neriifolia*, *Jatropha curcas* L., *Justicia gendarussa*, L., *Lawsonia inermis* L., *Melia composita* Willd, *Moringa oleifera* L., *Mimusops elengi* L., *Plumbago zeylanica* L., *Plumeria rubra* var. *acutifolia*, *Sesbania grandiflora* L., *Sesbania sesban*, *Spondias pinnata*, *Nyctanthes arbor-tristis* and many others.

Special emphasis should be given on the mass cultivation of some medicinally important plants endemic to this region such as *Andrographis paniculata, Aloe vera, Cestrus paniculatus, Dioscorea* species, *Withania somnifera, Tinospora cordifolia, Gloriosa superba, Pueraria tuberosa, Gymnema sylvestre, Centella asiatica, Urginea indica,* etc. This will form the source of continuous supply of raw materials for the pharmaceutical industry if developed in this region. The cultivation of ethnomedicinal plants and their utilisation by the industries may go a long way towards boosting the economic development in this State.

There is an urgent need to prepare a glossary of ethnomedicinal plants found and grown in this area with their botanical and local names, effective plant parts and specific medicinal uses with the help of local herbal practitioners, *ojhas* and *vaidyas*.

POLITICS OF BIODIVERSITY

Plant biodiversity is mostly located in limited areas in the developing countries, whereas the developed countries are rather poor in them. Some countries find themselves giving more than what they are receiving and *vice versa*. This problem is compounded by the question of ownership, particularly the current trend towards the private ownership of plants and plant products. The two issues, international inequalities in distribution and use of plant resources and private ownership of the fruits by using wild plant resources are distinct (Prescott-Allen, 1983).

In a sense, developing countries are conserving plant resources for the developed countries, which are enjoying the benefit of plant resources without having to sacrifice land for their conservation. The flow of germplasm from developing to developed countries is thus a one-way affair. The exchange of plant resources is rather informal and governed only by tacit recognition of two international principles. These are:

- Materials will be freely and fully available to all who can make use of it for the benefit of humanity.
- Duplicates of materials collected are always left in the country of origin.

However, the principle of free exchange of plant resources is at risk. There is a feeling that developing countries are being ripped off of almost all their plant resources. But the developed countries with their money and R & D skills are not just making use of them but rather exploiting the developing countries. Some countries have already started imposing restrictions on the movement of germplasm and others are threatening to do so. In recent years, this situation has been rather aggravated in view of the GATT Agreement and patent laws. Multinational companies are trying to patent plant species and plant products and even gene products. The patenting of neem, *Melia azadiracta* L. and our 'Basmati' rice by some companies in the U. S. A. may be cited as examples. This is a very dangerous trend which must be resisted by the developing countries led by India, China and Brazil.

CONCLUSION

Conservation of plant resources in general and ethnomedicinal plants in particular thus become imperative and the need of the hour. The 'hotspots' of ethnomedicinal plants must be fully protected and scientifically conserved otherwise it will be too late to take care of our rich ancient heritage. Both intensive and extensive search should be made by scientists to identify and locate valuable plant resources in Jharkhand. The Government and the NGOs, scientists and general public have a great task ahead towards achieving this goal.

REFERENCES

Anonymous. *Ethnobiology in India—A Status Report.* Ministry of Environment and Forest, Government of India, New Delhi, 1994.

Anonymous. *Medicinal Plants of India*, vol. I. New Delhi: ICMR, 1976.

Anonymous. *Medicinal Plants of India*, vol. II. New Delhi: ICMR, 1987.

Anonymous. *Traditional Medicine.* Geneva: WHO, 1977.

Basu, B .D. and Kirtikar, K. R. *Indian Medicinal Plants.* (2nd edn., revised in 1984), 4 vols., 1945.

Bodding, P. O. 'Studies in Santhal medicine and connected folklore, I and II'. *Mem. Asiat. Soc. Bengal* 10(2): 1-132, 133-426, 1925.

Bressers, J. *The Botany of Ranchi District, Bihar, India*, Ranchi: Catholic Press, 1951.

Chopra, R. N. and Verma, B. S. '*Chopra's Indigenous Drugs of India* (Revised by Chopra, R. N., Handa, K. L. and Kapur, L. H.). Kolkata: Academic Publ., 1958.

Chopra, R. N. and Verma, B. S. 'Supplement to the *Glossary of Indian Medicinal Plants.* New Delhi:CSIR, 1969.

Dayal, N. 'Conservation of genetic resources for crop improvement'. In *Phytodiversification and Human Welfare.* (Eds.). Roy, A. K., Dogra, J. V. V. and Verma, S. K. New Delhi: M. D. Publ., pp. 287-96, 1998.

Dayal, N. 'People's participation in biodiversity conservation'. Abstract. *Proc. Natl. Symposium on Environmental Applications of Biotechnology*, Bhagalpur (U. G. C. sponsored), 2002.

Dayal, N. 'Genetic conservation of tassar host plants in Chotanagpur region'. *Columban of Life Sci.* 1(1): 37-40, 1993.

Frankel, O. H. 'Genetic Conservation: Our Evolutionary Responsibility'. *XIII. Intern. Congr. Genet.* 78:53-65, 1974.

Hembrom, P. P. *Adivasi Ausadh* (Horopahy), vols. I-VII, Publ. Pahari Seva Samiti, Satia, Lilipara, Pakur (Bihar), 1995.

Hoffmann, J. S. J. *Encyclopaedia Moundarica.* Ranchi: Catholic Press, 1950.

Jain, S. K. *Dictionary of Indian Folk Medicine and Ethnobotany.* New Delhi: Deep Publ., 1991.

Jain, S. K. *Medicinal Plants.* New Delhi: National Book Trust, 1996.

Sinha, R. K. 'Legacy and ecology of the tribals: A gift to the modern civilisation'. In: *Indian Tribals.* Jaipur: Printwell Publ., 1995.

Sinha, R. K. 'Tribal Heritage: Their ecology and ecological significance'. In: *Studies in Tribal Development.* (Ed.). Gupta, G. P., vol. 1: 361-373. Jaipur: Arihant Publ., 1991.

Sinha, R. K. *Ethnobotany: The Renaissance of the Traditional Herbal Medicine.* Jaipur: Shree Publ., 1996.

Swaminathan, M. S. 'Genetic conservation: Microbes to man'. *Indian J. Plant Genet. Resources* 1: 1-22, 1983.

—oo(O)oo—

10

Observations on Medicinal Plant Richness and Associated Conservation Issues in District Kachchh, Gujarat

C. S. Silori, A. M. Dixit, Leena Gupta and Nisha Mistry

PLANTS containing medicinal and other beneficial properties have been known and used in some form or the other since time immemorial in the traditional system of medicines (Jain and Saklani, 1991). It has been estimated that out of about 17,500 flowering plants found in India, over 1,600 are used in traditional medicinal systems (BSI-MoEF, 1993). However, with the socio-economic development, the anthropogenic pressures have led to the degradation of natural resources, including medicinal plants, all over the globe. Habitat degradation, unsustainable harvesting due to over-exploitation to meet the demands of illegal trade in medicinal plants have led to the extinction of more than 150 species in the wild. At least 90 per cent of the plant species used in the herbal industry are extracted from the wild. Parallel to the decline of these resources in their natural habitats, population, distribution, availability and causes of decline for these resources have not been sufficiently documented, which otherwise could help in devising better conservation and management strategies of such resources. Such attempts are most required in the areas, which are inherently resource poor due to climatic conditions and other kinds of biophysical limitations. Moreover, any kind of disturbance may lead to the drastic reduction in the natural resources base of such areas.

District Kachchh in the western part of the country is one of such areas, which has predominance of arid climate with uncertainty of rainfall and frequent occurrence of droughts, making it prone to the degradation even in the face of low levels of anthropogenic pressure. Nonetheless, despite having extreme climatic conditions, the landscape variation all across makes it one of the most important areas in terms of biological diversity. The present paper, which is based on a study conducted during 2001-2002, describes the richness of medicinal plants in district Kachchh and also discusses issues of the conservation problems associated with these resources. Based on the field surveys on medicinal plant richness and existing threats to their conservation, certain forest areas have been prioritised, which can be brought under long-term conservation programme for medicinal plants in district Kachchh. The present study is also important in view of the totality of the information on the medicinal plant richness, as compared to the previous studies, which were restricted to certain parts of the district and lacked information on some of the important aspects such as abundance and threat to these resources (Thacker, 1926; Rao, 1983; Bhatt, 1993; Silori and Rana, 2000;, Ismail Master, 2000).

STUDY AREA

District Kachchh spreads over an area of 45,652 km^2 between 22°41' 11" to 24°41' 47" N. latitude and 68°9' 46" to 71°54' 47" E. longitude. It is predominantly an arid region covering about 73 per cent of the total arid region of Gujarat State. It experiences extremes of weather conditions with low and erratic rainfall (326 mm) with very high rate of annual variation in the rainfall (60-80 per cent). Because of such variability and uncertainty in the rainfall pattern, droughts are recurring phenomenon with variations only in the magnitude from year to year. Physiographically, district Kachchh exhibits a range of landscape diversity, which has provided the basis for diversity at habitat and species level. In the extreme north and south-east there are saline marshy plains of the Great and Little Rann of Kachchh, which together form about 50 per cent of total geographical area of the district. Rocky tablelands of moderate height and plains of Banni grasslands form the major landscape type further south, while mud flats, sandy beaches, creeks and mangrove patches form the coastal stretch of the district.

Such a large variation at landscape level has resulted in ecosystem diversity. Several major types of ecosystems and district transitional ecotones are evident in the district. Grassland, savannah, thorn forest and scrubland are the major productive terrestrial ecosystems. Of the total geographical area of the district, about 312,942.24 hectare area (16 per cent) is mentioned as forest cover in the records of the local forest department.

METHODOLOGY

The present article is an outcome of a rapid vegetation survey conducted during monsoon and post-monsoon seasons of year 2001, as a part of a three-year long study on the ethnobotanical resources of district Kachchh. The major aim of the rapid survey was to prepare an inventory of medicinal plants of district Kachchh and assess the distribution and abundance of medicinal plants in different forests of the study area. Based on these findings, forests were prioritised for conservation of medicinal plants in the region.

Based on the discussions with the officials of the local forest department and secondary information collected from published and unpublished studies, we selected about 30 forest areas in district Kachchh for vegetation sampling (Figure 1). While selecting forest areas, care was taken to represent variations in the ecosystem, landscape (terrain) and land use types (forest, non-forest and fallow agriculture lands) to capture the medicinal plant diversity of the entire study area.

In 30 forest areas, equal number of belt transects were laid for vegetation sampling. The width of each belt transect was fixed at 20 metres while the length varied from 1 to 6 km. In such a way, we covered a total distance of about 77 km across the sampled forest areas. Within the belt transect, a number of vegetation parameters such as name of plant species, habit, phenological stage, abundance based on the ocular observation and status of anthropogenic pressures were recorded. The specimens of all the plant species were collected for identification. The identification of plants

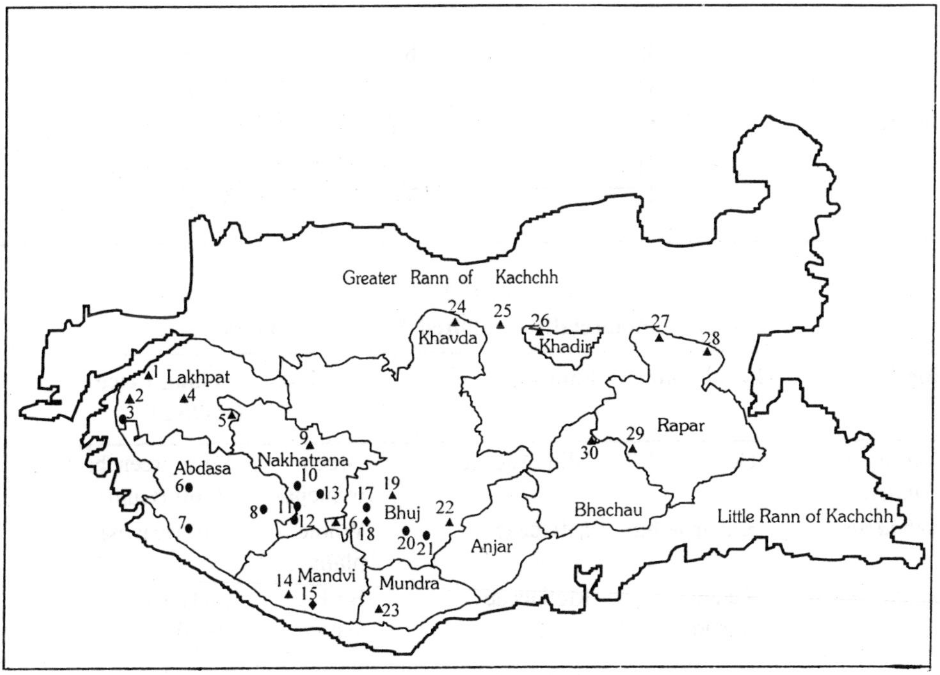

Figure 1. Location of the Surveyed Forest Areas in District Kachchh.

1. Kaiyari RF; 2. Lakshmirani RF; 3. Pipar Forest; 4. Mindhiyari RF; 5. Gugriyana RF; 6. Vengaber Grassland; 7. Lathedi Plantation Area; 8. Mothala Forest; 9. Dinodhar RF; 10. Roha Fort Forest; 11. Roha Nano Dungar; 12. Nanamo Dungar; 13. Mangwana Forest; 14. Lyza Coastal Forest; 15. Vijay Vilas Private Forest; 16. Nabhoi RF; 17. Samatra Forest; 18. Chadua Rakhal; 19. Nadibag Rakhal; 20. Kurgiriya Rakhal; 21. Tapkeshwari Rakhal; 22. Sumarai Wandh Rakhal; 23. Navinal RF; 24. Kalo Dungar; 25. Tragadi Bet; 26. Chhapariya Rakhal; 27. Jatavada RF; 28. Bela RF; 29. Badargarh RF; 30. Kanthkot Rakhal.

▲ Forest under Forest Department

● Forest under Revenue Department

◆ Forest under private ownership

TABLE 1
Distribution of Medicinal Plants Under Different Habit Categories

Habit	Total Plants	Medicinal Plants	% of Total Plants
Climbers & twiners	42	33	79
Grass	49	4	8
Herbs	280	186	67
Shrub	53	46	87
Undershrub	42	30	71
Trees	61	52	85
Total	527	351	67

TABLE 2
List of Commercially Exploited Medicinal Plants

Scientific Name	Local Name	Family	Part Used	Selling Price (Rs./Kg).
Acacia nilotica sub sp. *indica*	Desi baval	Mimosaceae	Green branches	1-1.5/green branch 40-60 (Gum)
Aloe barbadensis	Kuvarpathu	Liliaceae	Whole plant	5-10 (leaves)
Azadirachta indica	Kadavo Limado	Meliaceae	Bark leaves seeds	10-12 (bark) 30-40 (seeds)
Balanites aegyptiaca	Engariyo, Engoriyo	Balanitaceae	Flower seeds	NA
Capparis cartilaginea	Parvatrai, Kavari	Capparaceae	Root	100-150
Cassia italica sub sp. *micrantha**	Midhiaval	Caesalpiniaceae	Leaves	15-20 (dried leaves)
Commiphora wightii	Guggul/ Gugal	Burseraceae	Gum	150-200
*Emblica officinalis**	Amla	Euphorbiaceae	Fruit	20-30 (fruit)
*Lepidium sativum**	Aselio	Brassicaceae	—	20-30
*Ocimum sanctum**	Tulasi	Lamiaceae	Whole plant	NA
*Plantago ovata**	Isabgul	Plantaginaceae	Seeds	20-30

* Also cultivated in agriculture fields
NA- Not available

TABLE 3
List of Medicinal Plants Recorded from District Kachchh

No.	Botanical Name	Common Name	Family	Habit	Part Used	Ethnomedicinal Uses
1.	*Abelmoschus manihot*	Ran bhindi, Jangli bhindi	Malvaceae	Us	Bark	Emmennagogue
2.	*Abrus precatorius*	Chanothi	Fabaceae	Tw	Root, leaves	Cough, Rheumatism, Snake bite
3.	*Abutilion fruticosum*	Zini khapat Saneri dabliar	Malvaceae	Us	Root, leaves	Cough, Rheumatism, Snake bite,
4.	*Abutilon indicum*	Khapat, dabliar	Malvaceae	US	Root, leaves, seeds	Cough, Rheumatism, Snake bite, Boils, Ulcers
5.	*Abutilon theophrasti*	Nani khapat, Bhonykhanski	Malvaceae	Us	Root, leaves	Cough, Rheumatism, Snake bite
6.	*Acacia leucophloes*	Hermobaval, hiver, samadi	Mimosaceae	T	Bark	Inflammation, Bronchitis, Leprosy, Vomiting, Diseases of blood
7.	*Acacia nilotica* subsp. *indica*	Baval, bavar, bibarjo zad	Mimosaceae	T	Bark	Cough, Bronchitis,Diarrhoea, Dysentery, Biliousness, Burning sensation, Piles, Leucoderma
8.	*Acacia senegal*	Goradio baval, Desi baval	Mimosaceae	T	Gum	Intestinal inflammation, Cough
9.	*Acalypha ciliata*	Dadri, Runchalo, dadro	Euphorbiaceae	H	Root, Leaves	Constipation, Laxative, Sore throat, Skin disease
10.	*Acalypha indicum*	Dadari, Dadarjo, Vaichikato	Euphorbiaceae	H	Root, leaves	Diuretic, Bronchitis, Asthma, Pneumonia

Continued...

...Continued

No.	Botanical Name	Common Name	Family	Habit	Part Used	Ethnomedicinal Uses
11.	*Acanthospermum hispidum*	—	Asteraceae	H	Leaves	Swelling
12.	*Achyranthes aspera* var. *aspera*	Anghedi, Aghado	Amaranthaceae	H	Whole plant	Dropsy, Piles, Boils, Eruption of skin
13.	*Achyranthes aspera* var. *porphyristachya*	Sonar	Amaranthaceae	H	Whole plant	Diuretic, Astringent
14.	*Adhatoda zeylanica*	Ardusi	Acanthaceae	S	Whole plant	Diarrhoea, Bronchitis, Asthma, Cough
15.	*Aegle marmelos*	Bili	Rutaceae	T	Root, fruit, leaves	Fever, Digestive, Cough
16.	*Aerva lanata*	Kapuri	Amaranthaceae	H	Root	Diuretic, Demulcent
17.	*Aerva persica*	Bur, Gorakhganjo	Amaranthaceae	S	Whole plant	Swelling
18.	*Agave americana*	Ramban, Ketaki	Agavaceae	H	Leaves	Toothache, Rheumatism, Malaria, Antiseptic
19.	*Ailanthus excelsa*	Rukhdo, Moto arduso	Simaurubiaceae	T	Bark	Bronchitis, Asthma, Diarrhoea, Dysentery, Skin disease
20.	*Alangium salvifolium*	Ankol, Ankoli	Alangiaceae	T	Root, stem	Piles, Vomiting, Diarrhoea
21.	*Albizia amara*	Shirish	Mimosaceae	T	Root, bark, seeds, flowers	Piles, Diarrhoea, Boils, Swellings, Leprosy, Gums

Continued...

...*Continued*

No.	Botanical Name	Common Name	Family	Habit	Part Used	Ethnomedicinal Uses
22.	*Albizia odoratissima*	Dholosaras, Sasalozad	Mimosaceae	T	Bark, leaves	Leprosy, Ulcers, Cough
23.	*Aloe barbadensis*	Kunvarpato	Liliaceae	S	Whole plant	Fever, Spleen, Liver trouble, Constipation, Piles
24.	*Alternanthera sessilis*	—	Amaranthaceae	H	Stem, leaves	Eye wash, Skin disorder, Blisters
25.	*Alysicarpus longifolius*	Ghodasamaervo, Motosamervvo	Fabaceae	H	Root, leaves	Joint pain
26.	*Amaranthus lividus*	Tandaljo	Amaranthaceae	H	Whole plant	Cooling, Emollient
27.	*Amaranthus spinosus*	Kandharo tandarbhe	Amaranthaceae	H	Whole plant	Cooling, Gonorrhea, Blood diseases, Cough, Boils, Burns
28.	*Amaranthus tricolor*	—	Amaranthaceae	H	Whole plant	Diuretic, Ascaricide
29.	*Amaranthus viridis*	Rajgaro Adbau Rajgaro	Amaranthaceae	H	Whole plant	Cooling, Gonorrhea, Blood Diseases, Cough, Boils, Burns
30.	*Andrographis echioides*	Kariyatu	Acanthaceae	H	Whole plant	Dysentery, Dyspepsia, Constipation
31.	*Anethum graveolens*	Suwa	Apiaceae	H	Fruit	Flatulence, Disordered digestion
32.	*Anisomeles indica*	Chodharo	Lamiaceae	S	Whole plant	Carminative, Astringent, Tonic properties
33.	*Argemone mexicana*	Darudi	Papaveraceae	H	Whole plant	Skin diseases, Leprosy, Inflammations
34.	*Argyreia nervosa*	Samudrasok, Samadar, Sog	Convolvulaceae	C	Root	Aphrodisiac, Diuretic, Chronic Ulcer

Continued...

...Continued

No.	Botanical Name	Common Name	Family	Habit	Part Used	Ethnomedicinal Uses
35.	*Aristolochia bracteolata*	Kidamari	Aristolochiaceae	C	Whole plant	Fever, Cough, Joint pain
36.	*Asparagus racemosus*	Satvari	Liliaceae	S	Root	Blood diseases, Eye diseases, Dysentery, Leprosy, Epilepsy
37.	*Asphodelus tenuifolius*	Dungro	Liliaceae	H	Root	Aphrodisiac, Kidney, Liver, Diarrhoea
38.	*Asystasia gangetica*	—	Acanthaceae	H	Whole plant	Anthelmintic, Swelling, Rheumatism
39.	*Avicennia marina*	Cher	Avicenniaceae	S	Root, Seed	Aphrodisiace, Boils, Abscesses
40.	*Azadirachta indica*	Limdo	Meliaceae	T	Bark, leaves, seeds, flower	Blood impurities, Wounds, Gums, Antiseptic, Ulcers
41.	*Balanites aegyptiaca*	Ingorio, Angario Hingoriya	Balanitaceae	T	Flower, seeds	Cooling, Blood purification, Cough, Skin disease
42.	*Barleria acanthoides*	—	Acanthaceae	S	Whole plant	Wounds, Ear pain
43.	*Barleria prionitis*	Kadha aserio, Pilo kanta aserio	Acanthaceae	Us	Root, bark, leaf	Boils, Swelling, Whooping Cough, Fever, Toothache
44.	*Basella rubra*	Poi	Basellaceae	S	Whole plant	Leprosy, Dysentery, Ulcers,
45.	*Bouhinia racemosa*	Kasotri, Asotri, Apto, Asondaro, Rakta kachnar	Caesalpiniaceae	H	Bark, leaves	Urinary Discharge, Skin disease, Throat troubles, Tumours, Blood disease, Dysentery, Diarrhoea

Continued...

...Continued

No.	Botanical Name	Common Name	Family	Habit	Part Used	Ethnomedicinal Uses
46.	*Bergia ammannioides*	—	Elatinaceae	T	Whole plant	Ulcers, Blisters
47.	*Bergia suffruticosa*	Ropatri, Lavariyu, Vithi kharsan	Elatinaceae	H	Leaves	Headache—external use
48.	*Bidens biternata*	Karakokdi, Samarakokdi	Asteraceae	H	Whole plant	Chronic dysentery, Eczema
49.	*Blainvillea acmella*	Dholu Foldu	Asteraceae	H	Whole plant	Bronchitis, Asthma, Leucoderma, Anemia, Skin and heart diseases
50.	*Blepharis linariaefolia*	Gokhru kandho, Ubhera gokhru	Acanthaceae	H	Seed	Ear ache
51.	*Blepharis repens*	Zinku Utingan	Acanthaceae	H	Seed	Urinary Disorder, Diabetes
52.	*Blumea mollis*	Bhutaco, Chanchadmari	Asteraceae	H	Root, leaves	Anthelmintic, Febrifuge, Astringent, Diuretic
53.	*Boerhaavia chinensis*	Rafedi, Rafdial, Sanidhokriar	Nyctaginaceae	H	Leaves	Gums, Poisonous animal bite
54.	*Boerhaavia diffusa*	Satodi	Nyctaginaceae	H	Root, leaves	Diuretic, Jaundice, Ascites, Anasarca, Urinary Problems
55.	*Boerhaavia verticillata*	Zeri Satodo	Nyctaginaceae	H	Root, leaves	Diuretic, Jaundice
56.	*Bombax ceiba*	Savar, Shimlo	Bombacaceae	T	Root, bark, fruit, flower	Inflammation, Heat, Cough, Blood purification, Diarrhoea, Dysentery

Continued...

...Continued

No.	Botanical Name	Common Name	Family	Habit	Part Used	Ethnomedicinal Uses
57.	*Borreria articularis*	Ganthiyu, Kharsat Shankhalo	Rubiaceae	H	Root, seeds	Alterative
58.	*Borreria stricta*	—	Rubiaceae	H	Seed	Tooth worms
59.	*Butea monosperma*	Khakharo, Palash, Kesudo	Fabaceae	T	Root, bark, seed	Night blindness, Dysentery, Piles, Ulcers, Liver disorders, Fractures
60.	*Cadaba indica*	Batkani, Katikal	Capparaceae	S	Root, leaves	Uterine obstruction
61.	*Calotropis gigantea*	Akado	Asclepiadaceae	S	Whole plant	Leprosy, Leucoderma, Ulcers, Tumours, Piles, Diseases of spleen, liver and abdomen, Joint pain, Swellings
62.	*Calotropis procera*	Nano Akado	Asclepiadaceae	S	Whole plant	Leprosy, Leucoderma, Ulcers, Tumours, Piles, Diseases of spleen, liver and abdomen, Swellings, Toothache
63.	*Capparis decidua*	Kerdo, Kera	Capparaceae	S	Bark	Cough, Asthma, Ulcers, Vomiting, Piles, Inflammation
64.	*Capparis grandis*	Thikari, Dumro, Dumrejozado	Capparaceae	S	Bark, Leaves	Internal Swelling, Eruption
65.	*Capparis cartilaginea*	Kavari	Capparaceae	S	Root,	Rheumatism, Paralysis, Toothache
66.	*Cardiospermum halicacabum*	Trigharivel, Valfofiti	Sapindaceae	H	Root, leaves	Swelling, Tumour, Rheumatism, Fever

Continued...

...Continued

No.	Botanical Name	Common Name	Family	Habit	Part Used	Ethnomedicinal Uses
67.	*Carica papaya*	Papaiyu, Papita	Caricaceae	T	Fruit, seeds	Haemoptysis, Bleeding piles, Ringworm, Skin diseases, Psoriasis
68.	*Carissa congesta*	Karamada	Apocynaceae	S	Root, fruit	Fever, Biliousness, Cooling
69.	*Caryota urens*	Shivjata	Arecaceae	T	Nut	Biliousness, Flatulence, Hemicrania
70.	*Cassia absus*	Chimed, Chon	Caesalpiniaceae	T	Leaves, seeds	Asthma, Blood related, Eye diseases, Ulcers, Leucoderma
71.	*Cassia angustifolia*	Son-Makkai	Caesalpiniaceae	H	Whole, plant	Constipation, Dyspepsia, Typhoid, Jaundice, Anemia, Leprosy, Poisoning symptoms
72.	*Cassia auriculata*	Aval, Avali, Avar	Caesalpiniaceae	S	Root, bark, leaves	Urinary discharge, Tumours, Skin diseases, Asthma, Leprosy
73.	*Cassia fistula*	Garmalo	Caesalpiniaceae	T	Root, leaves	Skin diseases, Leprosy, Syphilis, Throat troubles
74.	*Cassia italica* sub sp. *micrantha*	Mindhi, Aval, Pataval	Caesalpiniaceae	H	Leaves	Influenza, Purgative
75.	*Cassia obtusifolia*	Kuvandio, Pochandio	Caesalpiniaceae	H	Leaves, seeds	Eye diseases, Liver complaints, Boils
76.	*Cassia pumila*	Nidhecholjozad, Chimediyo	Caesalpiniaceae	H	Seed	Purgative
77.	*Casuarina equisetifolia*	Saru	Casuarinaceae	T	Bark	Chronic Diarrhoea, Dysentery
78.	*Catharanthus pusillus*	Ubhi Shingani, Sheda Shingni	Apocynaceae	H	Leaves, stem	Joint pains

Continued...

...Continued

No.	Botanical Name	Common Name	Family	Habit	Part Used	Ethnomedicinal Uses
79.	*Cayratia carnosa*	Khat-Khatumbo	Vitaceae	C	Root	Blood purification, Liver and heart troubles
80.	*Celastrus paniculatus*	Malkagani, Malkankni	Celastraceae	Tw	Leaves, seeds	Blood enriching, Abdominal problems, Asthma, Cough, Joint pain, Paralysis
81.	*Celosia argentea*	Lambdi, Lampdi	Amaranthaceae	H	Whole plant	Aphrodisiac, Diarrhoea, Blood diseases, Mouth sores
82.	*Cenchrus ciliaris*	Dhaman	Poaceae	G	Leaves	Wound (cattle)
83.	*Ceropegia bulbosa*	Kundher, Kund, Kundjimath	Asclepiadaceae	Tw	Tuber	Cold, Eye diseases
84.	*Chenopodium album*	Chil, Chilni, Bhaji	Chenopodiaceae	H	Whole plant	Eye diseases, Throat pain, Piles, Blood diseases, Heart diseases
85.	*Chlorophytum tuberosum*	Karli, Karliji bhaji	Liliacee	H	Tuber	Cough, Cold
86.	*Chrozophora rottleri*	Kalo okharad	Euphoribaceae	H	Seeds	Cathartic
87.	*Cissampelos pareira*	Venivel, Karandhiu, Phadvel	Menispermaceae	Tw	Whole plant	Removes pain, Fever, Dysentery, Skin eruption, Heart trouble, Burning, Itching, Vomiting, Asthma
88.	*Cissus quadrangulare*	Hadsankal	Vitaceae	C	Stem, leaves	Broken bones, Back and Spine ache, Asthma
89.	*Cissus repanda*	Gandavelo	Vitaceae	C	Leaves, roots	Used in poisonous animal bite, Elephantiasis
90.	*Cistanche tubulosa*	Jogido	Orobanchaceae	H	Whole plant	Diarrhoea

Continued...

...Continued

No.	Botanical Name	Common Name	Family	Habit	Part Used	Ethnomedicinal Uses
91.	*Citrullus colocynthis*	Indravarna, Kokadavarna	Cucurbitaceae	H	Fruit	Leucoderma, Ulcers, Asthma, Bronchitis, Urinary discharge, Jaundice, Constipation
92.	*Citrus medica*	Bijoru	Rutaceae	S	Fruit	Constipation, Tumours, Asthma, Leprosy, Sore throat, Piles
93.	*Cleome burmanni*	—	Capparaceae	H	Seeds	Skin disease
94.	*Cleome gracilis*	—	Capparaceae	H	Leaves	Swelling
95.	*Cleome gynandra*	Ghandhatu	Capparaceae	H	Root	Tumours, Ulcers, Ear ache, Fever
96.	*Cleome viscosa*	Pilitilvan	Capparaceae	H	Whole plant	Tumours, Inflammation, Skin diseases, Itching, Ulcers
97.	*Clerodendrum inerme*	Tapvel, Tappan	Verbenaceae	S	Leaves	Venereal afflictions, Rheumatism
98.	*Clerodendrum phlomidis*	Arni	Verbenaceae	S	Whole plant	Inflammation, Dropsy, Diarrhoea, Worms, Stomach swells
99.	*Clitoria ternatea*	Garni, Gokaran, Koyal, Bibli	Fabaceae	Tw	Whole plant	Aphrodisiac, Cures dysentery, Severe bronchitis, Asthma, Consumption, Purgative, Diuretic, Ear-aches, Snake-bites
100.	*Coccinia grandis*	Ghiloda, Tindora, Tondili, Kadhvi Gholi	Cucurbitaceae	C	Whole plant	Aphrodisiac, Burning; Itching, Biliousness, Jaundice, Galactagogue, Leprosy, Diabetes, Gonorrhea, Psoriasis

Continued...

...Continued

No.	Botanical Name	Common Name	Family	Habit	Part Used	Ethnomedicinal Uses
101.	*Cocculus hirsutus*	Vevdi, Vevti, Vagval, Vadhi, Achipad	Menispermaceae	H	Roots, leaves	Tubercular glands, Rheumatic, Laxative, Bilious dyspepsia, Neuralgic pains, Gonorrhea, Spermatorrhoea, Cough
102.	*Cocculus pendulus*	Orad, Valur, Parwatti	Menispermaceae	Tw	Leaves	Intermittent fever
103.	*Coldenia procumbens*	Okhrad, Basario	Boraginaceae	H	Whole plant	Suppuration, Rheumatic swelling
104.	*Commiphora wightii*	Gugal	Burseraceae	S	Whole plant	Laxative, Stomachic, Aphrodisiac, Ulcers, Indigestion, Leucoderma, Tumours, Ascites, Asthma, Nervous disease
105.	*Convolvulus arvensis*	Khetrau Phudardi, Veldi, Nerivel	Convolvulaceae	H	Roots	Cathartic, Wounds
106.	*Convolvulus auricomus* var. *auricomus*	Ruchhad neri	Convolvulaceae	H	Whole plant	Purgative
107.	*Convolvulus auricomus* var. *volubilis*	—	Convolulaceae	H	Whole plant	Purgative
108.	*Convolvulus microphyllus*	Shankhavli, Mankhani, Biraval	Convolvulaceae	H	Whole plant	Purgative, Wounds, Diabetes, Fever, Blood-purification, Hysteria, Tonic to brain
109.	*Convolvulus rhyniospermus*	—	Convolvulaceae	H	Leaves	Wounds
110.	*Corallocarpus conocarpus*	—	Cucurbitaceae	H	Fruit	Fever

Continued...

...Continued

No.	Botanical Name	Common Name	Family	Habit	Part Used	Ethnomedicinal Uses
111.	*Corallocarpus epigeus*	—	Cucurbitaceae	H	Whole plant	Alexipharmic, Inflammation, Dysentery, Chronic, Rheumatism, Snake-bite
112.	*Corchorus aestuans*	Chunch, Chhadhari	Tiliaceae	H	Whole plant	Wounds, Removes tumours, Piles, Diuretic, Gonorrhea
113.	*Corchorus depressus*	Bahu phali	Tiliaceae	H	Whole plant	Tumours, Pain, Piles, Fever, Emollient, Gonorrhea
114.	*Corchorus olitorius*	Kagagisodo, Gunpatdjo zad	Tiliaceae	Us	Whole plant	Alexipharmic, Piles, Ascites, Visceral obstruction, Fever, Purgative
115.	*Corchorus tridens*	—	Tiliaceae	H	Whole plant	Cooling
116.	*Corchorus trilocularis*	Ubhi munderi	Tiliaceae	H	Whole plant	Demulcent, Fever, Astringent, Piles, Laxative, Astringent
117.	*Cordia dichotoma*	Moto Gundo	Ehretiaceae	T	Fruit	Biliousness, Cooling
118.	*Cordia gharaf*	Liar Gundi, Nani Gundi	Ehretiaceae	T	Whole plant	Diabetes, Ulcers, Wounds, Cough, Tuberculosis
119.	*Crateva nurvala*	Vayvarno, Varno, Tripanjojad	Capparaceae	T	Whole plant	Antilithic, Vesicant, Snake-bite, Scorpion sting, Wounds, Swelling
120.	*Cressa cretica*	Rudanti, Palio, Khariyu	Convolvulaceae	H	Whole plant	Pungent, Aphrodisiac, Anthelmintic, Consumption, Cough, Leprosy, Asthma, Biliousness
121.	*Crinum asiaticum*	Nagdaman	Amaryllidaceae	H	Bulb, leaves	Diaphoretic, Ear ache, Elephantiasis, Vomiting

Continued...

...Continued

No.	Botanical Name	Common Name	Family	Habit	Part Used	Ethnomedicinal Uses
122.	*Crotalaria burhia*	Kharshan, Vagdaushan	Fabaceae	Us	Branches, leaves	Vomiting, Stops bleeding
123.	*Crotalaria juncea*	Shun, Shan, Shaniyu	Fabaceae	Us	Leaves	Leucorrhoea, Blood diseases, Skin diseases
124.	*Crotalaria leptostachya*	—	Fabaceae	Us	Leaves	Laxative, Abortifacient, Analgaesic, Leucorrhoea, Blood diseases, Indigestion, Blood purification
125.	*Cucumis callosus*	Kothimdu Gaivasukadan	Cucurbitaceae	H	Root, leaves, Fruit	Fever, Wounds, Diabetes
126.	*Cucumis prophetarum*	Kanıalo Indran, Kantalan Indranan	Cucurbitaceae	H	Whole plant	Biliousness, Purgative, Vomiting, Fever, Snake-bite
127.	*Cuscuta chinensis*	Amarvel	Cuscutaceae	Tw	Whole plant	Eye diseases, Heart diseases, Biliousness
128.	*Cuscuta hyalina*	—	Cuscutaceae	H	Whole plant	Chest pain
129.	*Cuscuta reflexa*	Amarvel Anatvel	Cuscutaceae	Tw	Whole plant	Eye diseases, Heart diseases, Billiousness
130.	*Cyamopis tetragonoloba*	Gawar, Guwar	Fabaceae	H	Whole plant	Eye diseases, Biliousness, Carminative, Jaundice, Purgative, Paralysis, Lumbago, Diuretic, Chronic fever,

Continued...

...Continued

No.	Botanical Name	Common Name	Family	Habit	Part Used	Ethnomedicinal Uses
131.	*Cynodon dactylon*	Darabh	Poaceae	G	Whole plant	Burning sensation, Epileptic fits, Leprosy, Skin diseases, Fever, Cobra-bite, Catarrhal ophthalmic
132.	*Cyperus haspan*	Needanmoth, Meecho	Cyperaceae	G	Whole plant	Blood purification, Cough, Chronic rheumatism, cholera, Dyspepsia, Fever
133.	*Cyperus triceps*	—	Cyperaceae	G	Leaves	Wounds
134.	*Dalechampia scandens*	Yarval, Aajval	Euphorbiaceae	Tw	Leaves	Swelling
135.	*Datura innoxia*	Kantalo Dhanturo, Kalo daturo	Solanaceae	Us	Seeds, leaves	Epilepsy, Asthma, Ear-ache, Ophthalmic pain, Swelling
136.	*Datura metel*	Ganthovalo, Dhanturo	Solanaceae	H	Seeds, leaves	Asthma, Ear-ache, Swelling Tumours
137.	*Derris indica*	Karanj	Fabaceae	T	Whole plant	Eye diseases, Piles, Wounds, Ulcer, Itching, Keratitis
138.	*Digera muricata*	Kanjro Lolar	Amaranthaceae	H	Whole plant	Astringent, Laxative, Biliousness
139.	*Dipcadi erythraeum*	Jungli dongli	Liliaceae	H	Whole plant	Cough, Biliousness, Urinary discharge, Diabetes
140.	*Diplocylos palmatus*	Shivlingi	Cucurbitaceae	C	Leaves, fruit	Inflammation, Tonic
141.	*Dipteracanthus patulus*	Tutadi, Teetuli, Sisodi, Amblieje-Zad	Acanthaceae	H	Whole plant	Inflammation, Pungent, Fever

Continued...

...*Continued*

No.	Botanical Name	Common Name	Family	Habit	Part Used	Ethnomedicinal Uses
142.	*Echinops echinatus*	Shulio, Utkanto	Asteraceae	H	Whole plant	Heart diseases, Brain diseases, Ophthalmia, Chronic fever, Inflammation
143.	*Eclipta prostrata*	Bhangaro	Asteraceae	H	Whole plant	Cough, Asthma, Wounds, Joint pains, Brain diseases, Chronic fever, Opthalmia, Diuretic
144.	*Ehretia laevis*	Dantrango, Vadhwardi, Darar, Vedhigalo	Ehretiaceae	T	Whole plant	Anthelmintic, Hairs, Itching, Night blindness, Syphilis, Spleen, Ulcers, Conjunctivitis, Catarrhal Jaundice, Blood Purification
145.	*Enicostemma axillare*	Zinku Kariyatu, Kadvinai, Mamejevo	Gentianaceae	H	Whole plant	Carminative, Laxative, Vomiting, Thirst, Leprosy, Eye troubles, Gonorrhea, Dysentery, Blood purification,
146.	*Ephedra foliata*	—	Ephedraceae	S	Whole plant	Fever, Stomachic, Worms, Blood purification, Snake-bite
147.	*Eucalyptus globulus*	Nilgiri	Myrtaceae	T	Leaves	Antiseptic, Colic, Headache
148.	*Euphorbia caducifolia*	Thor	Euphorbiaceae	S	Whole plant	Snake-bite, Skin diseases, Ear ache, Rabies, Carminative, Rheumatism, Spleen, Syphilis
149.	*Euphorbia hirta*	Vadi dudhi, Vadi rati dudhi	Euphorbiaceae	H	Whole plant	Dysentery, destroy warts, Asthma, Worms, Gonorrhea, Vomiting, Sores, Snake-bite
150.	*Euphorbia thymifolia*	Chhapri dudhi, Chhirvel, Sani mduhdi, Patdudhi	Euphorbiaceae	H	Whole plant	Ring worm, Amenorrhoea, Diarrhoea, Snake-bite, Diabetes

Continued...

...Continued

No.	Botanical Name	Common Name	Family	Habit	Part Used	Ethnomedicinal Uses
151.	*Euphorbia tirucalli*	Kharsani	Euphorbiaceae	H	Whole plant	Joint pains, Leprosy, Spleen, Jaundice, Stone, Syphilis, Rheumatism, Neuralgia, Skin diseases, Snake-bite
152.	*Evolvulus alsinoides*	Kali Shankhavali, Zini Fudardi, Kari Buti	Convolvulaceae	H	Whole plant	Bronchitis, Leucoderma, Brain & Memory, Hair growth, Hemorrhages
153.	*Fagonia indica*	Dhamasha, Dharmau	Zygophyllaceae	H	Whole plant	Asthma, Liver trouble, Chronic bronchitis, Toothache, Vomiting, Leucoderma, Snake-bite, Tumours, Dropsy, Wounds
154.	*Fagonia schweinfurthii*	Dhamaso	Zygophyllaceae	H	Whole plant	Toothache, Biliousness
155.	*Farsetia jacquemontii*	Abdau aselio	Brassicaceae	Us	Whole plant	Rheumatism
156.	*Ficus benghalensis*	Vad	Moraceae	T	Whole plant	Biliousness, Ulcers, Vomiting, Leprosy, Piles, Toothache, Diabetes, Rheumatism
157.	*Ficus racemosa*	Umaro, Umbar, Gular	Moraceae	T	Whole plant	Diabetes, Blood purification
158.	*Ficus religiosa*	Piplo	Moraceae	T	Whole plant	Biliousness, Ulcers, Vomiting, Toothache, Swelling, Asthma, Inflammation, Bone fracture
159.	*Fumaria indica*	Pitapapdo	Fumariaceae	H	Whole plant	Fever

Continued...

...Continued

No.	Botanical Name	Common Name	Family	Habit	Part Used	Ethnomedicinal Uses
160.	*Glinus lotoides*	Mitho Okharad	Molluginaceae	H	Leaves	Ulcers
161.	*Glossocardia bosvallea*	Adbau, Suva	Asteraceae	H	Whole plant	Female complaints
162.	*Gmelina arborea*	Sivan	Verbenaceae	T	Whole plant	Stomachic, Piles, Leprosy, Anemia, Ulcers, Gonorrhea, Cough, Snake-bite, Scorpion sting
163.	*Gomphrena globosa*	—	Amaranthaceae	H	Whole plant	Cooling, Biliousness
164.	*Gossypium herbaceum* var. *acerifolium*	Kapas, Desi Kapas	Malvaceae	S	Whole plant	Skin diseases, Snake-bie, Scorpion sting, Orchitis, Galactogogue, Fever, Anti-dysenteric
165.	*Grewia abutilifolia*	—	Tiliaceae	S	Fruit	Cooling
166.	*Grewia flavescens*	Choghari gangi, Choghari gangani, Ruchhad gangi	Tiliaceae	S	Root	Polyurea
167.	*Grewia tenax*	Nagbala, Gangeti	Tiliaceae	S	Bark	Cough, Pains
168.	*Grewia tiliaefolia*	Dhaman	Tiliaceae	T	Whole plant	Cough, Throat complaints, Dysentery, Burning sensation
169.	*Helicteres isora*	Maradsing, Ati, Aiti, Atai	Sterculiaceae	T	Whole plant	Antigalactogogue, Diarrhoea, Dysentery
170.	*Heliotropium bacciferum*	—	Boraginaceae	H	Whole plant	Snake-bite

Continued...

...Continued

No.	Botanical Name	Common Name	Family	Habit	Part Used	Ethnomedicinal Uses
171.	*Heliotropium marifolium*	Zinku Okhard	Boraginaceae	H	Whole plant	Fever, Urticaria, Applied to ringworm, Rheumatism, Ulcers, Gonorrhea, Erysipelas, Snake-bite
172.	*Heliotropium paniculatum*	Zumkhadu	Boraginaceae	H	Whole plant	Skin disease, Ulcers, In ear drops
173.	*Hemidesmus indicus*	Durivel, Uplasari	Periplocaceae	H	Root	Leprosy, Leucoderma, Itching, Skin disease, Fever, Loss of appetite, Asthma, Bronchitis, Piles, Rat bite Thirst, Burning sensation
174.	*Hibiscus lobatus*	Tali	Malvaceae	H	Root, seed	Polyurea
175.	*Hibiscus ovalifolius*	Chanak bhindo	Malvaceae	H	Whole plant	Febrifuge
176.	*Hibiscus palmatus*	—	Malvaceae	H	Leaves	Wounds
177.	*Holoptelea integrifolia*	Kanjo, Papda, Audo-aodo	Ulmaceae	T	Bark	Rheumatism, Diabetes, Blood
178.	*Hygrophila auriculata*	Kantashelio, Akaro, Akharo, Talimkhana	Acanthaceae	Us	Whole plant	Diarrhoea, Dysentery, Inflammation, Biliousness, Disease of eye, Anemia, Cough, Joints pain, Gonorrhea
179.	*Indigofera caerulea* var. *monosperma*	Gado, Gudo, Jangli gali	Fabaceae	S	Root, leaves, seed	Bitter, Tonic, Seeds used in anthelmintic

Continued...

...Continued

No.	Botanical Name	Common Name	Family	Habit	Part Used	Ethnomedicinal Uses
180.	*Indigofera cordifolia*	Gadargari, Ridhgari	Fabaceae	H	Leaves	Gums, Ulcers
181.	*Indigofera linifolia* var. *linifolia*	Jinkigali, Nahnigali	Fabaceae	H	Whole plant	Febrile eruption
182.	*Indigofera linnaei*	Fatakiya, Bhongyal	Fabaceae	H	Whole plant	Juice of the plant used as antiscorbutic, Alterative and and Diuretic
183.	*Indigofera oblongifolia*	Zil, Ziladi, Zildo	Fabaceae	S	Whole plant	Rheumatism, Dysentery, Spleen, Liver, Antidote to poison, Mercurial salvation
184.	*Indigofera tinctoria*	Gali, Nil, Gudi	Fabaceae	H	Whole plant	Snake-bite, Rheumatism, Cough
185.	*Ipomoea aquatica*	Narivel	Convolvulaceae	H	Whole plant	Fever, Jaundice, Bronchitis, Liver complaints
186.	*Ipomoea dasysperma*	Dipad vel	Convolvulaceae	Tw	Seeds	Hydrophobia
187.	*Ipomoea eriocarpa*	Bodi Fudardi	Convolvulaceae	Tw	Leaves	Cure of Headache, Rheumatism, Leprosy, Ulcers, Epilepsy
188.	*Ipomoea muricata*	Bhamardi, Gulabi Gario	Convolvulaceae	Tw	Seeds	Inflammation, abdominal disease, In disease of liver, spleen, Joints pain, Leucoderma, Scabies, Biliousness,
189.	*Ipomoea nil*	Kalandana	Convolvulaceae	Tw	Leaves, roots	Abdominal disease, Fever, Headache, Disease of liver and spleen, In joints pain, Leucoderma, Remove bad humour

Continued...

...Continued

No.	Botanical Name	Common Name	Family	Habit	Part Used	Ethnomedicinal Uses
190.	*Ipomoea obscura*	Vad fudardi	Convolvulaceae	H	Leaves	Valuable application in aphthous affection
191.	*Ipomoea pes-caprae*	Maryad vel, Dariyani vel	Convolvulaceae	H	Leaves, roots	Diarrhoea, Vomiting, Rheumatism, Colic, Diuretic, in Dropsy, Inflammation of legs, Blennorrhagia and Piles
192	*Ipomoea pes-tigridis*	Photial Wagpadi	Convolvulaceae	H	Roots	As purgative, Treatment of dog bites
193.	*Ipomoea quamoclit*	Ganesh vel	Convolvulaceae	C	Leaves	Piles, Vomiting, Diarrhoea
194.	*Ipomoea triloba*	Nani fudardi	Convolvulaceae	Tw	Leaves	Wounds
195.	*Jatropha gossypifolia*	—	Euphorbiaceae	S	Leaves, seeds, bark	Boils, Itches, Headache, Cures fever
196.	*Justicia heterocarpa*	—	Acanthaceae	H	Whole plant	Bronchitis, Inflammation, Dyspepsia, Tympanitis, eye disease and fever, Chronic rheumatism, Eczema, Jaundice
197.	*Justicia procumbens*	Pittpapdo, Rati manjrado	Acanthaceae	H	Leaves	Ophthalmia
198.	*Justicia simplex*	—	Acanthaceae	H	Whole plant	Wounds
199.	*Kalanchoe pinnatum*	Panfuit, Life plant	Bryophyllaceae	H	Leaves	Diarrhoea, Snake-bite, Scorpion sting
200.	*Kickxia ramossisima*	Bhini ghilodi, Bhini chat, bhini val, Kanoti	Scrophulariaceae	H	Whole plant	Diabetes

Continued...

...Continued

No.	Botanical Name	Common Name	Family	Habit	Part Used	Ethnomedicinal Uses
201.	*Kohautia aspera*	—	Rubiaceae	H	Leaves	Fever
202.	*Lactuca runcinata*	—	Asteraceae	H	Whole plant	Used as substitute for Taraxacum
203.	*Lagenaria leucantha*	Duthie, Kadri tunedi	Cucurbitaceae	C	Whole plant	Leucorrhoea, Earache, Bronchitis, Inflammation, Cardiotonic, Antibilious, Cures asthma, Ulcers, Tonic to the brain, Cough, Fever, Headache
204.	*Lannea coromandelica*	Madhol, Modhad, Miniyo, Moyno	Anacardiaceae	T	Whole plant	Elephantiasis, Ulcers, Coma, Swelling, Toothache, Wounds
205.	*Lantana camara*	Indradhanu	Verbenaceae	S	Whole plant	Tetanus, Rheumatism, Malaria
206.	*Lantana salvifolia*	—	Verbenaceae	Us	Leaves, roots	Gums, Ulcers
207.	*Launaea procumbens*	Moti bhonpatri	Asteraceae	H	Leaves	In fever for children
208.	*Launaea sarmentosa*	Bhonpatri, Nani bhonpatri	Asteraceae	H	Whole plant	Used as a lactagogue , Substitute for Taraxacum
209.	*Lawsonia inermis*	Mehndi	Lythraceae	S	Whole plant	Leucoderma, Headache, Hemicrania, Lumbago, Bronchitis, Ulcers, Stomaties, Ophthalmia, Growth of the hair, Jaundice, Leprosy, Skin disease, Applied to burns
210.	*Lepidagathis cristata*	—	Acanthaceae	H	Whole plant	Fever, Itchy affection of skin

Continued...

...*Continued*

No.	Botanical Name	Common Name	Family	Habit	Part Used	Ethnomedicinal Uses
211.	*Lepidagathis trinervis*	Harancharo, Paniru	Acanthaceae	H	Whole plant	Fever, Gums, Ulcers, Ring worm
212.	*Leptadenia pyrotechnica*	Khip, Ranser	Asclepiadaceae	S	Latex	Removing thorn from the body
213.	*Leptadenia reticulata*	Dodi, Khirdodi, Nani Dodi	Asclepiadaceae	Tw	Whole plant	Stimulant tonic, Cough Asthma,
214.	*Leucaena latisiliqua*	Pardesi baval, Losobaval, Vilayati baval	Mimosaceae	S	Bark	Internal pain
215.	*Leucas aspera*	Kubi	Lamiaceae	H	Leaves	Chronic rheumatism, Psoriasis, Snake-venom
216.	*Leucas cephalotes*	Khetrau kubo, Dosinokubo	Lamiaceae	H	Whole plant	Stimulant, Diaphoretic, Scabies, Coughs, Colds, Scorpion bite
217.	*Leucas longifolia*	—	Lamiaceae	H	Whole plant	Cough, Fever, Headache, Snakebite, Ear pain
218.	*Leucas urticaefolia*	Kubo	Lamiaceae	H	Whole plant	Fever
219.	*Limonia acidissima*	Kotha	Rutaceae	T	Fruit	Blood purification, Asthma, Tumour, Ophthalmia, Leucorrhoea
220.	*Lindenbergia muraria*	Pirsadedi, Zamarval, Patharchati, Bhintchati	Scrophulariaceae.	H	Leaves	Gums, Fever, Poisonous animal bite
221.	*Lotus garcini*	Kamal	Fabaceae	H	Whole plant	Gums, Ulcers of animal

Continued...

...*Continued*

No.	Botanical Name	Common Name	Family	Habit	Part Used	Ethnomedicinal Uses
222.	*Luffa acutangula*	Jangli Turiya	Cucurbitaceae	C	Fruits, leaves	Biliousness, Asthma, Bronchitis, Leprosy, Conjunctivitis, Snake bite
223.	*Lycium barbarum*	Taleti	Solanaceae	S	Whole plant	Piles, Scabies, Ascites, Toothache, Improves eye sight
224.	*Lycopersicon lycopersicum*	Tameta, Tamata	Solanaceae	H	Fruit	Blood purification
225.	*Maerua oblongifolia*	Hemkand	Capparaceae	S	Whole plant	Alterative, Stimulant
226.	*Mangifera indica*	Aambo, Keri, Aam	Anacardiaceae	T	Fruit, bark	Leucorrhoea, Dysentery, Biliousness, Ulcer- Eye sores, Diarrhoea, Spleen, Cooling
227.	*Maytenus emarginata*	Vico, Vickdo	Celastraceae	T	Whole plant	Purifies the blood, Cures biliousness, Ulcers, Piles, Inflammation, Burning, Thirst, Snake bite
228.	*Medicago sativa*	Lachko, Rajko	Fabaceae	H	Leaves	Cooling
229.	*Melia azadirach*	Bakanlimdo, Bakan Nimb	Meliaceae	T	Whole plant	Vomiting, Leucoderma, Headache, Fever, Spleen, Piles, Blood purification, Dyspepsia Leprosy
230.	*Merremia aegyptia*	Panch pan ni fudardi	Convolvulaceae	H	Leaves	Blood purification, Vatta and Pitta, Snake bite
231.	*Merremia gangetica*	Undardi, Undarkani, Undari	Convolvulaceae	H	Leaves	Applied to poisonous animal bite, Ring worm, Skin disease

Continued...

...Continued

No.	Botanical Name	Common Name	Family	Habit	Part Used	Ethnomedicinal Uses
232.	*Merremia tridentata*	Bhinigario	Convolvulaceae	H	Whole plant	Tonic, Rheumatism, Piles
233.	*Mimosa hamata*	Kasi, Kaibaval	Mimosaceae	Us	Stem, root	Asthma, Cough
234.	*Mirabilis jalapa*	Gulbas, 4'clock plant	Nyctaginaceae	H	Root, leaves	Syphilitic sores, Boils, Phlegmons
235.	*Momordica denudata*	Kantol, Kantol jeeval	Cucurbitaceae	C	Whole plant	Head trouble, Urinary calculi, Jaundice, Fever, Asthma, Consumption, Leprosy, Bronchitis, Snake-bite, Elephantiasis
236.	*Moringa concanensis*	Jangli Sargu, Kharo Saragavo	Moringaceae	T	Root, seeds	Biliousness, Asthma, Inflammation
237.	*Moringa oleifera*	Saragvo, Mittho saragvo	Moringaceae	T	Whole plant	Burning sensation, Biliousness, Blood impure, Heart complaint, Eye disease, Fever, Inflammation, Dyspepia, Cough, Leucoderma
238.	*Mukia maderaspatana*	Chanak-Chibhdi	Cucurbitaceae	H	Fruit	Used in Ascariascis
239.	*Musa paradisiaca*	Kela	Musaceae	H	Whole plant	Anti dysenteric, Urinary discharge, Leprosy, Gonorrhea
240.	*Nelumbo nucifera*	Vado Kamalful, Suryakamal, Kamal, Motukamal	Nymphaceae	H	Whole plant	Cough, Biliousness, Vomiting, Leprosy, Piles, Fever, Inflammation, Eye diseases, Snake-scorpion venom
241.	*Nerium indicum*	Lal karen	Apocynaceae	S	Flower, root	Scabies, Leprosy, Ulcer, Swelling, Ophthalmia

Continued...

...*Continued*

No.	Botanical Name	Common Name	Family	Habit	Part Used	Ethnomedicinal Uses
242.	*Nicandra physaloides*	—	Solanaceae	H	Leaves, seeds	Toothache
243.	*Nymphaea pubescens*	Kamal, Kamudani, Poyana, Kamalful	Nymphaceae	H	Whole plant	Piles, Dysentery, Dyspepsia, Astringent, Cardio tonic
244.	*Ocimum americanum*	Tukmariya, Jungli tulsi, Ran Tulsi, Nasbo	Lamiaceae	H	Leaves, seeds	Malaria, Fever, Hemorrhage
245.	*Ocimum basilicum*	Damro, Maruo, Sbjo	Lamiaceae	H	Whole plant	Earache, Disease of heart and Brain, Asthma, Inflammation, Chronic, In joint pains, Headache, Snake-bite
246.	*Ocimum gratissimum*	Ram Tulsi, Mala Tulsi	Lamiaceae	H	Whole plant	Sin disease, Erysipelas, Disease of brain, Piles, Rheumatism, Paralysis, Headache, Neuralgia, Toothache
247.	*Ocimum sanctum*	Shyam Tulsi	Lamiaceae	H	Whole plant	Malaria fever, Bronchitis, In stomatic and gastic disorders, Hepatic affection, Earache, Cough, Bites of mosquitoes, Snake-bite
248.	*Oldenlandia corymbosa*	Parpat, Parpapti	Rubiaceae	H	Whole plant	Fever, Jaundice, Liver disease
249.	*Oligochaeta ramosa*	—	Asteraceae	H	Whole plant	Old fever, Cough, General debility

Continued...

...*Continued*

No.	Botanical Name	Common Name	Family	Habit	Part Used	Ethnomedicinal Uses
250.	*Opuntia elatior*	Fafda thor	Cactaceae	S	Whole plant	Cough, Asthma, Refrigerant, Gonorrhea, Inflammation, Ophthalmia
251.	*Pandanus odoratissimus*	Kevdo	Pandanaceae	H	Leaves	Tumours, Pruritus, Leprosy, Smallpox, Syphilis, Scabies, Leucoderma
252.	*Parkinsonia aculeata*	Rambaval	Caesalpiniaceae	T	Leaves	Eye diseases, Gums
253.	*Passiflora caerulea*	Krishna kamal	Passifloraceae	C	Leaves	Giddiness, Headache, Biliousness, Asthma
254.	*Pavetta crassicaulis*	Papat	Rubiaceae	S	Root	Dropsy
255.	*Pavonia arabica* var. *arabica*	Ratobalbuvaro	Malvaceae	Us	Root, Leaves	Vermifuge, Purgative, Inflammation
256.	*Pavonia ceratocarpa*	Karandia, Khatumbdejo	Malvaceae	Us	Leaves	Scorpion bite
257.	*Pedalium murex*	Ubhu gokharu	Pedaliaceae	H	Whole plant	Ulcers, Gonorrhea, Dysaria, Demulcent, Diuretic
258.	*Pentatropis spiralis*	Shingroti	Asclepiadaceae	Tw	Roots	In decoction of astringent
259.	*Pergularia daemia*	Chamar dudheli, Nagla dudheli, Amer dudheli	Asclepiadaceae	Tw	Whole plant	Used as anthelminitic
260.	*Periploca aphylla*	Singdi, Rati-khip, Hom, Dudhali-khip	Periplocaceae	H	Latex	Ringworm, Arthritis, Rabies
261.	*Peristrophe paniculata*	Adhedi, Lisi adhedi, Kali anghedi	Acanthaceae	H	Whole plant	Antidote for Snakebite, Cough, Swellings

Continued...

...Continued

No.	Botanical Name	Common Name	Family	Habit	Part Used	Ethnomedicinal Uses
262.	*Phyllanthus fraternus*	Bhonyamli	Euphorbiaceae	H	Whole plant	Swellings, Polyurea, Jaundice, Acidity
263.	*Phyllanthus virgatus*	Moti bhonyamli	Euphorbiaceae	H	Whole plant	Gonorrhea, Itch in children, External application
264.	*Physalis minima*	Popti, Parpopti	Solanaceae	H	Whole plant	Useful in inflammation, Ascites
265.	*Pithecellobium dulce*	Goras amli	Mimosaceae	T	Pod	Cooling
266.	*Pluchea arguta*	—	Asteraceae	H	Leaves	Fever
267.	*Plumbago zeylanica*	Chitrak, Chitro	Plumbaginaceae	Us	Root, Rootbark	Intestinal troubles, Dysentery, Leucoderma, Inflammation, Piles, Bronchitis, Itching, Disease of liver, Rheumatism, Ringworm, Scabies, Dyspepsia, Piles, Diarrhoea
268.	*Plumeria rubra*	Khadchampo	Apocynaceae	T	Latex, Root	Toothache, Blennorrhagia
269.	*Polycarpaea corymbosa*	Jangli soa, Rupa puli	Caryophyllaceae	H	Whole plant	Swelling, Ulcer, Jaundice
270.	*Polygala erioptera*	Patsan, Bhonysan	Polygalaceae	H	Whole plant	Migraine
271.	*Portulaca oleracea*	Ghol	Portulacaceae	H	Whole plant	Ulcer, Asthma, Diarrhoea, Dysentery, Leprosy, Piles, Scorpion sting
272.	*Portulaca quadrifida*	Zini luni, Patluni, Sunluni, Khati bhaji	Portulacaceae	H	Whole plant	Asthma, Eye & Skin diseases, Cough, Ulcer, Toothache

Continued...

...*Continued*

No.	Botanical Name	Common Name	Family	Habit	Part Used	Ethnomedicinal Uses
273.	*Portulaca tuberosa*	Idar	Portulacaceae	H	Whole plant	Erysipelas, Dysuria
274.	*Premna resinosa*	Kundher	Verbenaceae	S	Leaves	Laxative, Diuretic
275.	*Prosopis chilensis*	Gando Baval	Mimosaceae	S	Leaves	Wounds
276.	*Prosopis cineraria*	Khijado, Shami	Mimosaceae	T	Root	Appetite, Astringent to boils, Rheumatism, Pain in joints, in case of Ophthalmia
277.	*Psidium guajava*	Jamphal	Myrtaceae	T	Fruit, Leaves	Bronchitis, Sore eyes, Thirst, Colic, Bleeding gums, Diarrhoea
278.	*Psoralea corylifolia*	Gawar, Bavachi	Fabaceae	H	Whole plant	Teeth, Leprosy, Skin diseases, Vomiting, Asthma, Piles, Elephantiasis, Snakebite, Scorpion sting
279.	*Psoralea plicata*	Kapurio	Fabaceae	H	Root	Toothache, Migraine
280.	*Pupalia lappacea*	Bhurat, Gadar bhurat	Amaranthaceae	Us	Whole plant	Cough destroyer
281.	*Rhus mysuresis*	Dasan, Davan, Dasarni	Anacardiaceae	S	Leaves	Swelling
282.	*Rhynchosia minima* var. *laxiflora*	Dariavel	Fabaceae	H	Leaves	Abortifacient
283.	*Rhynchosia minima* var. *minima*	Nahnikamalvel	Fabaceae	H	Leaves	Abortifacient
284.	*Ricinus communis*	Diveli, Divelio	Euphorbiaceae	S	Root, Root bark	Inflammation, Pains, Ascites, Fever, Glands, Bronchitis, Leprosy, Night blindness, Elephantiasis, Cough, Tumours, Headache

Continued...

...Continued

No.	Botanical Name	Common Name	Family	Habit	Part Used	Ethnomedicinal Uses
285.	*Rivea hypocrateriformis*	Fang	Convolvulaceae	C	Root	Cough, Pioisonous animal bites, Swellings, Headache
286.	*Rubellia tuberosa*	Bandhukadi	Acanthaceae	H	Root	Gonorrhea, Syphilis, Sore eyes
287.	*Rungia repens*	—	Acanthaceae	H	Whole plant	Fever, Cough
288.	*Salicornia brachiata*	—	Chenopodiaceae	H	Whole plant	Mange, Itch, Emmenagogue
289.	*Salvadora oleoides*	Piludi	Salvadoraceae	T	Whole plant	Piles Tumours, Bronchitis, Disease of spleen, Ascites, Ulcers, Cough, Rheumatic affection
290.	*Salvadora persica*	Pilvo, Piludi	Salvadoraceae	T	Whole plant	Biliousness, Tonic to the liver, Piles, Scabies, Leucoderma, Lesion inflammation, Strengthen the teeth, Skin disease
291.	*Sapindus emerginatus*	Aritha	Sapindaceae	T	Fruits	Epilepsy, Fever, Skin diseases
292.	*Sarcostemma acidum*	Som	Asclepiadaceae	S	Whole plant	Cures Tridosha, Biliousness, Thirst
293.	*Securinega leucopyrus*	Chhini, Thumari, Shenvi	Euphorbiaceae	T	Leaves	Destroys worms in sores
294.	*Senra incana*	—	Malvaceae	H	Leaves	Gums
295.	*Sericostoma pauciflorum*	Karvas	Ehretiaceae	H	Whole plant	Very Nutritious, Thirst, Cough

Continued...

...Continued

No.	Botanical Name	Common Name	Family	Habit	Part Used	Ethnomedicinal Uses
296.	*Sesamum indicum*	Tal	Pedaliaceae	H	Whole plant	Promotes growth of hair, Inflammation, Scorpion sting, Snake bite, Spleen trouble, Asthma, Disease of lungs, Burning sensation, Disease of ear and eye, Scabies
297.	*Sesbania bispinosa*	Ikad	Fabaceae	H	Root, Seeds	Eye diseases, Ringworm, Skin diseases, Wounds, Vomiting
298.	*Sesbania cannabina*	Lisikad	Fabaceae	H	Leaves, Seeds	Skin disease
299.	*Sida acuta*	Bala	Malvaceae	Us	Whole plant	Fever, Burning, Intestinal worms, Snakebite, Scorpion sting
300.	*Sida alba*	Kantalobala	Malvaceae	Us	Leaves	Polyurea, Arthritis, Gums, Diarrhoea, Heart disease, Swelling
301.	*Sida cordata*	Bhoyabala, Nidhidhatuval	Malvaceae	H	Whole plant	Burning sensation, Diarrhoea
302.	*Sida cordifolia*	Bala, Baldana, Kharenti	Malvaceae	Us	Whole plant	Bleeding piles, Phthisis, Insanity Leucorrhoea, Paralysis, Tenesmus
303.	*Sida ovata*	—	Malvaceae	Us	Leaves	Swelling (external)
304.	*Siegesbeckia orientalis*	Pilibadkadi	Asteraceae	H	Whole plant	Ulcer
305.	*Solanum albicule*	—	Solanaceae	Us	Whole plant	Ulcer

Continued...

...*Continued*

No.	Botanical Name	Common Name	Family	Habit	Part Used	Ethnomedicinal Uses
306.	*Solanum incanum*	Ubhi Ringni	Solanaceae	S	Whole plant	Cough, Leucoderma, Fever, Vomiting, Asthma, Ascites, Heart disease, Acidity
307.	*Solanum indicum*	Ubhi Ringni, Vadringni, Dorili	Solanaceae	Us	Root	Cough, Fever, Leucoderma, Vomiting, Asthma, Heart disease, Acidity
308.	*Solanum nigrum*	Piludi	Solanaceae	H	Whole plant	To reduce swelling
309.	*Solanum surattense*	Bhoringni, Bhoyringni	Solanaceae	H	Whole plant	Cough, Asthma, Heart disease, Gastric trouble
310.	*Sphaeranthus senegalensis*	Gorakh mundi, Bhurandi	Asteraceae	H	Whole plant	Tuberculosis gland, Bronchitis, Elephantiasis, Anemia, Leucoderma, Dysentery, Hemicrania
311.	*Sterculia urens*	Kadai, Kadio Kadayo	Sterculiaceae	T	Leaves	Throat infection, Wounds, Fractures, Orchitis, Pseudo pneumonia in cattle
312.	*Striga gesneroides*	Rato agiyo	Scrophulariaceae	H	Whole plant	Gums, Animal ulcers
313.	*Suaeda nudiflora*	Moras	Chenopodiaceae	Us	Whole plant	Digestible
314.	*Syzygium cumini*	Jambu	Myrtaceae	T	Fruit, Bark	Asthma, Thirst, Dysentery, Heavy speech, Liver complaints
315.	*Tamarindus indica*	Amli	Caesalpiniaceae	T	Leaves	Used in preparation of medicine

Continued...

...Continued

No.	Botanical Name	Common Name	Family	Habit	Part Used	Ethnomedicinal Uses
316.	*Taverniera cuneifolia*	Jethimadh, Jethimal	Fabaceae	Us	Leaves	Ulcers
317.	*Tecomella undulata*	Ragat rohido, Roydo, Rohido	Bignoniaceae	T	Bark	Tubercular glands, Cough, Fever
318.	*Tephrosia pauciflora*	Vitho Sarpankho, Chhatro Sarpankho	Fabaceae	H	Whole plant	Spleen, Ringworm, Pruritis, On poisonous animal bites, Promotes hair groth
319.	*Tephrosia purpurea*	Sarpankho	Fabaceae	Us	Whole plant	Snakebite, Ulcer, Wound, Asthma, Bronchitis, Diarrhoea, Syphilis, Gonorrhea, Colic
320.	*Tephrośia strigosa*	Sani Sarpankhi, Asmani sarpankho	Fabaceae	H	Whole plant	Fever, Blood Purifier, Cough, Tightness of chest, Gonorrhea
321.	*Teramnus labialis*	—	Fabaceae	H	Whole plant	Inflammation, Blood disease, Fever, Consumption, Paralysis, Rheumatism, Catarrhs, Bronchitis
322.	*Thespesia populnea*	Paras piplo, Pardeshi bhindi	Malvaceae	T	Whole plant	Nutrients, Polyurea, Piles
323.	*Thevetia peruviana*	Pili Karen	Apocynaceae	S	Whole plnat	Skin diseases, Leucoderma, Piles, Itching, Rheumatism
324.	*Tinospora cordifolia*	Gulvel, Gadu, Gudaj	Menispermaceae	Tw	Root	Snakebite, Fever, Spleen pain,
325.	*Trianthema portulacastrum*	Satodo	Aizoaceae	H	Leaves	Gums, Eye disease, Jaundice

Continued...

...Continued

No.	Botanical Name	Common Name	Family	Habit	Part Used	Ethnomedicinal Uses
326.	*Trianthema triquetra*	Satodi	Aizoaceae	H	Root	Gums
327.	*Tribulus pentandrus*	—	Zygophyllaceae	H	Fruit	Inflammation, Uterine complaints
328.	*Tribulus terrestris*	Bethu, Gokhru, Mithu gokhru, Akanti	Zygophyllaceae	H	Whole plant	Cough, Asthma, Pain, Leprosy, Stones, Blood purification, Kidney diseases, Gonorrhea, Scorpion sting
329.	*Trichodesma amplexicaule*	Undha fuli, Agiya kharsan	Boraginaceae	H	Whole plant	Eye diseases, Snakebite, Swelling, Fever
330.	*Trichodesma indicum*	Undha fuli, Agiya kharsan	Boraginaceae	H	Whole plant	Applied on the poisonous animal bite, Snake and scorpion bite, Fever, Eye pains, Gums, Leucoderma
331.	*Tricholepis amplexicaulis*	—	Asteraceae	H	Leaves	Inflammation
332.	*Trichosanthes cucumerina*	Jangli parval	Cucurbitaceae	C	Whole plant	Used in fever
333.	*Tridax procumbens*	Pardesi bhangaro	Asteraceae	H	Leaves	Earache, Piles, Skin diseases, Reduce swellings
334.	*Trigonella foenum-graecum*	Bhaji, Methi	Fabaceae	H	Whole plant	Leprosy, Bronchitis, Piles, Vomiting, Chronic cough, External and internal swelling
335.	*Triumfetta pentandra*	—	Tiliaceae	H	Leaves	Swelling

Continued...

...Continued

No.	Botanical Name	Common Name	Family	Habit	Part Used	Ethnomedicinal Uses
336.	*Triumfetta rhomboidea*	Bhurati, Japati	Tiliaceae	Us	Root, Leaves	Dysentery, Diarrhoea, Gonorrhea, Diuretic, Tumours
337.	*Triumfetta rotundifolia*	Zipti, Gol zipti	Tiliaceae	H	Root, Leaves	Wounds, Blood clotting
338.	*Typha angustata*	Gha bajriyo, Bant, Band, Kalpan	Typhaceae	H	Leaves	Leprosy, Wounds, Ulcers, Dysentery, Gonorrhea
339.	*Urginea indica*	Jangli dungli, Jangli pyaz	Liliaceae	H	Tuber, Bulb	Vomiting, Paralysis, Bronchitis, Asthma, Dropsy, Leprosy, Headache, Catarrhs
340.	*Verbascum chinense*	Kalhar, Kolhala, Kutki	Scrophulariaceae	H	Whole plant	Useful in vata complaints and blood derangements, Chronic dysentery
341.	*Vernonia anthelmintica*	Kalijiri	Asteraceae	H	Seeds	Fever, Skin diseases, Leucoderma, Snakebite, Scorpion sting
342.	*Vernonia cinerascens*	Vadi sadebi	Asteraceae	Us	Whole plant	Sleepiness property
343.	*Vernonia cinerea*	Sahadevi, Sadedi	Asteraceae	H	Whole plant	Fever
344.	*Vicoa indica*	Sonasali	Asteraceae	Us	Whole plant	Sinus, Fever
345.	*Vigna trilobata*	—	Fabaceae	H	Leaves, Fruits	Good for eyes, Cures consumption, Inflammation, Fever, Burning sensation, Thirst, Piles, Dysentery, Cough, Biliousness

Continued...

...Continued

No.	Botanical Name	Common Name	Family	Habit	Part Used	Ethnomedicinal Uses
346.	*Viola cinerea* var *stocksii*	Banafsa	Violaceae	H	Whole plant	Asthma, Bronchitis, Fever
347.	*Wattakaka volubilis*	Dodi, Motidodi, Malti	Asclepiadaceae	Tw	Whole plant	Aphrodisiac, Piles, Leucoderma, Rat-bite, Asthma, Cold
348.	*Zizyphus mauritiana*	Bor, Boadi, Bordi, Borjo zad	Rhamnaceae	T	Fruits, Bark	Diarrhoea, Dysentery, Vomiting, Blood purification, Leucorrhoea Gums, Syphilitic ulcers, Asthma, Fever
349.	*Zizyphus nummularia*	Chani bor, Chania bor, Palia	Rhamnaceae	S	Fruit, Leaves	Joint pains, Gums, Bilious afflictions
350.	*Zornia gibbosa*	Samarapani	Fabaceae	H	Whole plant	Bends on swellings, Earache
351.	*Zygophyllum simplex*	Patlani, Atheli, Alethi	Zygophyllaceae	H	Leaves, Seeds	Ophthalmia, Eye pain

Habit: H = Herb; G = Grass; S = Shrub; T = Tree; Tw = Twiner; Us = Undershrub.

TABLE 4

Number of Medicinal Plants in the Surveyed Forests of Kachchh

Tauka	Name of Forest	Total Plants	Medicinal Plants
Abdasa	Lathedi Plantation	107	83
	Mothaala Forest	112	95
	Vegaber Grassland	90	74
Bhachau	Chhapariya Rakha*	151	129
	Kanthkot Rakhal	106	85
	Tragadi Bet	48	43
Bhuj	Chaduva Rakhal	131	117
	Kalo Dunger	118	104
	Kurgiriya Rakhal	173	142
	Nabhoi Rakhal*	128	104
	Nadi Bag Rakhal	72	56
	Samatra Forest	80	75
	Sumariwandh	118	102
	Tapkeshwari*	170	134
Lakhpat	Gugariyana Rakhal£	138	117
	Kaiyari RF	82	68
	Laxmirani RF	105	97
	Mindhiari RF	76	66
	Piper RF	108	93
Mandvi	Lyza Coastal Forest	42	37
	Vijay Vilas Palace Forest	124	116
Mundra	Navinal Rakhal	74	59
Nakhatrana	Dinodar Dungar*	155	132
	Mangawana Forest	102	88
	Nanamo Dungar*	195	160
	Roha Fort Forest	129	121
	Roha Nano Dungar	125	105
Rapar	Badargarh Forest*	148	122
	Bela Forest*	129	121
	Jatavada Rakhal	82	74

* Prioritised forests of medicinal plant conservation.

was done with the help of existing published literature in the form of flora (Kirtikar and Basu, 1933; Thacker, 1926; Bhandari, 1990; Shah, 1978; Blatter & McCann, 1984), research articles and theses (Rao 1970, 1983; Rao and Sabnis 1977, 1983; Bhatt, 1993). The herbariums of various universities and colleges were also visited frequently to accomplish the task of plant identification.

From the threat point of view, ocular observation based abundance assessment was done and plants were categorised in the following five major categories:

TABLE 5
List of Rare and Very Rare Medicinal Plants Recorded in the Present Study

No.	Botanical Name	Family	Local Name	Habit	Present Status
1.	*Alangium salvifolium*	Alangiaceae	Ankol, Ankoli	T	R
2.	*Crotalaria leptostachya*	Fabaceae	—	H	R
3.	*Ephedra foliata*	Ephedraceae	—	S	VR
4.	*Ficus racemosa*	Moraceae	Umaro, Umbar, Gular	T	R
5.	*Helicteres isora*	Sterculiaceae	Maradsing, Ati, Aiti, Atai	T	R
6.	*Holoptelea integrifolia*	Ulmaceae	Kanjo, Papda, Audo-aodo	T	VR
7.	*Impomoea dasysperma*	Convolvulaceae	Dipad vel	Tw	R
8	*Lannea coromandelica*	Anacardiaceae	Madhol, Modhad, Miniyo, Moyno	T	R
9.	*Lawsonia inermis*	Lythraceae	Mehndi	S	R
10.	*Lepidagathis cristata*	Acanthaceae	—	H	VR
11.	*Leucas longifolia*	Lamiaceae	—	H	R
12.	*Leucas urticaefolia*	Lamiaceae	Kubo	H	R
13.	*Lindenbergia muraria*	Scrophulariaceae	Pirsadedi, Zamarval, Patharchati, Bhintchati	H	R
14.	*Maerua oblongifolia*	Capparaceae	Hemkand	S	R
15.	*Melia azaderach*	Meliaceae	Bakanlimdo, Bakan Nimb	T	R
16.	*Nelumbo nucifera*	Nymphaceae	Vado Kamalful, Suryakamal, Kamal, Motukamal	H	R
17.	*Nicandra physaloides*	Solanaceae	—	H	R
18.	*Pandanus odoratissimus*	Pendanaceae	Kevdo	H	R
19.	*Pavetta crassicaulis*	Rubiaceae	Papat	S	R
20.	*Plumbago zeylanica*	Plumbaginaceae	Chitrak, Chitro	Us	R
21.	*Psoralea plicata*	Fabaceae	Kapurio	H	R
22.	*Rhus mysurensis*	Anacardiaceae	Dasan, Davan, Dasarni	S	R
23.	*Ruellia tuberose*	Acanthaceae	Bandhukadi	H	R
24.	*Rungia repens*	Acanthaceae	—	H	R
25.	*Sarcostemma acidum*	Asclepiadaceae	Som	S	VR
26.	*Senra incana*	Malvaceae	—	H	VR
27.	*Sericostoma pauciflorum*	Ehretiaceae	Karvas	H	R
28.	*Striga gesneroides*	Scrophulariaceae	Rato agiyo	H	VR
29.	*Tecomella undulata*	Bignoniaceae	Ragat rohido, Roydo, Rohido	T	VR

Habit: H=Herb; S=Shrub; T=Tree; Tw=Twiner; Us=Undershrub. Present Status: R=Rare; VR=Very Rare.

1. Abundant;
2. Common;
3. Uncommon;
4. Rare; and
5. Very Rare.

For such ranking, the frequency of occurrence of species in terms of their presence in a number of transects and their distribution in the field was also considered. The results obtained through the present study were compared with the existing lists on the conservation status of plants at various levels—International (IUCN, 2000), National (Nayar and Sastry, 1990) and local (Sabnis and Rao, 1983; Bhatt, 1993).

RESULTS

Medicinal Plant Richness

Based on the rapid assessment, the present study has listed a total of about 527 plant species from different forests of district Kachchh, while few more species are yet to be identified. The identified plant species belong to 95 families and about 230 genera. Of the total 527 plant species, the medicinal properties of as many as 351 (67 per cent) plant species are described in the literature (Table 3). The proportion of medicinal plants against total plants across different habitats was highest under shrub category (89 per cent) followed by trees and climber and twiner categories (Table 1). On the other hand, proportion of grasses with medicinal properties was least with only eight per cent species having medicinal value. However, of the total medicinal plants (n = 351), the herbs contributed maximum (53 per cent) followed by trees (15 per cent), shrubs (13 per cent) and undershrub and climbers (9 per cent each). Grasses contributed only one per cent to the total medicinal plants recorded in the study area.

Conservation Status of Medicinal Plants

The results on the abundance of medicinal plants revealed that of the total 351 medicinal plants, 22 species (six per cent were recorded under rare occurrence category, while seven species (two per cent) are recorded under very rare category. About 53 per cent plants were recorded as common while only 16 species were abundantly present and the rest were under uncommon category. The list of rare and very rare species is presented in Table 5. Of the 29 rare and very rare species, two species, *Holoptelea integrifolia* and *Tecomella undulata* are also listed as rare at the international level (IUCN, 2000), while only one species *Indigofera careulea* var. *monosperma*, recorded as uncommon in the present study, is listed as rare in the Red Data Book of Indian Plants (Nayar and Sastry, 1990). However, the medicinal use of this species has not been described in the literature. The status of only gymnosperm having medicinal value, *Ephedra foliata*, is unknown at the international level.

Other than these, the uncommonly found species in the present study, such as *Commiphora wightii* is also listed in the IUCN Red Data Book (2000), while species such as *Pavonia ceratocarpa* and *Dipcadi erythraeum* are listed as indeterminate at the international level. The earlier regional inventories by Rao and Sabnis (1983) have listed some of the rare and threatened plants of south-eastern Kachchh. Among these, species such as *Commiphora wightii*, *Heliotropium bacciferum*,

Indigofera caerulea var. *monosperma*, and *Pavonia ceratocarpa*, which were recorded as uncommon in the present study from the entire district, were rated under rare category by the authors.

Threats to the Conservation of Medicinal Plants

Similar to many parts of the country, the major threat to the abundance and distribution of medicinal plants in district Kachchh is posed because of anthropogenic activities, mainly in the form of large-scale grazing by resident as well as migratory livestock and cutting for fuel wood and timber for domestic and commercial needs. According to the latest Census (1997), the total livestock population of district Kachchh is around 15.75 million, which is about 12 per cent more than the previous Census of 1992. On top of this, every year 2-3 lakh livestock also migrate into the area during monsoon. Of the total resident population, sheep and goat together constitute about 69 per cent of total population, and similar is the case with migratory livestock also. The large proportion of sheep and goats in the area causes serious damage to the vegetation, particularly to the herbaceous flora, including new saplings and seedlings, thus hampering the regeneration process of the forests.

Some of the medicinal plants, which showed poor regeneration in the forests due to heavy livestock grazing include *Butea monosperma*, *Helicteres isora*, *Tecomella undulata*, *Commiphora wightii*, *Acacia nilotica* sub sp. *indica*, *Sterculia urens*, *Prosopis cineraria*, *Indigofera linifolia* var. *linifolia*, *Argemone mexicana*, *Acalypha indica*, *Chlorophytum tuberosum*, *Striga gesneroides*, *Ephedra foliata*, *Grewia obutilifolia*, *Grewia flavescens*, *Ceropegia bulbosa*, *Pavonia ceratocarpa* and *Plumbago zeylanica*. Some of these species are also used for firewood, timber for house construction and agricultural requirements, therefore, also face pressure due to cutting.

During rapid assessment through questionnaire survey, the villagers reported commercial exploitation of some of the medicinal plants (Table 2). However, this aspect of medicinal plant conservation needs further exploration and more concrete information is required to be more specific about the conservation of such species. Nevertheless, there are incidences of destructive collection of some of the species such as *Commiphora wightii* (Dixit and Rao, 2000), *Capparis cartilaginea* (whole plant) and *Ceropegia bulbosa* (tuber), which has drastically reduced the population of these species in the wild. Especially, the population of species such as *Commiphora wightii* and *Capparis cartilaginea*, which already have restricted distribution, is fast depleting in the natural habitat because of destructive harvesting methods.

The spread of woody species, *Prosopis juliflora,* in the region is another major conservation concern. Although its impact is more visible in the grassland areas, the forests areas, especially the rivulets and river courses, are also coming under its invasion, leading to the rapid loss of biodiversity, including some of medicinal plants also. It has been recorded that about 0.35 M ha of the total geographical area of the district is invaded by *Prosopis juliflora* (SAC, 2001). Other than these, the fast development of the industrial sector in the region is leading to the destruction of habitat, which is quantitatively a large-scale destruction and requires huge efforts for restoration. The rich mineral resources of Kachchh have attracted a large number of industrial houses in the region and thermal power plants, cement industry, mineral exploitation and port-based activities are increasing on a large scale in the region.

DISCUSSION

In terms of floral exploration, the present study is perhaps the first complete account of the medicinal plant richness and their abundance and distribution in district Kachchh, although on a subjective basis. Record of more than 350 species with medicinal properties is an important finding from the point of view of biodiversity conservation and sustainable use of these resources. Availability of such a large proportion of medicinal plants from Kachchh calls for conservation of these resources in view of several kinds of anthropogenic and other pressures operating in the area, mainly in the form of expansion of industrial and other kinds of developmental activities. These activities are accelerating the degradation of habitats, their fragmentation and finally lowering the population of natural resources (GEER and GUIDE, 2001).

The present study has been able to identify the important forest areas from medicinal plant richness point of view. Such forests will be taken up for detailed sampling in the future aiming at collecting quantified information on the distribution of medicinal plants, their abundance and threats they are facing in different forests in a more systematic way. Parallel to this, the work on the documentation of the traditional knowledge of local communities is also being taken up to complete the targeted programme of *in situ* conservation of medicinal plants with community participation and conservation of traditional knowledge of local communities in district Kachchh.

REFERENCES

Bhandari, M. M. *Flora of the Indian Desert.* Jodhpur: MPS Repros. (Revised Edition), 1990.

Bhatt, J. B. Studies on the flora of western Kachchh. Ph.D. Thesis. M. S. University, Baroda, 1993.

Blatter, E. and McCann, C. *The Bombay Grasses.* Dehradoon: Bishen Singh Mahendra Pal Singh, 1984.

BSI-MoEF *Conservation of Medicinal Plants of India.* Botanical Survey of India, Kolkata, and Ministry of Environment and Forests, Government of India, New Delhi, 1993.

Dixit, A. M. and Rao, S. 'Observation on distribution and habitat characteristics of Gugal (*Commiphora wightii*) in the arid region of Kachchh, Gujarat (India)'. *Tropical Ecology* 41(1): 81-88, 2000.

GEER and GUIDE *Ecological Status of Narayan Sarovar Wildlife Sanctuary with a Management Perspective.* Gujarat Institute of Desert Ecology (GUIDE), Bhuj, and Gujarat Ecological Education and Research (GEER) Foundation, Gandhinagar, 2001.

Ismail Master. *Pachchham Bet ni Vanaspatiyo* (in Gujarati). Bhuj: Sahjeevan, 2000.

IUCN 'Threatened plant species in Gujarat State'. IUCN Red Data Book, 2000.

Jain, S. K. and Saklani, A 'Observations on the ethnobotany of the Tons valley region in the Uttarkashi district of the northwest Himalaya, India'. *Mountain Research and Development*, vol. 11(2): 157-161, 1991.

Kirtikar, K. R., Basu, B. D. and an I. C. S. *Indian Medicinal Plants.* (in four volumes with plates). Lalit Mohan Basu, Allahabad and Manik Chandra Das, Prabasi Press, Kolkata, 1933.

Nayar, M. P. and Sastry, A. R. K. *Red Data Book of Indian Plants.* vols. 1-3. Botanical Survey of India. Kolkata, 1990.

Rao, K. S. S. Flora of south-eastern Kachchh. Ph.D. Thesis. S. P. University, Vallabh Vidya Nagar, 1983.

Rao, K. S. S. and Sabnis, S. D. 'Addition to Kutch flora'. *J. Bio. Sci.*, 20:1-6, 1977.

Rao, R. S. 'Studies on the flora of Kutch, Gujarat State (India) and their utility in the economic development of the semi-arid region'. *Annals of Arid Zone* 9: 125-142, 1970.

Sabnis, S. D. and Rao, K. S. S. 'Rare and endangered endemics of south-eastern Kachchh'. In: *Assessment of Threatened Plants of India*. (Eds.). Jain, S. K. and Rao, R. R.). Howrah: Botanical Survey of India, pp. 71-72, 1983.

SAC. Grassland mapping in Gujarat using remote sending and GIS techniques. Space Application Centre, ISRO, Ahmedabad, 2001.

Shah, G. L. *Flora of Gujarat State*, parts I & II. University Press, Sardar Patel University, Vallabh Vidyanagar, Gujarat, 1978.

Silori, C. S. and Rana, A. 'Indigenous knowledge on medicinal plants and their use in Narayan Sarovar Sanctuary, Kachchh'. *Ethnobotany* 12:1-7, 2000.

Thacker, J. I. *Plants of Kutch and their Utility* (in Gujarati), Rajkot, 1926.

—oo(O)oo—

11

Medicinal Plants: A Probe in the Forests of Rajasthan

Satish Kumar Sharma

It is not easy to define a medicinal plant. Every plant is medicinal at one place or the other. However, some plants are well known to various medicinal systems and many codified drugs are obtained from them. Many plants are known as source of traditional medicines. Our tribals and rural people procure indigenous medicines from them. A glimpse of the medicinal plants of Rajasthan can be had from the work of Bhandari (1990), Billore and Audichya (1978), Joshi (1981, 1989, 1993, 1995), Sebastian and Bhandari (1984a, 1984b, 1988), Sharma and Vyas (1985), Sharma and Tiagi (1979), Sharma (1998), Sharma (1997a, 1997b, 1997c, 1998a. 1998b, 1999a, 1999b, 2000, 2001a, 2001b, 2001c, 2003), Shetty and Pandey (1983), Shetty and Singh (1987-1993), Singh (1983), Singh and Pandey (1980), etc.

Forests are the major source of medicinal plants in Rajasthan, especially in the tribal and rural areas. A bird's eye view of different aspects of medicinal plants of this State is presented in fuller details below so that guidelines for their *in-situ* and *ex-situ* conservation can be decided.

IMPORTANT MEDICINAL PLANT AREAS OF RAJASTHAN

Different agro-climatic zones are there in Rajasthan *vis-à-vis* varied forms of micro-habitats are available here, resulting in availability of good number of medicinal plant species, useful in traditional as well as in codified medicines. Though every part of the State has medicinal plants, few spots are relatively rich in the occurrence of these plants. The important medicinal plant areas of the State are given in Table 1

Beside the areas mentioned in Table 1, Ratanpur, Vanjoi-ki-Nal (Dungarpur), Jeen Mata (Sikar), Borawas, Darrah (Kota), Shergarh (Bara), Kualji (Sawai Madhopur), Ramgarh Vishdhari (Bundi), Nal Mokhi (Udaipur), are also rich in the occurrence of medicinal plants and floral diversity.

TABLE 1
Important Medicinal Plants of Rajasthan

Locality	Situation	Plants Available
Tiger Project, Seriska	Alwar district, on Alwar-Jaipur road	*Gloriosa superba* *Adhatoda zeylanica* *Commiphora wightii* *Sarcostemma acidum* *Abrus precatorius* *Naringi crenulata* *Ceropegia bulbosa* *Urginea indica* *Asparagus racemosus*
Sirawas-ki-Rundh	Alwar district	*Adhatoda zeylanica* *Gloriosa superba* *Commiphora wightii* *Asparagus racemosus*
Jamwa Ramgarh Wildife Sanctuary	Jamwa Ramgarh tehsil of Jaipur district on Jaipur-Andhi road	*Adhatoda zeylanica* *Gloriosa superba* *Commiphora wightii* *Abrus precatorius* *Asparagus racemosus*
Nahargarh Wildlife Sanctuary and adjoining area	Jaipur district	*Adhatoda zeylanica* *Gloriosa superba* *Commiphora wightii* *Abrus precatorius* *Urginea indica* *Naringi crenulata* *Asparagus racemosus*
Nag Pahad	Ajmer district	*Commiphora wightii* *Abrus precatorius* *Urginea indica* *Asparagus racemosus*
Todgarh-Ravli Wildlife Sactuary	Pali, Ajmer, Rajasamand districts	*Commiphora wightii* *Abrus precatorius* *Urginea indica* *Tuberous* sp. *Asparagus racemosus*

Continued...

...Continued

Locality	Situation	Plants Available
Kumbhalgarh Wildlife Sanctuary	Pali, Rajasamand, Udaipur districts	*Sterculia urens* *Commiphora wightii* *Abrus precatorius* *Annona squamosa* *Plumbago zeylanica* *Urginea indica*
Gujri-ki-Nal forest, Nalsandol, Jhameri Forest blocks	Jhadol tehsil, Udaipur district	"*Shilajeet**" *Sterculia urens* *Eulophia ochreata* *Asparagus racemosus* *Feronia limonia* *Aegle marmelos* *Emblica officinalis* *Phyllanthus niruri* *Hemidesmus indicus* *Stereospermum colais* *Crateva nurvala* *Ensete superbum* *Urginia indica* *Bacopa monneri* (in Sandol anicut)
Harsh Nath	Sikar district	*Commiphora wightii* *Urginea indica*
Jarga Hills	Near Sayra village, Gogunda tehsil, Udaipur district	*Ensete superbum* *Sterculia urens* *Aegle marmelosa* *Abrus precatorius* *Plumbago zeylanica*
Kamal Nath Hills	Near Magwas village, Jhadol tehsil, Udaipur district	*Centella asiatica* *Putranjiva roxburghii* *Carissa congesta* *Terminalia bellirica* *Emblica officinalis* *Sterculia urens* *Gloriosa superba* *Ensete superbum* *Viteveria zizanoides*

Continued...

...Continued

Locality	**Situation**	**Plants Available**
Som I and Madri Forest blocks	Jhadol tehsil, Udaipur district	*Pueraria tuberosa* *Gloriosa superba* *Ensete superbum* *Carissa congesta*
Phulwari Wildlife Sanctuary	Kotra and Jhadol tehsils, Udaipur district	*Terminalia bellirica* *Terminalia arjuna* *Eulophia ochreata* *Momordica dioica*** *Ensete superbum* *Carissa congesta* *Sterculia urens* *Madhuca indica* *Pongamia pinnata* *Woodfordia fruiticosa* *Helicteres isora* *Nyctenthes arbortristis* *Phoenix sylvestris* *Centella asiatica* *Chlorophytum borivilianum*
Torna, Tinsara, Ladan, Ramkunda, Samoli, Khakharia-ki-Nal forest areas	Udaipur district	*Terminalia bellirica* *Terminalia arjuna* *Eulophia ochreata* *Momordica dioica*** *Ensete superbum* *Carissa congesta* *Sterculia urens* *Madhuca indica* *Pongamia pinnata* *Woodfordia fruiticosa* *Helicteres isora* *Nyctenthes arbortristis* *Phoenix sylvestris* *Centella asiatica* *Chlorophytum borivilianum*
Keora-ki-Nal	Udaipur district	*Stereospermum colais* *Hymenodictyon excelsum* *Aegle marmelos*

Continued...

...*Continued*

Locality	Situation	Plants Available
Jaisamand Wildlife Sanctuary	Udaipur district	*Tamarindus indicus* *Leptaedinia reticulata* *Sarcostemma acidum* *Gloriosa superba*
Sitamata Wildlife Sanctuary	Chittorgarh and Udaipur districts, near Pratapgarh	*Buchanania lanzan* *Selaginella rependa* *Leea macrophylla*
Mount Abu Wildlife Sanctuary	Sirohi district	*Berberis asiatica* *Eulophia ochreata*
Machiya Safari Park	Jodhpur district	*Asparagus racemosus* *Tridex procumbens*
Heera-ka-Wadia	Rajsamand (Beawar-Bhilwara road)	*Commiphora wightii*
Thar Desert	Districts west of Aravallis	*Calligonum polygonoides* *Ephedra foliata* *Capparis decidua* *Withania somniphera* *Withania coagulans*
Baghdarrh	Udaipur district	*Sterculia urens* *Commiphora wightii*
Sundamata Hills	Jalore	*Sterculia urens*
Area of Shahabad Forest Range	Baran district	*Buchanania lanzan* *Sterculia urens* *Terminalia bellirica*
Menal	Bhilwara district	Rich in ferns, bryophytes *Sterculia urens*
Morus Forest area near Pindwara	Sirohi district	*Sterculia urens* *Aegle marmelos* *Gloriosa superba* *Urgenia indica*
Ubheshwar and Kaileshwar forest area	Udaipur	*Bacopa monnieri* *Sterculia urens* *Chlorophytum borivilianum*

* Not a medicinal plant but medicinal material. Liquid flows on rocks near Sandol Mata temple, specially during winters. Folk medicine men of the area call it "Shilajeet".

** Large amounts of fruit are collected in the rainy season around Deola village and sold as vegetables.

THREATS TO MEDICINAL PLANTS IN THE FOREST AREAS OF RAJASTHAN

There are many threats existing in the State of Rajasthan which are responsible for declining of availability of medicinal plants. Few of them are listed in Table 2.

Unripe fruits of *Annona squamosa* are massively collected from Deola, Kumbhalgarh and Rajsamand area, ripened at home by the locals using indigenous techniques and marketed. Unripe fruits of *Momordica dioica* are massively collected and marketed to Ahmedabad, Falana and other cities. Unripe fruits of *Emblica officinalis* are collected and boiled to facilitate de-seeding. The de-seeded fruits obtained so are dried and marketed. Unripe fruits of *Mangifera indica* and *Carissa congesta* are collected from the wild and consumed locally. Sometimes surplus is marketed also.

Seeds of *Buchanania lanzan* and *Sterculia urens* are collected for domestic consumption. Seeds of *Sterculia urens* are used as substitute of groundnut and relished by the tribals. Many birds like Rufous Treepie (*Dendrocitta vagabunda*) is also very fond of seeds of *Sterculia* and it devours those seeds which are still present on trees even in inaccessible gradient. Massive debarking is done of *Sterculia urens* and *Helicteres isora* to get fibres for domestic use, specially for farm-fences.

Many plants like *Chlorophytum borivilianum, Pueraria tuberosa, Gloriosa superba,* etc. are harvested by destructive methods. Digging and extraction of their underground parts destroy them forever. *Chlorophytum borivilianum* is sold as *safed musli* in the market. *Chlorophytum tuberosum* is also extracted for adulteration in the tubers of *Chlorophytum borivilianum*. Tubers of male plants of *Momordica dioica* are extracted for traditional lice killing medicine. Though bulbs of *Urginea indica* are non-edible, they are dug out by the Kathodis, sliced, collected in bamboo baskets and kept under flowing water the whole night and then consumed. *Eulophia ochreata*, a terrestrial orchid, is collected and sold as aphrodisiac medicine (Sharma, 1997a). Tubers of *Corallocarpis epigeous* are extracted to make country barometers. Tubers of *Pueraria tuberosa* are collected by the Bhils on Makar Sankranti festival (January 14) every year and consumed.

Bombax ceiba is massively extracted by the local tribals from the wild and sold in the market or door-to-door in urban areas to perform the Holi Dhahan, a famous festival of the Hindus. This practice is in vogue especially in the Mewar region. Young plants of *Bombax ceiba* are also extracted to consume their tuberous roots as a delicacy.

Habitat destruction is a major problem in the state. Free grazing by cattle, trampling, encroachment, especially in the foothill zone and riverine banks are destroying many species. Canopy opening in closed canopy areas is changing nature of microhabitats. Mass scale earth works done during relief and other similar operations take a very heavy toll of propagules and perennating parts of many species. While making approach roads, existing farm fences and hedges and unattended edges of fields are destroyed which badly affects the hedge flora. The relief works affect *Momordica dioica, Abrus precatorius, Urginea indica, Leptadaenia reticulata, Ipomoea, Jatropha curcas, Baliospermum montanum, Cryptolepis buchanani, Cryptostegia grandiflora,* etc.

River and steam banks are encroached by the tribals and others for agriculture. Since water is available there in pockets for irrigation, hence riverine banks are deforested here and there. It takes heavy toll of *Terminalia arjuna, Pongamia, pinnata, Vitex negundo, Syzygium heyneanum, Syzygium jambos, Syzygium cumini,* etc. Agriculture encroached in the foot hills is responsible for destruction of many mesophytic forest species including large numbers of tuberous species. Poor

TABLE 2
Medicinal Plants of Rajasthan Under Threat

Under Threat	Species Affected
Over collection of fruit	*Annona squamosa*
	Momordica dioica
	Emblica officinalis
	Mangifera indica
	Carissa congesta
Unripe fruit collection	*Annona squamosa*
	Momordica dioica
	Emblica officinalis
	Mangifera indica
	Jatropha curcas
Over-collection of seed	*Buchnania lanzan*
	Sterculia urens
Fibre extraction (destructive harvesting)	*Sterculia urens*
	Helicteres isora
Harvesting of underground parts (destructive harvesting)	*Chlorophytum borivilianum*
	Chlorophytum tuberosum
	Pueraria tuberosa
	Gloriosa superba
	Momordica dioica
	Corallocarpus epigaeus
	Urginea indica
	Eulophia ochreata
	Plumbago zeylanica
	Asparagus racemosus
Selective extraction	*Bombax ceiba*
	Pterocarpus marsupium
	Plants of foothill zone like
	Terminalia arjuna
	Pongamia pinnata
	Tuberous plants
Poor fruit setting	*Oroxylum indicum*
	Stereospermum colais
	Pueraria tuberosa
	Sterculia urens

Continued...

...Continued

Under Threat	Species Affected
Low seed germination	*Chlorphytum borivilianum* *Oroxylum indicum* *Stereospermum colais* *Tinospora cordifolia* *Asparagus racemosus* *Celastrus peniculatus*
Habitat destruction	Different stages of degradation are prevalent in most parts of the State due to heavy anthropogenic and bovine pressure. Habitat destruction and alteration can be seen even in the protected areas. This is creating problems for most species

fruit setting in many species is also responsible for poor occurrence of many species like *Oroxylum indicum, Stereospermum colais, Sterculia urens, Pueraria tuberosa*. Pods of *Oroxylum indicum* are of huge size and look like sword. Pods of this species when still present on trees are collected and used as novelty for house decoration. Low seed germination and low establishment in *Chlorophytum borivilianum, Oroxylum indicum* and *Stereospermum colais* is responsible for their low occurrence. Premature extraction of tubers of *Chlorophytum borivilianum* by tribals is badly affecting seed production in this species. Collection of tubers as "seed" for agriculturisation of this species is dwindling its occurrence in the wild at a fast pace.

HILL PATTERN AND OCCURRENCE OF MEDICINAL PLANTS

Isolated, conical, small hill or single isolated long chain of hill generally remain more dry in nature due to massive run off. Soil cover on such hills either remains absent or very thin and patchy. The xerophytic vegetation clad such hills. *Commiphora wightii, Euphorbia* sp., specially *Euphorbia caducifolia, Acacia senegal, Adhatoda zeylanica, Anogeissus pendula, Dichrostachys cinerea,* etc. patronise such hills. Harsh Nath (Sikar,) Neemuch Mata, Thur Magra, Sajjangarh (Udaipur) are good example of isolated conical hills. Bichun hills in Jaipur district are examples of an isolated chain.

But isolated hill or hill chain, having concaving or cupping in their upper reaches, bear less dry vegetation. Water storage in their concave zone, increases moisture regime in whole or part of the hill. Similarly, valleys of multiple parallel hill chains have nallahs and chord of different moisture regime. Such moist hill systems have many mixed broad-leafed species and grasslands in foothills and along the nallahs (Harsvardhan, Pers. Comm.). Kamal Nath hills, Phulwari Wildlife Sanctuary (Udaipur), Mount Abu Wildlife Sanctuary (Sirohi), etc. are good examples of this pattern. Due to towering height, Mt. Abu possesses semi-evergreen forests at its upper reaches. Nakki Lake, Traverse Tank, etc. are good surface water reservoirs, situated at upper reaches of this hill station. These water bodies represent the atop cupping of this hill.

Kamal Nath hill also has a pond atop. Flat extensive area atop is equally good and allows massive percolation of water inside hills. The water so retained comes out in the farm of hill streams and surface oozing at places. All these factors increase water regime of habitat and such hills can sustain many mixed broad-leafed species in pockets. Presence of spongy rocks also responsible for high water regime. Similarly, multiple parallel chains of hills are also able to sustain mixed broad-leafed forest species. Phulwary is a good example where a network of stream enhancing water regime in valleys to support better kind of forest. The hill stream, present between long 'open tunnel' of two parallel hills provide suitable micro-climate to many ever-green and hygrophilous plant species. Presence of soil cover on such hills again is responsible for creating more congenial conditions for better type of forest. Due to soil cover and good water regime, these hills can sustain broad-leafed species like *Mangifera indica, Anogeissus latifolia, Mallotus philippensis, Bridelia retusa, Cissus rependa, Ampelocissus latifolia* and *Pongamia pinnata* along with xerophytic species. Xerophytes like *Anogeissus pendula, Commiphora wightii, Rhus mysurensis,* etc. are totally absent at Kamal Nath, Phulwari and upper reaches of Mt. Abu hills. Pheology of same species present in dry hills and moist hills is also different. The 'moist hills' are very rich in *Centella asiatica Eulophia ochreata, Leea macrophylla, Habenaria digitata, Habenaria marginata, Habenaria furcifera, Habenaria longicorniculata, Nervilia aragoana, Baccopa monneiri, Begonia tricarpa, Pueraria tuberosa,* etc. We should take utmost care not to change the hydrology and pedology of moist pockets of hills of southern Aravallis and Baran district of Hadoti zone. Both these places are 'mega medicinal plant diversity zone' of this State.

THE "NAL" FORESTS

The area present between two long narrow hill chains is locally called as "nal." The forest present in "nal" area is always more mesic in nature than the rest of the area. "Nal-Forest" is protected from two or three sides by the high hills itself. "Nal forests" of Rajasthan are rich in medicinal plants, especially in tuberous plants, climbers, lianas and broad-leafed tree species. Generally a seasonal or perennial stream is also associated with a "nal" (Figure 1). According to availability of moisture level, "nals" are of three types:

(a) Dry, (b) Moist, and (c) Wet

"Nals" of northern and central Aravallis are generally of dry type but in centro-southern and southern Aravallis, many "nals" are of moist and wet nature. Sometimes all the three main stages, namely, dry, moist and wet and their transition phases are seen within the same "nal." "Nal" forests are rich in medicinal plants as well as in other floral diversity including Bryophytes and Pteridophytes. Few notable "nal" forests of Rajasthan, rich in medicinal plants are given in Table 3.

"KHOLAS" OR "KHADRAS"

In northern Aravallis, specially in Alwar and Jaipur districts, an inward fold in a hill or a deep nallah present at the right angle of the long axis of the hill or a notch like appearance is called "khola"

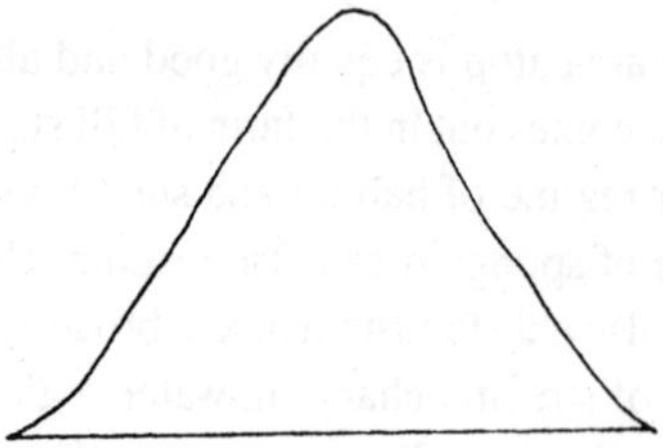

Convex hill

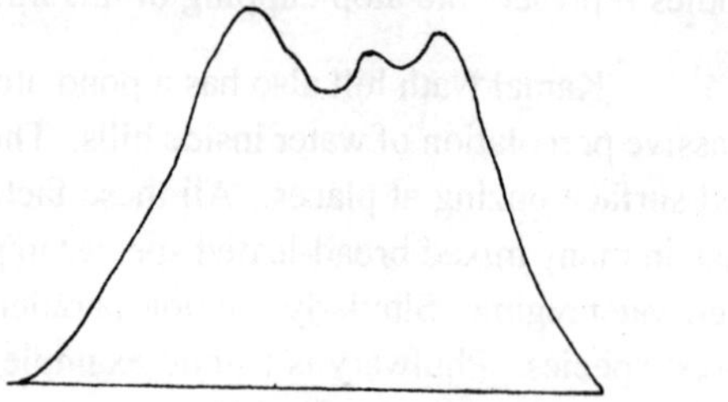

Concave hill

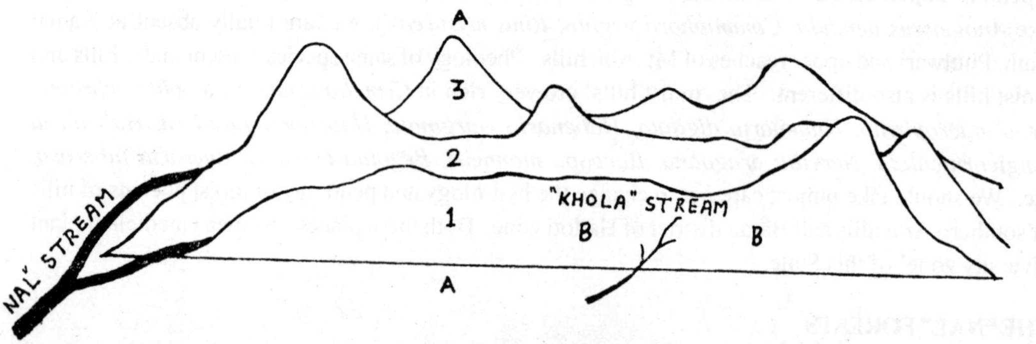

Parallel chains of three hills with two 'nals'

T.S. at A-A of middle diagram

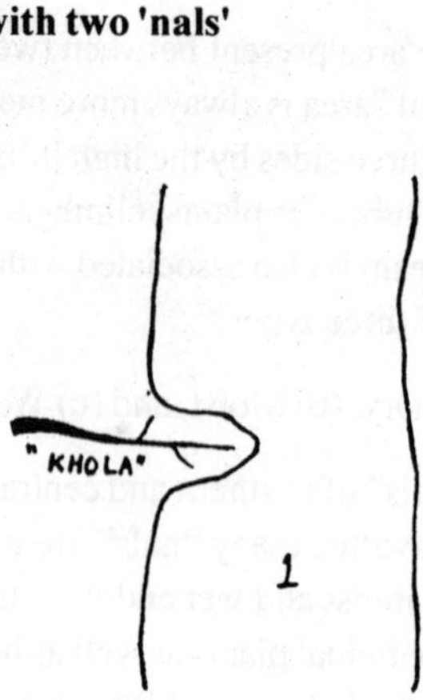

Horizontal section of hill no. 1 at B-B (Position is tilted)

Figure 1. Some hill features.

TABLE 3

Notable "Nal" Forests of Rajasthan Which are Rich in Medicinal Plants

No.	Name of "Nal" Forest	Location
1.	Digota-ki-Nal	Jamwa Ramgarh Wildlife Sanctuary, Jaipur
2.	Keora-ki-Nal	Near Keora village, Udaipur district
3.	Gujri-ki-Nal	Near Jhadol village, Udaipur district
4.	Desuri-ki-Nal	Near Desuri town, Pali district
5.	Menal	Bhilwara district
6.	Nal Mokhi	Near Gogunda, Udaipur district
7.	Magga-ki-Nal	Near Magga village, Kumbhalgarh Wildlife Sanctuary, Udaipur district
8.	Nal Sandol	Near Jhadol, Udaipur district
9.	Khokhariya-ki-Nal	Between Ukhaliyat and Deola villages, Udaipur district
10.	Phulwari-ki-Nal	Phulwari Wildlife Sanctuary, Udaipur district
11.	Jhanjhri-ki-Nal	Forest Range Khirwara, Udaipur district
12.	Ganwa (Garanwas)-ki-Nal	Forest Range Phalasia, Udaipur district
13.	Chakli-ki-Nal	Forest Range Bichhiwara, Dungarpur district
14.	Subri-ki-Nal	Forest Range Kotra, Udaipur district

(Figure 1). Actually "khola" is a shallow "nal" present on either lateral sides of the hill chain itself. Sometimes "kholas" have a water spring or water stream also. In the southern Aravallis, the "kholas" are called "khadras." Generally some ancient temple occurs in the "kholas" or "khadras" and its forest is protected as a sacred grove by the natives. Many medicinal plant species occur in such "khola" forests. Renagiri and Pehal villages in Mundawar Tehsil of Alwar district have good "khola" forests in the form of sacred groves.

CONSERVATION MEASURES

1. Little knowledge is available about status, local extraction and trade trends, use pattern of medicinal plants of Rajasthan. Hence, emphasis should be given on these aspects to bridge the gaps. A base live survey about status of different species is must for periodic evaluation and monitoring of the situation in future.
2. Many individuals, institutes and NGOs are working in isolation. Continuous networking is necessary among different agencies to achieve the common goal of medicinal plant protection, conservation, propagation, cultivation marketing and utilisation.
3. Continuous intensive and extensive habitat conservation measures are needed in medicinal species rich natural forests for *in-situ* conservation.
4. Medicinal plant gardens should be established in all typical habitats for *ex-situ* conservation and to promote the extension activities. The Forest Department of

TABLE 4-A
Survey of Medicinal Plants of Rajasthan

Family	Name of Plant	Hindi Name	Districtwise Present Status*												
			Sirohi	Udaipur	Rajasamand	Banswara	Dungarpur	Chittorgarh	Bhilwara	Ajmer	Kota	Baran	Jhalawar	Bundi	Tonk
Annonaceae	*Annona squamosa*	Sitaphal		3	4	+	+	+	+	+	2	+	+	+	+
Menispermasceae	*Tinospora cordifolia*	Neem giloy	2	2	2	2	2	2	2	2	+	+	+	+	+
Berberidaceae	*Berberis asiatica*	Daru haldi	1	+	+	+	+	+	+	+	+	+	+	+	+
Nymphaeceae	*Euryale ferox*	Talmakhani	+	+	+	+	+	+	+	1	+	+	+	+	+
	Nelumbo nucifera	Kamal	+	3	1	+	+	+	2	+	+	+	2	2	2
Papaveraceae	*Argemone mexicana*	Satyanasi	4	4	4	4	4	4	4	4	3	3	4	3	4
	*Papaver somnifera***	Afeem	+	2	+	+	+	3	+	+	3	+	+	+	+
Capparidaceae	*Capparis decidua*	Kair	4	1	2	1	1	2	2	3	1	1	1	2	3
	Creteva nurvala	Barna		3	1	2	+	2	+	+	2	+	2	+	+
	Maerua arenaria		+	+	+	+	+	+	+	3	2	+	+	2	2
Stercaliaceae	*Helicteres isora*	Marorphali	3	3	2	2	2	2	2	2	2	+	+	+	+
	Sterculia urens	Kadhaya	2	2	2	2	2	2	2	2	2	2	2	2	2
Zygophallaceae	*Peganum harmala*	Harmal	+	+	+	+	+	+	+	+	+	+	+	+	+
Averrhoaceae	*Averrhoa cammbola***	Kamrak	+	1	+	+	+	+	+	+	+	+	+	+	+
Rutaceae	*Aegle marmelos*	Belpatra	2	2	2	2	2	2	2	2	+	+	2	+	+
	Feronia limonia	Kaith	+	3	2	+	+	+	+	2	2	+	+	+	+
Balanitaceae	*Balanites aegyptiaca*	Hingore	3	3	3	3	3	3	3	3	3	+	+	+	3

Continued...

...Continued

Family	Name of Plant	Hindi Name	Districtwise Present Status*												
			Sirohi	Udaipur	Rajsamand	Banswara	Dungarpur	Chittorgarh	Bhilwara	Ajmer	Kota	Baran	Jhalawar	Bundi	Tonk
Burseraecae	*Boswellia serrata*	Salar	4	4	4	4	4	4	4	4	3	2	2	3	3
	Commiphora wightii	Gugal		2	2	+	2	2	2	2	+	+	+	+	+
	C. aglocha	Badi gugal	+	1	+	1	+	+	+	+	+	+	+	+	+
Meliaceae	*Azadirachta indica*	Neem	4	3	4	2	3	4	4	4	3	4	2	4	4
Celastraceae	*Celastrus paniculata*	Mal makangni	4	4	4	2	2	2	2	2	+	+	2	+	+
Sapindaceae	*Sapindus imarginatus*	Areetha	2	2	2	+	+	+	+	1	+	1	+	+	+
	Schliechera oleosa	Kusum	+	+	+	+	+	+	+	+	+	1	1	+	+
Anacardiaceae	*Buchaniana lanzan*	Chironji	1	1	+	+	+	2	+	+	2	+	2	+	+
	Mangifera indica	Aam	4	3	3	3	3	2	3	1	3	3	3	1	1
	Moringa concanensis	Sehajna	+	+	+	+	+	+	+	+	+	+	+	2	2
	M. oleifera	Sehajna	2	2	2	+	+	+	+	+	2		+	+	+
Fabaceae	*Abrus precatorius*	Rati	4	4	4	3	3	3	3	3	3	3	3	3	3
	Desmodium gangeticum	Salmani	4	4	3	3	3	3	2	2	3	3	3	2	2
	Mucuna pruriens	Koch	4	4	4	3	3	3	3	2	3	3	3	2	2
	Pongamia pinnata	Karanj	3	4	3	3	2	2	3	+	3	+	+	+	+
	Psoralea corylifolia	Vavchi	1	1	+	1	+	+	1	+	+	+	1	+	+

Continued...

...Continued

Family	Name of Plant	Hindi Name	Districtwise Present Status*												
			Sirohi	Udaipur	Rajsamand	Banswara	Dungarpur	Chittorgarh	Bhilwara	Ajmer	Kota	Baran	Jhalawar	Bundi	Tonk
	Pterocarpus marsupium	Beeja	1	1	+	+	+	+	+	1	+	+	+	+	+
	Puerana tuberosa	Ghodabel, Modi	1	1	+	+	+	+	+	1	+	+	+	+	+
Caesalpinaceae	*Caesaplinia banduc*	Katakranj	+	2	+	+	2	+	2	1	+	+	+	+	+
	Cassia fistula	Amaltas	3	3	3	2	2	2	2	2	2	2	2	2	2
	C. angustifolia	Sanay	+	1	+	+	+	+	+	+	+	+	+	+	+
	Tamarindus indicus	Imli	2	2	2	2	2	2	2	2	2	2	2	+	+
Mimosaceae	*Acacia catechu*	Khair	+	3	3	3	3	3	3	3	3	3	3	3	3
	Acacia senegal	Kumti	3	3	3	2	2	2	3	2	2	2	2	2	2
Combretaceae	*Anogeissus latifolia*	Ghavra	3	4	3	3	3	3	3	2	3	3	3	+	+
	Terminalia arjuna	Arjun	+	2	+	+	+	+	+	2	2	2	+	+	+
	Terminalia bellirica	Baheda	3	4	3	3	3	2	+	+	2	2	3	+	2
Myrtaceae	*Syzygium cumini*	Jamun	3	2	2	2	2	2	2	2	2	2	2	2	2
	S. heyneanum	Makhania jamun	3	4	+	+	+	+	+	+	+	+	+	+	+
Lythraceae	*Ammania baccifera*		4	4	2	3	2	2	3	2	3	4	4	2	2

Continued...

...*Continued*

Family	Name of Plant	Hindi Name	Districtwise Present Status*												
			Sirohi	Udaipur	Rajsamand	Banswara	Dungarpur	Chittorgarh	Bhilwara	Ajmer	Kota	Baran	Jhalawar	Bundi	Tonk
Cucurbitaceae	*Citrullus colocynthis*	Gartumba	+	+	+	+	+	+	+	2	+	+	+	+	2
	Cucumis melo	Kachri	+	+	+	+	+	+	+	2	+	+	+	+	2
	Diplocyclos palmatus	Shivlingi	3	4	3	3	3	3	3	3	3	3	3	3	+
	Momordica dioca	Kikoda	3	4	3	3	3	3	3	2	3	2	2	2	3
Ficoidaceae	*Trianthema portulacastrum*	Santi	3	3	3	3	3	3	3	3	3	3	3	3	3
Apiaceae (Umbelliferae)	*Centella asiatica*	Mandukpani	2	1	+	+	+	2	2	+	2	+	2	+	+
Asteraceae	*Artemisa scoparia*	Bana	+	1	+	+	+	+	+	+	+	+	+	+	1
	Eclipta alba	Bhrungraj	4	3	3	3	3	2	2	2	4	3	3	2	2
	Spilanthes calva	Akarkari	1	+	+	+	+	+	+	+	+	+	+	+	+
	Vernonia cinerea	Sehdevi	4	4	4	4	4	4	3	3	4	3	4	3	3
Plumbaginaceae	*Plumbago zeylanica*	Chitrak	3	3	3	3	2	2	2	2	3	2	2	2	+
Sapotaceae	*Manikara hexandra*	Rayan	+	1	+	1	2	+	+	+	+	2	1	+	+
Ebenaceae	*Diospyros melanoxylon*	Beedi pata	3	4	3	3	3	3	2	2	4	2	2	2	2
Oleaceae	*Nyctanthes arbortristis*	Haarsinghar	4	4	4	1	1	5	3	2	4	4	2	+	+

Continued...

...Continued

Family	Name of Plant	Hindi Name	Districtwise Present Status*												
			Sirohi	Udaipur	Rajsamand	Banswara	Dungarpur	Chittorgarh	Bhilwara	Ajmer	Kota	Baran	Jhalawar	Bundi	Tonk
Apocynaceae	*Carissa congesta*	Karonda	2	2	2	2	2	2	2	+	2	2	+	+	+
	Holarehena antidysenterica	Indoji	2	4	3	3	2	2	2	2	3	2	+	+	+
Gentianaceae	*Enicostema axillare*	Nami	3	3	3	3	3	3	3	3	3	3	3	3	3
Ehretiaceae	*Cordia dichotoma*	Lisoda	3	3	3	3	3	3	3	3	3	3	3	2	2
Convolvulaceae	*Evolvulus alsinoides*	Shankpushpi	2	2	2	2	2	2	2	2	2	2	2	2	2
Solanaceae	*Datura stramonium*	Datura	3	2	2	2	2	+	+	+	+	+	+	+	+
	Solanum nigrum	Makoya	4	4	4	3	4	4	4	4	4	4	4	4	4
	S. virginianum (S. xanthocarpum)	Bhrungni	3	3	3	3	3	3	3	3	3	3	3	3	3
	Withania somnifera	Ashwaganda	2	+	+	+	2	+	+	+	+	+	+	2	+
	W. coagulans	Ashwaganda	+	+	+	+	+	+	+	1	+	+	+	+	+
Scrophulariaceae	*Bacopa monnieri*	Brahmi	4	4	3	4	3	3	3	2	4	4	4	3	3
Bignoniaceae	*Oroxylum indicum*	Tentu, Phari	+	1	+	+	+	+	+	+	+	+	+	+	+
	Stereospermum colais	Padal	+	1	+	+	+	+	+	+	1	+	+	+	+
Pedaliaceae	*Pedalium murex*	Gokhru	2	1	2	2	+	+	+	+	+	+	3	+	+
Acanthaceae	*Adhatoda zeylanica*	Adusa	2	2	2	3	2	2	2	2	2	2	2	2	2
	Andrographis paniculata		+	+	+	+	+	2	+	+	+	+	2	+	+

Continued...

...*Continued*

Family	Name of Plant	Hindi Name	Districtwise Present Status*												
			Sirohi	Udaipur	Rajsamand	Banswara	Dungarpur	Chittorgarh	Bhilwara	Ajmer	Kota	Baran	Jhalawar	Bundi	Tonk
Verbenaceae	*Clerodendrum phlomidis*	Arbi	2	3	3	3	2	2	2	3	3	2	2	2	2
	Vitex negundo	Negad	2	4	3	3	3	3	3	2	+	+	+	+	2
Lamiacea (Labiatae)	*Leucas aspera*	Dronpushpi	4	4	4	4	4	4	4	4	3	3	3	3	4
Nyctaginaceae	*Boerrhavia diffusa*	Santi	4	4	4	4	4	4	4	4	4	4	4	4	4
Amaranthaceae	*Achyranthes aspera*	Chirachita	4	4	4	4	4	4	4	4	4	4	4	4	4
	Amaranthus spinosus	Cholai	4	4	4	4	4	4	4	4	4	4	4	4	4
Chenopodiaceae	*Chenopodium album*	Bathua	3	3	3	3	3	3	3	4	4	4	4	4	4
Aristolochiaceae	*Aristolochia bracteolata*	Keedamaar	+	1	2	2	+	+	+	2	2	+	+	+	+
Santalaceae	*Santalum album*	Chandan	+	1	1	+	+	1	1	1	+	+	1	+	+
Euphorbiaceae	*Acalypha indica*		3	3	3	3	3	3	3	3	3	3	3	3	3
	Chrozophora rottlieri		+	3	+	3	+	+	+	+	+	+	3	+	3
	Jatropha curcas	Ratanjot	4	4	4	4	4	4	4	2	4	+	+	+	+
	J. gossypifolia	Jamalgota	3	4	4	3	3	3	4	3	3	3	4	3	3
	Mallotus philippensis	Rohini	4	4	2	2	2	2	2	+	2	2	2	2	2
	Emblica officinalis	Amla	3	3	2	3	3	2	2	2	+	+	+	+	+
	Phyllanthus nirurie	Bhumi amla	3	3	3	3	3	3	3	3	3	3	3	3	3

Continued...

...Continued

Family	Name of Plant	Hindi Name	Districtwise Present Status*												
			Sirohi	Udaipur	Rajsamand	Banswara	Dungarpur	Chittorgarh	Bhilwara	Ajmer	Kota	Baran	Jhalawar	Bundi	Tonk
Gnetaceae	*Ephedra ciliata*	Oontfog	+	+	+	+	+	+	+	1	+	+	+	+	+
Orchidaceae	*Eulophia ochreata*	Saalam mishri	2	2	+	+	+	+	+	+	+	+	+	+	+
Zingiberaceae	*Curcuma indora*	Jungli haldi	1	1	+	+	+	+	+	+	+	+	+	+	+
	C. amada	Jungli haldi	+	+	+	+	+	+	+	+	1	+	+	+	+
Hypoxidaceae	*Curculigo orchiodes*	Kali musli	2	2	2	2	+	2	+	2	2	+	+	+	+
Dioscoreaceae	*Discorea bulbifera*		3	3		2	+	+	2	+	2	+	+	2	+
Liliaceae	*Aloe vera*	Gwarpata	2	2	2	2	2	2	2	2	2	2	2	2	2
	Asparagus racemosus	Shatavar	3	3	3	3	3	3	3	3	3	3	3	3	3
	Chlorophytum borivilianum	Safed musli	2	3	3	2	2	+	+	+	+	+	+	+	+
	Gloriosa superba	Kalihari	3	3	3	3	3	3	3	3	3	3	3	3	3
	Urgenia indica	Kaili kanda	4	4	4	4	4	4	4	3	3	3	3	3	3
Pandanaceae	*Pandanus fascicurlaris*	Kewra	1	1	1	+	+	+	+	+	1	+	+	+	1
Araceae	*Colocasia esculenta*	Jungli arbi	1	1	+	+	+	1	+	+	1	+	+	+	+
Cyperaceae	*Cyperus rotundus*	Nagar Motha	3	3	3	3	3	3	3	3	3	3	3	+	+
Poaceae	*Cympopogon martinii*	Gadheli	1	4	3	3	3	3	3	3	3	3	3	3	+
	Vetiveria zizanioides	Khus khus	3	3	3	3	3	3	3	2	3	3	3	3	3

\+ 1 = Rare 2 = Common 3 = Fairly common 4 = Abundan; ++ Cultivated; (+) No data is available about status of species

TABLE 4-B
Survey of Medicinal Plants of Rajasthan

Family	Name of Plant	Hindi Name	Districtwise Present Status*												
			Pali	Barmer	Jaisalmer	Jodhpur	Bikaner	Ganganagar	Hanumangarh	Churu	Nagaur	Sikar	Jhunjhunu	Sawai Madhopur	Karauli
Annonaceae	*Annona squamosa*	Sitaphal	+	+	+	+	+	+	+	+	+	+	+	+	+
Menispermasceae	*Tinospra cordifolia*	Neem giloy	2	+	+	+	+	+	+	1	+	+	+	+	+
Berberidaceae	*Berberis asiatica*	Daru haldi	+	+	+	+	+	+	+	+	+	+	+	+	+
Nymphaeceae	*Euryale ferox*	Talmakhani	+	+	+	+	+	+	+	+	+	+	+	+	+
	Nelumbo nucifera	Kamal	+	+	+	+	+	+	+	+	+	+	+	2	2
Papaveraceae	*Argemone mexicana*	Satyanasi	4	3	2	2	2	2	2	2	3	4	4	3	3
	*Papaver somnifera***	Afeem	+	+	+	+	+	+	+	+	+	+	+	+	+
Capparidaceae	*Capparis decidua*	Kair	3	3	4	4	4	3	3	4	4	4	4	3	3
	Creteva nurvala	Barna	+	+	+	+	+	+	+	+	+	+	+	+	+
	Maerua arenaria		2	2	+	+	+	+	+	+	+	+	+	2	2
Sterculiaceae	*Helicteresisora*	Marorphali	+	+	+	+	+	+	+	+	+	+	+	+	+
	Sterculia urens	Kadhaya	2	+	+	+	+	+	+	+	+	+	+	2	+
Zygophallyceae	*Peganum harmala*	Harmal	+	+	2	2	2	2	2	2	2	2	2	2	2
Averrhoaceae	*Averrhoa cammbola***	Kamrak	+	+	+	+	+	+	+	+	+	+	+	+	+
Rutaceae	*Aegle marmelos*	Belpatra	+	+	+	+	+	2	+	+	+	+	+	+	+
	Feronia limonia	Kaith	+	+	+	1	1	+	+	+	+	+	+	+	+

Continued...

...*Continued*

Family	Name of Plant	Hindi Name	Districtwise Present Status*												
			Pali	Barmer	Jaisalmer	Jodhpur	Bikaner	Ganganagar	Hanumangarh	Churu	Nagaur	Sikar	Jhunjhunu	Sawai Madhopur	
Balanitaceae	*Balanites aegyptiaca*	Hingore	+	+	+	3	+	+	+	+	+	+	+	+	+
Burseraeceae	*Boswellia serrata*	Salar	4	3	2	2	+	+	+	2	2	+	+	4	4
	Commiphora wightii	Gugal	+	+	2	2	+	+	+	+	+	+	+	+	+
	C. aglocha	Badi gugal	+	+	+	+	+	+	+	+	+	+	+	+	+
Meliaceae	*Azadirachta indica*	Neem	4	3	3	4	3	3	3	2	3	4	4	3	3
Celastraceae	*Celastrus paniculata*	Mal makangni	+	+	+	+	+	+	+	+	+	1	+	+	+
Sapindaceae	*Sapindus imarginatus*	Areetha	+	+	+	1	+	+	+	+	+	+	+	+	+
	Schliechera oleosa	Kusum	+	+	+	+	+	+	+	+	+	+	+	+	+
Anacardiaceae	*Buchanaina lanzan*	Chironji	+	+	+	+	+	+	+	+	+	+	+	+	+
	Manigifera indica	Aam	1	+	1	+	+	+	+	+	+	+	+	2	2
Moringaceae	*Moringa concanensis*	Sehajna	2	+	1	+	+	+	+	1	+	+	+	+	+
	M. oleifera	Sehajna	2	1	1	+	+	+	+	+	+	+	+	+	+
Fabaceae	*Abrus precatorius*	Rati	3	+	+	+	+	+	+	+	2	2	2	3	3
	Desmodium gangeticum	Salmani	3	+	+	+	+	+	+	+	+	+	+	2	+
	Mucuna pruriens	Koch	2	+	+	+	+	+	+	+	+	+	+	3	2
	Pongamia pinnata	Karanj	+	+	1	+	+	+	+	+	+	+	+	+	+
	Psoralea corylifolia	Vavchi	+	+	+	+	+	+	+	+	+	+	+	+	+

Continued...

...*Continued*

Family	Name of Plant	Hindi Name	Districtwise Present Status*												
			Pali	Barmer	Jaisalmer	Jodhpur	Bikaner	Ganganagar	Hanumangarh	Churu	Nagaur	Sikar	Jhunjhunu	Sawai Madhopur	Karauli
	Pterocarpus marsupium	Beeja	+	+	+	+	+	+	+	+	+	+	+	+	+
	Puerana tuberosa	Ghodabel, Modi	+	+	+	+	+	+	+	+	+	+	+	+	+
Caesalpiniceae	*Caesaplinia banduc*	Katakranj	+	+	+	+	+	+	+	+	+	+	+	+	+
	Cassia fistula	Amaltas	2	+	+	2	+	2	+	+	+	+	+	2	2
	C. angustifolia	Sanay	+	+	2	3	+	+	+	+	+	+	+	+	+
	Tamarindus indicus	Imli	2	+	+	2	2	+	+	+	+	+	+	+	2
Mimosaceoe	*Acacia catechu*	Khair	+	+	+	+	+	+	+	+	+	+	+	3	3
	Acacia senegal	Kumti	4	4	4	4	4	3	3	4	4	4	4	3	3
Comfretaceae	*Anogeissus latifolia*	Ghavra	2	+	+	+	+	+	+	+	+	+	+	+	+
	Terminalia arjuna	Arjun	+	+	1	+	+	+	+	+	+	+	+	+	+
	Terminalia bellirica	Baheda	+	+	+	+	+	+	+	+	+	+	+	+	+
Myrtaceae	*Syzygium cumini*	Jamun	2	+	+	+	+	+	+	+	+	+	+	2	2
	S. heyneanum	Makhania jamun	+	+	+	+	+	+	+	+	+	+	+	+	+
Lythraceae	*Ammania baccifera*		2	+	2	+	+	+	+	+	+	+	+	2	+

Continued...

...*Continued*

Family	Name of Plant	Hindi Name	Districtwise Present Status*												
			Pali	Barmer	Jaisalmer	Jodhpur	Bikaner	Ganganagar	Hanumangarh	Churu	Nagaur	Sikar	Jhunjhunu	Sawai Madhopur	Karauli
Cucurbitaceae	*Citrullus colocynthis*	Gartumba	4	4	4	4	4	4	4	4	4	4	4	+	+
	Cucumis melo	Kachri	2	3	4	4	4	4	4	4	4	4	4	+	
	Diplocyclos palmatus	Shivlingi	+	+	+	+	+	+	+	+	+	+	+	+	+
	Momordica dioca	Kikoda	2	+	+	2	+	+	+	+	+	+	+	2	2
Ficoidaceae	*Trianthema portulacastrum*	Santi	2	+	3	+	+	+	+	2	2	3	3	3	3
Apiaceae (Umbelliferae)	*Centella asiatica*	Mandukpani	+	+	+	+	+	+	+	+	+	+	+	+	+
Asteraceae	*Artemisia scoparia*	Bana	+	+	+	+	+	3	+	3	2	3	3	+	+
	Eclipta alba	Bhrungraj	2	+	+	+	+	+	+	1	+	+	+	3	2
	Spilanthes calva	Akarkari	+	+	+	+	+	+	+	+	+	+	+	+	+
	Vernonia cinerea	Sehdevi	2	2	2	2	+	+	+	+	+	+	+	3	3
Plumbaginaceae	*Plumbago zeylanica*	Chitrak	+	+	+	+	+	+	+	+	+	+	+	+	+
Sapotaceae	*Manikara hexandra*	Rayan	+	+	+	+	+	+	+	+	+	+	+	+	+
Ebenaceae	*Diospyros melanoxylon*	Beedi pata	+	+	+	+	+	+	+	+	+	+	+	3	2
Oleaceae	*Nyctanthes arbortristis*	Haarsinghar	3	+	+	+	+	+	+	+	+	+	+	2	2

Continued...

...Continued

Family	Name of Plant	Hindi Name	Districtwise Present Status*												
			Pali	Barmer	Jaisalmer	Jodhpur	Bikaner	Ganganagar	Hanumangarh	Churu	Nagaur	Sikar	Jhunjhunu	Sawai Madhopur	Karauli
Apocynaceae	*Carissa congesta*	Karonda	+	+	+	+	+	+	+	2	+	+	+	+	+
	Holarehena antidysenterica	Indoji	3	+	+	+	+	+	+	+	+	+	+	+	3
Gentianaceae	*Enicostema axillare*	Nami	3	3	2	2	2	2	2	2	2	2	2	3	3
Ehretiaceae	*Cordia dichotoma*	Lisoda	2	2	2	2	+	+	+	+	+	+	2	2	3
Convolvulaceae	*Evolvulus alsinoides*	Shankpushpi	3	3	3	3	3	3	3	3	3	3	3	2	2
Solanaceae	*Datura stramonium*	Datura	2	2	2	3	2	2	2	2	2	2	2	+	+
	Solanum nigrum	Makoya	4	2	2	2	2	2	2	2	3	3	3	4	4
	S. virginianum (S. xanthocarpum)	Bhrungni	3	2	3	2	3	3	3	4	4	3	4	4	3
	Withania somnifera	Ashwaganda	+	2	2	2	2	2	2	2	2	2	2	2	2
	W. coagulans	Ashwaganda	+	+	1	1	+	+	+	+	+	+	+	+	+
Scrophulariaceae	*Bacopa monnieri*	Brahmi	2	+	+	2		3	3	+	+	+	+	4	4
Bignoniaceae	*Oroxylum indicum*	Tentu, Phari	+	+	+	+	+	+	+	+	+	+	+	+	+
	Stereospermum colais	Padal	1	+	+	+	+	+	+	+	+	+	+	+	+
Pedaliaceae	*Pedalium murex*	Gokhru	+	+	+	3	2	3	2	2	2	2	2	2	3

Continued...

...Continued

Family	Name of Plant	Hindi Name	Districtwise Present Status*												
			Pali	Barmer	Jaisalmer	Jodhpur	Bikaner	Ganganagar	Hanumangarh	Churu	Nagaur	Sikar	Jhunjhunu	Sawai Madhopur	Karauli
Acanthaceae	*Adhatoda zeylanica*	Adusa	2	2	2	2	2	+	+	+	+	+	+	2	2
	Andrographis paniculata		+	+	+	+	+	+	+	+	+	+	+	+	+
Verbenaceae	*Clerodendrum phlomidis*	Arbi	2	3	2	3	3	3	3	3	3	4	4	2	2
	Vitex negundo	Negad	3	+	+	2	+	+	+	+	+	+	+	+	+
Lamiaceae (Labiatae)	*Leucas aspera*	Dronpushpi	4	4	4	4	4	4	4	4	3	3	3	3	4
Nyctaginaceae	*Boerrhaavia diffusa*	Santi	4	4	4	4	4	4	4	4	4	4	4	4	4
Amaranthaceae	*Achyranthes aspera*	Chirachita	4	4	4	4	4	4	4	4	4	4	4	4	4
	Amaranthus spinosus	Cholai	4	4	4	4	4	4	4	4	4	4	4	4	4
Chenopodiaceae	*Chenopodium album*	Bathua	3	3	3	3	3	3	3	4	4	4	4	4	4
Aristolochiaceae	*Aristolochia bracteolata*	Keedamaar	+	1	2	2	+	+	+	2	2	+	+	+	+
Santalaceae	*Santalum album*	Chandan	+	1	1	+	+	1	1	1	+	+	1	+	+

Continued...

...Continued

Family	Name of Plant	Hindi Name	Districtwise Present Status*												
			Pali	Barmer	Jaisalmer	Jodhpur	Bikaner	Ganganagar	Hanumangarh	Churu	Nagaur	Sikar	Jhunjhunu	Sawai Madhopur	Karauli
Euphorbiaceae	*Acalypha indica*		3	3	3	3	3	3	3	3	3	3	3	3	3
	Chrozophora rottlieri		+	3	+	3	+	+	+	+	+	+	3	+	3
	Jatropha curcas	Ratanjot	4	4	4	4	4	4	4	2	4	+	+	+	+
	J. gossypifolia	Jamalgota	3	4	4	3	3	3	4	3	3	3	4	3	3
	Mallotus philippensis	Rohini	4	4	2	2	2	2	2	+	2	2	2	2	2
	Emblica officinalis	Amla	3	3	2	3	3	2	2	2	+	+	+	+	+
	Phyllanthus nirurie	Bhumi amla	3	3	3	3	3	3	3	3	3	3	3	3	3
Gnetaceae	*Ephedra ciliata*	Oontfog	+	+	+	+	+	+	+	1	+	+	+	+	+
Orchidaceae	*Eulophia ochreata*	Saalam mishri	2	2	+	+	+	+	+	+	+	+	+	+	+
Zingiberaceae	*Curcuma indora*	Jungli haldi	1	1	+	+	+	+	+	+	+	+	+	+	+
	C. amada	Jungli haldi	+	+	+	+	+	+	+	+	1	+	+	+	+
Hypoxidaceae	*Curculigo orchiodes*	Kali musli	2	2	2	2	+	2	+	2	2	+	+	+	+
Dioscoreaceae	*Dioscorea bulbifera*		3	3		2	+	+	2	+	2	+	+	2	+
Liliaceae	*Aloe vera*	Gwarpata	2	2	2	2	2	2	2	2	2	2	2	3	2
	Asparagus racemosus	Shatavar	3	2	2	2	2	2	2	2	2	2	2	3	3
	Chlorophytum borivilianum	Safed musli	+	+	+	+	+	+	+	+	+	+	+	+	+

Continued...

...Continued

Family	Name of Plant	Hindi Name	Districtwise Present Status*												
			Pali	Barmer	Jaisalmer	Jodhpur	Bikaner	Ganganagar	Hanumangarh	Churu	Nagaur	Sikar	Jhunjhunu	Sawai Madhopur	Karauli
	Glonosa superba	Kalihari	3	3	+	+	+	+	+	+	+	+	+	3	3
	Urgenia indica	Kaili kanda	3	2	2	2	2	2	2	3	2	2	2	3	3
Pandanceae	*Pandanus fascicurlaris*	Kewra	1	+	+	1	+	+	+	+	+	+	1	+	+
Araceae	*Colocasia esculenta*	Jungli arbi	+	+	+	+	+	+	+	+	+	+	+	+	+
Cyperaceae	*Cyperus rotundus*	Nagar Motha	+	+	3	+	+	3	+	+	+	+	+	3	3
Poaceae	*Cymbopogon martinii*	Gadheli	+	2	+	+	+	+	+	+	+	+	+	3	3
	Vetiveria zizanioides	Khus khus	+	+	+	+	+	3	3	+	+	+	+	3	3

\+ 1 = Rare 2 = Common 3 = Fairly common 4 = Abundant
++ Cultivated
(+) No data is available about status of species

TABLE 4-C
Survey of Medicinal Plants of Rajasthan

Family	Name of Plant	Hindi Name	Districtwise Present Status*					
			Jalore	Jaipur	Dausa	Alwar	Bharatpur	Dholpur
Annonaceae	*Annona squamosa*	Sitaphal	+	+	+	+	+	+
Menispermaceae	*Tinospra cordifolia*	Neem giloy	+	4	4	4	4	1
Berberidaceae	*Berberis asiatica*	Daru haldi	+	+	+	+	+	+
Nympheaceae	*Euryale ferox*	Talmakhani	+	+	+	+	+	+
	Nelumbo nucifera	Kamal	+	+	+	+	+	+
Papaveraceae	*Argemone mexicana*	Satyanasi	4	4	4	4	4	4
	*Papaver somnifera***	Afeem	+	+	+	+	+	+
Capparidaceae	*Capparis decidua*	Kair	3	3	3	3	3	3
	Creteva nurvala	Barna	+	+	+	+	+	+
	Maerua arenaria		+	2	1	1	1	1
Sterculiaceae	*Helicteres isora*	Marorphali	+	+	+	+	+	+
	Sterculia urens	Kadhaya	+	1	+	1	+	+
Zygophyllaceae	*Peganum harmala*	Harmal	+	+	+	+	+	+
Averrhoaceae	*Averrhoa cammbola***	Kamrak	+	+	+	+	+	+
Rutaceae	*Aegle marmelos*	Belpatra	+	1	+	1	+	+
	Feronia limonia	Kaith	+	+	+	+	+	+
Balanitaceae	*Balanites aegyptiaca*	Hingore	2	2	2	2	1	1
Burseraceae	*Boswellia serrata*	Salar	+	3	2	+	1	1
	Commiphora wightii	Gugal	+	2	1	2	1	1
	C. aglocha	Badi gugal	+	+	+	+	+	+

Continued...

...*Continued*

Family	Name of Plant	Hindi Name	Districtwise Present Status*					
			Jalore	Jaipur	Dausa	Alwar	Bharatpur	Dholpur
Meliaceae	*Azadirachta indica*	Neem	2	2	2	2	2	2
Celastraceae	*Celastrus paniculata*	Mal makangni	+	+	+	+	+	+
Sapindaceae	*Sapindus imarginatus*	Areetha	+	+	+	1	+	+
	Schliechera oleosa	Kusum	+	+	+	+	+	+
Anacardiaceae	*Buchanania lanzan*	Chironji	+	+	+	+	+	+
	Manigifera indica	Aam	+	1	+	1	+	1
	Moringa concanensis	Sehajna	+	+	+	+	+	+
	M. oleifera	Sehajna	+	1	1	1	1	1
Fabaceae	*Abrus precatorius*	Rati	1	1	1	1	1	1
	Desmodium gangeticum	Salmani	+	+	+	+	+	+
	Mucuna pruriens	Koch	+	+	+	+	+	+
	Pongamia pinnata	Karanj	+	+	+	+	+	+
	Psoralea corylifolia	Vavchi	+	+	+	+	+	+
	Pterocarpus marsupium	Beeja	+	+	+	+	+	+
	Puerana tuberosa	Ghodabel, Modi	+	+	+	+	+	+

Continued...

...*Continued*

Family	Name of Plant	Hindi Name	Districtwise Present Status*					
			Jalore	Jaipur	Dausa	Alwar	Bharatpur	Dholpur
Caesalpiniceae	*Caesaplinia banduc*	Katakranj	+	+	+	+	+	+
	Cassia fistula	Amaltas	+	1	1	1	1	1
	C. angustifolia	Sanay	+	+	+	+	+	+
	Tamarindus indicus	Imli	+	1	1	1	2	1
Mimosaceoe	*Acacia catechu*	Khair	+	+	+	1	+	1
	Acacia senegal	Kumti	+	+	+	1	+	1
Comfretaceae	*Anogeissus latifolia*	Ghavra	+	+	+	+	+	+
	Terminalia arjuna	Arjun	+	+	1	+	+	+
	Terminalia bellirica	Baheda	+	+	+	+	+	+
Myrtaceae	*Syzygium cumini*	Jamun	+	+	+	+	+	+
	S. heyneanum	Makhania jamun	+	+	+	+	+	+
Lythraceae	*Ammania baccifera*		+	+	+	+	+	+
Cururbitaceae	*Citrullus colocynthis*	Gartumba	1	1	1	1	1	
	Cucumis melo	Kachri	1	1	1	1	1	1
	Diplocyclos palmatus	Shivlingi	+	+	+	+	+	+
	Momordica dioca	Kikoda	+	+	+	+	+	+
Ficoidceae	*Trianthema portulacastrum*	Santi	1	2	2	3	4	2

Continued...

...*Continued*

Family	Name of Plant	Hindi Name	Districtwise Present Status*					
			Jalore	Jaipur	Dausa	Alwar	Bharatpur	Dholpur
Apiaceae (Umbelliferae)	*Centella asiatica*	Mandukpani	+	+	+	+	+	+
Asteraceae	*Artemisa scoparia*	Bana	+	3	3	3	3	+
	Eclipta alba	Bhrungraj	+	1	1	1	1	1
	Spilanthes calva	Akarkari	+	+	+	+	+	+
	Vernonia cinerea	Sehdevi	+	2	2	2	3	3
Plumbaginacea	*Plumbago zeylanica*	Chitrak	+	+	+	+	+	+
Sapotaceae	*Manikara hexandra*	Rayan	+	+	+	+	+	+
Ebenaceae	*Diospyros melanoxylon*	Beedi pata	+	1	+	1	+	+
Oleaceae	*Nyctanthes arbortristis*	Haarsinghar	+	+	+	+	+	+
Apocynaceae	*Carissa congesta*	Karonda	+	+	+	+	+	+
	Holarehena antidysenterica	Indoji	2	+	+	1	+	+
Gentianaceae	*Enicostema axillare*	Nami	3	+	+	+	+	+
Ehretiaceae	*Cordia' dichotoma*	Lisoda	3	2	2	2	2	1
Convolvulaceae	*Evolvulus alsinoides*	Shankpushpi	3	2	2	2	2	2
Solanaceae	*Datura stramonium*	Datura	2	1	1	1	1	1
	Solanum nigrum	Makoya	2	4	4	4	4	3

Continued...

...*Continued*

Family	Name of Plant	Hindi Name	Districtwise Present Status*					
			Jalore	Jaipur	Dausa	Alwar	Bharatpur	Dholpur
	S. virginianum (S. xanthocarpum)	Bhrungni	2	4	4	4	4	2
	Withania somnifera	Ashwaganda	2	2	2	2	2	+
	W. coagulans	Ashwaganda	+	+	+	+	+	+
Scrophulariaceae	*Bacopa monnieri*	Brahmi	+	2	2	2	2	2
Bignoniaceae	*Oroxylum indicum*	Tentu, Phari	+	+	+	+	+	+
	Stereospermum colais	Padal	1	+	+	+	+	+
Pedaliaceae	*Pedalium murex*	Gokhru	+	4	4	4	4	+
Acanthaceae	*Adhatoda zeylanica*	Adusa	+	3	3	3	2	+
	Andrographis paniculata		+	+	+	+	+	+
Verdenaceae	*Clerodendrum phlomidis*	Arbi	2	4	4	4	4	1
	Vitex negundo	Negad	+	1	1	1	1	+
Lamiacea (Labiatae)	*Leucas aspera*	Dronpushpi	3	3	3	3	3	2
Nyctaginaceae	*Boerrhavia diffusa*	Santi	4	4	4	4	4	4
Amaranthaceae	*Achyranthes aspera*	Chirachita	4	4	4	4	4	4
	Amaranthus spinosus	Cholai	4	4	4	4	4	4

Continued...

...Continued

Family	Name of Plant	Hindi Name	Districtwise Present Status*					
			Jalore	Jaipur	Dausa	Alwar	Bharatpur	Dholpur
Chenopodiaceae	*Chenopodium album*	Bathua	3	4	4	4	4	3
Aristolochiaceae	*Aristolochia bracteolata*	Keedamaar	+	+	+	+	+	+
Santalaceae	*Santalum album*	Chandan	+	+	+	+	+	+
Euphorbiaceae	*Acalypha indica*		2	3	3	3	3	2
	Chrozophora rottlieri		+	+	+	+	+	+
	Jatropha curcas	Ratanjot	+	+	+	+	+	+
	J. gossypifolia	Jamalgota	+	+	+	+	+	+
	Mallotus philippensis	Rohini	+	+	+	+	+	+
	Emblica officinalis	Amla	+	+	+	+	+	+
	Phyllanthus nirurie	Bhumi amla	+	3	3	3	4	4
Gnetaceae	*Ephedra ciliata*	Oontfog	+	+	+	+	+	+
Orchidaceae	*Eulophia ochreata*	Saalam mishri	+	+	+	+	+	+
Zingiberaceae	*Curcuma indora*	Jungli haldi	+	+	+	+	+	+
	C. amada	Jungli haldi	+	+	+	+	+	+
Hypoxidaceae	*Curculigo orchiodes*	Kali musli	+	+	+	+	+	+
Dioscoreaceae	*Dioscorea bulbifera*		+	+	+	+	+	+
Liliaceae	*Aloe vera*	Gwarpata	2	1	1	1	1	1

Continued...

...Continued

Family	Name of Plant	Hindi Name	Districtwise Present Status*					
			Jalore	Jaipur	Dausa	Alwar	Bharatpur	Dholpur
	Asparagus racemosus	Shatavar	2	2	2	2	2	3
	Chlorophytum borivilianum	Safed musli	+	+	+	+	+	+
	Gloriosa superba	Kalihari	2	1	1	1	1	1
	Urgenia indica	Kaili kanda	2	1	1	1	1	1
Pandanceae	*Pandanus fascicurlaris*	Kewra	+	+	+	+	+	+
Araceae	*Colocasia esculenta*	Jungli arbi	+	+	+	+	+	+
Cyperareae	*Cyperus rotundus*	Nagar Motha	+	1	1	1	3	2
Poaceae	*Cymbopogon martinii*	Gadheli	+	+	+	+	+	+
	Vetiveria zizanioides	Khus khus	+	2	2	2	4	2

\+ 1 = Rare 2 = Common 3 = Fairly common 4 = Abundant
++ Cultivated
(+) No data is available about status of species

Rajasthan has taken a good start in this direction. Medicinal herbal gardens have been established at Nal Sandol (Jhadol), Makodia (Ogna), Banki Forest Research Centre (Sisarma), all in Udaipur district, Bhimana and Mt. Abu in Sirohi district, Sarvan Deri in Banswara district and World Forestry Arboretum in Jaipur district. An *Aloe vera* reservoir is being developed near Ubheshwar in Udaipur district. Medicinal plants are now planted in routine plantations also to increase their availability in nature. A medicinal plant cell has been established in the department for conservation and preservation of medicinal plant species in natural forests.

5. A public awareness campaign is necessary to protect the medicinal plants in the wild. Village Forest Protection and Management Committees (VFPMC) can prove good in this work.
6. Agriculturisation of certain species should be promoted to minimise pressure on forests. There is a great scope in this field. Scientific agriculture of certain medicinal species can uplift the socio-economic status of many families of rural areas.
7. Negative factors, responsible for decrease and destruction of medicinal plants in nature should be identified, analysed and suitable measures should be adopted to minimise them. Our target should be forests, fallow lands, grasslands and all other known habitats.

STATUS OF MEDICINAL PLANTS IN VARIOUS PARTS OF RAJASTHAN

Two plants, namely *Commiphora wightii* and *Rosa involucreta* are Red Data Book species in Rajasthan. *Rosa involucreta* is confined to upper reaches of Mt. Abu hills in a very restricted area while *Commiphora wightii* is widely distributed in the State. This species is present in Haldighati, Jagat, Chirwa Ghata (Amberi), Thur Magra, Sajjangarh Wildlife Sanctuary, Kurabad (all in Udaipur district), Jhalana Kukas, Jamwa Ramgarh Wildlife Sanctuary, Nahargarh Wildlife Sanctuary (all in Jaipur district), Sirawas-Ki-Rundh, Tiger Project Sariska, Jindoli-Ki-Ghati, Renagiri (all in Alwar district), Bagdi (Jassakheda-Sojat Road), Machind (near Nathdwara), forest areas near Jawaja (Ajmer district), Todgarh-Ravli Wildlife Sanctuary, Kumbhalgarh Wildlife Sanctuary, Heera-Ka-Wadia (Beawar-Bhilwara Road, Rajsamand district), forest areas of Dholpur and Tonk districts, etc. This species is also present on hills of Thar desert zone. This species is so important, so widely distributed that it can be declared as "State Medicinal Plant of Rajasthan."

Rajasthan is rich in other medicinal plants also. A list of a few of them with their status is given in Table 4.

REFERENCES

Bhandari, M. M. *Flora of the Indian Desert*, pp. 1-435, 1990.

Billore, K. V. and Audichya, K. C. 'Some oral contraceptives—family planning tribal ways'. *Jour. Res. Ind. Med. Yoga & Homoeo*. 13: 104-109, 1978.

Joshi, P. 'Herbal drugs in tribal Rajasthan—from child birth to child care'. *Ethnobotany* 1:77-87, 1989.

Joshi, P. 'The forest herbal resources and Bhil medicine'. In: *Social Forestry in Tribal Development*. (Ed.). Vyas, N. N. *Tribe* (Spl. No.) 13 (2-4): 129-136, 1981.

Joshi, P. 'Tribal remedies against snake bite and scorpion stings in Rajasthan'. In: *Glimpses in Plant Research,* vol. 10. *Medicinal Plants—New Vistas in Research.* (Eds.). Singh, V. K. and Vovil, J. N. New Delhi: Today and Tomorrow's Printers and Publishers, 1993.

Joshi, P. *Ethnobotany of the Primitive Tribes in Rajasthan.* Jaiur:Printwell Publishers,1995.

Sebastian, M. K. and Bhandari, M. M. 'Medicinal plant lore in Udaipur district, Rajasthan'. *Bull. Medico. Ethno. Bot. Res.* 5(3-4): 133-134, 1988.

Sebastian, M. K. and Bhandari, M. M. 'Medico-ethnobotany of Mt. Abu, Rajasthan'. *Journal of Ethnopharmacology* 12: 223-230, 1984a.

Sebastian, M. K. and Bhandari, M. M. 'Some plants used as veterinary medicines by Bhils'. *Intern. J. Trop. Agric.* 11(4): 307-310, 1984b.

Sharma, B. D. and Vyas, M. S. 'Ethnobotanical studies on the ferns and fern allies of Rajasthan'. *Bull. Bot. Surv. India* 29(1-4): 90-91, 1985.

Sharma, K. L. Survey of medicinal plants in Aravallis in Jhadol Tehsil with special reference to their pharmacogonosical studies. M.D. (Ayurveda) Dissertation. M. M. Malaviya Govt. Ayurvedic College, Udaipur, 1998.

Sharma, S. and Tiagi, B. *Flora of North-East Rajasthan,* pp. 1-540. Ludhiana: Kalyani Publishers, 1979.

Sharma, S. K. 'Addition to fish stupefying plants employed by tribals of southern Rajasthan'. *J. Econ. Tax. Bot.* 21(1): 249, 1997c.

Sharma, S. K. 'Dependency of the tribals of southern Rajasthan on plants'. *Vijnana Parishad Anusandhan Patrika* 44(1): 54-67, 2001c.

Sharma, S. K. 'Distribution of Wild Plantain (*Ensete superbum*) in Rajasthan'. *Indian Journal of Environmental Science* 5(1): 97-100, 2001a.

Sharma, S. K. '*Eulophia ochreata*: A useful plant for tribals of southern Rajasthan'. *J. Econ. Tax. Bot.* 21(3): 721, 1997a.

Sharma, S. K. 'Henna of Bhils'. *J. Econ. Tax. Bot.* 21(1): 250, 1997b.

Sharma, S. K. 'New record of *Nervilia aragoana* in Rajasthan'. *JBNHS* 98(3): 493, 2001b.

Sharma, S. K. 'On the occurrence of *Leea macrophylla* Roxb. (Vitaceae) in Rajasthan'. *JBNHS* 97(3): 46-57, 2000.

Sharma, S. K. 'Plants used as henna dye by Bhils of southern Rajasthan'. *J. Econ. Tax. Bot.* 23(2): 257, 1999a.

Sharma, S. K. 'Rajasthan: Some plant specialities'. *Vijnana Parishad Anusandhan Patrika* 46(2): 175-184, 2003.

Sharma, S. K. 'Tuberous plants of Sitamata, Phulwari and Sajjangarh Sanctuaries'. *Vijnana Parishad Anusandhan Patrika* 42(4): 278-285, 1999b.

Sharma, S. K. 'Use of bamboo by tribals of Rajasthan'. *Vijnana Parishad Anusandhan Patrika* 41(2): 127-143, 1998b.

Sharma, S. K. 'Use of *Lindenbergia muraria* leaves and *Impatiens balsamina* flowers as a substitute for henna'. *JBNHS* 95(1): 150, 1998a.

Shetty, B. V. and Pandey, R. P. *Flora of Tonk District.* Botanical Survey of India, pp. 1-253. 1983.

Shetty, B. V. and Singh, V *Flora of Rajasthan*, vols. I to III, 1987-1993.

Singh, V. *Flora of Banswara, Rajasthan*. Botanical Survey of India, pp. 1-312, 1983.

Singh, V. and Pandey, R. P. 'Medicinal plant-lore of the tribals of Eastern Rajasthan'. *J. Econ. Tax. Bot.* 1:137-147, 1980.

—oo(O)oo—

12

Important Diseases of Medicinal and Aromatic Plants and Their Management Practices

Anand Singh, Rakesh Pandey and H. B. Singh

AROMATIC PLANTS

1. *Mentha* Species

Mints (*Mentha* species), belonging to the family Lamiaceae, are a group of aromatic herbs of considerable economic importance. The economically important products of mints are the essential oils obtained by steam distillation of their herbage. These essential oils are used in the food, pharmaceutical, cosmetic and perfumery industries. In recent years, interest in the cropping of mints has increased because of increasing demand for their oils and specific fractions thereof in the international market. The herb itself is used in its fresh, dried and processed forms for flavouring the items of food and in the preparation of traditional medicines. Mints are widely cultivated on almost all types of soils and climates. The major commercially produced species are Japanese or menthol mint (*Mentha arvensis* L. var. *piperascens*), peppermint (*Mentha piperita* L.), common or native spearmint (*Mentha spicata* L.), scotch spearmint (*Mentha cardiaca* Baker), garden mint (*Mentha viridis* L.) and bergamot mint (*Mentha citrata* Ehrh.). China, India, the U. S. A., Japan, France, Italy, Russia and Bulgaria are some of the major producers of mint oils.

As with most agricultural crops, diseases impose significant production constraints affecting both yield and overall quality of mint oils. Mints have been reported to be susceptible to a variety of diseases. Some of these reduce the yield from mint crops, especially when virulent forms of one or more of them attack the monoclonal mint crops spread over wide areas.

Among the 30 or more pathogens recorded on mints, about a dozen are of major economic importance. Some important diseases of mints are given below.

Diseases in Mints

Fungal Diseases: The most economically serious diseases of mints are caused by fungi.

The major fungal pathogens of mints are *Alternaria alternata* (leaf spot), *Erysiphe cichoracearum* (powdery mildew), *Phoma strasseri* (stem rot), *Puccinia menthae* (rust), *Rhizoctonia solani/ Rhizoctonia bataticola* (root and stolon rot), *Sclerotium rolfsii* (collar rot) and *Verticillium dahlia*. The intensity of damage caused by them has been found to vary according to specific location and genotypes. The wilt rust and stem rot are more common in the U. S. A. while leaf blight, powdery mildew and root rot have been found to cause more severe diseases in India.

(i). Rust (*Puccinia menthae*)

The disease has been reported from all the mint-growing countries and is believed to be present on most of the cultivated species of mint. Peppermint, however, appears to be relatively more sensitive. The rust was first recorded in the beginning of this century in Germany on *Mentha arvensis* and *Mentha piperita* (Cruchet, 1907; Das and Sultana, 1979) and India on leaves of *Mentha sylvestris* from Kashmir and Himachal Pradesh (Butler and Bisby, 1931). This disease in recent years has assumed importance in India after it appeared in epidemic proportions on *Mentha arvensis* in the Terai region of the Uttar Pradesh, now in Uttaranchal, a prime area for mint cultivation (Anonymous, 1997). The leaves of the affected plants show characteristic dark brown uredial pustules (Plate I g and j) and consequent leaf fall is common. In a study, about 20 per cent of *Mentha arvensis* leaves were found to fall off due to rust attack (Ganguly and Pandotra, 1962). In Bulgaria, the severity of the disease is much more as the resultant losses can surpass 50 per cent (Margina and Zheljazkov. 1994).

Puccinia menthae is a macrocyclic autoecious rust. Uredosori are produced on leaves, stems and runners. Uredospores (17-28 × 14-19 μm) are borne singly. The aecial stage has not been observed in India (Ganguly and Pandotra, 1962). Teliospores (37 × 20 μm) are brown, two-celled, pedicillate, obtuse to slightly pointed.

High degree of physiological specialisation has been observed (Bruckner, 1972; Walker and Corroy, 1969). Rust isolates from *Mentha spicata* have been found to infect *Mentha cardiaca* but not *Mentha piperita*. The biotypes that infected *Mentha piperita* were avirulent on *Mentha spicata* (Roberts and Horner, 1981). Eight races of *Puccinia menthae* were identified in France during the early part of the century (Cruchet, 1907). Six races were found in North Eastern United States (Neiderhauser, 1945), 9 races in England (Fletcher, 1963) and 3 races in New Zealand (Bressford, 1982). A total of 15 physiological races have been observed on mints in the U. S. A. (Baxter and Cummins, 1953). In another study, a high degree of physiologic specialisation was found within the 17 collections of *Puccinia menthae* on mint hosts (Johnson, 1995).

Rust has been found to persist on the runners of the host as uredospores (Wheeler, 1969). In another study on disease cycle of rust carried out on peppermint in Oregon, the fungus was found to overwinter only as teliospores (Horner, 1963). The main agents of dissemination of the disease appear to be uredospores; the sporidia and aeciospores seem to be involved only marginally (Dietz *et al,* 1951; Stone and Green, 1967). Maximum germination of uredospores occurs at 20°C (El-Zayat *et al,* 1994). The bottom and middle leaves of the mint plant are more prone to rust disease (Bhardwaj *et al,* 1995). The disease increases in severity when cultivation is continued in the same area for several years (Kral, 1977). The rust pathogen produces symptoms on leaves, which appears as elliptical blisters or pustules on leaves, stem and runners. These blisters develop parallel with long axis of leaf, stem and runners. The epidermis covering the pustules is later ruptured irregularly and pushed back revealing a powder mass of brick red coloured uredospores (Plate 1a). Later in the

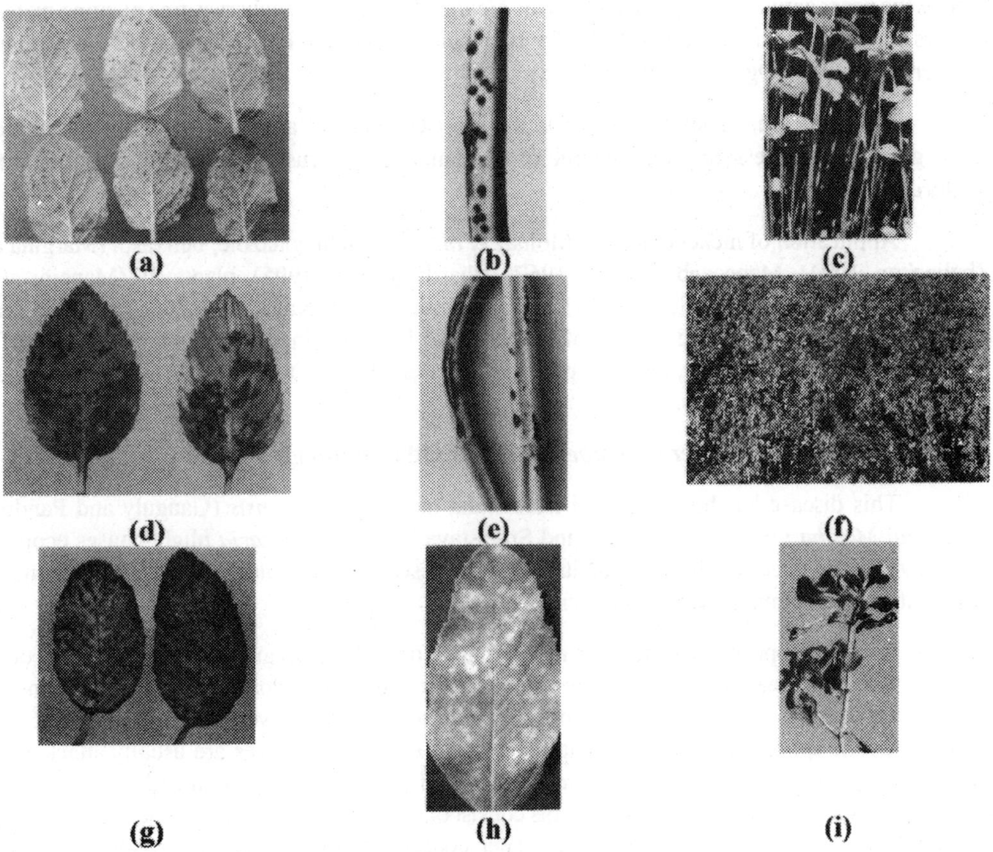

Plate I.

(a). Rust symptoms (uredial pustules) on *Mentha arvensis* leaves; (b). Telial pustules on stem of *Mentha arvensis*; (c). Defoliation of lower leaves of *Mentha arvensis* by rust pathogen; (d). Leaves of *Mentha arvensis* showing blight symptom caused by *Alternaria alternata;* (e). *Alternaria* infection on stem of *Mentha arvensis;* (f). A portion of field view showing severe blight due to *A. alternata* on *Mentha arvensis;* (g). *Curvularia* leaf spot of *Mentha arvensis*; (h). Powdery mildew of *Mentha arvensis;* (i). Aerial blight of *Mentha arvensis* caused by *Rhizoctonia solani.*

season, as the plant approaches maturity, the rusty colour of pustules turns black and fungus produces teliospores (37 × 20 μm) which are brown coloured, two-celled, pedicillate and obtuse to slightly pointed (Plate 1b). The aecial stage has not been observed in India. In severe conditions, defoliation can be seen in the field (Plate 1c).

The disease can be avoided by using the disease-free planting material; this is especially important in *Mentha piperita, Mentha spicata* and *Mentha cardiaca,* where aboveground parts are used as the propagative material. In the case of *Mentha arvensis,* to obtain rust-free planting material, runners are treated with hot water at 112°F for 10 minutes (Staniland, 1947) or at 44.4°C for 10 minutes (Neiderhauser, 1945; Ogilvie and Brian, 1935).

Planting clones resistant to rust is the most economical approach to check rust disease. Some genotypes possessing a high degree of resistance against rust have recently been identified (Kalra *et al,* 1997).

Application of nickel chloride (Molnaz *et al,* 1960), tebuconazole, belixasol (Margina and Zheljazkov, 1994), Mancozeb (Melian, 1967), Bhardwaj *et al,* 1995), plantavax (Mancini *et al,* 1976), propiconazole and diclobutazol (Nagy and Szalay, 1985; Kalra *et al,* 2001) permit reliable protection against rust. Good control of rust has also been obtained by spraying the soil surface with denitoroamine (Campbell, 1956), at pre-emergence and Krezonit–E (DNOC) at shoot emergence (Suab and Nagy, 1972) stages.

(ii). Leaf Spot (*Alternaria alternata*) and Other Pathogens

This disease has been reported from India on *Mentha arvensis* (Ganguly and Pandotra, 1962) and *Mentha piperita* (Srivastava and Srivastava, 1971). *Alternaria* blight causes economic losses by inflicting heavy defoliation on its host. The disease is particularly severe during monsoon, though it is also common during summer months.

Infection appears in the form of round to oval or slightly irregular dark brown spots on the upper surface of the leaf. The leaf spots developed as a result of infection of *Alternaria* are generally dark brown to black, often numerous and enlarging and usually developing in concentric rings which gives the spots a target-like appearance (Plate 1d). Lower, leaves are usually attacked first but the disease progresses upwards and makes affected leaves turn yellowish and senescent which either dry up and droop or fall off. These spots consist of concentric rings/zones, which are surrounded by pale yellow margin (Jain, 1995). Spots later coalesce forming large dark patches leading to defoliation, which is often heavy, with a marked decrease in essential oil content (Ganguly and Pandotra, 1962). The stem may also be infected (Plate 1e) and after severe infection the severely affected fields may show blighted appearance (Plate 1f).

Conidia (22.8–74.8 × 9.8–16.3 mm) are found in chains of up to six with a short apical beak, mostly 3-5 septate with slight constriction at the cross septa.

Sometimes, the disease is also found to be associated with uredia of mint rust *(Puccinia menthae)* on *Mentha arvensis,* the *Alternaria* spots occurring on the upper surface and the uredia on the undersurface (Shukla *et al,* 1997).

Spraying of copper fungicides provides an effective control of the disease (Sastry *et al,* 1982).

TABLE 1
Minor Leaf Spot Diseases of Mint (*Mentha* sp.)

Pathogen	Host	References
Corynespora cassicola	*M. arvensis*	Sattar *et al,* 1981; Singh & Husain, 1993.
Cercospora menthicola	*M. canadensis,* *M. sylvestris.* *M. arvensis*	Stone *et al,* 1962; Shukla, 1995; Munjal *et al,* 1961.
Septoria menthae	*Mentha* sp. *M.cardiaca*	Green & Savada, 1960; Hemmi & Kurata, 1933; Savada & Green, 1961.

(iii). *Curvularia lunata*

The disease was first reported by Thakur and Husain (1974) on *Mentha arvensis.* The first symptoms of the disease appear as minute dirty brownish spots scattered all over the leaves. Later, with the advance of the disease, the spots increase in size becoming spherical or irregular patches of larger sizes. Though the symptoms may appear at any stage of growth of the plant but larger spots usually occur on lower leaves only (Plate 1g). The remaining portions of the infected leaves become chlorotic and finally wither away.

The leaf spots on mints are also caused by several other fungal species, some of which are listed in Table 1.

(iv). Anthracnose (*Sphaceloma menthae*)

This disease causes stunting, defoliation and loss in economic yield in peppermint, spearmint and menthol mint. It is common in mint-growing areas of the U. S. A. (Baines, 1938) and Yugoslavia (Dermelj, 1960). The fungus grows well at temperatures of 14-28°C while temperatures of 21-28°C appear favourable for the disease development. Saturation of the atmosphere for 48 hours at >15°C promoted infection, which did not take place at 80 per cent R.H. (Dermelj, 1960). Over-wintering of the fungus was shown to occur on infected mint debris (Baines, 1938). Use of planting material from healthy crop helps to prevent this disease. Application of Ferbam and copper oxychloride checks the disease to some extent (Dermelj, 1960).

(v). Powdery Mildew *(Erysiphe cichoracearum)*

This disease has been reported from Argentina (Ramallo, 1992), the USSR (Byzova, 1961) and India (Ganguly and Pandotra, 1962). Powdery mildew is severe during the months of April-May. The yield of essential oil is reduced up to 20 per cent due to defoliation. The disease first appears on young leaves as slightly raised blister like areas that soon become covered with greyish, white and powdery growth of the pathogen on mature leaves (Plate 1h), though the fungal growth appears but there is little distortion. The white patches of fungal growth similar to those observed on the leaves may also be seen on green stolons and stems, which may coalesce and cover the entire surface. Dusting of wettable sulphur (Ganguly and Pandotra, 1962) or application of Karathane effectively checks the disease.

(vi). Aerial Blight *(Rhizoctonia solani)*

This disease causing moderate to severe aerial blight has been reported from India on *Mentha viridis* (Sharma and Mahmud, 1951), *Mentha citrata, Mentha piperita* and *Mentha sylvestris* (Sharma and Munjal, 1978). Maximum loss of herbage has been found to occur in *Mentha arvensis* and *Mentha spicata,* which are relatively more prone to *Rhizoctonia* aerial blight than other species of *Mentha.* The infected plants show typical blight symptoms (Plate 1I). The disease is particularly damaging after the first harvest (Bhardwaj *et al,* 1980) and when the crop is closely planted (Bhardwaj and Garg, 1986).

The disease first appears on leaf surfaces as faded patches, which generally start from the margin and extend inwards under moist and humid weather. Later the blight extends towards twigs/stem causing necrosis of the above-ground parts (Bhardwaj *et al,* 1980). In the case of severe infection, fungal webs can be seen on aerial portion. Sometimes sclerotia of the pathogen are also seen on dark brown coloured bodies in fungal webs.

Early planting of the crop to avoid rainy months during maturity reduces the resultant losses. One or two applications of Mancozeb or Carbendazim are also quite helpful in restricting aerial blight.

(vii). Stolon Rot (Multiple agents)

Stolon rot or stolon decay caused by *Rhizoctonia bataticola* was first recorded on *Mentha cardiaca* (Green, 1961) and subsequently on *Mentha arvensis* and *Mentha spicata* (Husain and Janardhanan, 1965). Singh (1991) reported that stolon rot is a complex of *Rhizoctonia solani* and *Rhizoctonia bataticola.* The initial symptoms of the disease are yellowing followed by the death of the whole plant. Underground stolons exhibit pinkish brown lesions in the earlier stages, which gradually turn into dark brown or black patches (Plate IIb). These patches increase in size and finally result in decay of a portion or entire stolon. The disease can be checked if healthy planting material is used and practices like deep summer ploughing and crop rotation are followed (Jain, 1995). Treatment of the stolons before planting with Zineb or Mancozeb or Captan is quite effective in reducing the losses caused by this disease (Sastry, 1969).

Thielavia basicola has also been reported to cause stolon and root rot in *Mentha arvensis* (Sattar and Husain, 1976). The incidence of *Thielavia* rot was found to be severe in soils of high moisture and low aeration. The stolons show typical wilting symptoms (Plate IIc). To avoid the spreading of disease through stolons, healthy stolons should be multiplied in a disease-free plot.

(viii). Collar Rot *(Sclerotium rolfsii)*

This disease so far reported from Japan (Goto, 1933) and India (Ganguly and Pandotra, 1962; Singh *et al,* 1999), is serious only in rich and heavy soils. White mycelial strands develop around the infected collar portion resulting in yellowing and wilting of the plant. In advanced stages, white mustard like sclerotial bodies develop around the collar portion and the plant topples down (Plate IIe). *Mentha spicata* and *Mentha arvensis* are relatively tolerant to this disease (Pandotra and Sastry, 1968). Singh *et al* (1999) reported two new species of *Mentha* as hosts of *Sclerotium rolfsii.* Deep summer ploughing and an effective and proper drainage help in reducing the incidence of the disease (Jain, 1995). Singh (1996) reported that use of different species of *Trichoderma* and *Gliocladium* can effectively control the disease.

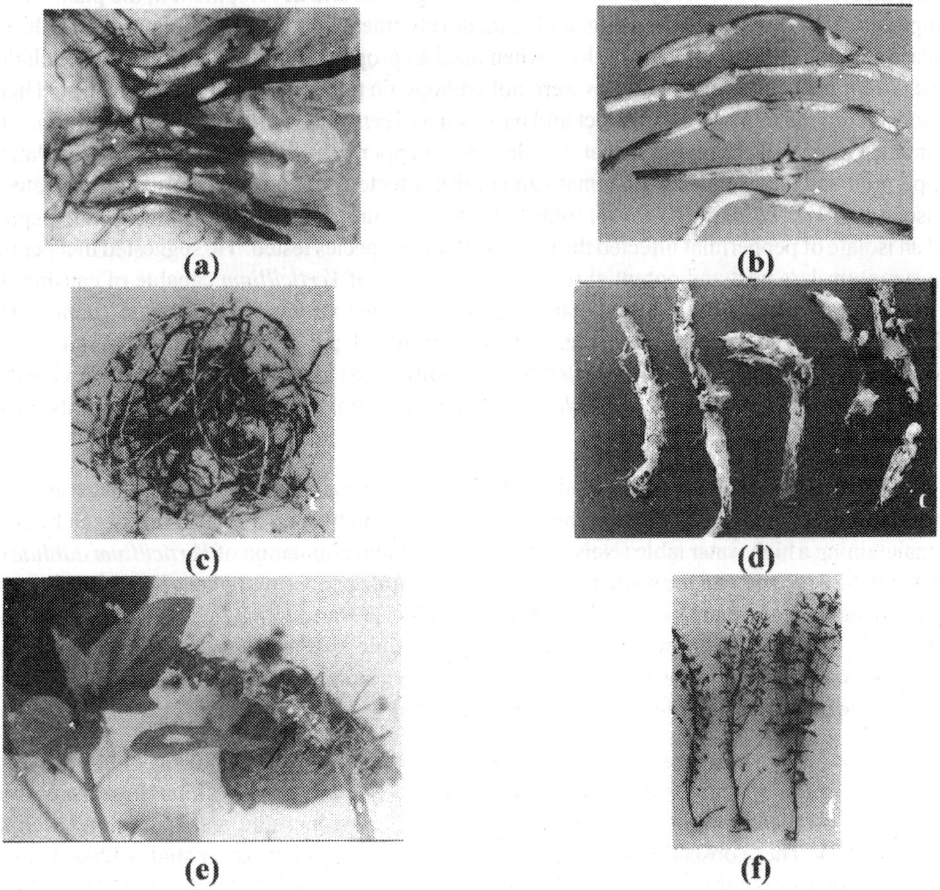

Plate II.

(a). Stolon decay of *Mentha arvensis* caused by *Fusarium* species; (b). Stolon rot and decay of *Mentha arvensis* caused by *Rhizoctonia solani;* (c). Stolon rot and decay of *Mentha arvensis* caused by *Thielavia basicola;* (d). Stolon rot caused of *Mentha arvensis* caused by *Sclerotinia sclerotioru;.* (e). Collar rot of *Mentha arvensis* caused by *Sclerotium rolfsii.* Note brown coloured sclerotia on the surface of infected stem (arrow); (f). Fusarial wilt symptoms of *Mentha spicata* (left) and healthy (right).

(ix). Wilt (*Verticillium* and *Fusarium* Species)

Verticillium wilt had been a serious problem in mints, especially peppermint, in the U. S. A. from the early part of this century. *Verticillium dahliae* and *Verticillium albo-atrum* are the causing organisms in *Mentha piperita* and *Mentha cardiaca* (Nelson, 1926). The pathogen is soil-borne, infects the roots thereby affecting the normal growth and development in the plant. The main symptoms of the disease are dwarfing, unilateral development of branches, etiolation and wilting. The disease spreads through infected stolons when used as propagating material. Nelson concluded that *Verticillium* isolates from other hosts were not pathogenic to peppermint and vice-versa. Therefore, he considered the mint fungus distinct and named it as *Verticillium albo-atrum* var. *menthae.* On the contrary, Green (1951) reported that eggplant and pepper were hosts of *Verticillium* isolates from peppermint and that isolates from tomato and radish infected peppermint. Horner (1954) later tested 17 isolates of *Verticillium albo-atrum* from 11 hosts and found that these were infectious to peppermint and an isolate of peppermint infected the roots of all plant species tested. He suggested that peppermint is a symptom-less host and potential reservoir for strains of *Verticillium* capable of causing disease in other crops. Green (1977) found that isolate pathogenic to mints is *Verticillium. dahliae* (micro-sclerotial). He further suggested that host specificity of peppermint and spearmint isolates of *Verticillium dahliae* has changed under field conditions as potato cv. Superior previously non-susceptible to mint isolate of *Verticillium dahliae* has shown increased susceptibility in a near mono-culture.

Soil moisture influences the development of disease and excessive drainage and drought have increased the destructiveness of the disease and acceptable commercial control can be achieved by maintaining a high water table (Nelson, 1937). Maximum population of *Verticillium dahliae* occurs in the top 0-30 cm soil and the rooted cuttings of susceptible peppermint plants have shown maximum infection incidence in samples taken from 0-15 cm and 15-30 cm depth (Green, 1937). The number of propagates of *Verticillium* recovered from the susceptible species, *Mentha piperita* exceeded the number recovered from resistant species, *Mentha crispa* indicating that proliferation of *Verticillium dahliae* is faster in susceptible host (Brandt *et al,* 1984).

Verticillium. nigrescens was also isolated from peppermint plant showing mild wilt symptoms. Inoculation of this species on different plant species revealed that *Verticillium nigrescens* colonises the roots of all plant species and is weakly pathogenic to peppermint and spearmint (Melouk and Horner, 1974). These observations, however, differ from those of an earlier study of Skotland (1971) who found that *Verticillium nigrescens* is non-pathogenic to peppermint and spearmint. Protective effects in mints (*Mentha spicata* and *Mentha piperita)* by inoculation with mild pathogen *Verticillium nigrescens* to subsequent inoculations with a virulent strain of *Verticillium dahliae* (cross protection) have been observed (Melouk and Horner, 1975). Cross-protection effects were maximum when inoculation with *Verticillium nigrescens* preceded *Verticillium dahliae* by 7-9 days.

Soil inversion during summer and use of healthy planting material (Jain, 1995) reduces the incidence of disease. Heat treatment of mint rhizomes at 47°C for 55 minutes or 48°C for 35 minutes results in production of greatest percentage of viable disease-free rhizomes (Porter and Himmelick, 1952). Fumigation of soil (Green, 1958, 1964) and five years of maize or reed canary grass rotation (Green, 1967; Horner and Dooley, 1966) are also effective ways of reducing the wilt severity. Singh *et al* (2001) used *Trichoderma harzianum* and *Gliocladium virens* to control wilt and rot of mints and found significant reduction in the disease incidence.

TABLE 2
Other Fungal Diseases of Mints

Disease	Pathogen	Host	Reference
Downy mildew	*Perenospora stigmaticola*	*M. arvensis*	Bai *et al,* 1991; Cheng and Bai, 1986; Saville, 1951.
Typhula root rot	*Typhula itoana*	*M. piperita*	Steenland & Burke, 1950.

In India, a wilt of *Mentha arvensis* caused by *Fusarium oxysporum* has also been recorded (Sattar and Husain, 1978). The stolons show typical wilting symptoms accompanied with the yellowing of leaves (Plate IIa & f).

(x). Rhizome or Stem Rot *(Phoma strasseri)*

Phoma strasseri causes the common rot disease in peppermint (Horner, 1971; Paizs and Nagy, 1975) and spearmint (Melouk *et al,* 1975), in the U. S. A. and Japan (Mano *et al,* 1964). Disease symptoms consist of reddening of leaves, wilting and stunting of plants. On above-ground stem, infection occurs near the soil-surface forming sunken cankers, which later girdle the stem and plant collapses. On rhizome, black lesions can be observed which later coalesce causing general necrosis of rhizome. Losses as high as 90 per cent have been recorded (Melouk *et al,* 1975). Rhizome rot is the most serious aspect of the disease and losses of 50 per cent in rhizome production have been observed in the field (Melouk and Horner, 1972). The fungus *(Phoma strasseri)* grows best in culture at 20-25°C and rhizome rot develops faster over a temperature range of 15-25°C (Melouk and Horner, 1972).

Tolerance of peppermint plants to *Phoma strasseri* increases with age but development of disease is extensive in wounded plants (Melouk and Horner, 1972). Benomyl as soak treatment for shoot tip cutting greatly reduces the losses caused by *Phoma strasseri* and results in weight increase of 46 per cent in spearmint and 78 per cent in peppermint (Melouk *et al,* 1975).

(xi). Sclerotinia Blight

The disease is caused by *Sclerotinia sclerotiorum* (Singh *et al,* 1999). The disease is characterised by the appearance of symptoms on the stem as white cottony growth of the mycelium of the pathogen in the collar zone. After some time, small water soaked lesions appear on the stem. Later on, the fungal mycelium moved both upwards and downwards resulting in stolon decay and decay of aerial plant parts, respectively. Under moist conditions, the pathogen produces white fluffy mycelia on different plant part (Plate IId). With the advance of disease, the infected parts show chocolate brown discoloration and watery symptoms of soft also develop resulting in die back of the branches of infected plants.

Some of the other mint diseases caused by fungal pathogens are listed in Table 2.

Nematode Diseases of Mint

Nematodes belonging to different species and genera have been reported to cause significant losses to mint crop (Pandey, 1994, 1998, 2000). The first account of association of a nematode with mint diseases was reported by Buhrer in 1938. After that, a lot of work has been done on the various aspects of nematode disease of mints. Root knot and root lesion nematodes have been regarded as the most important ones as far as disease of *Mentha* species is concerned.

(i). Root Knot Nematode

Buhrer (1938) for the first time reported *Mentha arvensis* as a host of *Meloidogyne.* In India, Pandey (1989) reported severe damage of this crop by *Meloidogyne incognita.* Haseeb and Pandey (1989) surveyed mint-growing areas of India and observed that *Meloidogyne incognita* was more prevalent than *Meloidogyne javanica.* Peppermint and spearmint have also been reported to be infected by *Meloidogyne.* Horner and Jenson (1954) found *Meloidogyne hapla* on these mints while Gokte and Mathur (1990) and Pandey (1998) reported *Meloidogyne incognita* and *Meloidogyne javanica* affecting *Mentha spicata* and *Mentha piperita.*

The root knot infested plants are stunted with smaller and chlorotic leaves. Such plants, when uprooted, had fewer rootlets and root-hairs and roots bear small knots/galls.

A comprehensive study was carried out by Pandey (1989) to determine the pathogenicity of *Meloidogyne incognita* on six genotypes of Japanese mint and maximum loss in oil yield was observed in genotypes MA-3 and MAS-1. Reduction in the content of 1-menthol was also observed in *Mentha arvensis* because of *Meloidogyne incognita* infection (Singh and Kumar, 1995).

Application of neem oil, seed cake and dried leaves of *Adhatoda vasica* and *Murraya koenigii* to the soil have been suggested to be useful in managing *Meloidogyne incognita* in Japanese mint (Pandey, 1995; Pandey *et al,* 1992) and spearmint (Khan and Khanna, 1992). Hot water treatment at 48°C for 30 minutes or at 50°C for 10 minutes could also completely eradicate *Meloidogyne incognita* from *Mentha spicata* roots (Gokul and Mathur, 1990).

(ii). Root-Lesion Nematode

Mentha spicata, Mentha piperita and *Mentha citrata* have been found to be particularly prone to root lesion nematodes like *Pratylenchus penetrans. Pratylenchus minus, Pratylenchus scribneri* and *Pratylenchus thornei* (Esmenjaud *et al,* 1990; Faulkner, 1962; Haseeb and Shukla, 1994, 1995; Pandey, 1997; Skotland and Menzies, 1957).

Infested plants show stunted growth, burning of leaves and lesions on the root system. Losses of up to 39 and 66 per cent in herbage and suckers have been observed (Bergenson, 1963). Apart from this *Pratylenchus penetrans* and *Pratylenchus minus* play a significant role in enhancing the infection of *Verticillium albo-atrum* and *Verticillium dahliae* on peppermint (Bergenson, 1963; Faulkner and Bolazaer, 1969; Faulkner and Skotland, 1965).

While *Pratylenchus penetrans* was found to be the main cause of reduction in herbage in spearmint and peppermint in Indiana, U. S. A. (Bergenson, 1979), *Pratylenchus scribneri* caused maximum damage to spearmint in Central Florida (Rhoades, 1983). In India, however, *Pratylenchus thornei* is the major pathogen of spearmint and peppermint. The population of *Pratylenchus thornei* in the rhizosphere of *Mentha spicata* and *Mentha piperita* was found to be maximum in February and minimum in June (Pandey, 1997). Peppermint grown in Russia was found to be severely affected by *Pratylenchoides laticuda* (Esmenjaud *et al,* 1990) and no significant differences in severity were observed between three peppermint sub-species tested *(Mentha piperita sylvestris, Mentha piperita officinalis* and *Mentha piperita vulgaris).* Pandey (1988) studied the comparative potentiality of *Pratylenchus thornei* on four mint species and found spearmint and peppermint as most susceptible hosts.

Pinkerton (1984) based on his greenhouse studies reported that *Pratylenchus penetrans* significantly reduced crop yield of *Mentha spicata* and found cv. Murroy Mitchem to be highly susceptible. Bergeson and Green (1979) found that cultivars of peppermint in Indiana were susceptible to this parasite.

The pathogen can be well managed by the application of pesticides. Rhoades (1984) got a good control of *Pratylenchus scribneri* on *Mentha spicata* with the use of Carbofuran, Fenamiphos and Terbufos though Fenamiphos was the most effective followed by Terbufos. An inverse relationship between nematode population and total foliage yield was also observed by him. Reduction in *Pratylenchus penetrans* population and increase in herb yield of peppermint was achieved by single treatment of Oxamyl or Carbofuran or Aldicarb in early April but fall application neither reduced the nematode population nor enhanced the spring growth (Pinkerton *et al,* 1988). Ingham *et al* (1988) controlled the *Pratylenchus penetrans* of peppermint by using Oxamyl or Ethophos. Aldicarb, applied three months prior to harvest improved the yields of *Mentha piperita* by 20 per cent (Esmenjaud *et al,* 1989).

A number of other plant parasitic nematodes are also known to affect mints (Table 3).

AROMATIC GRASSES

Aromatic grasses belong to the *Cymbopogon* species. They are known to suffer from a number of diseases caused by fungi, bacteria, viruses and nematodes. Though many of the diseases have only academic importance, several diseases cause extensive damage to these grasses. Many diseases besides reducing the oil yield also affect the quality of the oil as they interfere with the biosynthetic pathway of the oils. The successful cultivation of *Cymbopogon* species can only be achieved when the crop remains free from the attack of different pathogens.

(a). Palmarosa (*Cymbopogon martinii*)

Palmarosa oil grass or Rosha grass is a tall perennial herb grown in different States of India. The herb when distilled along with flower tops and foliage yields a colourless to pale (greenish) yellow essential oil with a sweet scented rose-like aroma. The oil is very rich in geraniol (75-90 per cent). Thus the oil is a source of high-grade geraniol for cosmetics and perfumery industry.

(i). Leaf Spot

Leaf spot caused by *Colletotrichum caudatum* during rainy season is an important disease of palmarosa (Sarwar and Parmeshwaran, 1981). Initially, small brownish spots appear on the lower leaves. The ventral surface of the leaves is infected first and later the infection spreads to the leaf sheath and midrib (Plate IIIa). In severe cases, the leaves dry out. The mature lesions caused by the pathogen release black fruiting bodies in warm weather conditions helping in the spread of disease.

The leaf blight caused by *Curvularia andropogenis* is another economically important disease, which may result in losses of 31 per cent in oil content and 17.8 per cent of geraniol in the oil.

TABLE 3
Nematode Diseases of *Mentha* sp.

Mentha/Nematode Species	Reported by
Mentha arvensis	
Meloidogyne sp.	Buhrer,1938
Meloidogyne hapla	Horner & Jensen, 1954
Meloidogyne incognita	Haseeb & Pandey, 1989
Meloidogyne javanica	Haseeb & Pandey, 1989
Pratylenchus thornei	Pandey, 1994; Pandey *et al*, 1992
Ditylenchus destructor	Henderson, 1951
Tylenchus sp.	Pandey, 1998; Pandey *et al*, 1992
Tylenchorhynchus vulgaris	Pandey, 1998; Pandey *et al*, 1992
Hoplolaimus sp.	Pandey, 1994; Pandey *et al*, 1992
Rotylenchulus reniformis	Pandey, 1998; Pandey *et al*, 1992
Helicotylenchus sp.	Pandey, 1998; Pandey *et al*, 1992
Helicotylenchus indicus	Pandey, 1988
Paratylenchus sp.	Pandey 1988
Criconemoides sp.	Pandey, 1988
Hirschmanniella sp.	Pandey, 1988
Xiphinema sp.	Pandey, 1994; Pandey *et al*, 1992
Longidorus pisi	Pandey, 1998; Pandey *et al*, 1992
Mentha cardiaca	
Meloidogyne chitwoodi	O'Bannon *et al*, 1982.
Meloidogyne hapla	Horner & Jensen, 1954
Meloidogyne incognita	Haseeb & Pandey, 1989
Pratylenchus thornei	Pandey, 1988
Pratylenchus minus	Skotland & Menzies, 1957
Pratylenchus penetrans	Skotland & Menzies, 1957
Pratylenchus hamatus	Skotland & Menzies, 1957
Tylenchus sp.	Pandey, 1994
Tylenchorhynchus vulgaris	Pandey, 1994
Hoplolaimus sp.	Pandey, 1994
Rotylenchulus reniformis	Pandey, 1994
Helicotylenchus sp.	Pandey, 1994
Longidorus pisi	Pandey, 1994
Xiphinema sp.	Pandey, 1994

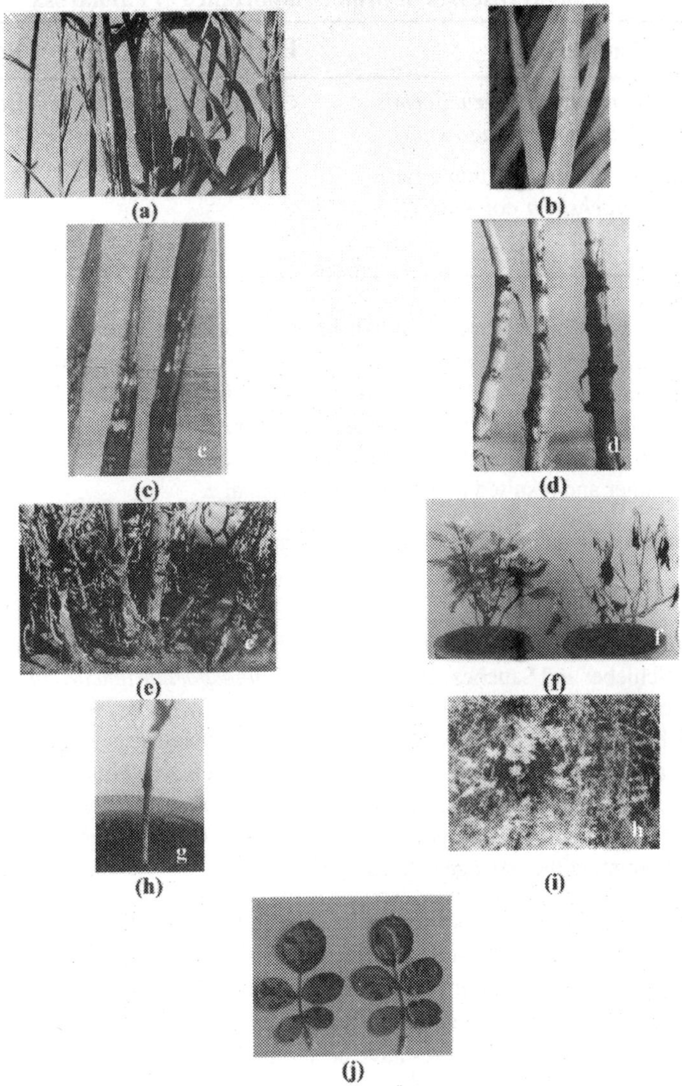

Plate III.

(a). Curvularia leaf spot of palmarosa; (b). Curvularia leaf spot of lemongrass; (c). Helminthosporium leaf blight of palmarosa; (d). Sheath rot and blight of *Java citronella* caused by *Rhizoctonia solani;* (e). Sclerotinia blight of *Tagetes minuta;* (f). Patchouli wilt and root rot caused by *R. solani;* (g). Collar rot of patchouli caused by *Sclerotium rolfsii*; (h). Alternaria blight of geranium; (i). Diploidia leaf spot of damask rose.

TABLE 4
Fungal Diseases of Minor Importance of Palmarosa

Disease	Pathogen	Host	Reported By
Leaf spot	*Curvularia verruciformis* *Curvularia eragrostidis*	*Curvularia flexuous*	Barua & Bordoloi, 1952
Grey blight	*Pestalotiopsis mangiferae*		Anonymous, 1981
Leaf spot and Clump rot	*Drechslera colocasia*		Anonymous, 1981

The disease appears as circular and reddish brown spots mostly on the leaf margins and tips (Janardhanan *et al,* 1980). *Colletotrichum graminicola* has also been reported to cause leaf spot on lemongrass (Thakur and Husain, 1975). The disease initially appeared as small brownish spots scattered all over the leaf during rainy season. The spots later enlarged to develop into brown patches (Plate IIIa). The pathogen formed black fruiting bodies on the necrotic lesions of the leaves during humid weather and resulted in extensive crop damage.

A number of fungal diseases of minor importance (Table 4) also affect the crop.

(ii). Leaf Spot

Two different species of *Helminthosporium* (Plate IIIc), namely, *Helminthosporium sacchari* (Bourne, 1941; Schieber and Sanchez, 1960) and *Helminthosporium leucortylum* (Santara, 1981) and two of *Dreschlera,* namely, *Dreschlera victoriae* and *Dreschlera helmi* have been reported to be associated with leaf spot disease. But as the symptomatology suggests, the causal organism appears to be the same, namely, *Helminthosporium saccharia* as *Dreschlera sacchari* by Verma (1987). Some other species of *Dreschlera victoriae* and *Dreschlera helmi* have also been associated with leaf spot disease. Some resistant cultivars of lemongrass RRL-59, RRL-18 and RRL-14 have been reported which help in eliminating the damage caused by pathogens.

C. flexuous is the indigenous species of lemongrass in India. Its oil has strong lemon-like odour, which is responsible for its name and due to this property only the oil is extensively used for scenting soaps, detergents and an array of other products. Citral extracted from the oil forms an important raw material for perfumery, confectionery, beverages and the starting material for manufacture of ionones. Though a number of diseases have been reported on lemongrass, none has been reported to cause significant reduction in oil yield.

(iii). Leaf Blight

Leaf blight caused by *Ellisiella caudata* is a serious disease of palmarosa to the extent that it leads to epiphytotics in all palmarosa growing areas. The disease first appears in the form of small greenish brown spots scattered on the leaf lamina. Later on the spots enlarge and coalesce with one another; the result is severe blight symptoms. In the mature necrotic lesions, profuse spore mass of brownish colour are produced by the pathogen. The leaf sheath is also affected. The experimental studies have pointed to the fact that the disease is either perpetuated through plant debris or self sown plants.

(c). Java Citronella (*Cymbopogon winterianus*)

(i). Leaf Blotch (*Curvularia andropogenis*)

Curvularia andropogenis is the causal agent of leaf blotch disease of *Java citronella* (Alam and Husain, 1976, 1983). The symptoms of the disease appeared as small pink coloured spots of 1-2 × 8.5-1 mm size, which were scattered on the leaf blade in the initial stages. Later on, the spots coalesced resulting in blotch symptoms. A loss of more than 31 per cent oil and 11.8 per cent geraniol content has been reported due to leaf blotch disease. This may be due to the production of a toxin by the pathogen (Alam *et al*, 1997). *Curvularia andropogenis* infected leaves of *Java citronella* showed discoloration due to changes in phenol metabolism of host. At later stages, typical browning symptoms were observed on leaves.

The disease control in the field can be achieved by the spraying of Mancozeb (0.1 per cent) and Benlate (0.1 per cent) at an interval of 15 days. Turn brown, shrink and finally disintegrate. The young seedlings may be attacked before the emergence at any point from which the infection spreads rapidly and the seedling is over run by the fungus and dies (pre-emergence damping-off). The seedlings, which have already emerged, are usually attacked at the roots and sometimes stem at or just below the soil line. The invaded areas become water soaked and discoloured and they soon collapse with basal part of the seedling stem becoming softer and much thinner than the unaffected parts of the plant. In older plants, the pathogens may kill rootlets or induce lesions on the roots and stems. The lesions result in plants becoming stunted and ultimately to wither and die; drenching of 0.1 per cent Dithane M-45 is recommended for controlling damping off. Some other fungal diseases of *Cymbopogon* species are given in Table 5.

(ii). Sheath Rot and Blight

The disease is caused by *Rhizoctonia solani.* The symptoms initially developed on the leaves and sheaths in the form of concentric spots covering large areas of sheaths and leaves (Singh *et al,* 1997). Discoloured lesions first appeared on the leaf sheaths near the soil surface and gradually spread around the sheath arm inwards in to sheath tissues. Rotting remains restricted to lower side of the plant and in advanced cases, a weft of greyish mycelium develops within the sheath. Numerous small, round to irregular, dark-brown coloured sclerotia develop over the mycelial mat and inside the leaf sheath (Plate IIId).

(d). Khus (*Vetiveria zizanioides*)

Khus is a widely distributed perennial grass native to Indian sub-continent. The spongy and aromatic roots of vetiver are traditionally employed for household goods, for example, mats, fans, door-screens, which emit sweet fragrance imparting a cooling effect during summer months when sprinkled with water. The aerial parts are used as thatching of roofs in countryside. Roots are also the source of a highly fragrant and viscous volatile oil, which has high demand both in India and abroad for its use in perfumery, cosmetics, toiletry and related industries.

(i). *Curvularia* Leaf Spot and Blight

Although a number of fungal diseases have been reported on vetiver plants, the leaf blight caused by *Curvularia trifolii* is the most important (Sarwar, 1969). The infected leaves show tan to dark spots, which later on turn black in colour. The roots of infected plants become yellow and

TABLE 5
Other Fungal Diseases of *Cymbopogon* sp.

Disease	Pathogen	Host	Reported By
Leaf blight	*Rhizoctonia solani*	*C. winterianus*	Singh *et al,* 1999
Wilt	*Fusarium moniliforme*	*C. citratus*	Alam *et al,* 1994
		C. winterianus	Carrera, 1969
Wilt	*Fusarium oxysporum*	*C. winterianus*	Alam & Hussain, 1983
Eye spot	*Himantia stellifera*	*C. citratus*	Storey & McClean, 1930
Eye spot	*Helminthosporium ocellum*	*C. citratus*	Bourne, 1941
Leaf spot	*Khuskia oryzae*	*C. citratus*	Allen, 1971
Leaf spot	*Monochaetiella cymbopogonis*	C. *winterianus*	Preston, 1984
Leaf spot	*Colletotrichum ciliatum*	*C. caesium*	Govindu &
		C. polyneuros	Thirumalachar, 1954
			Ramkrishan &
			Ramakrishnan, 1947
Leaf spot	*Cochliobolus nodulosus*	*C. flexuosus*	Santra, 1981
Leaf spot	*Psilocybe winterianus*	*C. jwaarancusa*	Abraham, 1995

ultimately dry out. Two to three sprayings of copper fungicide (0.3 per cent) having 50 per cent metallic copper at the rate of 120-160 gallons/ha is found to give good control of the disease.

(ii). *Gloecospora sorghi*

Gloecospora sorghi was reported from Delhi by Puranik and Suryanarayan (1966). The symptoms of the disease include the appearance of small, diffused brown spots on leaf margins.

(iii). *Helminthosporium*

Helminthosporium species has also been reported to cause leaf spot on vetiver (Jain, 1995). The diseased plants show spots, which were scattered throughout the leaf and sheath. The spots are oblong, oval and have a dark brown colour.

(iv). *Heterodera zeae*

Lal and Mathur (1982) reported the nematode infestation of the roots by *Heterodera zeae* for which hot water treatment is effective. The removal of this nematode infestation is important before transit of the planting materials from one place to other.

TAGETES MINUTA

Marigolds (*Tagetes* species) are mainly cultivated for ornamental purposes all over the world. The leaves and flowers of this genus are characterised by the presence of distinct odoriferous oil. However, the oil of African marigold (*Tagetes minuta),* a native of South America, is valued for its characteristic essential oil. The oil produced at the higher altitudes of Himachal Pradesh has been found to be rich in ketonic constituents while the one cultivated in places like Uttar Pradesh and Punjab have low olfactory value. The oil is mainly used in perfumery industry. It also has broncho dilatory, tranquillising and anti-inflammatory properties (Chandhoke and Ghatak, 1969).

(i). Sclerotinia Blight

Sclerotinia sclerotiorum is the causal agent of this disease. The initial symptoms of the disease comprise of water soaked lesions on the stem near the soil surface, which later on move upwards to cause stem rot leading to decaying of the whole plant system. The stems shred easily exposing large (5-15 mm) dark coloured sclerotia (Plate IIIe). In advanced stages, the inflorescences of the plant are also affected producing typical blight symptoms. Such blooms fall down prematurely and white cottony growth of the fungus can be seen on these blooms (Singh *et al,* 1998).

PATCHOULI *(POGOSTEMON PATCHOULI/POGOSTEMON CABLIN)*

Patchouli is a native of the Philippines and grows wild in South-East Asian countries. The oil of patchouli, though rarely used as a dominant source of fragrance in its own right, is widely used to give solid foundation and lasting character to a fragrance. It has strong fixative properties and helps to prevent rapid evaporation of a perfume and thereby promotes tenacity. Dry patchouli leaves are used for scenting wardrobes. The leaves and tops are added to bath water for their anti-rheumatic action. In Chinese medicine, decoction from the leaves is used with other drugs to treat nausea, vomiting, diarrhoea, cold and headaches (Leung, 1980).

(i). Leaf Blight

Leaf blight of patchouli is caused by *Cercospora* species. Brown spots appearing near the leaf margin or tip, enlarge irregularly leading to drying of leaves. It can be controlled by giving two sprays of Dithane Z-78 (0.5 per cent) at monthly intervals (Sarwar *et al,* 1983).

Parameswaran *et al* (1987) observed severe leaf blight of patchouli during summer months. This caused defoliation and premature death of plants. The fungus was identified as *Alternaria alternata* (Fr.) Keissler. Pathogenicity tests were confirmed and more than 50 per cent fungal growth inhibition was achieved in the laboratory by using three fungicides, namely, Febam, Dithane M-45 and Captan.

(ii). Wilt

Wilt disease of patchouli is caused by *Rhizoctonia solani* Kuhn and has been reported in Karnataka (Narayanappa *et al,* 1984). Wilt incidence with characteristic symptoms of blackening of roots and collar region of fully-grown plants (Plate IIIf) has been recorded at Bangalore (Roopali Singh and Angadi, 1992). In a study, Java and Singapore cultivars showed resistance to this disease complex caused by *Fusarium solani* and *Pythium aphanidermatum,* the Johore, Malaysian and Indonesian cultivars were found highly susceptible.

(iii). Collar Rot and Wilt

The causal agent of this disease is *Sclerotium rolfsii.* The most apparent symptom of the disease is the yellowing of leaves, followed by severe wilt. The affected plants show typical rotting symptoms at the collar region on which numerous yellowish brown coloured, mustard seed like sclerotia can be seen (Plate IIIg).

DAVANA

Davana is an important aromatic crop of India and is commercially cultivated in Karnataka and to a lesser extent in Maharashtra, Tamil Nadu and Andhra Pradesh. The essential oil of davana (*Artemisia pallens)* has attained an important place in international trade of essential oils, especially in the U. S. A. India has monopoly in its world trade. The leaves and flowers are fragrant and are used in floral decoctions and religious offerings in India. They also contain an essential oil valued for its exquisite and delicate aroma and used in high-grade perfumes and cosmetics.

(i). Damping Off Disease

The disease is caused by *Rhizoctonia solani,* particularly in cloudy weather conditions. The disease leads to premature death of seedlings. The disease cane by minimised by the seed treatment with Dithane M-45 and by reducing the frequency of irrigation.

Nematodes of Davana

Haseeb and Pandey (1990) started the nematological studies on this crop in India. They reported that *Meloidogyne incognita* and *Meloidogyne javanica* are the most important pests of this crop. The plants infested with root knot nematodes show gradual decline characterised by stunted growth of plants followed by yellowing of leaves. The number of tillers is also reduced. The severely infested plants produce lesser number of flower buds than healthy ones. Pandey (1994), Haseeb and Butool (1991) found that Aldicarb, Ethoprofos and neem cake were effective in controlling the disease.

GERANIUM

Scented geranium or rose geranium (*Pelargonium graveolens)* is a highly adaptable, drought tolerant and perennial aromatic herb. It is cultivated mainly for rose scented essential oil extracted from leaves and tender shoots. The geranium oil contains large quantities of rose alcohol including individual components such as citronella and geraniol. These are collectively known as 'rhodionol' fraction and responsible for its suitability to a wide range of higher grade perfume compounds. Being stable and lasting, even in a slightly alkaline medium, the oil is used in scenting of soaps, talcum powders and hand creams. The tannins are important by products from geranium. Several diseases affect the geranium crop (Kalra *et al,* 2000).

(i). Alternaria Leaf Blight

The disease is caused by *Alternaria alternata* and reaches its maximum severity during the months of April–June. The symptoms first appear on the leaf margins as brown necrotic spots, which later on spread towards the midrib resulting in inward curling, complete necrosis and chlorosis of leaves (Plate IIIh). The typical disease syndrome directly affected the crop herbage and essential oil yield through the destruction of oil gland and defoliation.

(ii). Anthracnose Disease

The causal agent of this disease is *Colletotrichum acutatum.* Sometimes, the disease appears in epidemic form during the monsoon months. First symptoms of the disease is the appearance of minute pinhead and circular dark brown spots on the young leaves and twigs of infected plants which enlarge later on and coalesce to form large typical anthracnose necrotic lesions. These lesions are of unlimited growth and lead to premature drying and death of infected plants. The severely infected plants fail to regenerate in the next cropping season.

(iii). Wilt

The wilt disease of geranium is one of the major constraints in its cultivation. Several fungi have been reported to be associated with wilt disease but *Rhizoctonia solani* is the most important pathogen causing maximum damage (Kalra *et al,* 1992). The disease starts as yellowing of lower leaves, which move upwards simultaneously infecting the stem, which ultimately dry and topple down. The disease can by controlled by dipping the cuttings in Bavistin (0.03 per cent) before sowing and the spraying of Bavistin (0.03 per cent) about two weeks before harvest and repeating the spray after harvest.

(iv). Rhizoctonia Blight

The disease is caused by *Rhizoctonia solani* and is also known as web blight. In the infected parts of the plant, weft of fungal mycelia can be seen intermingled with orange sclerotia of the pathogen. The disease is prevalent in the *terai* region of former Uttar Pradesh (now Uttaranchal).

Nematodes of Geranium

The crop is attacked by *Meloidogyne incognita, Meloidogyne hapla* and *Helicotylenchus dihystera.* The plant infected with root knot nematodes show stunting, burning of lower leaves, yellowing and severe galling on the root system by *Meloidogyne incognita* and *Meloidogyne hapla* are the most important nematodes associated with the decline in geranium yield (Arumugam and Kumar, 1979). They reported up to 50 per cent reduction in oil yield of geranium due to these pathogens. Application of Aldicarb, Phorate and Quinapholes at the rate of 2 or 3 kg/ha after four months of transplanting proved to be effective in controlling the disease (Kumar and Nanjan, 1985).

MEDICINAL PLANTS

1. Belladonna

Atropa belladonna is the main source of atropine, one of the three major alkaloids used in the pharmaceutical industry. The roots are used for external application to relieve neuralgic and other pain, whereas leaves and their alkaloids are given for internal administration. Atropine and hyoscyamine are used mainly as pre-anaesthetic agents to check infection in throat and respiratory passages. Hyoscine constituting only 5 to 11 per cent of the total alkaloids is used as a truth confessor in criminological investigations.

(i). Damping-off

The seedlings of *Atropa belladonna* are affected by the damping off disease caused by *Pythium* species. Primarily the seeds when sown in an infested field fail to germinate, become shrunken, and ultimately die.

(ii). Leaf Spot

A leaf spot caused by *Cercospora atropae* causing leaf spot in belladonna has been reported by Singh and Singh (1984). The pathogen forms rounded or angular spots on the upper surface of leaves whereas brownish to roasted spots were restricted to leaf lamina. Six sprays of 0.1 solution of Blitox–50 at an interval of 15 days effectively controlled the disease.

(iii). Fusarium Root Rot

The fusarium rot of belladonna has been reported by Janardhanan and Husain (1974). The symptoms of the disease started as yellowing of leaves followed by wilting, dehydration and death of the infected plants. Root and stem of the infected plants show intensive degradation of the cortical tissues. Fully-grown and mature plants are more susceptible to infection and thus cause severe damage to the crop.

2. Foxglove *(Digitalis purpurea)*

It is cultivated commercially for three glycosides, namely, cligitoxin, gelatin and gitoxin, which are found in leaves. These glycosides have cadiotonic properties (Anonymous, 1973).

(i). Leaf Blight

The leaf blight caused by *Alternaria* species has been occasionally reported on the crop. The disease is characterised by the formation of brown spots on the leaves, which enlarge in size. Covering a larger part of the leaf, the disease can be effectively controlled by spraying of copper fungicides at he rate of 0.1-0.2 per cent.

3. Senna (*Cassia angustifolia* Vahl.)

Senna is a native of Yemen and Hadramaunt province of Saudi Arabia. The leaves and pods of Senna contain sennosides, which have laxative properties with the pods having slightly higher sennosides than leaves. Senna has a nauseous taste and a tendency to gripe, griping is prevented by combining some aromatics. Pods do not cause griping. However, leaves are preferred as ingredient of herbal tea in Europe. The calcium salts of sennosides in granulated form remain stable for long in storage and this is a popular form of dispensation useful in constipation in modern medicine.

(i). Damping–off

In north-western India, the crop is affected by damping-off disease at the seedling stage. The causal organism is *Rhizoctonia bataticola*. The presence of stagnating water in the field helps in the rapid spread of disease. Seed treatment with Thiram or Captan (2.5g/kg) is an effective preventive measure.

Drenching of soil with Bavistin (1 per cent) is effective in disease control. At a later stage *Macrophomina phaseoli* is known to attack the senna crop causing dry rot. The dry rot disease can be partially controlled by soil drenching with 0.2 per cent brassicol or 0.5 per cent rhizoctol. It is better not to grown senna again in the same field as the fungus perennates in the soil.

(ii). Leaf Spot

Occasionally, the leaf spots caused by *Phyllosticta* species and *Cercospora* species have been reported on the crop mainly during the cloudy weather (Gupta, 1984). The leaf spot pathogens can be controlled by the spraying of 0.15 per cent Dithane M-45.

Colletotrichum gloeosporioides is another pathogen causing leaf spot of senna (Gupta *et al*, 1997). Initially small pinhead and brown to dark brown spots develop on the leaf lamina, which later expand towards the margins leading to larger necrotic spots and drying of entire leaf. Subsequently, severe defoliation occurs resulting in heavy losses of leaves. The severely affected plants produce fewer flowers and pods thereby reducing the economic yield.

(iii). Wilt

The wilt disease of senna is caused by *Fusarium semitectum* (Singh and Chourasia, 1995). The infected plants show yellowing and marginal necrosis of leaves. The root system is reduced with the discoloration of vascular tissues and dark brown coloured bands on stem starting from the root zone to the later stages of disease development.

4. Safed Musli

A number of species belonging to genus *Chlorophytum* (Family Liliaceae) are grouped under one trade name 'safed musli', which is extensively used in Ayurvedic preparations. The roots of safed musli after drying are well known for their properties as a tonic and aphrodisiac drug given to persons with general debility.

(i). Collar Rot

Collar rot disease, caused by *Sclerotium rolfsii* is also an economically important disease of *Chlorophytum borivilianum* (Singh *et al*, 2001). The pathogen attacks stem just above the soil line during seeding stage. No control measures have yet been developed for collar rot of safed musli.

Under storage conditions the fleshy roots of safed musli were found to become hollow and are the infection of *Aspergillus* and *Fusarium* observed, but on inoculation of the fresh plants these fungi did not produce any disease (Anonymous, 1990).

The roots when treated with Thiram and Captan at the rate of 4g/kg before storage reduced rotting of roots in addition to enhancing the sprouting percentage.

5. Opium Poppy

Opium poppy (*Papavar somniferum* L.) is historically most important medicinal plant and is the chief source of commercial opium. The opium is known as the oldest and probably the best known pain killer since time immemorial. The alkaloids of opium have analgesic, anti-turic and anti-spasmodic properties and have been used in modern medicinal systems in different formulations. The oil extracted from opium seed and the seeds itself are edible.

Opium poppy is susceptible to several diseases but root rot, downy mildew and powdery mildew disease and Sclerotinia rot and blight are economically most important.

(i). Downy Mildew

The epiphytic form of this disease has been reported from different parts of the world though its first record is from India in 1918 (Pandey, 1995). Thakore *et al* (1983) reported that the secondary infection of the disease reduced latex yield (17-22.8 per cent), morphine content and seed yield (12.9-14.9 per cent) significantly. The infection spreads upwards from lower leaves. The entire leaf surface is covered with downy mildew coating which is comprised of conidiophores and conidia of the pathogen *(Peronospora arborescens)*. The symptoms are either localised (leaf spots) or systemic. The systemically infected plants have two distinct parts, the lower healthy and upper diseased. In the healthy part, the placement and size of the leaves is normal while the leaves are small, chlorotic, curling downward at the edges and closely placed in the disease parts. Heavy sporulation occurs on the entire lower surface of the diseased leaves. The capsules are shrunken, wrinkled and dries gradually after infection. Heavy sporulation develops on peduncle buds and capsules. More often than not, rudimentary brownish black structures develop in place of normal seeds. Such capsules are devoid of any latex and the heavily infected plants die prematurely.

The localised infection shows chlorotic spots which gradually turn necrotic and these spots coalesce to form larger spots. Sporulation may occur on the lower surface of the infected leaves but it is not heavy and consistent. In spite of the spots, the plants do not die prematurely.

Crop rotation, wide spacing, avoidance of low-lying damp sites for cultivation reduces the disease incidence. Spraying of Dithane Z-78, Ferbam or Bisdithane are effective in controlling the downy mildew disease of opium poppy.

(ii). Powdery Mildew

Powdery mildew of opium poppy is caused by *Erysiphe polygoni* and has been reported to occur in a severe form in Rajasthan, Madhya Pradesh and Uttar Pradesh. After 14-16 weeks of sowing, that is, nearly at or after flowering stage, the crop is affected by the powdery mildew disease. Late sown crops develop heavy infection whereas early sown crops almost escape the disease. The first attack of the pathogen is at the base of the stem where it appears as a small circular patch consisting of radially arranged mycelium. After seven to 10 days of initiation of infection, blackening develops in the affected parts. When mildew infection is at its peak, stem appears black interspersed with green patches. This spreads all over the leaves and their growth is checked. The buds on such branches remain rudimentary and wither away.

One application of wettable sulphur using 0.5 per cent concentration at the time of first appearance of the disease in the field or when the crop has reached the age of 80 days or when maximum daily temperatures in the poppy growing area have reached 27°C or above is effective in controlling powdery mildew of opium poppy.

(iii). Root Rot

The disease is caused by combination of fungi including *Fusarium semitectum, Macrophomina phaseolina* and *Rhizoctonia* species (Butler, 1918) and is very serious disease of seedling stage. The disease is characterised by the rotting of roots, and the leaves turn yellow leading ultimately to premature death of the plants. The disease can be effectively checked by removal of infected plants and spraying of Bavistin (1 g/l of water) or streptocycline (4-6 g/600-800 litres of water).

(iv). Sclerotinia Blight

Recently, a severe rot and blight disease of opium poppy caused by *Sclerotinia sclerotiorum* (Lib.) de Bary has been reported from Lucknow, Uttar Pradesh (Singh and Singh, 2003). Although the disease has yet not been reported from anywhere in India but it has earlier been reported from different parts of the world, namely, former USSR (Masalab, 1938), Poland (Fulara, 1971), Japan (Fujioka, 1952) and the U. S. A. (Shaw, 1972).

The disease is characterised by the appearance of symptoms on the stem as white cottony growth of the mycelium of the pathogen in the collar zone. After some time small water soaked lesions appear on the stem. Later on, the fungal mycelium moved both upwards and downwards resulting in root decay and decay of aerial plant parts, respectively. Under moist conditions, the pathogen produces white fluffy mycelia on different plant parts. In the stem and flower buds, embedded sclerotia of *Sclerotinia sclerotiorum* also develop. With the advance of disease, the infected parts show chocolate brown discoloration and watery symptoms of soft also develop resulting in die back of the branches of infected plants. Under severe conditions, the growth of the fungus can also be observed in the pith of the stem as well as heavily infected capsules replacing the seeds.

The spray of Bavistin, Dithane M-45 and Kavach (0.2 per cent) at the time of first appearance of the disease is quite effective. Different strains of *Trichoderma* have also been found to be effective in disease management (Singh, 2002).

Other fungal diseases of opium poppy reported from different parts of the world are given in Table 6.

6. Sarpagandha (*Rauvolfia serpentina*)

Rauvolfia serpentina is prone to infection by different groups of fungi causing various diseases.

(i). Leaf Spot and Blight

The disease is caused by *Cercospora rauvolfia* and *Mycosphaerella rauvolfiae.* The symptoms of the disease are the development of dark brown spots on the upper surface of the leaf and yellowish brown on the lower surface. These spots subsequently increase in size (up to 1 cm) and causes yellowing and drying of affected leaves leading to defoliation. The lowermost leaves are attacked first and the disease progresses upwards. The other fungi reported to be associated with the disease are *Cercospora serpentine* and *Saisootia coffeae.* Spraying of 0.2 per cent Dithane M-45 at an interval of 10-15 days has been found to be effective in controlling the diseases.

(ii). Corynespora Leaf Spot

The disease is caused by *Corynespora cassicala.* It produces dark brown spots on the upper and yellowish brown spots on the lower surface of the leaves throughout the growing season. These spots gradually enlarge into circular spots (2-20 mm in diameter) with concentric zones due to which the disease is named 'target spot.' Lower leaves are infected first and the disease progresses upwards. Heavily infected leaves turn yellow and are shed prematurely. Defoliation occurs throughout the season, only few top tender leaves remain on the plant. Spraying of 0.25 per cent Captan solution in water in early June before monsoon and repeated at monthly intervals until November, is most effective in controlling the diseases.

(iii). Anthracnose

The disease is caused by *Colletotrichum gloeosporioides* (Penz.) Sacc. and appears as tiny spots of the aceruvli scattered all over but confined to the upper leaf surface. Several spots coalesce

TABLE 6
Fungal Diseases of Opium Poppy Reported From Different Parts of the World

Disease	Pathogen	Reported By
Downy mildew	*Peronospora arborescens*	Cunningham, 1897
Collar rot	*Rhizoctonia solani*	Sattar *et al,* 1999
Root rot	*Fusarium semitectum*	Gupta *et al,* 1986
	Macrophomina phaseoli	Butler, 1918
	Rhizoctonia bataticola	Despandey *et al,* 1969
White rot	*Sclerotium rolfsii*	Patel *et al,* 1949
Charcoal rot	*Pelicularia filamentosa* (= *Corticium solani*)	Butler & Bisby, 1931
Leaf blight	*Helminthosporium* sp.	Girzitska, 1928
	Alternaria phragmospora	Gupta *et al,* 1989
Leaf spot	*Pleospora calvescens*	Zogg, 1945
	Alternaria alternata	Kishore *et al,* 1987
	Alternaria papaveris	Udit Narayan, 1991
	Entyloma fuscum	Savulescue, 1932
	Cercospora papaveri	Pavgi & Upadhyay, 1964
	Alternaria brassicae	Grummer, 1953
Capsule rot	*Macrosporium papaveris*	Parisi Rosa, 1921
	Fusarium scripi	Christoff, 1934
	Dendryphion penicillatum	Sehgal *et al,* 1971
Wilt	*Verticillium* sp.	Saxena *et al,* 1987
	Fusarium martii or *F. oxysporum* var. *cubense*	Vander Meer, 1925
Damping off	*Pythium dissoctocum*	Alam *et al,* 1996
	Pythium ultimum	Angell, 1950
	Pythium manillatum	

and cause drying of the lamina resulting in defoliation. Spraying of dithiocarbamates such as Fermate or Dithane M-45 (0.2 per cent) at intervals of 10-15 days has been recommended for controlling the disease. Cutting and burning of the infected shoots is also an effective mode of disease control.

Another species of *Colletotrichum,* namely, *Colletotrichum dematium* has also been reported to be associated with the disease. The pathogen infects the twigs, leaves and flowers and numerous spots bearing aceruvli scattered all over the leaf. The twigs are the most affected part most often killing the entire shoot. Sometimes, smaller lesions coalesce to form large and circular necrotic patches resulting in complete destruction of lamina and defoliation. Spraying of Dithane Z-78 (0.2 per cent) at initial stage of infection with 10-15 days of interval has been found to be effective. The pruning of the affected parts partially controls the spread of the disease.

(iv). Fusarium Wilt

The disease is caused by *Fusarium oxysporum* f. sp. *ravolfii* (Janardhanan *et al*, 1964). The initial symptoms of the disease consist of wilting of individual branches. The foliage symptoms are characterised by drooping of the leaves followed by upward curling. As the disease advances, the entire plant is affected resulting in drying of the leaves and the death of the plant.

The other diseases reported to cause damage to this crop are leaf blight and bud-rot caused by *Alternaria tenuis, Macrophomina phaseolina* and *Pellicularia filamentosa* and powdery mildew caused by *Laveillula taurica.* Root knot nematode (*Meloidogyne* sp.) is also known to attack the crop. However, the crop is not damaged severely by these pathogens. Dutta and Virmani (1964) and Sarin (1982) have presented an account of major diseases and pests attacking the sarpagandha crop at Lucknow and Jammu, respectively.

7. *Ocimum basilicum*

Different species of the genus *Ocimum* are popularly called as basil. *Ocimum basilicum* is variously called as 'sweet basil', 'French basil' or common basil and the mint smelling, linalool rich, *Ocimum canum* is known as mint basil.

The leaves and tender shoots of basil yield essential oils, which contain a heterogeneous group of aromatic compounds having immense value as flavour as well as fragrance.

(i). Leaf Spot

Leaf spot is caused by a number of pathogens. The important ones are *Cercospora canescens, Cercospora ocimicola, Glomerella cingulata* and *Phyllosticta ocimicola. Cercospora canescens* and *Glomerella cingulata* cause irregular to circular and sometimes hemispherical dark brown spots on the leaves. Due to heavy infection, a large number of leaves fall prematurely.

Phyllosticta ocimicola attacks *Ocimum sanctum* in Jammu area. In this disease, spherical to irregular spots on leaf surface with serrated purple and distinct margins are some of the characteristic symptoms. In advanced stage, they form shot holes. No control measures work out.

Some other pathogens like *Corynespora cassicala* and *Colletotrichum capsici* are also associated with leaf spot and anthracnose of basil, respectively. Initially, the spots are small, irregular and in advanced stage of infection. These spots enlarge, coalesce, necrotic giving blighted appearance during rainy season. Spraying of Dithane M-45 (0.3 per cent) at 15 days interval controls the disease effectively.

8. Damask Rose (*Rosa damascena*)

Scented roses are grown is several countries of the world for extraction of volatile roses. The major growing countries are Bulgaria, France, Italy, Turkey, USSR, China and India.

Rosa damascena was introduced in 1680 in Middle East countries and its cultivation was very successful in the Balkans. The oil of damask rose is extracted mainly from flower petals. Besides oil, rose water, rose attar, gulkand, gul-roghan, punkhuri and otto of rose are some other products of damask rose cultivation in India.

The rose family enjoys the greatest adoration for its colour and fragrance. Apart from its aesthetic importance, the roses have high economic value due to the presence of rose oil in the petals. The oil obtained from *Rosa damascena* is given high importance in the perfumery industry for its high quality essential oil. Besides oil, other important products from damask rose are rose water, rose attar, gulkand, gul-rogan, punkhuri and otto of roses.

(i). Black Spot Disease

This disease is caused by *Diplodia rosarum.* Initially growing twigs, leaves and flowers are affected by this disease. The twigs are the most affected resulting in the killing of the entire shoot. Sometimes the cut ends of the shoot turn black and die (Plate III-I). Immediately after pruning the cut ends of shoots should be treated with (0.2 per cent) copper fungicide.

(ii). Leaf Spot

The disease is caused by *Diplocarpon rosae.* Leaf spots occur on the upper surface, rarely on the lower surface and dark brown to black with radiating dark purplish margin. The fully developed spots are 7-12 mm in size, circular, separate and distinct from each other. In advanced stage of infection, the entire leaf turns yellow and defoliation takes place. Numerous bodies of aceruvli can be seen as slightly raised small dark dots on the leaf lesions. Spraying of chlorothalonil (0.1 per cent) at 15 days interval has been found effective.

(iii). Rose Mildew

The disease is caused by *Sphaerotheca pannosa* var. *rosae.* Small chlorotic spots appear on the upper surface and corresponding powdery mass is observed on the lower surface of the leaves. Spraying of triforine or chlorothalonil (0.1 per cent) at 15 days interval is effective in disease control.

(iv). Rust

The rust disease of rose is caused by several species of *Phragmidium mucronatum* (Dodov and Tanev, 1963). The initial symptoms of the disease appear on the lower surface of infected leaves in the form of raised pustules having orange to brown colour. In case of severe infection, the young twigs and the calyx of flower buds are also affected by the pathogen and show symptoms of the disease akin to those on the leaves. The disease can be effectively controlled by spraying of Bycor (0.2 per cent), Folicur Plus (0.05 per cent) and Saprol (0.2 per cent).

REFERENCES

Abraham, S. P. 'Notes on occurrence of an unusual agaric on *Cymbopogon* in Kashmir Valley'. *Nova Hedwigia.* 60: 227-232, 1995.

Alam, M. and Husain, A. 'Leaf blight and leaf spot of *Java citronella* caused by *Curvularia andropogenis* (Zimm.) Boed.' *New Bot.* 3: 54-56, 1976.

Alam, M. and Husain, A. 'Leaf blight and leaf spot of *Java citronella* caused by *Curvularia andropogenis*'. *Indian Phytopath.* 35: 480-483, 1983.

Alam, M., Chaurasia, H. K., Sattar, A. and Janardhanan, K. K. 'A new disease of *Java citronella* caused by *Fusarium moniliforme*'. *Plant Pathology*. 43: 1057-1061, 1994.

Alam, M., Sattar, A., Chaudhri, P. K.,, Janardhanan, K. K. and Husain, A. 'Isolation, purification and characterisation of a phytotoxin produced by *Curvularia andropogenis*'. *Plant Science*. 123: 47-55, 1997.

Alam, M., Sattar, A., Chourasia, H. K. and Janardhanan, K. K. 'Damping-off: a new disease of opium poppy caused by *Pythium dissoctocum*'. *Indian Phytopathology* 49: 94-97, 1996.

Allen, D. J. 'Some newly recorded diseases of minor horticultural crops in Tanzania'. *E. Afr. For. J.* 37: 22-25, 1971.

Angell, H. R. 'Seedlings blight. II. Soil in relation to seedling blight of opium poppy and peas'. *Aust. J. Agric. Res.* 1: 132, 1950.

Anonymous. Annual Progress Report of Scheme (ICAR) on development of suitable culture of safed musli (*Chlorophytum* sp.) for root yield and acceptable medicinal quality. Rajasthan College of Agriculture, 1990.

Anonymous. Annual Report of 1980-1981. Central Institute of Medicinal and Aromatic Plants, p. 98, 1981.

Anonymous. *British Pharmaceutical Codex*. London: Pharmaceutical Press, 1973.

Anonymous. *CIMAP Newsletter*. Lucknow: CIMAP, 1997.

Arumugam, R. and Kumar, N. 'Geranium cultivation in Kodaikanal hills'. *Indian Perfumer* 23(2): 128-130, 1979.

Bai, H. C., Chen, X. Y. and Wang. S. G. 'A preliminary study on Peronosporaceae in Gansu Province'. *Gansu Nongye Daxue Xue bao*. 26: 180-183, 1991.

Baines, R. C. 'Mint anthracnose'. *Phytopathology* 28: 1-3-113, 1938.

Barua, A. and Bordoloi, D. N. 'Records of a new disease of lemongrass (*Cymbopogon flexuosus* Stapf.) caused by *Curvularia verruciformis* Agarwal & Sahni'. *Curr. Sci.* 52: 640-641, 1952.

Baxter, J. W. and Cummins, G. B. 'Physiologic specialisation in *Puccinia menthae* and notes on epiphytology'. *Phytopathology* 43: 178-180, 1953.

Bergenson, G. B. and Green, R. J. 'Damage to cultivars of peppermint by the lesion nematode *Pratylenchus penetrans* in Indiana'. *Pl. Dis. Reptr*. 63: 91-94, 1979.

Bergeson, G. B. 'Influence of *Pratylenchus penetrans* alone or in combination with *Verticillium albo-atrum*'. *Phytopathology* 53: 1164-1166, 1963.

Bhardwaj, L. N., Sen, S., Sharma, R. C. and Malhotra, R. 'Effect of weather parameters on the development of mint rust under sub-temperate region of Himachal Pradesh'. *Indian Perfum*. 40: 83-87, 1996.

Bhardwaj, L. N., Sharma, R. C. and Rastogi, J. S. 'Studies on management of *Mentha* rust in sub-temperate'. *Indian Perfum*. 39: 16-18, 1995.

Bhardwaj, S. D. and Garg, R. C. 'Effect of row spacing on incidence of blight caused by *Rhizoctonia solani* in different *Mentha* species'. *Indian Perfum*. 30: 453-456, 1986.

Bhardwaj, S. D., Katoch, P. C., Kaushal, A. N. and Gupta, R. 'Effect of blight caused by *Rhizoctonia solani* on herb yield and oil content of some important collections of *Mentha* species'. *Indian J. Forestry* 3: 27-34, 1980.

Bourne, B. A. Eye spot of lemongrass'. *Phytopathology* 31(2): 186-189, 1941.

Brandt, W. H., Lacy, M. L. and Horner, C. E. 'Distribution of *Verticillium* in stems of resistant and susceptible species of mint'. *Phytopathology* 74: 567-591, 1984.

Breesford, R. M. 'Races of mint rust on cultivated peppermint and other hosts in New Zealand'. *New Zealand J. Agril. Res.* 25: 431-434, 1982.

Brejcha, U., Neubauer, J. and Stary, F. 'Experiences with protection of some officinale plants'. *Preslia.* 31:331-332, 1959.

Bruckner, K. 'Studies on the problem of physiological specialisation of mint rust'. *Archieves fur Pflanzenschutz.* 8: 15-27, 1972.

Buhrer, E. M. 'Addition to the list of plants attacked by root-knot nematode'. *Pl. Dis. Reptr.* 22: 216-234, 1938.

Butler, E. J. *Fungi and Diseases in Plants.* Calcutta: Thacker Spink and Co., 1918.

Butler, E. J. and Bisby, G. R. The fungi of India'. *Imp. Coun. of Agr. Res. India Sci.* Mono. I, XVIII, 1931.

Byzova, Z. M. 'On the mycoflora of Chu-Ili mountains'. *Trudent Institut Botank Nauk Kazakh SSR.* 11: 210-240, 1961.

Campbell, L. 'Control of plant disease by soil surface treatment'. *Phytopathology* 46: 635, 1956.

Carrera, C. J. M. 'A new disease of lemongrass'. *Hoja Inf INTA.* 34:2, 1969.

Chandhoke, N. and Ghatak, B. J. R. 'Studies on *Tagetes minuta*: some pharmacological action of essential oil'. *Ind. J. Med. Res.* 57(5): 864-876, 1969.

Cheeran, A. 'Leaf and stem blight of Japanese mint caused by *Corynespora cassicola*'. *Agril. Res. J., Kerala* 6:141, 1968.

Cheng, X. Y. and Bai, H. C. 'A new species of *Peronospora, Peronospora menthae*'. *Acta Mycologia.* 5: 135-137, 1986.

Christoff, A. Some plant diseases new to Bulgaria'. 2nd contribution. *Bull. Soc. Bot. de Bulgaria* 6: 37, 1934.

Cruchet, P. 'Contribution a letude biologique et quelques Puccinies sur Labiees Zentralblatt fur Baeriologie, Parasilenkunde und Infekions'. *Krankherten.* 17: 212-224, 1907.

Cunningham, D. D. 'On certain disease of fungal and algal origin affecting economic plants in India'. *Sci. Mem. Officer Army of India* 10: 95-130, 1897.

Das, V. M. and Sultana, S. 'Five new species of genus *Pratylenchus* from vegetable crops in Hyderabad'. *Indian J. Nematol.* 9: 5-14, 1979.

Dermelj, V. 'Studies on *Sphaceloma menthae,* the agent of peppermint anthracnose'. *J. Phytopathol.* 40: 151-186, 1960.

Deshpandey, A. L., Agarwal, J. P. and Mathur, B. N. '*Rhizoctonia bataticola* causing root rot of opium in Rajasthan'. *Indian Phytopathology* 22: 510.

Dietz, S. M., Steenland, A. P. and Horner, C. E. 'Mint rust epiphytotic in the North West'. *Phytopathology* 41: 938, 1951.

Dodov, D. N. and Tanev, I. 'Rust in oil bearing roses: Biology and means of control'. *Information of the Institute of Plant Protection*, Kostinbrod 4: 5-39, 1963.

Dutta, S. C. and Virmani, O. P. '*Rauvolfia serpentina*'. *Bull. Natl. Bot. Garden*, Lucknow. 107: 1-20, 1964.

El-Zayat, M. M., Elewa, I. S., Ahmed, M. A. and Zaky, W. H. 'Mint rust disease, species reaction chemical control and mint oil content'. *Annals of Agril. Sci.*, Cairo. 39: 397-406, 1994.

Esmenjaud, D., Minot, J. C., Voisin, R. and Gurian, G. De. 'Yield response and residues in the soil of field peppermint treated with Aldicarb'. *Mededelingen van de Faculteit Landbonwweten Schappen*. 54: 193-198, 1989.

Esmenjaud, D., Voisin, R., Minot, J. C. and Gurian, G. De. '*Pratylenchus laticauda* on peppermint in southern Alps: host range, population densities and host susceptibility of three mint sub species'. *Mededelingen van de Faceulteit Land bonwetenzschappen*. 55: 779-786, 1990.

Faulkner, L. R. 'Pathogenicity and population dynamics of *Pratylenchus hamatus* on *Mentha* species'. *Phytopathology* 52: 731, 1962.

Faulkner, L. R. and Bolazaer, W. J. 'Interaction of *Verticillium dahliae* and *Pratylenchus minus* in *Verticillium* wilt of peppermint: effect of soil temperature'. *Phytopathology* 59: 868-870, 1969.

Faulkner, L. R. and Skotland, C. B. 'Interaction of *Verticillium dahliae* and *Pratylenchus minus* in *Verticillium* wilt of peppermint'. *Phytopathology* 55: 583-586, 1965.

Fletcher, J. R. 'Experiments on the control of mint rust'. *Pl. Pathol.* 11: 115-120, 1963.

Fujioka, Y. List of crop diseases in Japan. General Headquarters, Supreme Commander Allied Powers, Tokyo. Economic and Scientific Section Natural Resources Division, Preliminary Study. 73: 1-212, 1952.

Fulara, A. *Poppy Culture*. Panstivowe Wydawnictwo Rolniczei Lesne, Warsaw (in Polish), 1971.

Ganguly, D. and Pandotra, V. R. 'Some of the commonly occurring disease of important medicinal and aromatic plants in Jammu and Kashmir'. *Indian Phytopathol.* 15: 50-54, 1962.

Girzitska, M. Z. K. 'Conidial stage of *Pleospora papaveracea* (Sacc.) Protc. Pan'. *Soviet* Congress *Botanisk*, Leningrad, January 1928, p. 172, 1928.

Goffart, H. 'Beobachtungen an Pflanzen schaidlichen nematodes'. *Nachrichtenblatt des Pflschutzdiensts*, Stuttgart. 5: 150-153, 1953.

Gokte, N. and Mathur, V. K. 'Thermal therapy for the eradication of *Mentha spicata* roots infected with *Meloidogyne incognita*'. *FAC Plant Protection Bulletin* 8: 213-215, 1990.

Goto, K. '*Sclerotium rolfsii* Sacc. in perfect stage'. *Trans. of Nat. Hist. Soc.*, Formosa 23: 37-43, 1933.

Govindu, H. C. and Thirumalachar, M. J. 'Notes on some Indian Cercosporae. IV. Sydowia'. 8: 221-230, 1954.

Green , R. J. 'Control of *Verticillium* wilt of peppermint by soil fumigation in muck soils'. *Pl. Dis. Reptr.* 48: 960-963, 1964.

Green, J. J. 'Control of *Verticillium* wilt of peppermint by crop rotation'. *Pl. Dis. Reptr.* 51: 449-453, 1967.

Green, R. J. 'Alteration of pathogenicity of *Verticillium dahliae* from *Mentha* sp. under field conditions'. *Pl. Dis. Reptr.* 61: 373-374, 1977.

Green, R. J. 'Deep ploughing for controlling *Verticillium* wilt of mint in muck soils'. *Phytopathology* 48: 575-577, 1958.

Green, R. J. '*Septoria* leaf spot disease of scotch spearmint'. *Pl. Dis Reptr*. 45: 696, 1961.

Green, R. J. 'Studies on host range of *Verticillium* that cause wilt of *Mentha piperita*'. *Science* 113: 207-208, 1951.

Green, R. J. 'The vertical distribution of *Verticillium albo-atrum* in muck soils and its control'. *Phytopathology* 47: 522, 1937.

Green, R. J. and Savada, K. '*Septoria* leaf spot disease of *Mentha* spp;. *Proc. Indian Acad. Sci*. 69: 128-130, 1960.

Grummer, G. 'The influence of *Alternaria* infection of poppy capsules on promptitude of germination by their seeds'. *Floro Fauna* 140: 298, 1953.

Gupta, M. L., Janardhanan, K. K. and Husain, A. '*Fusarium* root rot of opium poppy'. *Indian Phytopathology* 34(4): 108, 1986.

Gupta, M. L., Sattar, A., Janardhanan, K. K. and Husain, A. 'Leaf blight of opium poppy caused by *Alternaria phragmospora*'. *Indian Journal of Plant Pathology* 7(1): 83-84,1989.

Gupta, M. L., Singh, H. B., Kalra, A., Pandey, R. and Singh, S. P. 'A leaf spot of senna caused by *Colletotrichum gloeosporioides*'. *Indian J. Pl. Pathol*. 15(1 & 2): 95-96, 1997.

Gupta, R. 'Senna cultivation in India'. *Indian Hortic*. 28(4): 19-21, 1984.

Haseeb, A. and Butool, F. 'Evaluation of different pesticides and oil cake on the control of root knot nematode (*Meloidogyne incognita*) infecting Davana (*Artemisia pallens*)'. *Current Nematology*. 2(2): 204-210, 1991.

Haseeb, A. and Pandey, R. 'Observation of *Meloidogyne* spp. affecting Japanese mint: New host records'. *Nematropica*. 19: 93-97, 1989.

Haseeb, A. and Pandey, R. 'Root knot nematode, a constraint in cultivation of Davana, *Artemisia pallens*'. *Tropical Pest Management* 36(3): 317-319, 1990.

Haseeb, A. and Shukla, P. K. 'Effect of *Pratylenchus thornei* on growth, physiology and oil yield of *Mentha spicata*'. *Afro-Asian J. Nematol*. 4: 51-53, 1994.

Haseeb, A. and Shukla, P. K. 'Influence of *Pratylenchus thornei* on growth, photosynthetic rate, chlorophyll, total sugar and oil yield in *Mentha citrata*'. *Nematologia Mediterranea*. 23: 89-91, 1995.

Hemmi, T. and Kurata, S. 'Studies on septorioses of plants. V. Septoria disease of cultivated mint in Japan'. *Forschug demgeb Pflanzenkrankhoton*. 2: 10-19, 1933.

Henderson, V. R. 'Some host relationships of potato rot nematode, *Ditylenchus destructer* Thorne, 1905'. *Nature* 167(4295): 592, 1951.

Horner, C. E. 'Field disease cycle of peppermint rust'. *Phytopathology* 53: 1063-1067, 1963.

Horner, C. E. 'Pathogenicity of *Verticillium* isolates to peppermint'. *Phytopathology* 44: 239-242, 1954.

Horner, C. E. and Dooley, H. L. 'Control of *Verticillium* wilt of peppermint by soil fumigation'. *Pl. Dis. Reptr*. 50: 97-100, 1966.

Horner, C. E. and Jenson, H. J. 'Nematodes association with mint in Oregon'. *Pl. Dis. Reptr.* 38: 39-41, 1954.

Horner, C. F. 'Rhizome and stem rot of peppermint caused by *Phoma strasseri*'. *Pl. Dis. Reptr.* 55: 814-816, 1971.

Hurst, R. R. 'The potato rot nematode, *Ditylenchus destructer* in PE1'. *Proc. Can. Phytopathol. Soc.* 15: 17, 1948.

Husain, A. and Janardhanan, K. K. 'Stolon rot of Japanese mint'. *Curr. Sci.* 34: 156-157, 1965.

Ingham, R. E., Newcomb, G. B. and Morris, N. A. 'Spring nematicide application for control of root lesion and pin nematodes of peppermint'. *Fungicide and Nematicide Tests* 43: 70, 1988.

Inserra, R. N. and Rhoades, H. L. 'Some nematode problems of spearmint in Florida'. *Nematology Circular* 167: 3, 1989.

Jain, N. K. 'Disease management of aromatic plants'. In: *Advances in Horticulture, Medicinal and Aromatic Plants*, vol. 11. (Ed.). Chadha, K. L. New Delhi: Malhotra Publishing House, pp. 271-282, 1995.

Janardhanan, K. K. and Husain, A. 'Fusarium root rot of belladonna'. *Plant Science* 6:79, 1974.

Janardhanan, K. K., Ganguly, D. and Husain, A. 'Fusarium wilt of *Rauvolfia serpentina*;. *Curr. Sci.* 33(10): 313, 1964.

Janardhanan, K. K., Gupta, M. L. and Husain, A. 'Effect of *Curvularia* leaf blotch disease on the essential oil content of palmarosa'. *Indian J. Exp. Biol.* 18(4): 439-440, 1980.

Johnson, D. A. 'Races of *Puccinia menthae* in the pacific North West and interaction of latent period of mints infected with rust races'. *Plant Dis.* 79: 20-24, 1995.

Kacharmazov, U. and Tanev, I. 'Cure of mint variety maritsa by a filiform virus by combined use of thermotherapy and tissue culture'. *Rasternievdni Nauki.* 14: 114-118, 1977.

Kalra, A. and Singh, H. B. 'Evaluation of *Trichoderma harzianum* isolates for promoting growth in *Mentha arvensis* (Abstract), p. 133. *Symposium on Plant Science Research*, 2-3 April, 1996, Hisar, India, 1996.

Kalra, A., Parameswaran, T. N., Ravindra, N. S. and Singh, H. B. 'Disease problems, varietal resistance and chemical control in scented geranium'. *Proceedings IPS Golden Jubilee International Conference on Integrated Plant Disease Management for Sustainable Agriculture*, vol. 2, pp. 1237-1238, 2000.

Kalra, A., Parameswaran, T. N., Ravindra, N. S. and Singh, H. B. 'Influence of leaf blight on yields in geranium (*Pelargonium graveolens*)'. *Journal of Horticultural Sciences & Biotechnology* 74(6) 694-697,1999.

Kalra, A., Parmeshwaran, T. N. and Ravindra, N. S. 'Influence of data on plant losses and yield response of geranium (*Pelargonium graveolens*)'. *Indian J. Plant Pathol.* 6(1): 82-83, 1992.

Kalra, A., Singh, H. B. and Singh, H. P. 'Enhancement of growth of mints in presence of biocontrol agent *Trichoderma harzianum*'. (Abstract). *First International Symposium on Microbial Exploitation*, 13-16 March, 1996, Varanasi, India, 1996.

Kalra, A., Singh, H. B., Patra, N. K., Pandey, R., Shukla, R. S. and Kumar, S. 'The effect of leaf spot, rust and powdery mildew on yield components of nine Japanese mint (*Mentha arvensis*) genotypes'. *Journal of Horticultural Science & Biotechnology* 76(5): 546-548, 2001.

Kalra, A., Singh, H. B., Patra, N. K., Shukla, R. S. and Kumar, S. 'Severity of leaf spot, rust and powdery mildew and their effect on yield components on nine Japanese mint genotypes'. *Journal of Horticultural Science & Biotechnology* 76(5): 546-548, 1997.

Khan, M. L. and Khanna, A. S. 'Effect of organic amendment and nematicide on the population of *Meloidogyne hapla* and yield of *Mentha spicata*'. *Indian J. Hill Farming*. 5: 141-143, 1992.

Kishore, R., Tripathi, R. D., Johri, J. K. and Shukla, D. S. 'Some new fungal diseases of opium poppy (*Papavar somniferum* L.)'. *Indian Journal of Plant Pathology* 3(2): 213-217, 1987.

Kral, J. 'Protection of peppermint against mint rust'. *Agril. Lit. of Czechoslovakia*. 2: 291, 1977.

Kumar, S. and Nanjan. K. 'Increasing geranium yield'. *Indian Perfumer*. 29(1/2): 121-124, 1985.

Lal, A. and Mathur, V. K. 'Occurrence of *Heterodera zeae* on *Vetiveria zianioides*'. *Indian J. Nematol.* 12(2): 485-507, 1982.

Leung, A. Y. *Encyclopaedia of Common Natural Ingredients Used in Food, Drugs and Cosmetics*. John Wiley and Sons, Inc., 1980.

Lovisolo, O. and Luisoni, E. 'A new virosis of peppermint and the presence in this plant of a virus inhibitor'. *Att. Academic Torino*. 98: 213-225, 1963.

Maia, N. B., Malavolta, V. A., Carvalho, R. V. and Francelli, M. and Carmello, Q. A. C. 'Occurrence of *Pseudomonas cichorri* in *Mentha arvensis* Summa'. *Phytopathologica* 22: 185-188, 1996.

Mancini, G., Moretti, F. and Cotronea, A. 'A control trial against mint rust'. *Fitopathologica* 26: 9-11, 1976.

Mano, Y., Takakuwa, M. and Narita, T. 'Notes on black rot of peppermint'. *Annals of Phytopathol. Soc.*, Japan 29:91, 1964.

Margina, A. and Zheljazkov, V. 'Control of mint rust on mints with fungicides and their effect on essential oil content'. *J. Essen. Oil Res.* 6: 607-615, 1994.

Masalab, N. A. 'Diseases of medicinal and of some industrial plants caused by species of *Sclerotinia*'. *Sovetskaya Botanika* 6: 67-83, 1938.

Melian, L. 'Peppermint cultivation and control of rust'. *Boln Institute Invest Agronomi*. 27: 223-267, 1967.

Melouk, H. A. and Horner, C. E. 'Cross-protection in mints by *Verticillium nigrescens* against *V. dahliae*'. *Phytopathology* 65: 767-769, 1975.

Melouk, H. A. and Horner, C. E. 'Growth in culture and pathogenicity of *Phoma strasseri* to peppermint'. *Phytopathology* 62: 576-578, 1972.

Melouk, H. A. and Horner, C. E. '*Verticillium nigrescens* from peppermint'. *Phytopathology* 64: 1267-1268, 1974.

Melouk, H. A., Perkins, V. Q. and Horner, C. E. 'Control of *Phoma* stem and rhizome rot of mints with Benomyl'. *Pl. Dis. Reptr.* 59: 88-90, 1975.

Mishra, R. C., Singh, R., Shahi, S. K., Singh, H. B. and Dixit, Anupam. 'Biological management of patchouli (*Pogostemon cablin*) wilt caused by *Rhizoctonia solani*. *Current Science* 78 (3): 230-232, 2000.

Mishra, R. C., Singh, R., Singh, H. B. and Dixit, A. '*In situ* efficacy of *Trichoderma harzianum* as mycoparasite on *Sclerotium rolfsii* and *Rhizoctonia solani*'. *Tropical Agriculture* (Trinidad) 77(3): 205-206, 2000.

Molnaz, G., Farkas, G. and Kiraly, Z. 'Control of mint rust with Ni salts'. *Novenytermeles*. 9: 175-180, 1960.

Munjal, R. L., Lal, G. and Chona, B. L. 'Some *Cercospora* species from India. VI'. *Indian Phytopath.* 14: 179-190, 1961.

Nagy, F. and Szalay, P. 'Development of modern control methods against mint rust and terragon rust'. *Herba Hungarica* 24: 97-110, 1985.

Narayanappa, M., Chacko, C. I. and Vasantha Kumar, T. 'Wilt of patchouli—A new disease caused by *Rhizoctonia solani*'. *Curr. Sci*., 53(3): 707, 1984.

Neiderhauser, J. S. The rust of green house grown mint and its control'. *Nemers Cornell Agricultural Research Station* 263:30, 1945.

Nelson, R. 'Present status of wilt resistant hybrid mints'. *Proceedings Nich. Muck Association*. 25: 38, 1943.

Nelson, R. '*Verticillium* wilt of peppermint'. *Phytopathology* 27: 137, 1937.

Nelson, R. '*Verticillium* wilt of peppermint'. *United States, Department of Agriculture. Pl. Dis. Reptr. Suppl*. 50: 474, 1926.

Newton, H. C. F and Dulhoit, C. 'Stem and bulb eelworm of potato'. *Pl. Pathol*. 3: 139-140, 1954.

Ogilivie, L. and Brian, P. W. 'Hot water treatment for mint rust'. *Gardners Chronologicals* 2535: 65, 1935.

Paizs, L. and Nagy, F. '*Phoma strasseri*: a new pathogen of mint in Hungary'. *Herba Hungarica* 14: 65-75, 1975.

Pander, R. Studies on root-knot nematode, *Meloidogyne incognita* (Kofoid and White) Chitwood infesting Japanese mint (*Mentha arvensis* L. sub sp. *haplocalyx* Briquet var. *pipaeascens* Holmes and its control. Ph.D. Thesis. Kanpur University, Kanpur, 1988.

Pandey, G. N. 'Disease management of medicinal plants'. In: *Advances in Horticulture, Medicinal and Aromatic Plants*, vol. 11. (Ed.). Chadha, K. L. New Delhi: Malhotra Publishing House, New Delhi, pp. 271-282, 1995.

Pandey, R. 'Application of oil seed cake, pesticides and dry leaf matter on the reproduction potential of *Meloidogyne incognita* in Japanese mint'. *Indian J. Nematol*. 25: 12-13, 1995.

Pandey, R. 'Bionomics of phytonematodes in relation to medicinal and aromatic plants'. *Indian J. Pl. Pathol.* 12(1 & 2): 16-23, 1994.

Pandey, R. 'Nematode pests of medicinal and aromatic plants and their management'. In: *Phytonematology—Aspects and Prospects*. (Ed.). Trivedi, P. C. New Delhi: CBS, pp. 177-216, 1998.

Pandey, R. 'Phytopathological impact of root-knot nematodes on some medicinal and aromatic plants'. *J. Med. Arom. Pl. Sci.* 20: 67-84, 1998a

Pandey, R. 'Season variation in population of phytonematodes associated with peppermint (*Mentha piperita* L.) and spearmint (*Mentha spicata* L.), 1997.

Pandey, R. 'Seasonal variation in population of phytonematodes associated with peppermint and spearmint'. *J. Spices and Aromatic Crops* 6: 149-151, 1997.

Pandey, R. Studies on root knot nematode infesting Japanese mint (*Mentha arvensis*) and its control. Ph.D. Thesis. Kanpur University, Kanpur, 1989.

Pandey, R., Haseed, A. and Husain, A. 'Distribution, pathogenicity and management of *Meloidogyne incognita* on *Mentha arvensis* cv. MAS 1.' *Afro-Asian J. Nematol.* 2: 27-34, 1992.

Pandey, R., Sikora, R. A., Kalra, A., Singh, H. B. and Pandey, S. 'Plants and their products act as major nematode inhibitory agents'. In: *Nematode Management in Plants.* (Ed.). Trivedi, Trivedi. Jodhpur: Scientific Publishers, pp. 103-131, 2003.

Pandey, R., Singh, H. B. and Gupta, M. L. 'Antagonistic impact of vesicular-arbuscular mycorrhizal fungi on *Meloidogyne incognita* population development in Japanese mint'. *International Journal of Tropical Plant Diseases* 15: 237-245, 1998.

Pandey, R., Singh, H. B. and Kalra, A. 'Microbial management of plant parasitic nematodes'. *International Journal of Tropical Plant Diseases* 18: 1-23, 2000.

Pandotra, V. R. and Sastry, K. S. M. 'Studies on *Sclerotium* root of mints'. *Proc. Indian Acad. Sci.* 68: 9-10, 1968.

Parameswaran, T. N., Ravindra, N. S. and Sarwar, M. 'Alternaria blight: A new disease of patchouli'. *Curr. Sci.* 56(9): 408-409, 1987.

Parisi Rosa. 'Notes on some parasites of medicinal and aromatic plants'. *Bull. Osto. Bot. Napoli* 6: 285, 1921.

Sarwar, M. and Parmeshwaran, T. N. 'Fungus associated with leaf spot of *C. motia*'. *Indian J. Botany* 4(2): 228-229, 1981.

Sarwar, M., Narayana, M. R. and Virmani, O. P. 'Patchouli and its cultivation in India'. *Farm Bulletin* No. 17, CIMAP, Lucknow, 1983.

Sastry, K. S. M. 'Investigation and control of some important diseases of medicinal and aromatic plants'. *Indian Phytopath* 22: 140-142, 1969.

Sastry, K. S. N., Thakur, R. N. and Pandotra, V. R. 'Diseases of medicinal and aromatic plants and their control'. In: *Cultivation and Utilisation of Medicinal Plants.* (Eds.). Atal, C. K. and Kapur, B. M. Jammu: RRL, pp. 711-733, 1982.

Sattar, A. and Husain, A. 'Chemical control of *Thielavia basicola* causing stolon and rust rot of Japanese mint'. *Indian Phytopath.* 35: 106-110, 1982.

Sattar, A. and Husain, A. '*Fusarium* wilt of Japanese mint'. *New Botanist* 5: 9-10, 1978.

Sattar, A. and Husain, A. 'Stolon and rust rot of Japanese mint in Uttar Pradesh'. *Indian Phytopath* 29: 442-444, 1976.

Sattar, A., Alam, M., Janardhanan, K. K. and Husain, A. 'A new leaf disease of Japanese mint caused by *Corynespora cassicola*'. *Indian Phytopath.* 34: 404, 1981.

Sattar, A., Dhawan, O. P., Saini, S., Trivedi, M., Shahabuddin, S. and Alam, M. 'Collar rot, a new disease of opium poppy caused by *Rhizoctonia solani.*' *Indian J. Plant Pathol.* 17: 99-101, 1999.

Savada, K. and Green, R. J. 'Studies on *Septoria* leaf spot disease of *Mentha* spp.' *Pl. Dis. Reptr.* 47: 208-212, 1961.

Savile, D. B. O. '*Pernospora stigmaticola* in Canada'. *Mycologia*. 43: 113-114, 1951.

Savulescu, T. 'Phytosanitary conditions in Rumania during the year 1930-31'. *Inst. Cerc Agron. Al Romaniei. Publ.* 8: 31, 1932.

Saxena, R. N., Thakore, B. B. L. and Doshi, A. 'Capsule rot of opium poppy'. *FAO Plant Protection Bulletin* 35(2): 65, 1987.

Scheiber, E. and Sanchez, A. 'Eye spot of lemongrass'. *Plant Disease Reporter* 44(9): 72, 1960.

Sehgal, S. P., Gupta, I. J. and Agrawal, J. M. 'Capsule rot of opium poppy (*Papavar somniferum* L.)'. *Raj. J. Agric. Sci.* 2: 61-62, 1971.

Sether, D. N., Deangelis, J. D. and Rossignol, P. A. 'First report of tomato spotted wilt virus on peppermint'. *Plant Dis*. 75: 644, 1991.

Sharma, A. D. and Munjal, R. D. 'Blight of some commercial species on *Mentha* in Himachal Pradesh'. *Indian Forester* 104: 238-239, 1978.

Sharma, O. P. and Mahmud, K. A. 'A leaf spot of *Mentha viridis* caused by *Rhizoctonia solani*'. *Magazine Agric. College*, Nagpur 26:23, 1951.

Shaw, C. G. 'Host fungus index for the Pacific Northwest 1'. *Washington Agricultural Experiment Station Bulletin* No. 765, 1972.

Shukla, R. S. '*Cercospora menthicola* causing leaf spot disease of Japanese mint in India'. (Abstract). 47th Annual Meeting of Indian Phytopathological Society. Faizabad, pp. 34-35, 1995.

Shukla, R. S., Singh, H. B. and Kumar, S. 'Pathogenic response of *Cercospora menthicola* on different cultivated mint species'. *Indian Jour. Pl. Path.* 16: 76-77, 1998.

Shukla, R. S., Singh, H. B., Kalra, A., Singh, V. P. and Kumar, S. 'Occurrence of a new isolate of *Alternaria alternata* infecting rust pustules of *Mentha arvensis*'. *Journal of Medicinal and Aromatic Plant Sciences* 21: 311-315, 1999.

Shukla, R. S., Singh, H. B., Kalra, A., Singh, V. P. and Sushil Kumar. 'Occurrence of dual infection by *Puccinia menthae* and *Alternaria alternata* on *Mentha arvensis* in Tarai region of Uttar Pradesh'. *Journal of Medicinal and Aromatic Plant Sciences* 21: 311-315, 1999.

Singh, A. Studies on the collar rot of *Mentha* spp. with special emphasis on biological control. M.Sc. Thesis. GBPUA&T, Pantnagar, 1996.

Singh, A., Chaturvedi, C. and Singh, H. B. 'Anti-fungal efficacy of some essential oils against *Sclerotium rolfsii*'. *Indian Perfumer*. 44(2): 71-73, 2000.

Singh, A., Chaturvedi, C., Kalra, A. and Singh, H. B. 'Two species of *Mentha* as new hosts of *Sclerotium rolfsii*'. *EPPO/OEPP Bulletin*, France 29(2): 211, 1999..

Singh, G. and Singh, R. N. 'Leaf spot disease of *A. belladonna*'. *Indian Phytopathology* 37(3): 585, 1984.

Singh, H. B. and Chourasia, H. K. 'Outbreak and management of wilt disease of senna caused by *Fusarium semitectum*'. In: *National Symposium on Detection of Plant Pathogens and Their Management*, 18-20 January, 1995. NDUA&T, Faizabad. (Abs.), 1995.

Singh, H. B., Kalra, A. and Patra, N. K. 'Potential for biological control of wilt and rot in mints by *Trichoderma harzianum* and *Gliocladium virens*'. *Kavaka* 28 & 29: 45-48, 2001.

Singh, H. B., Kalra, A. and Patra, N. K. 'Sheath rot and blight—a new disease of *Java citronella* caused by *Rhizoctonia solani'*. *OEPP/EPPO Bulletin* 27: 269-271, 1997.

Singh, H. B., Kalra, A., Patra, N. K. and Kumar, S. 'African marigold—a new host of *Sclerotinia sclerotiorum'*. *J. Mycol. Pl. Pathol.* 28(3): 365-366, 2000.

Singh, H. B., Kalra, A., Patra, N. K. and Kumar, S. 'Stolon decay of menthol mint caused by *Sclerotinia sclerotiorum* and its biological control'. *Proceedings IPS Golden Jubilee International Conference on Integrated Plant Disease Management for Sustainable Agriculture,* vol. 1, pp. 386-388, 2000.

Singh, H. B., Kalra, A., Patra, N. K. and Kumar, S. 'Stolon decay of menthol mint caused by *Sclerotinia sclerotiorum'*. *International Conference on Integrated Plant Disease Management for Sustainable Agriculture,* New Delhi, (Abstract, p. 244), 1997.

Singh, H. B., Kalra, A., Patra, N. K. and Sushil Kumar. 'African marigold, a new host of *Sclerotinia sclerotiorum'*. *Jour Mycology and Pl. Pathology* 28: 365-366, 1998.

Singh, H. B., Patra, N. K., Kalra, A., Singh, H. P., Tanveer, H. and Sushil Kumar. 'Identification of resistant and susceptible alleles for reaction to the rust (*Puccinia nakanishikii*) in lemongrass (*Cymbopogon flexuosus*)'. *Journal of Medicinal and Aromatic Plant Sciences* 29(3): 695-699, 1999.

Singh, H. B., Singh, A., Tripathi, A., Tewari, S. K. and Johri, J. K. 'Collar rot of *Chlorophytam borivilianum* caused by *Corticium rolfsii*, a new disease'. *EPPO Bulletin* 31:112-113, 2001.

Singh, K. P. and Husain, A. 'Studies on *Corynespora* leaf spot of Japanese mint'. In: *Recent Trends in Plant Disease Control.* (Eds.). Singh, H. B., Upadhyaya, D. N. and Saha, L. R. New Delhi: Today and Tomorrow Publisher, pp. 327-331, 1993.

Singh, P. and Singh, H. B. '*Sclerotinia sclerotiorum*—A new disease report in opium poppy'. *Journal of Mycology and Plant Pathology*, 2003.

Singh, Priya. Studies on *Sclerotinia* rot of opium poppy (*Papavar* spp.). Ph.D. Thesis. V.B.S. Purvanchal University, Jaunpur, 2003.

Singh, R. 'Stolon rot of *Mentha arvensis*. *Indian Perfum*. 35: 192, 1991.

Singh, R. N. 'Leaf spot disease of *A. belladonna'*. *Indian Phytopathology* 37(3): 585, 1984.

Singh, R. V. and Kumar, U. 'Effect of different inoculum levels of *Meloidogyne incognita* on oil quality of Japanese mint'. *Annals of Pl. Prot. Sci*. 3: 187-188, 1995.

Skotland, C. B. 'Pathogenic and non-pathogenic *Verticillium* species from Central Washington'. *Phytopathology* 61: 435-436, 1971.

Skotland, C. B. and Menzies, J. D. 'Two peppermint diseases found in the Yakima valley of Washington'. *Pl. Dis. Reptr*. 41:493, 1957.

Srivastava, A. K. and Srivastava, R. '*Mentha piperita*: A new host of *Alternaria tenuis'*. *Indian Forester* 97: 34, 1971.

Staniland, L. N. 'Hot water treatment of plants'. *J. Minnesota. Agril. Univ*. 6: 278-282, 1947.

Steenland, A. and Burke, E. '*Typhula* pathogenic on mint'. *Pl. Dis. Rptr*. 34: 322, 1950.

Stone, W. J. H. and Green, R. J. 'The epiphytology of spearmint rust in Indiana'. *Mycopath. Mycol. Appl.* 31: 17-26, 1967.

Stone, W. J., Mink, G. I. and Bergeson, G. B. 'A new disease of American spearmint caused by tobacco ring spot virus'. *Pl. Dis. Reptr*. 46: 623-624, 1962.

Storey, H. H. and McCleand, A. D. P. The transmission of streak disease between maize, sugarcane and wildgrass'. *Ann. Appl. Bio*. 17: 691-719, 1930.

Suab, J. and Nagy, F. 'Results of mint rust control experiments'. *Herba Therparica*. 11: 66-67, 1972.

Sultana, S. '*Hirschmanella orycrena* n. sp and *H. oryzae* (Nematoda–Tylenchida) from Hyderabad, India'. *Indian J. Nematol*. 8: 174-176, 1978.

Tehon, R. and Daniels, E. 'Notes on parasitic fungi in Illinois'. *Mycologia*. 240-249, 1925.

Thakore, B. B. L., Jain, J. P., Singh, R. B., Khandelwal, G. L. and Mathur, S. 'Loss due to downy mildew of opium and its reduction by fungicides'. *Indian Phytopath.* 8:77, 1983.

Thakur, R. M. and Hussain, A. 'A new leaf spot disease of lemongrass'. *Indian Phytopathology* 28: 100-102, 1975.

Thakur, R. N., Singh, K. P. and Hussain, A. '*Curvularia* leaf spot of Japanese mint in India'. *Indian J. Mycol. Pl. Pathol*. 4: 199, 1974.

Thomas, J. 'Lemongrass'. In: *Advances in Horticulture,* vol. II, *Medicinal and Aromatic Plants.* (Eds.). Chand, K. L. and Gupta, Rajendra. New Delhi: Malhotra Publishing House, pp. 717-734, 1995.

Udit Narayan. 'New record of *Alternaria papaveris* from India'. *Indian Phytopathology* 44 (1): 147, 1991.

Vander Meer, J. H. H. '*Verticillium* wilt of herbaceous and woody plants'. *Meded Landbouw hoogescool. Wageningen* (Holland) 28: 82, 1925.

Verma, S. 'Diseases of lemongrass and vetiver'. *Proceedings of 7th All India Co-ordinated Workshop on Aromatic and Medicinal Plants*, RCA, Udaipur, November, 1987, 1987.

Walker, J. and Corroy, R. J. '*Puccinia menthae* in Australia'. *Aust. J. Agril. Sci*. 32: 164-165, 1969.

Wheeler, B. E. J. *An Introduction to Plant Disease*. London: John Wiley, 1969.

Zogg, H. 'Contribution to the knowledge of plant defence reactions: The influence of the temperature on the development of the gummous demarcation zone'. *O. Ber. Schweiz. Bot. Ges*. 4: 507, 1945.

—oo(O)oo—

13

Plants of Potential Medicinal Value From Thar Desert, India

Pawan K. Kasera, Sher Mohammed and Jitendra K. Shukla

THE discovery of medicine is an effort of mankind over-millions of years of search for eternal health, longevity and remedies to relieve pain and discomfort, which prompted early man to explore his natural surroundings and try many plants, animal products, minerals and develop a variety of therapeutic agents. The systematic record and incorporation into a regular system of medicine, which was refined and developed, became a part of the *Materia Medica* of many eastern cultures including those of India, China and the Arab/Persian world. The ancient civilisations of India, China, Greece, Arabia and other countries of the world developed their system of medicine independent of each other, but all of them were predominantly plant based. But the theoretical foundation and the insight and in-depth understanding of the practice of medicine that we find in Ayurveda is much superior among all the organised ancient systems of medicine. It is perhaps the oldest (6000 BC) among the organised traditional systems of medicine. It spread with Vedic, Hindu and Buddhist cultures and reached as far as Indonesia in the east and to the west it influenced the ancient Greeks who developed a similar form of medicine (Report of the Task Force on Conservation and Sustainable Use of Medicinal Plants, 2000).

About 80 per cent of the world population depends on traditional medicines for primary health care (Krishna *et al,* 2000). Interest in traditional medicine is renewed nowadays. Demand of more and more drugs from plant sources is increasing specially from developed countries during the past decade. This is because of the wide belief that 'green medicine' is safe and more dependable than the costly synthetic drugs, many of which have adverse side effects. The revival of interest in plant-based drugs has necessitated and increased demand of medicinal plants leading to over-exploitation, unsustainable harvesting and finally to the virtual decimation of several valuable plant species in the wild. Moreover, the habitat degradation due to increased human activities (human settlements, agricultural and other developmental programmes), illegal trade in rare and endangered medicinal plants and loss of regeneration potential of the degraded forests have further accelerated the current rate of extinction of plants, particularly medicinal plants. The user groups at various levels are now conscious of the decline in availability and factors like short supply, high prices and forced substitution of certain species. In fact, the survival of many of these plants is threatened all over the world (Gupta and Chaddha, 1995; Gupta, 1996).

India is rich in medicinal plant diversity and is considered a treasure house of valuable medicinal and aromatic plants. The unique biogeographical position of India makes possible the existence of all known types of ecosystems. India is rich in all the three levels of biodiversity, namely, species diversity, genetic diversity and habitat diversity. Due to varied topography and altitudinal variations from sea level to the highest mountain ranges and the vast coastal line in peninsular India, desert in the west, coolest desert in the eastern regions, the plant diversity is quite versatile in the Indian subcontinent (Sharma and Goel, 1990). Nearly 426 biomes representing different habitat diversity give rise to one of the richest centres in the world for plant genetic resources. Out of 17,000 flowering plants, the classical systems of medicine like Ayurveda, Siddha and Unani make use of only about 2,000 plants in various formulations. The traditional village physicians of India are using about 4,500 to 5,000 species of plants for medicinal purposes. The oral tradition of the villagers uses about 5,000 plants for medicinal purposes. A survey conducted by the All India Co-ordinated Research Project on Ethnobiology (AICRPE) during the last decade recorded over 8,000 species of wild plants used by the tribal and other traditional communities in India for treating various health problems (Report of the Task Force on Conservation and Sustainable Use of Medicinal Plants, 2000). The Indian systems of medicine have identified 1,500 medicinal plants, of which 500 species are commonly used in the preparation of ISM and H drugs. The World Health Organisation's (WHO) forecast is that the global market for herbal products is expected to be US $ 5 trillion by 2050 (NMPB, 2002). Herbal medicines are in great demand in both developed and the developing countries in primary health care because of their great efficacy and little or no side effects (Narula *et al,* 2000). Atul *et al* (2002) reported that the knowledge of status of existing resources of medicinal plants is the prerequisite for their efficient conservation in its broad sense.

As a result of continuous exploitation of these plants in forests and absence of regular developmental programmes, some plant species have become vulnerable to extinction due to lack of cultivation and also due to unscrupulous collection of these plants by unskilled persons (Gupta and Chadha, 1995; Kasera *et al,* 2002). Presently, the forest area in the Indian desert is only 2.41 per cent of the total geographical area extending from the western Indo-Pak border to the dry deciduous mixed forest of the Aravalli hills and the southeast plateau (Tripathi and Arya, 2002). The introduction of medicinal plants in the cropping patterns, especially in dry land and wasteland areas, could provide a strong thrust to the present need (Farooqi and Sreeramu, 2001). Medicinal plants of the arid region are well reputed and mostly used in a crude form. It is estimated that about one fourth of the total plants of the Indian Thar Desert is useful for the welfare of human beings and domestic animals for food, fuel, fodder, medicine and other requirements (Saxena, 1995; Sen, 1982). The arid zone experiences chronic water deficit along with high temperature. The erratic rainfall and poor soil fertility have marked effects on the vegetation (Kasera, 1988; Mohammed, 1988; Sen, 1982; Sen and Kasera, 1994). Despite the prevailing harsh climatic conditions, the Indian Thar desert comprises the richest plant diversity among the other deserts of the world. Recently, the National Medicinal Plants Board had prioritised 31 plant species for encouraging their cultivation during 2002. Out of the prioritised species, a few of them grow very well in desert conditions, which include *Asparagus racemosus* (shatawar), *Cassia angustifolia* (senna), *Chlorophytum borivillianum* (safed musli), *Commiphora wightii* (guggal), *Glycyrrhiza glabra* (mulhatti), *Plantago ovata* (isabgol), *Tinospora cordifolia* (gilioe), *Withania somnifera* (asgand), etc. Besides, there are many other species of medicinal importance such as *Abutilon indicum* (kanghi), *Achyranthes aspera* (andhi jhara), *Aristolochia bracteolata* (kiramar), *Balanites aegyptiaca* (hingoto), *Caesalpinia cristata* (karanju), *Cymbopogon jwarancusa* (lemongrass), *Evolvulus alsinoides* (shankhpushpi), *Pedalium murex* (bara-gokhru), *Peganum harmala* (harmal), *Prosopis cineraria* (khejri), *Salvadora persica* (khara jhal), *Sida cordifolia* (kungyi), *Tecomella undulata* (rohira), *Tribulus terrestris* (chhota-gokhru), etc. which are distributed among the desert vegetation. The present communication deals with the medicinal properties and economic utility of some important medicinal plants growing well in the Indian Thar Desert. The details of each plant species are as follows.

(i). *Achyranthes aspera* (Latjeera, Andhi Jhara; Amaranthaceae)

It is an annual rainy season herb (Figure 1). It is widely used by the tribal and traditional healers of India. The stem is quadrangular and hairy. Leaves are variable in shape, often bearing red-coloured blotches. The inflorescence is an elongated terminal spike. The seedlings appear after 2-3 showers of rain during the rainy season, but the flowering takes place in winter. Flowers are green and purple when young and become deflexed when the fruit is formed. Fruit is a single seeded, indehiscent, enclosed by a persistent and hardened perianth, bracts and bracteoles. The fruits easily stick into the skin of animals or the clothes of human beings and get dispersed (Sen, 1981). It is used as a laxative to improve appetite and also in treatment of heart diseases, mental problems, bronchitis, piles, dyspepsia, diseases of blood, etc. When administered with anti-leprosy drug DDC (Diamino diphenyl sulphone) chances of adverse reaction become less and fast improvement takes place, which shows the contributory role in the treatment of leprosy. The dried plant is given to children for colic. It is also diuretic, digestive and protective to the kidneys (Chemexcil, 1992). Bhatt *et al* (2002) documented that decoction of the whole plant is useful in renal calculi. Vyas (2001) documented the use of fruit powder along with jaggery for treatment of cough. Young leaves and flowers are used in fever, boils, cuts and wounds. Fruits are used in stomach complaints, toothache and treatment of pyorrhoea. It is used in primary syphilitic sores. In large doses, it produces abortion or labour pains. Aqueous extract of root is used for stones in the bladder. Singh and Pandey (1983) observed that the ash of the plant yields a dye which is used in the textile industry, calico printing, varnishes, paints, etc. The seeds are boiled in milk or 'chhach' and taken as tonic during winters.

(ii). *Blepharis sindica* (Unt-kantalo; Family: Acanthaceae)

Blepharis sindica is a common plant of rocky to sandy habitats in the western Rajasthan desert. The plant is an annual herb and also perennates through rootstocks (Figure 2). It may be used for reclamation of dry areas. The seeds are used as diuretic, expectorant and aphrodisiac (Singh *et al*, 1996). The seeds are boiled in milk and taken as tonic. It is also given to cattle to increase milk production (Bhandari, 1990). Seeds are used as a cure for earache (Sastry and Kavathekar, 1990).

(iii). *Boerhaavia diffusa* (Punarnava, Santhi; Family: Nyctaginaceae)

It is a fairly common rainy season weed (Figure 3) in mixed habitats throughout the State. It is a useful lithophytic for eroded rocky surfaces. It is relished by sheep and goats and given to

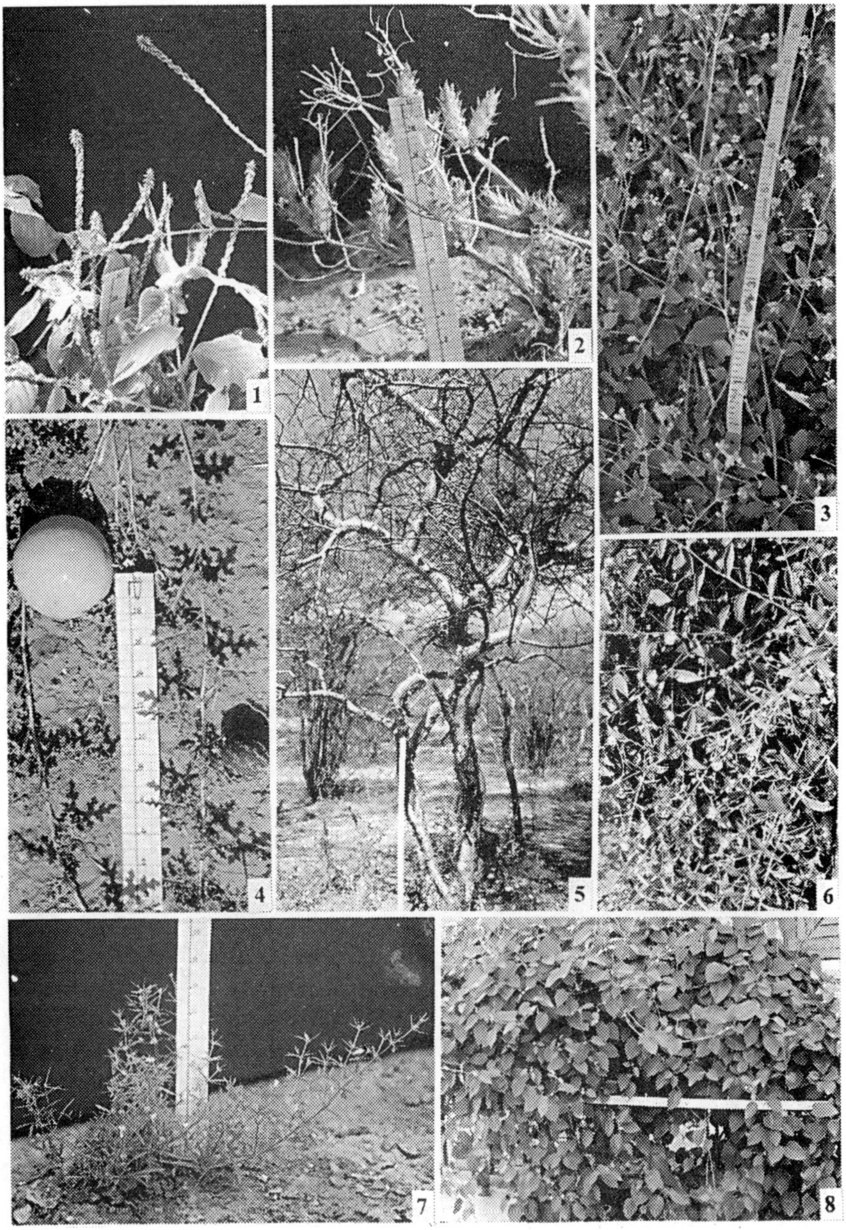

Figure I. Plants growing in natural habitats.

1. ***Achyranthes aspera*** **2.** ***Blepharis sindica;*** **3.** ***Boerhaavia diffusa;*** **4.** ***Citrullus colocynthis;*** **5.** ***Commiphora wightii;*** **6.** ***Evolvulus alsinoides;*** **7.** ***Fagonia indica;*** **8.** ***Leptadaenia reticulata.***

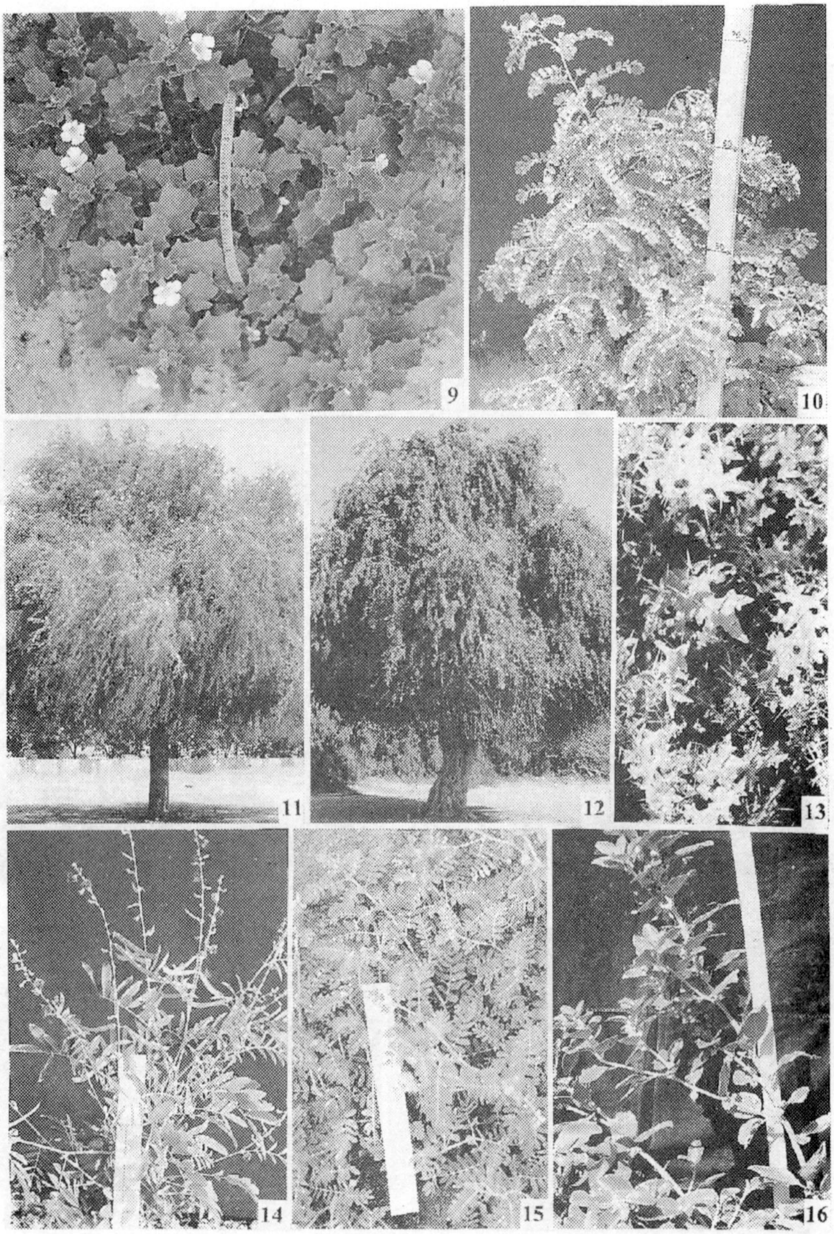

Figure II. Plants growing in natural habitats.
9. *Pedalium murex;* 10. *Phyllanthus amarus;* 11. *Prosopis cineraria;* 12. *Salvadora persica;* 13. *Solanum surattense;* 14. *Tephrosia purpurea;* 15. *Tribulus terrestris;* 16. *Withania somnifera.*

milch cows to increase milk production. Plant yields drug 'punarnava', which possesses diuretic and anti-inflammatory activities. The plant is also recommended for asthma. Roots are used to cure acidity, flatulence, rheumatism, eye diseases and credited with anticonvulsant, analgesic, laxative, diuretic and expectorant properties (Sastry and Kavathekar, 1990). Leaves are used as diuretic in jaundice and leaf juice in chronic renal failure and dropsy. Tender leaves are eaten and a garland made of root pieces is worn to cure jaundice. Decoction is prescribed for patients suffering from jaundice, where it helps and protects the liver and also for patients suffering from kidney troubles, where it helps in the kidney function and promotes urination. Ash of leaves and crushed and boiled roots are useful in night blindness (Singh and Pandey, 1983).

(iv). *Citrullus colocynthis* (Tumba; Family: Cucurbitaceae)

It is a perennial trailing herb (Figure 4) native to Asia and Africa, but found in North India, Madhya Pradesh, Gujarat, South India, Rajasthan, etc. Bitter fruits are used as purgative and roots in urinogenital disorders and jaundice. Extract form pulp is highly effective against bacteria (Singh *et al,* 1996). Paste of root applied in enlarged abdomen of children. It is used in cerebral congestion, dropsy, cough and rheumatism. Seed oil blackens grey hair. Fruit juice contains a-elatrine, citrulluin, citrullene and citrulluic acid. Bitter oil, that is, citbittol is isolated from the peel-free flesh of ripe fruit, while colocynth drug from the dried pulp of the fruit, which is used in indigenous medicine such as drastic hydragogue, cathartic and provides large watery evacuations. Small fruits are collected during the rainy season, stuffed with salt and ajwain and then used as a cure for acute stomach ache (Singh and Pandey, 1983). Bitter seeds are buried in common salt to wash-off their bitter principles, dried and mixed with bajra seeds and flour of the mixed seeds is taken in the time of scarcity (Bhandari, 1990).

(v). *Commiphora wightii* (Guggal; Family: Burseraceae)

It is a perennial shrub/small medium-sized tree, reaching a height of 5-8 metres. It is a slow growing plant with crooked and knotty branches ending in sharp spines (Figure 5). It grows on the foothills of the Aravalli range and also in arid/semi-arid lands including desert areas. In India it occurs in Rajasthan, Gujarat, Maharashtra, Madhya Pradesh and Karnataka States. The plant is polymorphic in nature, that is, one having bisexual and male flowers, while others having female flowers with staminodes (apparently look like well-developed stamens but contain only sterile pollen (Dalal and Patel, 1995). A third category of plants with only male flowers has also been reported by Rao *et al* (1984). Yadav *et al* (1999) reported the occurrence of only female plants from Rajasthan. It is the main source of the drug guggulu in India. The oleogum resin is moist, fragrant and of golden colour. It is a complex mixture of diterpenes, aliphatic esters, steroids, carbohydrates, inorganic ions, essential oils, etc. (Chadha, 2001). It acts as an astringent and antiseptic on the abraded skin and mucous membrane. When taken internally it is reported to possess appetising carminative, antispasmodic, diaphoretic, ecbolic, anti-suppurative, aphrodisiac and emmenagogue properties. The gum solution is used as a gargle for spongy gums, chronic tonsillitis and caries in the teeth (Raghunathan and Mitra, 1999). The ethyl acetate fraction of gum-resin gives different constituents, namely, Z-guggulsteron, E-guggulsteron and Guggulsterol-I, II and III, which are useful in lowering cholesterol levels (Gupta and Chadha, 1995). The Central Drug Research Institute, Lucknow, has developed 'Guggulip', a drug for lowering the cholesterol level (Anonymous, 1987). Essential oil is anthelmintic and antibiotic (Sastry and Kavathekar, 1990). The oleo-gum resin causes an increase of leucocytes in the blood and stimulates phagocytosis.

Inhalation of the fumes of burnt guggal is recommended in hay fever, acute chronic catarrh, chronic bronchitis, etc. (Farooqi and Sreeramu, 2001).

(vi). *Evolvulus alsinoides* (Shankhpushpi, Vishnukranta; Family: Convolvulaceae)

Evolvulus alsinoides is recorded throughout India in open and rocky areas, gardens, lawns, along roadsides and also in cultivated fields. The plant is slow growing and the growth becomes restricted after the environmental conditions become dry (Sen, 1973). It is an annual/perennial herb with spreading branches in all directions, arising from a small woody rootstock (Figure 6). The roots are fairly deep with radiating branches up to a distance of 25 cm or more. The whole plant and especially the leaves are densely clothed with white appressed and long spreading hair. Seed germination takes place during the rainy season after two or three showers of rain under field conditions. Flowering takes place from August to November and fruit formation in the last week of August, while the flowering still continues. Saharan *et al* (2002) reported three types of flower colour variations, that is, dark blue, light pink and white. The whole plant is used medicinally. The important alkaloids present are: evolvine, betaine and β-sitosterol (Chemexcil, 1992). It is used in bronchitis, biliousness, epilepsy, leucoderma, teething of infants, loss of appetite, etc. This plant is also used as a febrifuge and as an alternative to oil for promoting the growth of hair (Kirtikar and Basu, 1994). Girach *et al* (2001) mentioned that it is useful as a blood purifier, bleeding piles, eye diseases and management of diabetes. The fresh flowers with sugar are eaten as a brain tonic. This is the real Ayurvedic drug 'Shankhpushpi' (Singh and Pandey, 1998; Bhatnagar *et al,* 2000; Sinha and Sinha, 2001). The plant is useful in internal haemorrhages. The leaves are made into cigarettes and smoked in chronic bronchitis and asthma (Singh and Pandey, 1983). It improves complexion, voice and cure intestinal worms, animal poisoning and uterine disorders (Sivarajan and Balachandran, 1999). It is a digestive, carminative and also possesses cooling and calming properties and above all promotes 'medha', the power of memory. It is also known as 'wisdom plant' with potential to accelerate brain function in children and prevents loss of memory in the aged. It has also gained exceptionally high reputation in the medical world (Sinha and Sinha, 2001).

(vii). *Fagonia indica* (Dhamaso; Family: Zygophyllaceae)

It is a short erect spiny undershrub with slender branches, terete striates, a glabrous or sparsely glandular puberulous growing almost throughout the year. A peculiar phenomenon of leaf surface reduction in response to increasing aridity has been observed by Mohammed and Sen (1987) and Lekhak *et al* (1992). Seedlings produce long-petiolated trifoliate leaves having thin leaflets (Figure 7). The degree of reduction in total transpiring area of this plant is regulated directly by the intensity of decrease in soil moisture. The plant is suitable for growing in gypsum and lime rich areas. Twigs are used as tooth-brushes (Sastry and Kavathekar, 1990). The plant is used as bitter tonic, diuretic, astringent, prophylactic against smallpox, etc. It is employed in the preparation of Kumari Asava, an indigenous medicinal preparation known for its stimulant and laxative properties. Singh and Pandey (1998) reported that plant decoction is used by the Bhils to cure fever, dropsy and disorders caused by poisoning. In Barmer district, its powder is mixed with fruits and leaves of *Terminalia chebula* and *Cassia italica* and taken orally to cure abdominal pain. Boiled residue of the plant in water is used for abortion (Singh and Pandey, 1983).

(viii). *Leptadaenia reticulata* (Jivanti; Family: Asclepiadaceae)

Leptadaenia reticulata is a climber/liana having stem with cork like deeply cracked bark with numerous branches. It flourishes well in humid and shady places (Figure 8). In India, it is found in Gujarat, Punjab, Himalayan ranges, Khasia hills, Konkan, Nilgriris, South India, Sikkim, etc. Seed germination takes place from June to September after one or two showers of rain under field conditions. Flowering takes place throughout the year, but does not lead to fruit formation up to December. Fruit formation takes place in December to February. Dispersal of seeds takes place during June-July.

Jivanti is considered a stimulant and tonic in Ayurvedic literature. The medicinal use dates back to about 4500 to 1600 BC as mentioned in the *Atharva Veda,* Kanda 8, Sukta 2. The *Atharva Veda* also mentions its uses as a life and strength giver, propagator of milk and useful in many other ailments. Charaka described it as an important rasayana drug, capable of maintaining the youthful vigour and strength and Vagbhata incorporated it among the 10 drugs that constitute the *Jivaniya gana* or the vitalising group. Jivanti is cold, sweet, aphrodisiac, rejuvenative and easy to digestion. It promotes health and vigour, improves voice, alleviates the three *dosas*—vata, pitta and kapha—and cures eye diseases, haemetemesis, emaciation, cough, dyspnoea, fever, burning sensation, dysentery, night blindness, poisonous affections and tuberculosis. Mostly the whole plant with leaves and stem branches is used. Anjaria *et al* (1997) mentioned it as a stimulant, galactagogue, oestrogenic, eye tonic, astringent, agalactia and decreased milk after parturition to increase milk, prolapse of uterus, vagina, controlling habitual abortion, maintain pregnancy, repeat breeders, induce heat, soothe hard milkers and induce milk letting. Its restorative property makes it an important ingredient in preparation of Chyawanprash (an Ayurvedic tonic). The leaf paste and roots are taken orally with water to cure gangrene by the Bhils of southern Rajasthan (Singh and Pandey, 1998). Kirtikar and Basu (1994) mentioned it as a stimulant and tonic.

(ix). *Pedalium murex* (Bara-gokhru; Family: Pedaliaceae)

It is mostly distributed in Northern India. It is much branched, erect or sub-prostrate, annual, succulent herb. Stem is rough with glandular protuberances. Leaves are simple, opposite, fleshy, elliptica-obovate with grooved glandular petiole. Flowers are pale yellow, solitary, axillary and zygomorphic (Figure 9). The important chemicals present are: Triterpenoida; ursolic acid; steroid: sitosterol and miscellaneous compounds such as vinillin, phenolic acid, fatty acid and oils, resins, etc. Leaves are consumed as vegetable. It is used to treat urinary disorders, incontinuance of urine, sexual impotency, spermatorrhoea, nocturnal emission and impotency. The mucilaginous water produced from the fresh leaves is taken as a remedy for gonorrhoea and dysuria. Juice of fruit is used in puerperal diseases and to promote lochial discharges. Decoction of whole fruit or infusion of whole plant is used in treatment of renal calculi (Bhatt *et al*, 2002). Fruits and seeds are also used in reducing blood sugar and controlling diabetes (Sinha and Sinha, 2001).

(x). *Phyllanthus amarus* (Bhumi-amalaki, Jar-amala; Family: Euphorbiaceae)

It grows abundantly throughout India during the rainy season; however it is less frequent in the southern part of the country. It is well adapted to a variety of soils, at pH ranging from alkaline to neutral and acidic soil. It prefers calcareous, well-drained light textured soils. It rarely survives under dry or very low temperature conditions, but water logging does not show any lethal effects. It grows as an erect or ascending annual herb. Stem is smooth, terete and stipulate at base of branches bearing leaves arranged on 15-30 leafed branchlets, which are 4-8 cm long. The flowering and fruiting take place almost throughout the year but more profusely during rains

(Figure 10). Its leaves and roots are used in jaundice. The plant is also used as a diuretic in oedema. It is also used to increase appetite and locally to relieve inflammations (Chemexcil, 1992). Drug from *Phyllanthus niruri* can cure even Hepatitis-B for which there is no curative treatment to date but only preventive vaccine (Sinha and Sinha, 2001).

(xi). *Prosopis cineraria* (Khejri; Family: Mimosaceae)

It is an important leguminous multipurpose tree species of the Indian Thar Desert and is a very slow growing tree species (Figure 11). In nature, it reproduces by seeds only. However, this tree can be raised through air-layering. It has deep root system with low water and nitrogen requirements. New leaves appear on the fully mature tree twice in a year, that is, during March-April and July-October and thereafter new leaves develop slowly. The leaf fall is observed from November onwards. The initiation of flowering begins in January and this tree is in full blooming stage in February-March. The fruit setting takes place from April onwards. The fruits attain maximum length in May.

Prosopis cineraria is a vital component of a traditional agro-forestry system and is grown together with field crops to provide dry season fodder and fuel. The wood is suitable for interior construction work such as columns of huts, roofs, doors, windows, wheels and hubs of carts, small agriculture implements, tool handles, small turnery articles and well curbs (Anonymous, 1969). It does not compete with the crops/plants grown near it for water and minerals because of its deep root system. Purohit *et al* (2002) observed more fungal biomass and population and soil nutrients in under canopy soil of this tree as compared to open habitat. This quality is ideal for its introduction in silvipastoral and agro-forestry systems. The leaves locally called 'loong' are highly palatable and used as a nutritious top feed for cattle and livestock. The protein-rich pods provide considerable amount of moisture to the animals during the peak summer months of May-June. A moderately grown tree yields nearly 25-30 kg of dry leaf forage per year (Bohra and Ghosh, 1980). The immature pods are used as fodder for livestock and are rich in sweetish farinaceous pulp, which is consumed as food. The pods are eaten green or dried after boiling and serve as green and dry vegetable for rural masses locally known as 'sangari'. The dry pods are fed to milch cattle and one tree gives at least five kg of ripened pods. The dry pods reduce the quest for water in summer months and generally farmers eat them in dry periods. The ground inflorescence mixed with sugar in water is used for cooling effect, as a blood purifier and for prevention of boils and skin diseases (Purohit and Khan, 1980; Singh and Pandey, 1998). Flowers are pounded, mixed with sugar and eaten by women during pregnancy as a safeguard against miscarriage (Singh and Pandey, 1983). The bark is dry, acrid, bitter with sharp taste, cooling and anthelmintic, tonic, cures leprosy, dysentery, bronchitis, asthma, leucoderma, piles, tumours of the muscles, wandering of mind and scorpion and snake bites (Kirtikar and Basu, 1994). The gum oozing out in February–March, is used by rural folk with sweet balls at the time of delivery and considered nutritive. The firewood makes a better charcoal among local plants of the arid zone and gives better heat and energy. The wood ash contains 31 per cent soluble potassium salts, which may be used as source of potash (Purohit and Khan, 1980). Ash is also rubbed over the skin to remove hair (Memon *et al,* 1988). Besides increasing soil fertility, it acts as a soil binder and lowers the speed of hot wind. Khan and Harsh (2000) reported an effective and commercial plant growth regulator, that is, triacontanol (0.012 per cent) in the leaves of *Prosopis cineraria,* which is responsible for better grass yield under and in the vicinity of this tree.

(xii). *Salvadora persica* (Khara Jhal; Family: Salvadoraceae)

It is a typical desert species, which grows as a mangrove perennial tree as well as under extreme saline (salt stress) and drought conditions. The flowering takes place during September–October (Figure 12). The plants produce fruits with and without seeds. The seedless fruits are purple red to creamy white and semi-transparent. The seedless fruit formation takes place in November. The seeded fruits are formed from December onwards. The plant produces three types of fruits, that is, pink, purple and white. The purple fruit bearing plants showed better seed traits, namely, seed weight, size, thickness, volume, density, viability and germination percentage as compared to other two types of fruit bearing plants (Prakash *et al,* 2001). The average seed production is abut 20-30 kg plant^{-1}. The fruits are marked by NGOs for the oil extraction (Bhansali and Jindal, 2000).

The root contains steam-distillable oil, which has 90 per cent Benzylisothiocyanate, a compound responsible for decreasing dental caries and used in the preparation of Meswak toothpaste (Zodape and Indusekhar, 1997). The virucidal activity of *Salvadora persica* due to the presence of Benzylisothiocyanate against Herpes Simplex virus (HSV) seems to support the use of Meswak as preventive measure in controlling the oral infection (Al-Bagieh, 1992). Singh and Pandey (1998) observed that tender branches are used as hygienic and medicated toothbrush, probably due to presence of sodium and potassium chloride and sulphate with traces of ethereal oil. Two-three year-old fruits are crushed in water and given orally against snakebite for inducing vomiting. The dried seeds contain 30-40 per cent oil, which is of a great economic value (Anonymous, 1964; Sen and Chawan, 1969; Prakash, 2001). Seeds are purgative, diuretic, tonic and yield fatty oil applied on rheumatic swelling. The fruit is sweet in taste, aphrodisiac, alexiteric, stomachic, improves appetite and useful in biliousness. Formation of insect galls on stem and leaf is commonly observed. The aqueous extract of these insect galls possesses some growth-promoting principles (Sen and Chawan, 1969). It is a good fodder for camels. Stem bark is used for gastric troubles and as an ascarifuge. Decoction of leaves used in asthma and cough.

(xiii). *Solanum surattense* (Kateli; Family: Solanaceae)

It is distributed all over India and also in the Thar Desert. It may be termed as winter-summer weed as the plants flower and produce fruits with viable seeds in both the seasons. The plant is very prickly, diffuse, procumbent, often becomes perennial reaching a spread of a metre or so under luxurious conditions (Sharma, 1970; Sen, 1981). The plants appear after rains and start bearing fruits in the following winter. Fruits are large and have a very firm leathery pericarp and spongy mesocarp. The fruit turns yellow when ripe with cream coloured stripes (Figure 13). The part used is the dried roots. The chief chemical compound is solasodine alkaloid. It is used traditionally to cure cough, asthma, chest and muscular pain, bronchitis and diuretic to remove bladder stone. It has gained importance in recent years for the treatment or removal of bladder stones. Jain (1968) reported the antibacterial property in its fruits. The chemical 'solasodine' is important in preparation of a steroid that helps the body adapt to stress and balance the body fluids. It also controls inflammation and promotes tissue regeneration. Root is an expectorant, forming an ingredient of Ayurvedic medicine 'Dasamula'. Juice of fruits is used in sore throat and juice of leaves mixed with black pepper is recommended in rheumatism. Fruit yields glycol-alkaloids, which can be source material for cortisone and sex hormone preparation. A decoction of plant is used in gonorrhoea and it is also said to promote conception in females (Chemexcil, 1992). The buds and flowers with salt solutions are good for watery eyes. The roots of white-flowered plants are used to increase fertility in women (Singh and Pandey, 1983).

(xiv). *Tephrosia purpurea* (Biyani, Sarpankho, Dhamasia; Family : Papilionaceae)

It is a branched, erect, perennial herb, assuming a shrubby growth (Figure 14) and found throughout India. It is also grown as green manure and cover crop. Stem is stout and hairy. Leaves are pinnately compound. Leaflets are hairy on both the surfaces, density being more on lower surface. Flowers are reddish purple on terminal or leaf opposed peduncles with 6-20 in number. The seedlings appear within 48 hours of first shower. The plant produces flowers during the monsoon season (August-September) and fruiting occurs in late September.

Singh and Pandy (1983) reported that leaves are useful in leprosy. Roots are bitter and useful in dyspepsia, chronic diarrhoea, enlarged liver, asthma, urinary disorders and stomach troubles. The seeds are used as cooling agent. The plant is tonic and laxative, used as anthelmintic for children and internally as blood purifier. A decoction in water is used against a disease locally called 'dhamasia' (cough with black phlegm). The plant with *Cannabis sativa* is used in piles and cholera. The plant is also used as a digestive, diuretic and antitussive in Ayurvedic practice. It has undergone clinical trials in viral hepatitis and is claimed to improve liver function (Chemexcil, 1992). The dried herb is used for boils, pimples and bleeding piles. Leaves are useful in jaundice (Sharma and Prajapati, 2002).

Leaves have rutin alkaloid and also yield dye (Singh *et al,* 1996). The roots, leaves and seeds contain tephrosin, deguelin and quercetin. The roots also contain isotephrosin and rotenoneand 2.5 per cent rutin is found in roots and leaves (Chemexcil, 1992).

(xv). *Tribulus terrestris* (Chhota-gokhru; Family: Zygophyllaceae)

It is a common weed which comes up soon after the rains from seeds and also regenerating from the stumpy rootstocks of the earlier season. It is common on sandy soil and wasteland. The stem is woody with compound leaves in 5-6 opposite pairs and short stalks. Flowers are light pink to purplish red (Figure 15). White coloured petals have also been reported by Sen (1981). Fruit is a flat pod with 4-8 seeds. The seeds are cylindrical pale-yellow to dark brown or mottled and very hard. It is used traditionally in treatment of haematuria. It has a cooling effect and used for promotion of urination and as a nervine tonic. It can be grown for stabilising the arid sandy regions and hills. The green parts are highly palatable to livestock. Leaf and tender parts are rich in calcium. Paste prepared from leaves is used for treatment of stones in bladder. Powdered fruit made into bread and eaten; fruits are diuretic and tonic and used for treatment of calculous affections and painful micturition. Root is a constituent of Dasmoolarista and Amritaprasagritha (Sastry and Kavathekar, 1990).

(xvi). *Withania somnifera* (Ashwagandha, Asgand; Family: Solanaceae)

It is branched erect perennial undershrub with more or less tuberous root. Branches are terete, clothed with stellate hairy tomentum and at length somewhat glabrous. Leaves are ovate, obovate or oblong and entire rounded. Flowers are greenish-yellow and sessile axillary in 4-6 flowered cymes. Fruits are orange-red berry. The dried roots and fresh leaves are useful (Figure 16). Several biologically active principles are reported in it. Traditionally, it has been used as a rejuvenator and restorative. The varieties from Nagaur and Pali districts of Rajasthan are more effective. Ashwagandha oil is soothing to the body and induces sound sleep. The herb is a boon for children suffering from rickets. Traditional healers use it is treatment of sexual impotency, respiratory and urinogenital disorders, male sterility, general debility, leucorrhoea, rheumatoid arthritis, as anti-inflammatory, diuretic, promote urination and for purification of blood. In modern uses, it has found wide acceptance as an anabolic, rejuvenator and as an adaptogen against stress. It is called 'Indian Ginseng' and a 'wonder drug' of the 21st century. Bark has withaniols group of alkaloids (0.13–0.68 per cent), out of which withanine and pseudo-withanine are therapeutically important. The roots of cultivated crop contain up to 50 per cent of these alkaloids (Chadha, 2001). For growing children, it is an elixir to accelerate growth, improve their health and vitality (Sinha and Sinha, 2001). Extract of roots can be used as an adjuvant to local tumour excision and may increase the overall survival rate. The roots and leaves possess antibiotic and antibacterial activities. Farooqi and Sreeramu (2001) reported that fruits and seeds are diuretic in nature. An ointment prepared by boiling the leaves is useful for bed-sores and wounds. The fresh leaf juice is also applied on anthrax pustules. An infusion of the bark is given for asthma.

CONCLUSION

The knowledge of medicinally important plant species which is the outcome of the experiences passed on to the successive generations make the desert dwellers not only to remain healthy but also to overcome prolonged illness. Some of these plant species are part of the product/process of commercial exploitation. In recent times with an increase in the use of fast-acting allopathic drugs on one hand, the peoples are returning back to the use of drugs derived from locally available plant materials, because of least side effects. Medicinal plants are an integral part/component of research and development in the pharmaceutical industry with a research focus on isolation and direct use of active medicinal constituents. The biodiversity of plant species, coupled with the chemical diversity found within each plant, leads one to the conclusion that plants are perhaps the most valuable source of new bioactive chemical entities. Only a small fraction of plants has been systematically investigated for the presence of bioactive compounds. A single plant can serve as a source for a variety of chemical structures having different pharmacological indications. India is ranked among the major exporters of medicinal plants and vegetative/sap extracts, but when compared to developed countries it stands nowhere with regard to the export of more specific products, that is, the bioactive like alkaloid, hormones, glycosides, etc. in the world (Saxena and Kumar, 2002). The indigenous plant species of the arid zone need special attention in this matter as they have a large therapeutic and medicinal value. The above-mentioned 16 medicinal plants are well adapted in our area. Hence, these plants need priority attention for commercial cultivation and sustainable use in different agro-climatic conditions. Thus, the cultivation of economically important species should be intensified to reduce the burden on the nature habitat.

REFERENCES

Al-Bagieh, N. H. 'Anti-herpes simplex virus type-1, activity of Benzylisothiocyanate'. *Biomed Lett.* 47:67-70, 1992.

Anjaria, J. V., Parabia, M., Bhatt, G. and Khamar, R. *Nature Heals: A Glossary of Selected Indigenous Medicinal Plants of India.* Ahmedabad: Sristi Innovations, 1997.

Anonymous. 'Guggul lipid technology developed by C.D.R.I., commercialised in India (News)'. *The Eastern Pharmacist* 30: 107-108, 1987.

Anonymous. *Non-Edible Oil and Soap Industry.* Bombay: Khadi & Village Industry Commission Publication, 1964.

Anonymous. *The Wealth of India.* vol. III. New Delhi: CSIR, pp. 247-249, 1969.

Atul, Punam and Sharma, S. 'The medicinal wealth of western Himalayan agro-ecological region of India. I. An inventory of herbs'. *Annals of Forestry: Special Issue Focus on Medicinal and Aromatic Plants* 10: 28-61, 2002.

Bhandari, M. M. *Flora of the Indian Desert.* MPS Repros, Jodhpur: Scientific Publishers, 1990.

Bhansali, R. R. and Jindal, S. K. 'Role of farmers in promotion of eco-friendly multipurpose trees of arid zone'. In: *Environmental Protection.* (Eds.), Chaudhary, V., Singh, K. and Kakralya, B. L. Jaipur: Pointer Publishers, pp 92-102, 2000.

Bhatnagar, M., Shukla, S. D., Jain, S. and Mundra, A. 'Cytoprotective effects of Shankhpushpi, an *E. alsinoides* preparation on hippocampal cells in mice'. *Indian Drugs* 37: 280-285, 2000.

Bhatt, D. C., Mitaliya, K. D., Patel, N. K. and Ant, H. M. 'Herbal remedies for renal calculi'. *Ad. Plant Sci.* 15: 1-3, 2002.

Bohra, H. C. and Ghosh, P. K. 'The nutritive value and digestibility of loong [*P. cineraria* (Khejri)] leaves'. In: *Khejri (Prosopis cineraria) in the Indian Desert—Its Role n Agroforestry.* (Eds.). Mannem, H. S. and Saxena, S. K. CAZRI Monograph No. 11, pp. 45-50, 1980.

Chadha, K. L. (Ed.). *Handbook of Horticulture.* New Delhi: ICAR, 2001.

Chemexcil *Selected Medicinal Plants of India: A Monograph of Identity, Safety and Clinical Usage.* Bombay: Pharmaceuticals & Cosmetics Export Promotion Council, 1992.

Dalal, K. C. and Patel, M. A. 'Guggal'. In: *Advances in Horticulture: Medicinal and Aromatic Plants.* (Eds.), Chadha, K. L. Gupta, R. vol. II, New Delhi: Malhotra Publishing House, pp. 491-501, 1995.

Farooqi, A. A. and Sreeramu, B. S. *Cultivation of Medicinal and Aromatic Crops.* Hyderabad: Universities Press (India) Ltd, 2001.

Girach, R. D., Brahmam, M., Misra, M. K. and Ahmed, M. 'Some less known medicinal plants in relation to Unani system of medicine from District Bhadrak, Orissa'. *Hamdard Medicus* 44: 51-56, 2001.

Gupta, R. 'Medicinal and aromatic crops'. In: *50 Years of Crop Science Research in India.* (Eds.). Paroda, R. S. and Chadha, K. L. New Delhi: ICAR, pp. 724-737, 1996.

Gupta, R. and Chadha, K. L. 'Medicinal and aromatic plants research in India'. In: *Advances in Horticulture: Medicinal and Aromatic Plants.* (Eds.). Chadha, K. L. and Gupta, R. vol. 11. New Delhi: Malhotra Publishing House, New Delhi, pp. 1-43, 1995.

Jain, S. K. *Medicinal Plants.* New Delhi: National Book Trust of India, 1968.

Kasera, P. K. Arid agro-ecosystem: Weed biology and weed management. Ph.D. Thesis. University of Jodhpur, India, 1988.

Kasera, P. K., Saharan, P., Prakash, J. and Chawan, D. D. 'Agrotechniques for cultivation and multiplication of some important medicinal plants of the That desert'. In: *Advances in Resource Management of the Indian Desert.* (Eds.). Kapoor, B. B. S., Ali, A., Mathur, S. K. and Kaushik, S. Bikaner: Madhu Publications, pp. 201-214, 2002.

Khan, H. A. and Harsh, L. N. 'Role of minor forest products (MFP) producing plants in governmental protection'. In: *Environmental Protection.* (Eds.). Chaudhary, V., Singh, K. and Kakralya, B. L. Jaipur: Pointer Publishers, pp. 240-243, 2000.

Kirtikar, K. R. and Basu, B. D. *Indian Medicinal Plants* (2nd edn.). Dehradun: Bishen Singh Mahendra Pal Singh, vols. 1-4, 1994.

Krishna, A., Singh, A. K., Srivastava, R. K., Tomar, V. K. S. and Kumar, S. 'Need for large scale production and quality control of medicinal herbs'. In: *National Seminar on Frontiers of Research and Development in Medicinal Plants.* Lucknow: CIMAP. Abst. p. 81, 2000.

Lekhak, H. D., Mohammed, S. and Sen, D. N. 'Drought induced leaf abortion in *Fagonia cretica* Linn.' *Sci. & Cult.* 58: 235, 1992.

Memon, M. I. A., Shahani, N. M. and Syed, G. M. *Glimpses of Medicinal Plants of Sind.* Sind Agriculture Univ., Tandojam Sind, Pakistan, pp. 79-80, 1988.

Mohammed, S. Comparative studies of saline and non-saline vegetation in India arid zone. Ph.D. Thesis. University of Jodhpur, Jodhpur, India, 1988.

Mohammed. S. and Sen, D. N. 'Antholysis in *Fagonia cretica* L.' *Sci. & Cult.* 53: 219-220, 1987.

Narula, A., Srivastava, P. S. and Rangaswamy, N. S. '*In-vitro* culters studies on *Dioscorea* species' *J. Trop. Med Plants* 1:60-74, 2000.

National Medicinal Plants Board (NMPB). *Cultivation Practices of Some Commercially Important Medicinal Plants.* New Delhi: Government of India, 2002.

Prakash, J. Biology of some medicinal plants in Indian arid zone. Ph.D. Thesis. J. N. Vyas University, Jodhpur, India, 2001.

Prakash, J., Chauhan, A., Kasera, P. K., Mohammed, S. and Chawan, D. D. 'Studies on seed variability in *Salvadora persica* in Indian arid zone'. *Indian Jour. Environ. Sci.* 5: 27-32, 2001.

Purohit, M. L. and Khan, W. 'Socio-economic dimensions of Khejri [*Prosopis cineraria* (Linn.) MacBride]. In: *Khejri (Prosopis cineraria) in the Indian Desert—Its Role in Agroforestry.* (Eds.). Mann, H. S. and Saxena, S. K. CAZRI Monograph No. 11, pp. 56-63, 1980.

Purohit, U., Mehar, S. K. and Sundaramoorthy, S. 'Role of *Prosopis cineraria* on the ecology of the soil fungi in Indian desert'. *Jour. Arid Environ.* 52:17-27, 2002.

Raghunathan, R. and Mitra, R. (Eds.). *Pharmacognosy of Indigenous Drugs.* vol. I. New Delhi: CCRAS, pp. 354-375, 1999.

Rao, K. S. S., Patel, D. H. and Dalal, K. C. 'Occurrence of *Commiphora stocksiana* (mitha guggal) in Kutch'. *Indian Drugs* 21: 541-543, 1984.

Report on the Task Force on Conservation & Sustainable Use of Medicinal Plants. Government of India, Planning Commission, New Delhi, 2000.

Saharan, P., Kasera, P. K. and Chawan, D. D. 'A new report on variations in flower colours of *Evolvulus alsinoides* (Shankhpushpi) from the Indian Thar desert'. *J. Econ. Taxon. Bot.* 26: 21-24, 2002.

Sastry, T. C. and Kavathekar, K. Y. (Eds). *Plants for Reclamation of Wastelands.* New Delhi: Publications & Information Directorate, CSIR, 1990.

Saxena, S. and Kumar, D. 'Tailoring biodiversity for development of new therapeutics'. *Natural Product Radiance* 1(3): 18-25, 2002.

Saxena, S. K. 'Economic plants of the Indian arid zone'. In: *Sustainable Development of the Indian Arid Zone.* (Eds.). Singh, R. P. and Singh, S. Jodhpur: Scientific Publishers, pp. 65-85, 1994.

Sen, D. N. 'Ecology of Indian desert. III. Survival adaptations of vegetation in dry environment'. *Vegetatio* 27: 201-265, 1973.

Sen, D. N. *Ecological Approaches to Indian Weeds.* Jodhpur: Geobios International, 1981.

Sen, D. N. *Environment and Plant Life In Indian Desert.* Jodhpur: Geobios International, 1982.

Sen, D. N. and Chawan, D. D. 'Search for supplementary useful plants in Indian desert and their ecology. I. *Salvadora persica* Linn. and *S. oleoides* Druce.' *Indian Forester* 95: 681-688, 1969.

Sen, D. N. and Kasera, P. K. 'Weed biology and chemical weed control in the Indian arid zone'. In: *Sustainable Development of the Indian Arid Zone—A Research Perspective.* (Eds.). Singh, R. P. and Singh, S. Jodhpur: Scientific Publishers, pp. 303-318, 1994.

Sharma, B. B. L. and Prajapati, P. 'Phytogeographical distribution of medicinal plants of western Rajasthan'. In: *Advances in Resource Management of the Indian Desert.* (Eds.) Kapoor, B. B. S., Ali, A., Mathur, S. K., Kaushik, S. Bikaner: Madhu Publications, pp. 151-164, 2002.

Sharma, K. D. Ecophysiological studies on human in relation to some desert weeds and cultivated plants. Ph.D. Thesis. University of Jodhpur, Jodhpur, India, 1970.

Sharma, S. C. and Goel, A. K. 'The need for *ex-situ* conservation of endangered plants from tropical India'. *Botanic Gardens Conservation News* (U.K.) 1: 16-19, 1990.

Singh, U., Wadhwani, A. M. and Johri, B. M. *Dictionary of Economic Plants in India.* New Delhi: ICAR, 1996.

Singh, V. and Pandey, R. P. (Eds.). *Ethnobotany of Rajasthan,. India.* Jodhpur: Scientific Publishers, 1998.

Singh, V. and Pandey, R. P. 'Economic and medicinal plants of Indian desert'. In: *Desert Resources and Technology.* (Ed.), Singh, Alam. vol. I. Jodhpur: Scientific Publishers, pp. 307-368, 1983.

Sinha, R. K. and Sinha, S. *Ethnobiology (Role of Indigenous and Ethnic Societies in Biodiversity Conservation, Human Health Protection and Sustainable Development).* Jaipur: Surabhi Publications, Jaipur, 2001.

Sivarajan, V. V. and Balachandran, I. *Ayurvedic Drugs and their Plant Sources.* New Delhi: Oxford & IBH Publishing Co. Pvt., Ltd., pp. 425-428, 1999.

Tripathi, Y. C. and Arya, R. 'Floral resources of Indian That desert'. In: *Bioresources Technology.* (Ed.). Tripathi, G. New Delhi: CBS Publishers & Distributors, pp 16-33, 2002.

Vyas, S. P. 'Ethno-medicinal plants of Kachchh'. *Indian Jour. Environ. Sci.* 6: 91-94, 2001.

Yadav, B. B. L., Billore, K. V., Joseph, T. G. and Chaturvedi, D. D. *Cultivation of Guggulu.* New Delhi: CCRAS, 1999.

Zodape, S. T. and Indusekhar, V. K. '*Salvadora persica*, a boon to wasteland development'. *Jour .Scientific & Industrial Res.* 56: 657-661.

—oo(O)oo—

14

Medicinal Pteridophytes—An Overview

R. D. Dixit and Shweta Singh

PLANTS have always been the source of food, medicine, shelter, etc, and other necessities of man's life since time immemorial. The primitive human societies of the world even today depend for all their medical and other necessities of life on the surrounding plant wealth. In the 20th century, field studies on edible, economic and medicinal plants have advanced enormously. But such studies have been mainly confined on flowering plants and no serious efforts have been made so far to explore the medicinal properties of pteridophytes. The ferns and their allies are also known as *botanical snakes* or *plant reptiles*. These pteridophytes have always been at the centre of attraction to botanists, horticulturists, and naturalists due to the presence of beautiful foliage since the olden days. Such handsome plants of this fascinating group of Pteridophyta are well-distributed in the Himalayan ranges, Western Ghats, Nilgiri Hills, Vindhyan ranges, hills ranges of Bihar, Orissa, Madhya Pradesh and Chhattisgarh States of the Indian region as well as in the Aravalli ranges, particularly in Mount Abu in the desert land of Rajasthan. Many important contributions about taxonomy, ecology, and distribution of these plants have already been published, but their useful aspects are largely ignored.

Keeping in view the occurrence of the large number of Pteridophytic species, that is, about 1200 in India. The attempts have also been made by various workers to work out the medicinal importance of such plants in India also and stray publications have also been made. The present paper consolidates all such information available on medicinal Pteridophytes in condensed tabular form to enable and to assess all available publications at one place as far as practicable (Table 1).

TABLE 1
Medicinal Values of Indian Pteridophytes

No.	Botanical Name	Family	Vernacular Name	Uses	Area	References
1	*Acrostichum aureum* L	Acrostichaceae	Leather fern	Fertile fronds used for syphlitic ulcers and . emollient topically. Rhizome is vulnerary used in healing inveterate ulcers and in wounds and boils.	Coastal regions (Goa, Karnataka, Kerala Anadaman & Nicobar)	Quisumbing, 1955. Usher, 1971
2.	*Actiniopteris radiata* (Sw.) Link	Actinopteridaceae	Morpankhi	Fronds chewed for sore throat. Rhizome styptic anthelminthic and its decoction used in cure of dandruff.	Drier regions (Kumaun, Haryana, Panjab, U.P, Central & S. India)	Dymock, 1890. Lloyd, 1964. Dixit, 1975.
3.	*Adiantum aethiopicum* (L.) Syst.	Adiantaceae	——	Leaves and rhizome smoked for cold and chest disease in South India. Fronds chewed for sore throat. Rhizome boiled cured dandruff.	S India N. E India	Watt, 1962. Vasudeva, 1999. Manickam, 1999
4.	*Adiantum capillus veneris* L.	Adiantaceae	Southern maiden hair fern	Whole plants used in cure of ricketts in children and steamed for curing smallpox. It is used as diuretic, tonic, febrifuge expectorant, demulcent and astringent.	Mountainous regions	Scully, 1970. Remero, 1954 Dixit, 1975 Vasudeva, 1999

Continued...

...Continued

No.	Botanical Name	Family	Vernacular Name	Uses	Area	References
5	*Adiantum caudatum* L	Adiantaceae	Mayur Shikha	Leaves externa remedy for skin disease, internally for diabetes.	Mountainous region	Quisumbing, 1955
				Also used in cure of chest complaints, cough and fever.		Vasudeva, 1999 Manickam, 1999
6.	*Adiantum edgeworthii* Hook	Adiantaceae	Adhe-sir-di-jar	Paste of fronds used in cure of headache	N. W. Himalayas	Kirn & Kapahi, 2001
7.	*Adiantum flabellulatum* L	Adiantaceae	——	Herbs used for cure of cough and rhizomes are anthelminthic	Eastern India	Vasudeva, 1999
8.	*Adiantum incisum* Forssk.	Adiantaceae	——	Fronds used in cure of skin disease, cough and diabetes.	Throughout India	Vasudeva, 1999
				Fronds are chewed to cure mouth blisters and juice used to cure bronchitis		Pande *et al*, 1994
9.	*Adiantum pedatum* L	Adiantaceae	Northern maiden hair fern	Fronds used to stop bleeding, in chest and stomach troubles. Also used as tonic, demulcent, expectorant, astringent, catarrhal and pectoral.	N. W. Himalayas to Sikkim	Vasudeva, 1999
				Rhizome used in respiratory ailments.		Smith, 1924

Continued...

...Continued

No.	Botanical Name	Family	Vernacular Name	Uses	Area	References
10.	*Adiantum philippense* L.	Adiantaceae	Kali-Jhant	Fronds used in fever, asthama, bronchitis, dysentery, epileptic fits, leprosy and erysipelas.	Throughout India	Dixit, 1975 Vasudeva, 1999
				Rhizomes used against dog-bite and snake-bite as an antidote.		Manickam, 1999
11.	*Adiantum tenerum* Sw.	Adiantaceae	Brittle maiden hair fern	Plants used as expectorant and demulcent	Throughout India	Vasudeva, 1999
12.	*Adiantum venustum* D. Don	Adiantaceae	Hansraj	Fronds used in biliousness, disease of chest, cold, headache, ophthalmia, hydrophobia, inflammation and tumours.	N. E. Himalayas	Dixit, 1975
				Vapour bath of leaves is done in fever.		Asolkar *et al*, 1992
				Used as tonic, diuretic, emetic, resolvent, expectorant and against wounds, piles, and scorpion sting		Vasudeva, 1999
13.	*Asplenium adiantum-nigrum* L.	Aspleniaceae	Black spleen wort	Plant bitter, laxative, diuretic, useful in jaundice, opthalmia, cold, chest pain and diseases of spleen.	N. E. Himalayas	Vasudeva, 1999 Kirn & Kapahi, 2001

Continued...

...Continued

No.	Botanical Name	Family	Vernacular Name	Uses	Area	References
14.	*Asplenium falcatum* Lam.	Aspleniaceae	Spleen wort	Fronds used in malaria, jaundice, enlargement of spleen, urine trouble and calculus.	S. India, Sikkim, Andaman Nikobar	Dixit & Sinha, 2001 Chopra, 1956
15.	*Asplenium nidus* L	Aspleniaceae	Ruai-mangma	Leaves juice given to cure labour pain Extraction of leaves are useful in removal of lice.	N. W. Himalayas	Dixit, 1975 Singh *et al*, 2001
16.	*Asplenium rutamuraria* L.	Aspleniaceae	Wall Rue	Fronds expectorant and used as cure for rickets. Rhizome anthelmintic and astringent.	Kashmir, Kumaun, Arunachal Pradesh	Vasudeva, 1999 Chopra, 1959 Jacobs, 1968
17.	*Asplenium trichomanes* L	Aspleniaceae	Common spleen wort	Plant bitter, laxative, expectorant used in pulmonary disease and in abscess of uterus. Rhizome used as anthelminthic and for hypochondriac infections Whole plant extract is used against enlargement of spleen	N. E. Himalayas, Central India, Rajasthan, Sikkim, South India, Eastern Himalayas	Kirn & Kapahi, 2001 Vasudeva, 1999 Asolkar *et al*, 1992 Bir *et al*, 1983
18.	*Athyrium filix-faemina*	Athyriaceae	Lady fern	Rhizome vermifugal and used as anthelminthic.	Mountainous regions	Vasudeva, 1999 Chopra, 1959

Continued...

...*Continued*

No.	Botanical Name	Family	Vernacular Name	Uses	Area	References
19.	*Alsophila albosetacea*		——	Leaves are locally applied on wounds	Andaman & Nicobar	Manickam, 1999
20.	*Alsophila spinulosa* Wall. ex Hook.	Cyatheaceae	——	Leaves are locally applied on wounds.	Andaman & Nicobar	Manickam, 1999
21.	*Blechnum orientale* L.	Blechnaceae	Hastajori	Whole plant used as medicine for diarrhoea and stomach disorders. Plants used as poultice for boils. It is used in impotency in men, urinary disorders, cure of sanipat (delirium).	Central India, N. W Himalayas, Sikkim, South India	Dixit, 1975. Vasudeva, 1999 Quisumbing, 1951 Kaushik & Dhiman, 1995
22.	*Botrychium lunaria* (L.) Sw.	Botrychiaceae	Moon wort	Fronds are good vulnerary, used in dysentery ruptures, for healing cuts and wounds. Rhizome juice used in treatment of breast cancer.	N. W. Himalayas, Sikkim, S. India	Vasudeva, 1999 Dixit, 1975 Kaushik & Dhiman 1995 Asolkar *et al*, 1992
23.	*Botrychium ternatum* (Thumb.) Sw	Botrychiaceae	China-yin -tichuch	Flashy rhizomes are applied on cuts and bruises. Also used in dysentery.	N. W. Himalayas, Sikkim, Rajasthan	Vasudeva, 1999 Cauis, 1935 Dixit, 1975

Continued...

...*Continued*

No.	Botanical Name	Family	Vernacular Name	Uses	Area	References
24.	*Botrychium virginianum* (L.) Sw.	Botrychiaceae	Rattle snake	Flashy rhizomes are applied on cuts and . bruises. Also used in dysentery.	N. W. Himalayas, Sikkim, Rajasthan	Vasudeva, 1999 Dixit, 1975
25.	*Cheilanthes albomarginata* Clarke	Cheilanthaceae	Nanha	Whole plants used against tuberculosisand as tonic.	Mountainous region	Vasudeva, 1999 Vays & Sharma, 1988
26.	*Cheilanthes bicolor* (Roxb.) Griff.ex Fras-Jenk.	Cheilanthaceae	Silver fern	Fronds are useful in seasonal and cold fever.	Mountainous region	Asolkar *et al*, 1992 Vasudeva, 1999
27.	*Cheilanthes tenuifolia* (Burm. f.) Sw.	Cheilanthaceae	Dodhari	There is a superstition among the tribals that preparation made from roots is given for sickness attributed to "evil eye" or "witch craft". Also used as tonic.	Mountainous region	Vasudeva, 1999 Caius, 1935 Manickam, 1999
28.	*Cephalomanes javanicum* (Bl.) v.d. Bosch	Hymenophyl-losidaceae	——	Whole plant with garlic and onion smoked to cure headache.	Eastern India (Assam)	Dixit & Sinha, 2001
29.	*Ceratopteris thalictroides* (l.) Ad. Brongn.	Parkeriaceae	Water fern	Whole plant used as tonic and styptic. Fronds are used as poultice in skin complaints.	N. W Himalayas, Rajasthan, Central India, N. E. India, S. India	Vasudeva, 1999 Dixit, 1975

Contiued...

...Continued

No.	Botanical Name	Family	Vernacular Name	Uses	Area	References
30.	*Cibotium assamicum* Hook.	Dicksoniaceae	Kow chiak	Young stem sore starchy, pith are eaten in times of famine.	Eastern India (Assam)	Dixit, 1999
31.	*Cibotium barometz* (L.) J. Sm	Dicksoniaceae	Mini tree fern	Stem used as styptic and tonic. Rhizome vermifuge, treats tropical wounds, ulcers, stimulating to liver, kidneys and "Old man's remedy". It is said to exercise a special action on genitourinary organs.	Eastern India (Assam) Central India.	Vasudeva, 1999 Usher, 1971 Quisumbing, 1951 Kaushik & Dhiman, 1995
32.	*Ceterach officinarum* Willd.	Aspleniaceae	Finger fern	Whole plant used as astringent and diuretic. It is used in infirmities of spleen, helps in strangely, anal wastes, stones in bladder and hiccough. Decoction of plant used in melancholia.	N. W Himalayas	Vasudeva, 1999 Caius, 1935 Kaushik & Dhiman, 1995
33.	*Cystopteris fragilis* (L.) Bernh.	Athyriaceae	Bladder fern	The decoction of rhizome is used as anthelminthic enema. It is pectoral, mucilaginous, expectorant and refrigeration tonic.	Himalayan regions	Kaushik & Dhiman, 1995 Vasudeva, 1999

Continued...

...Continued

No.	Botanical Name	Family	Vernacular Name	Uses	Area	References
34.	*Cyrtomium falcatum* (L. f.) Presl	Aspleniaceae	Holy fern	Rhizomes have anthelminthic properties and chiefly used for expulsion of tapeworm.	Himalayan regions, S. India	Vasudeva, 1999
35.	*Christella arida* (D. Don) Holtt.	Thelypteridaceae	——	Rhizome decoction is useful in veterinary larval infections.	Sikkim, Central India, N. W. Himalayas	Manickam, 1999
36.	*Christella parasitica* (L.) Lev.	Thelypteridaceae	——	Fronds are useful against rheumatism.	N. W. Himalayas, Goa, Lakshadeep, Andaman, Nicobar	Manickam, 1999
37.	*Dicranopteris liearis* (Burm. f.) Underw.	Gleicheniaceae	Thicket fern	Fronds are useful in cure of asthma, also having antibacterial properties. Young fronds with cow's milk given in woman's sterility. Rhizome anthelminthic. Spores used as favourite remedy for diarrohea in children.	Eastern, Central and S. India, N. W. Himalayas	Vasudeva, 1999 Asolkar *et al*, 1992 Dixit, 1975 Kaushik & Dhiman, 1995

Continued...

...Continued

No.	Botanical Name	Family	Vernacular Name	Uses	Area	References
38.	*Diplazium esculentum* (Retz.) Sw.	Athyriaceae	Lingra or Kheri	Young tips of fronds are used as tonic for health. Decoction of rhizome and young leaves are useful for haemoptysis and constipation	Throughout India	Kaushik & Dhiman, 1995 Quisumbing, 1951
39.	*Diplazium dilatatum* Bl.	Athyriaceae	——	The extraction of fronds is diuretic.	South and N. E. India, N. W. Himalayas, U.P.	Vasudeva, 1999
40.	*Drymoglossum carnosum* (Wall.) J. Sm	Polypodiaceae	Polypody	Fronds used as astringent, diuretic and pectoral. Whole plant is useful in urinary trouble and rheumatism.	South . and N. E. India, N. W. Himalayas, U.P.	Vasudeva, 1999 Caius, 1935 Kaushik & Dhiman, 1995
41.	*Drymoglossum piloselloides* (L.) Presl.	Polypodiaceae	——	Whole plant is useful against itching and relieving pain. Leaves are used as antiseptic. Used in cure of healing eczema, cough, constipation and gonorrhea.	Throughout hilly regions of India	Dixit & Sinha, 2001

Continued...

...Continued

No.	Botanical Name	Family	Vernacular Name	Uses	Area	References
42.	*Drynaria quericifolia* (L.) J. Sm.	Drynariaceae	Ashvakatri	Whole plant used in hectic fever, dyspepsia, cough, poulticing swelling and typhoid fever. Rhizome anthelminthic, expectorant, pectoral and astringent.	Throughout India	Vasudeva, 1999 Kirtikar and Basu, 1918 Dixit, 1975 Chopra, 1956
43.	*Dryopteris barbigera* (Moore ex Hook.) O. Ktze	Dryopteridaceae	——	Rhizomea have anthelminthic properties. Substitute for the European male fern. Rhizome vermifuge	Himalayas regions	Vasudeva, 1999 Kaushik & Dhiman, 1995 Chopra, 1956
44.	*Dryopteris blanfordii* (Hope) C.Chr.	Dryopteridaceae	——	Rhizomes have . anthelminthic properties chiefly used for expulsion of tapeworm.	Himalayan regions	Vasudeva, 1999 Kaushik & Dhiman, 1995 Usher, 1971
45.	*Dryopteris chrysocoma* (Christ.) C. Chr.	Dryopteridaceae	——	Rhizomes have anthelminthic properties. Substitute for the European male fern. Fronds are good source of "Filcin".	Himalayan regions	Vasudeva, 1999 Bir *et at*, 1983 Kaushik & Dhiman, 1995

Continued...

...Continued

No.	Botanical Name	Family	Vernacular Name	Uses	Area	References
46.	*Dryopteris cochleate* (Ham. ex D.Don.) C.Chr.	Dryopteridaceae	Jatashankari	Juice extract is given in epilepsy and leprosy. Whole plant paste used against snake bite. Rhizomes are used in swellings and pain and have antifungal properties.	Himalayan region, Central India, S. India	Kaushik & Dhiman, 1995 Verma *et al*, 1995 Asolkar *et al*, 1992
47.	*Dryopteris filix-mas* (L.) Schott	Dryopteridaceae	Male fern	Rhizomes and stipes yield the drug known as "Male fern". This is an oleo resinous substance that has been used since long for expelling tapeworms.	Cosmopolitan	Vasudeva, 1999 Vasudeva, 1999, 1995
48.	*Dryopteris juxtaposita* Christ.	Dryopteridaceae	——	Rhizome used as anthelminthic.	N. W. Himalayas, Sikkim, W. B., Assam, S. India	Vasudeva, 1999
49.	*Dryopteris marginata* (Wall. ex Christ) Christ	Dryopteridaceae	——	Rhizomes have anthelminthic properties.	N. W. Himalayas, Eastern India	Vasudeva, 1999 Kaushik & Dhiman, 1995
50.	*Dryopteris odontoloma* (Moore) C. Chr.	Dryopteridaceae	——	Rhizomes used as anthelminthic.	N. W. Himalayas	Kaushik & Dhiman, 1995

Continued...

...*Continued*

No.	Botanical Name	Family	Vernacular Name	Uses	Area	References
51.	*Dryopteris sparsa* (Ham. ex D.Don) O. Ktze.	Dryopteridaceae	——	Rhizomes have anthelminthic properties.	Sikkim, W. B., Bihar, Orissa, Central India, S. India	Manickam, 1999
52.	*Davallia trichomanoides* Bl.	Davalliaceae	——	Whole plant is antidote for food poisoning.	Andaman, Nicobar, Eastern Himalayas	Manickam, 1999
53.	*Equisetum arvense* L.	Equisetaceae	Gold rush	Dried plant useful in dropsy, navel and kidney infections.	Himalayan regions	Vasudeva, 1999 Asolkar *et al*, 1992
				Decoction used in nasal polypus and breast cancers.		
				Ashes are useful in acidity of stomach and dyspepsia.		Lloyd, 1964 Kirn & Kapahi, 2000
				Also used for washing tumours and cancerous lesions of bones.		
				Stems used for treatment of bone fracture.		Burkill, 1966
54.	*Equisetum diffusum* D. Don	Equisetaceae		Whole plants are useful in acidity and dropsy.	Central India. Himalayan regions	Manickam, 1999

Continued...

...Continued

No.	Botanical Name	Family	Vernacular Name	Uses	Area	References
55.	*Equisetum ramossissimum* Desf. Sub sp. *debile* (Roxb ex Vauch) Hauke	Equisetaceae	Horsetail	The plant is useful in cure of gonorrhoea and treatment of fracture.	Himalayan regions	Kaushik & Dhiman, 1995 Das, 1997 Kirn & Kapahi, 2000 Bir *et al*, 1983 Vasudeva, 1999
56.	*Helminthostachys zeylanica* (L.) Hook.	Helminthostachyaceae	——	Frond juice is used for relieving from blisters. Plant is intoxicant, aperients and anodyne used in sciatica. Rhizome powder used as a brain tonic for vitality and as a cure for waist pain. Rhizome paste with cow's urine is used in cure of skin disease.	Bengal Plains to Assam, Himalayas, U.P., South India	Vasudeva, 1999 Kaushik & Dhiman, 1995 Dixit, 1975 Singh *et al*, 1989 Dixit & Sinha, 2001
				It is also useful is spermatorrhea and for improving memory. Also useful in cure of malaria. Is given to promote strength and vitality in male.		Singh & Maheshwari, 1992 Quisumbing, 1951 Upnof, 1968

Continued...

...Continued

No.	Botanical Name	Family	Vernacular Name	Uses	Area	References
57.	*Hypodematium crenatum* (Forssk.) Kuhn	Hypodemataceae	Bhootkesri	Whole plants is used for gynecological disorders and against insect bite.	Central and S. India, Himalayan regions	Vyas & Sharma, 1988 Kaushik & Dhiman, 1995
				Scales of this fern are used against the effect of "Witch craft or evil eye".		Vasudeva, 1999
58.	*Lycopodium clavatum* L.	Lycopodiaceae	Club Moss	Plant decoction is anti-spasmatic, useful in rheumatism, diseases of lungs and kidneys.	Throughout India in hilly regions	Vasudeva, 1999
				Spores are used as water repellant and protective dusting powder for tender skin.		Watt, 1932
59.	*Lygodium flexuosum* (L.) Sw.	Lygodiaceae	Kalijar	Fronds boiled with mustard oil useful as local application to carbuncles externally in rheumatism, sprains, scabies, ulcers and cutwounds.	Throughout India	Vasudeva, 1999 Dixit, 1975 Chopra *et al*, 1956
				Rhizome cures gonorrhea and paste applied on piles.		Dixit, 1975 Dixit & Sinha, 2000
				Spores cure high fever.		Manickam, 1999

Continued...

...Continued

No.	Botanical Name	Family	Vernacular Name	Uses	Area	References
60.	*Lygodium japonicum* (Thunb.) Sw.	Lygodiaceae	Climbing fern	Plant used as expectorant. Used in cure of haematuria and an amulet of this plant is tied round the neck of patient suffering from . malaria. It is diuretic or cathartic. Rhizome decoction taken by ladies to regularise menstruation.	N. E. India, Western Himalayas, S. India	Vasudeva, 1999 Das, 1997 Dixit, 1975 Kirn & Kapahi, 2000 Manickam, 1999
61.	*Lygodium circinatum* (Burm.) Sw	Lygodiaceae	——	Stipe chewed and applied against bite of venomous snake or insect. Fronds used in external application for wounds. Leaves used in rheumatic pain in gynecological disorders.	N. E. India, Andaman and Nicobar	Quisunbing, 1951 Dixit & Sinha, 2000
62.	*Lygodium microphyllum* (Cav.) R. Br.		——	Decoction of leaves used in dysentery and also useful in skin disorders. Leaves cure hiccoughs. Rhizome used as astringent.	Sikkim, S. India, Central India, N. E India	Dixit, 1975 Bouquest, 1974 Dixit & Sinha, 2001

Continued...

...Continued

No.	Botanical Name	Family	Vernacular Name	Uses	Area	References
63.	*Lygodium pinnatifidum* Sw.	Lygodiaceae	Kathikund	Its rhizome paste is applied on the site of snake bite and about 20 gm of dried rhizome power is given orally after every half an hour till recovery.		Jha & Verma, 1996 Dhiman, 1998
64.	*Lygodium longifolium* (Willd.) Sw.	Lygodiaceae	——	Fronds chewed with ash salt to cure stomach ache and diaorrhea.	South India	Holdsworth & Giheno, 1975
65.	*Leucostigia immersa* (Wall. ex Hook.) Presl	Davalliaceae	——	The leaves cure constipation.	Throughout India	Dixit & Das, 1978
66.	*Marsilea minuta* L.	Marsileaceae	Water clover	Decoction of leaves mixed with ginger given in bronchitis, spastic condition of legs, cough sedative and insomnia. Fresh young leaves are in form of juice, is effectivein urinary disorder. Leaves extract with sugar or fishes is useful in migraine. Drops of juice are very effective in eye disease	Throughout India except Kashmir	Vasudeva, 1999 Roy & Gupta, 1965 Dixit, 1975 Dixit & Sinha, 2001 Dadhich & Sharma, 2002 Jha & Sharma, 1996 Dhiman, 1998 Vyas and Sharma, 1988

Continued...

...*Continued*

No.	Botanical Name	Family	Vernacular Name	Uses	Area	References
67.	*Marsilea quadrifolia* L.	Marsileaceae	——	Whole plans is useful in bone fracture.	North India	Manickam, 1999
68.	*Marattia fraxinea* Smith	Marattiaceae	——	Young leaves are used as remedy for bronchial and intestinal catarrh.	South India	Dixit, 1975
69.	*Microlepia speluncae* (L.) Moore	Dennstaedtiaceae	——	Leaves are effective in curing high fever.	Himalayan regions, S. India, Andaman, Nicobar	Dixit & Sinha, 2001 Manickam, 1999
70.	*Microsorium punctatum* (L.) Copel.	Dennstaedtiaceae	——	Whole plant used for curing snake bite. Used as purgative, diuretic and wound healer.	Andaman, Nicobar, S. India	Dixit & Sinha, 2001 Bouquest, 1974
71.	*Nephrolepis cordifolia* (L.) Presel	Nephrolepidaceae	Sanay	Rhizomes and tubers are used in intestinal and kidney disorders. Extract of rhizome is used in permanent curing of sterility in women. Decoction used for cough. Rhizome stock is applied locally in skin disease.	Throughout India	Dixit, 1975 Jamir, 1997 Henry *et al*, 1996 Quisumbing, 1951 Dhiman, 1998

Continued...

...Continued

No.	Botanical Name	Family	Vernacular Name	Uses	Area	References
72.	*Nephrolepis auriculata* (L.) Trimen	Nephrolepidaceae	Banu	A decoction of fresh tubers and fronds are given in cough.	N. E. Himalayas, W.B., S. India	Singh, 1993
73.	*Nephrolepis biserrata* (Sw.) Schott.	Nephrolepidaceae	——	Haemostatic treatment for wounds.	N. E. India, S. India.	Bouquest, 1974
74.	*Ophioglossum costatum* R. Br.	Ophioglossaceae	Sheambli	Dried tubers are crushed in the form of powder mixed with mustard oil used in skin disease.	N. E. Himalayas, W.B., S. India, Maharashtra.	Dadhich & Sharma, 2002
75.	*Ophioglossum pendulum*	Ophioglossaceae	——	Spores given to babies at birth to purge meconium.	Arunachal Pradesh, Andaman, Nicobar, N. E Himalayas	Fosberg, 1942
76.	*Ophioglossum reticulatum* L.	Ophioglossaceae	Vanpalak	Fronds are used in preparation of tonic. It is useful in relief of headache. Paste of fresh leaves and tubers applied on boils.	Throughout India	Vasudeva, 1999 Singh *et al*, 1989

Continued...

...*Continued*

No.	Botanical Name	Family	Vernacular Name	Uses	Area	References
77.	*Ophioglossum vulgatum* L	Ophioglossaceae	Adder's Tongue	Fronds used as tonic and styptic. Antidote for snake bite.	N. E. Himalayas	Vasudeva, 1999
				Whole plants vulnerary, in cuts and wounds.		Caius, 1935
				Decoction of fronds used in angina and as lotion for boils.		Kaushik & Dhiman, 1995
78.	*Osmunda claytoniana* L.	Osmundaceae	Interrupted fern	Rhizome used as adulteration for male fern	N. E. Himalayas	Vasudeva, 1999 Kaushik & Dhiman, 1995
79.	*Osmunda regalis* L.	Osmundaceae	Royal fern	Plants used as tonic and styptic. Young fronds cure toothache, rheumatism and internally for intestinal gripping.	N. E. Himalayas, U.P., Central India, S. India	Vasudeva, 1999 Dixit, 1975 Chopra *et al*, 1956 Manickam, 1999
80.	*Onychium siliculosum* (Desv.) C.Chr.	Cryptogrammaceae	——	Fronds used for dysentery and to check/ prevent falling hair.	N. E. Himalayas, Andaman, Nicobar	Dixit & Sinha, 2001 Manickam, 1999
81.	*Ophioderma pendula* (L.) Presl	Ophioglossaceae	——	Fronds mixed with coconut oil prevent falling hair.	N. E. Himalayas, Andaman, Nicobar	Dixit & Sinha, 2001

Continued...

...Continued

No.	Botanical Name	Family	Vernacular Name	Uses	Area	References
82.	*Palhinhaea cernua*	Lycopodiaceae	——	Leaves are effective in skin eruptions, beri-beri.	Throughout India	Dixit & Sinha, 2001
83.	*Pellaea calomelanos* (Sw.) Link	Sinopteridaceae	——	Rhizomes are anthelmintic used in cold and headache.	N. E. Himalayas	Vasudeva, 1999 Caius, 1935
84.	*Pityrogramma calomelanos* (L.) Link	Hemionitidaceae	——	Whole plant decoction remedy for kidney trouble. Tea prepared by its fronds useful in flu, fever and hypertension.	Throughout India	Quisumbing, 1951 Jim Croft, 1982
85.	*Phlegmariurus phegmaria*	Hemionitidaceae	——	Rhizomes are useful in dropsy, emmenogogue.	Andaman, Nicobar	Manickam, 1999
86.	*Psilotum nudum* (L.) P. Beauv.	Psilotaceae	——	Whole plant used as purgative.	Throughout India in hilly region	Dixit & Sinha, 2001
87.	*Polypodium vulgare* L.	Polypodiaceae	Polypody	Rhizomes are anthelmintic and purgative.	Himalayan regions	Vasudeva, 1999 Manickam, 1999
88.	*Pleopeltis macrocarpa* (Bory ex Willd.) Kaulf	Polypodiaceae	Polypody	Whole plants used in form of tea to cure itching.	N. E. Himalayas, Central & S. India, W.B.	Vasudeva, 1999 Kaushik & Dhiman, 1995 Manickam, 1999

Continued...

...Continued

No.	Botanical Name	Family	Vernacular Name	Uses	Area	References
89.	*Phymatosorus scolopendria* (Burm.) Pic.-Ser.	Polypodiaceae	——	Fronds used for curing chronic diarorhea, dysentery and gonorrhea.	South India Nicobar	Dixit & Sinha, 2001
90.	*Pteris biaurita* L.	Pteridaceae	——	The paste of stipe and stem is useful in wounds	Sikkim, W.B., Bihar, Orissa	Manickam, 1999
91.	*Pteris ensiformis* Burm. f.	Pteridaceae	Laich ang khrang	Leaf juice used as an astringent to cure dysentery. It is also used as diuretic and cooling agent and to cure malaria. Decoction of fresh fronds given in the glandular swelling of neck.	Throughout India	Dixit & Sinha, 2001 Singh *et al*, 2001 Burkill, 1966 Quisumbing, 1951
92.	*Pteris tripartita* Sw.	Pteridaceae	——	Fronds are used during parturition.	South India	Dixit & Sinha, 2001
93.	*Pteris vittata* L.	Pteridaceae	Jasumba	Rhizome used as demulcent. It used in glandular swelling	Throughout India	Dixit & Sinha, 2001 Dadhich & Sharma, 2002

Continued...

...Continued

No.	Botanical Name	Family	Vernacular Name	Uses	Area	References
94.	*Pteris wallichiana* Agardh	Pteridaceae	Unio	Fresh leaves are crushed and applied on cuts to stop bleeding and also on wounds for healing.	N. E. Himalayas	Dixit *et al*, 1978
95.	*Pteridium aquilinum* (L.) Kuhn	Pteridiaceae	Bracken fern	Rhizome have astringent and anthelminthic properties. The decoction of rhizome and fronds is given in chronic disorders arising from obstructions of viscera and spleen.	Throughout India	Dixit, 1975 Chopra *et al*, 1956 Manickam, 1999
96.	*Pteridium aquilinum* var. *wightianum* (Wall.) Trayon	Pteridiaceae	Kakaie	Plants boiled with mustard oil are locally applied on wounds and skins affections of cattle.	N. E. Himalayas	Kirn & Kapahi, 2000 Chopra *et al*, 1956
97.	*Pyrossia adnascens* (Sw.) Ching	Polypodiaceae	——	Fronds used in skin burn and in dysentery.		Dixit & Sinha, 2001 Manickam, 1999
98.	*Selaginella bryopteris* (L.) Bak.	Selaginellaceae	Sanjivani	Whole plant diuretic and anti-gonorrhea. Dried plants with tobacco smoked for hallucination.	Throughout India	Vasudeva, 1999 Singh *et al*, 2001 Shah & Singh, 1990 Kaushik & Dhiman,

Continued...

...Continued

No.	Botanical Name	Family	Vernacular Name	Uses	Area	References
				Plants and leaves with sugar is taken in stomachache, inflammation of urinary tract and in some venereal diseases. A popular strength tonic amongst local people. Effective in spermatorrhoea and leucorrhoea.		Dixit, 1992 Manickam, 1999
99.	*Selaginella ciliaris* (Retz.) Spring	Selaginellaceae	——	Plant extract is used in stopping bleeding	Throughout India	Singh *et al*, 2001
100.	*Selaginella willdenovii* (Desv. ex Poir) Bak.	Selaginellaceae	——	Whole plant is useful in backache and rheumatism.	Andaman, Nicobar	Manickam, 1999
101.	*Sphenomeris chinensis* (L.) Maxon	Lindsaeaceae	Farsley fern	Fronds paste used internally for chronic enteritis.	Throughout India	Vasudeva, 1999 Caius, 1935 Manickam, 1999
102.	*Schizaea dichotoma* (L.) Sm	Schizaeaceae	——	Juices of fronds to cure cold and cough. It is useful in child birth.	South India	Dixit & Sinha, 2001
103.	*Stenochlasna palustris* (Burm. f.) Bedd.	Stenochlaenaceae	——	Whole plants used for stomachache and remittent fever. Cooling agent and for the treatment of burns and ulcers.	Western Ghats, W.B., Orissa, Sikkim	Dixit & Sinha, 2001 Manickam, 1999

Continued...

...*Continued*

No.	Botanical Name	Family	Vernacular Name	Uses	Area	References
104.	*Taenitis blechnoides* (Willd.) Sw.	Taenitidaceae	——	Whole plants used as tonic for postpartum prospective medicine.	Nicobar, S. India	Dixit & Sinha, 2001
105.	*Tectaria cicutaria* (L.) Copel.	Aspidiaceae	Harishakarr pattor	10 gm rhizome along with seven fruits of black pepper mixed with cow's milk given once daily as tonic and to purify blood and also in blood dysentery.	Throughout India	Brahman & Saxena, 1990
				About 10 gm of rhizome paste with *Zingiber purpureum* Rosc. and *Croton roxburghii* Balak. in equal proportion is given in menstrual problems. About 15 gm. of rhizome power with root of *Cissampelos pareira* L. and *Smilax ovalifolia* Roxb. in equal proportion is given in leucorrhoea and body temperature.		Brahman & Saxena, 1990
106.	*Tectaria coadunate* (Wall. ex Hook et Grev) C.Chr.	Aspidiaceae	——	The decoction of rhizome is given in stomachache of children.	Eastern India, S. India	Pande *et al*, 1994 Manickam, 1999

Continued...

...Continued

No.	Botanical Name	Family	Vernacular Name	Uses	Area	References
107.	*Tectaria macrodonta* (Fee.)C.Chr.	Aspidiaceae	——	The rhizome has anthelmintic properties. Used in asthma, bronchitis and in getting relief from bites and stings by insect and centipedes.	Throughout India	Vasudeva, 1999 Vyas & Sharma, 1988
108.	*Tectaria polymorpha* (Wall.ex Hook.) Copel	Aspidiaceae	——	Rhizome used as anthelminthic.	N. India, S. India, M.P.	Vasudeva, 1999 Kaushik & Dhiman, 1995
109.	*Vittaria elongata* Sw.	Vittariaceae	——	Leaf juice used for curing rheumatic pain and stiffness.	Throughout India in hilly region	Dixit & Sinha, 2001 Manickam, 1999
110.	*Vittaria zosterifolia* Willd.	Vittariaceae	——	Whole plant is useful in skin disease.	Eastern India (Assam)	Manickam, 1999

REFERENCES

Anand, R. K. and Srivastava, R. B. 'Ethnopharmacological study of *Adiantum lunulatum* Burm. F'. *Indian Fern J.* 11: 137-141, 1994.

Asolkar, L. V., Kakkar and Chakae, P. *Glossary of Indian Medicinal Plants with Active Principles.*

Bir, S. S., Satija, C. K., Vasudeva, M. and Goyal, Pramod. *Pteridophytes Flora of Garhwal Himalaya Jungle.* Dehradun: Kishore & Co. 1983.

Bouquet, A. *Plantes Medicinales de la cote d' Ivoire Oratom. Peris,* 1974.

Brahaman, M. A. Saxena, H. O. 'Ethnobotany of Gandhamardan Hills—Some noteworthy folk medicinal uses'. *Ethnobotany* 2: 71-79, 1990.

Burkill, I. H. *A Dictionary of the Economic Products of the Malaya Peninsula*, Government of Malaysia and Singapore, 1996.

Caius, J. F. 'The medicinal and poisonous ferns of India'. *J. Bombay Nat. Hist. Soc.* 38: 341-361, 1935.

Chopra, R. N., Nayar and Chopra, L. C. *Glossary of Indian Medicinal Plants.* New Delhi: CSIR, 1956.

Copeland, E. B. 'Edible Ferns'. *Amr. Fern J.* 32: 121-126, 1942.

Croft, Jim. 'Ferns and Man in New Guinea'. Centre for Plants Biodiversity Research based on a paper presented to Papua New Guinea Botany Society, 1982.

Dadhich, L. K. and Sharma, A. P. 'Biodiversity strategies for conservation'. In: *Dr. S. K. Agarwal Commemoration Volume.* New Delhi: A P H Publishing Corporation, pp. 223-235, 2002.

Das, A. K. 'Less known uses of plants among the aids of Arunachal Pradesh'. *Ethnobotany* 9: 90-93, 1997.

Dixit, R. D. 'Fern—a much neglected group of medicinal plants-I'. *J. Res. Indian Med.* 9 (4): 59-68, 1975.

Dixit, R. D. 'Fern—a much neglected group of medicinal plants–II'. *J. Res. Indian Med.* 10 (2): 74-90, 1975.

Dixit, R. D. 'Fern—a much neglected group of medicinal plants–III'. *J. Res. Indian Med.* 10 (3): 68-76, 1975.

Dixit, R. D. 'Studies on Ethnobotany-III on some less known edible, economic and medicinal ferns of Darjeeling District. W. B.' In: *Rep. from Nagarjun*—June, 1978, vol. XXI: 10. 1-4, 1956.

Dixit, R. D. and Sinha, B. K. 'Pteridophytes of Andaman Nicobar'. Dehradun: Bishan Singh Mahendra Pal Singh, 2001.

Fosberg, F. R. 'Uses of Hawaiian Ferns'. *Amer. Fern J.* 32: 15-23, 1942.

Henry, A. N., Hosagoudor and Kumar, R. 'Ethnomedicobotany of the Southern Western Ghats of India'. In: *Ethnobiology in Human Welfare.* (Ed.). Jain, S. K., pp. 173-86, 1996.

Holdsworth, D. K and Giheno, J. 'A preliminary survey of highland medicinal plants'.. *Sci. in New Guinea* 3::198, 1975.

Jacobs, Marion Lee. *Index of Plants of North Carolina with Reputed Medicinal Uses.* North Carolina, U. S. A.: Chapel Hill, 1958.

Jamir, N. S. 'Ethnobiology of Naga tribe in Nagaland, medicinal herbs'. *Ethnobotany* 9: 101-104, 1997.

Jha, R. R. and Verma, S. K. 'Ethnobotany of Sauria Paharis of Santhal Pargana Bihar. I. Medicinal plants'. *Ethnobotany* 8: 31-35, 1996.

Joshi, Pramila 'Ethnobotany of Pteridophytes of hilly district of Uttar Pradesh, India'. *Indian Fern J.* 14: 14-18, 1997.

Kapur, S. K. and Sarin, Y. K. 'Useful medicinal ferns of Jammu and Kashmir State'. *Indian Drugs* 14(7): 136-140, 2001.

Kaushik, Purshotum and Dhiman, Anil Kumar. 'Common medicinal Pteridophytes'. *Indian Fern J.* 12: 139-145, 1995.

Kirn and Kapahi 'Ethnobotanical notes of some ferns and ferns allies of Jammu and Kashmir State, India'. *Indian Fern J.* 18: 35-38, 2001.

Kirtikar, K. R. and Basu, B. D. *Indian Medicinal Plants*. Allahabad: Lalit Mohan Bose, 1918.

Lloyd, Robert M. 'Ethnobotanical uses of California Pteridophytes by Western Indian'. *Am. Fern J.* 54: 76-82, 1964.

Manicham, V. S. ;Medicinal ferns of India'. *Amruth* (Feb.) pp. 3-9, 1999.

May, L. W. 'The economic uses and associated folklore of ferns and fern allies'. *Botanical Review* 44(4): 491-528, 1978.

Nand Lal, Singh, S. P. and Roy, S. K. 'Some medicinal ferns from South Andaman Island'. *Bull. Medi. Eth. Bota. Res.* III. No. 2-4, 178-185, 1982.

Nayar, B. K. 'Medicinal ferns of India'. *Bull. Nat. Bot. Garden* 29: 1-36, 1957.

Niranjan, A. K. S and Dudey, J. P. 'Some medicinal ferns from Pithoragarh Hills'. *J. Sci. Res.* (B.H.U.) 29(10): 183-189, 1978.

Pande, H. C. 'Observation on the distribution of tree ferns in Western Himalayas'. *Indian Fern J.* 10: 73-74, 1993.

Pande, P. C. and Pangtey, Y. P. S. 'Studies on the Ethnobotany-I. On some less known edible, medicinal and economic ferns of Kumaun region of W. Himalayas'. *J. Eco. Tax. Bot.* II(i): 81-85, 1987.

Pande, P. C., Joshi, Pramila and Pande, H. C. 'Studies on the ethnobotany-II. On some less known edible, medicinal and economic ferns of Kumaun region of W. Himalayas'. (Eds.). Sharma, T. A., Saini, S. S., Trivedi, M. L. and Sharma, M. *Current Researches Plants Science*. Dehradun: Bishan Singh Mahendra Pal Singh, 1994.

Pt. 1. New Delhi: CSIR, 1992.

Puri, G. S. and Arora, R. K. 'Some medicinal ferns from Western India'. *Indian Forester* 87: 179-188, 1961.

Quisumbing, Eduardo 'Medicinal plants of Philippines'. *Manila Dept. of Agr. and Nat. Resources Bulletin* ,Manila, 1951.

Remero. *The Botanical Lore of California Indians*. New York, U. S. A.: Vantage Press, 1954.

Roy, P. and Gupta, H. N. *Charaka Samhita* (A scientific synopsis). History of Science in India Publication. *Natn. Inst. Sci. India*. 1-120, 1965.

Scully, Virginia. *A Treasury of American Indian Herbs*. New York, U. S. A.: Crown, 1970.

Shah, N. C. and Singh, S. C. 'Hitherto unreported phytotherapeutical uses from tribal pockets of M. P. (India)'. *Ethnobotany* 2: 91-95, 1990.

Simith, Huron, H. 'Ethnobotany of Menomini Indians'. *Bulletin of Public Museum of the City of Milwaukee* 4: 1-174. Westport, U. S. A.: Greenwood Press, 1924.

Singh, J. B. 'Some medicinal ferns of Sikkim Himalayas'. *Indian. J. Medi. Res.* 3: 71-73, 1969.

Singh, K. K. and Maheshwari, J. K. 'Folk medicinal uses of some plants among the Tharus of Gorakhpur District, Uttar Pradesh, India'. *Ethnobotany* 4: 39-43, 1992.

Singh, K. K. and Maheshwari, J. K. 'Traditional herbal remedies among the Tharus of Bahraich District, U. P.' *India Ethnobotany* 1: 51-56, 1989.

Singh, K. K., Saha, S. and Maheshwari, J. K. 'Ethnobotanical uses of some ferns amongst the tribals of Uttar Pradesh'. *Indian Fern J.* 6: 63-67, 1992.

Singh, L. S. 'Ethnobotanical uses of some Pteridophytes species in Manipur'. *Indian Fern J.* 18: 14-17, 2001.

Singh, S. 'Some edible ferns and fern allies of North-West Himalayas having promising food value'. *Indian J. For.* 16(2): 174-176, 1993.

Turner, Nancy and Bell Marcus, A. M. 'The ethnobotany of the Coast Salish Indians of Vancouver Islands' *Economic Botany* 25: 63-99, 1971.

Upnof, J. C. Rh. *Dictionary of Economic Plants*. New York, U. S. A.: Stechert Hafner, 1968.

User, George. *A Dictionary of Plants Used by Man*. New York, U. S. A.: Hafner Press, 1971.

Vasudeva, S. M. 'Economic importance of Pteridophytes'. *Indian Fern J.* 16: 130-152, 1999.

Verma, P., Khan, A. A. and Singh, K. K. 'Traditional phytotherapy among the Baiga tribe of Shadol District of Madhya Pradesh. India'. *Ethnobotany* 7: 69-73, 1995.

Vyas, M. S. and Sharma, B. D. 'Ethnobotanical importance of ferns of Rajasthan. Indigenous medicinal plants including microbes and fungi. (Ed.). Kaushik, P. New Delhi: Today and Tomorrow Printers and Publications, pp. 61-66, 1988.

Watt, John Mitchell and Maria Gerdina Breyer-Brandwijk. *The Medicinal and Poisonous Plants of South and Eastern Africa*. 2nd. edn. Edinburgh, U. K.: E. & S. Livingstone.

—oo(O)oo—

15

PROPAGATION OF IMPORTANT MEDICINAL PLANTS WITH SPECIAL REFERENCE TO ARAVALLIAN ECO-REGION

U. R. SIYOL AND SATISH KUMAR SHARMA

PLANTS are one of the most important sources of medicine. The application of plants as medicine dates back to prehistoric period. With the development of synthetic drugs, plant products lost their significance for some time. In the last few decades, however, there has been an awakening all over the world for use of organic medicaments in place of synthetic drugs. This has given rise to large-scale collection of several plants from the wild, which resulted in several serious problems such as depletion of resources, extinction of rare and endangered species, etc.

The Aravallian eco-region of Rajasthan is having a number of medicinal plant species growing naturally. Among these, some are rare, endangered and threatened, while some are on the verge of extinction, due to over exploitation, exploitation in unscientific manner, uprooting of entire plants, collection of fruits and seeds before maturity, habitat destruction, erratic rainfall and repeated droughts, poor regeneration, poor establishment, unawareness, etc. Some of the rare, endangered and threatened species of the Aravalli region of southern Rajasthan are *Abrus precatorius, Acacia sinuata, Adhatoda beddomei, Commiphora wightii, Celastrus paniculatus, Gloriosa superba, Oroxylum indicum, Sapindus emarginatus, Stereospermum suaveolens, Pterocarpus marsupium, Sterculia urens, Chlorophytum borivilianum*, etc.

Anticipating the importance of medicinal plants, study to develop low cost suitable propagation techniques of some rare and important species of Aravallian eco-region of southern Rajasthan, has been carried out in field conditions at Forest Research Farm, Banki, Udaipur, for mass multiplication of these plants and restocking of the forest areas with these species. About 50-60 species of different rare, endangered and important medicinal plants are propagated here in nursery to distribute these plants to various government and non-government organisations as well as the general public for further mass multiplication. Among these, some are having standard propagation techniques and for some species studies have been done, while for others it is yet to be done.

TABLE 1
Results of Germination Trials

No.	Plant/Species	Pre-treatment of Seeds for Better and Quick Germination	Time of Seed Sowing	Germination Percentage
1.	*Abrus precatorius* (Fm: Papilionaceae)	Seeds soaked in boiled water and allowed to cool for 24 hrs. Swollen seeds were sown,	Feb.-March July-Aug.	70-80
		unswollen were treated again	Feb.-March	40-50
2.	*Abutilon indicum* (Fm: Malvaceae)	Seeds dipped in H_2SO_4 for 10 minutes, then washed with tap water		
3.	*Acacia sinuata* (Fm: Mimosaceae)	Seeds soaked in boiled water and allowed to cool for 24 hrs. Swollen seeds were sown	Feb.-April	65-75
4.	*Adansonia digita* (Fm: Bombacaceae)	Seeds soaked in boiled water and allowed to cool for 24 hrs. Swollen seeds were sown	Feb.-March July-Sept.	25-30
5.	*Alangium salvifolium* (Fm: Alangiaceae)	No treatment	May-June Immedately after seed collection	40-50
6.	*Argyreia nervosa* (Fm: Convolvulaceae)	Seeds soaked in hot water and kept for 12-24 hours	Feb.-April	70-80
7.	*Asparagus racemosus* (Fm: Liliaceae)	Seeds soaked in cold water for 12 to 24 hours	Feb.-April	70-80
8.	*Balanites aegyptiaca* (Fm: Simaroubaceae)	Seeds kept in cowdung for 2-3 days	Feb.-March	50-60
9.	*Caesalpinia bonduc* (Fm: Caesalpiniaceae)	Seeds soaked in hot water and allowed to cool for 24 hours	Feb.-April	85-90
10.	*Erythrina suberosa* (Fm: Papilionaceae)	Seeds soaked in cold water for 12 hours	June-July	70-80
11.	*Gloriosa superba* (Fm: Liliaceae)	Seeds soaked in cold water for 6-8 hours	July	60-70
12.	*Mucuna pruriens* (Fm: Papilionaceae)	No treatment	June-July	75-85
13.	*Plumbago zeylanica* (Fm: Plumbaginaceae)	No treatment	Feb.-March July-Sept.	70-80

Continued...

...*Continued*

No.	Plant/Species	Pre-treatment of Seeds for Better and Quick Germination	Time of Seed Sowing	Germination Percentage
14.	*Pterocarpus marsupium* (Fm: Papilionaceae)	Hard, impervious fruit wall removed manually and then soaked in cold water for 48 hours	Feb.-March July-Sept.	60-70
15.	*Putranjiva roxburghii* (Fm: Euphorbiaceae)	Seeds soaked in cold water for 24 hours	Feb.-March July-Sept.	60-80
16.	*Rauwolfia serpentina* (Apocynaceae)	Fresh collected fruit were washed to depulp, dried in shade for 2-3 days, soaked in cold water for 24 hours and sown	Aug.-Sept.	20-40
17.	*Sapindus emarginatus* (Fm: Sapinadaceae)	Seeds soaked in boiled water, allowed to cool for 24 hours. Only swollen seeds were sown.	Feb.-April	50-60
18.	*Stereospermum suaveolens* (Fm: Bignoniaceae)	Seeds soaked in cold water for 24 hours	March-April	40-50
19.	*Terminalia arjuna* (Fm: Combretaceae)	Hard, impervious fruit wall removed manually and then soaked in cold water for 3-5 days	Feb.-April	70-80
20.	*Terminalia bellirica* (Fm: Combretaceae)	Fruits cracked mechanically, soaked in cold water for 24 hours	Feb.-April	65-85

MATERIALS AND METHODS

To carry out studies on low cost propagation techniques, propagation by seeds and vegetative means have been tried in field conditions.

For propagation by seeds, fresh seeds were collected from different localities and they were given different sets of treatment like cold water treatment, boiling water treatment, acid treatment, mechanical scarification, etc. before sowing and these treated seeds were sown in polythene bags filled with potting medium in mother-beds under field conditions at Forest Research Farm, Banki, Udaipur. Observations were made on germination of these treated seeds for different treatments and better pre-treatment for a particular species for quick and more germination were found out.

For species which are difficult to propagate by seeds like *Commiphora wightii, Celastrus paniculatus, Barleria prionitis,* etc. propagation by vegetative means were tried. For vegetative

TABLE 2
Regeneration by Cuttings

No.	Plant/Species	Average Size of Cuttings Length	Diameter	Direction for Treatment to Cuttings	Time of Cutting Planting	Sprouting/ Rooting Percentage
1.	*Barleria prionitis* (Fm: Acanthaceae)	12-15 cm	5-7 mm	Dip lower end in IBA 500 ppm solution for 5 sec.	Feb.-March	20-30
2.	*Celastrus paniculatus* (Fm: Celastraceae)	25-30 cm	10-15 mm	Dip lower cut end in IBA 500 ppm solution for about 12 hours	Feb.-March July-Aug.	20-25
3.	*Commiphora wightii* (Fm: Burseraceae)	25-30 cm	15-20 mm	Dip lower cut end in IBA 500 ppm solution for about 12 hours	Feb.-May	65-75
4.	*Tinospora cordifolia* (Fm: Menispermaceae)	15-20 cm	8-12 mm	No treatment	Feb.-March	60-70
5.	*Tylophora asthmatica* (Fm: Asclepiadaceae)	10-15 cm	5-7 mm	No treatment	Jan.-Feb.	70-80

propagation, branch cuttings with different length and diameter were tried with different treatments of root hormones. For this, branch cuttings of required size were prepared with sharp secateur and upper cut end of these cuttings were dipped in melted wax to prevent fungal attack and drying and lower cut end were dipped in hormone solution for quick and more rooting. These treated cuttings were planted in polybags placed in sunken beds in nursery, under field conditions and observations were made on sprouting and rooting of these cuttings.

RESULTS AND DISCUSSION

A list of species and results of trials carried out at Forest Research Farm, Banki, Udaipur, are depicted in Tables 1 and 2.

Table 1 indicates that most of hard coat seeds of forest plant species require boiling water treatment and mechanical scarification treatment to induce fast germination. Also, these treatments provide better germination percentage.

Table 2 highlights that *Barleria prionitis, Commiphora wightii, Celastrus paniculatus, Tinospora cordifolia* and *Tylophora asthmatica* which are difficult to propagate by seeds can be propagated by using stem cuttings, however for standardisation of propagation techniques of these species, some more studies with different sets of treatment are being carried out at this Research Farm.

—oo(O)o—

16

Conservation and Production of Medicinal Plants by Cultivation I. *Chlorophytum borivilianum* Sant. et Fernand

Vinita Sharma and Sandhya Tyagi

THE science of medicinal plants, Ayurveda, flourished during the Vedic period (2000-800 BC) when people lived in caves whereas the study of medicinal plants in Europe was seriously made only during the 'Age of Herbals' which according to Arber (1938) lasted from 1407 to 1670 AD. Thus, there appears to be a gap of some 3,500 years or so in the study of the science of medicinal plants in India and Europe. *Vrikshayurveda* (science of medicinal plants) was compiled by Parasara (Core, 1955) which was a textbook for pre-medical students. During the last few decades, people the world over have evinced much greater interest in herbal medicine which is generally believed to have no side effects. This, coupled with the population explosion and over-exploitation, has endangered the very existence of several species of medicinal plants. Several species of medicinal plants such as *Tylophora indica, Acorus calamus, Aristolochia bracteata, Basella rubra,* etc. are extremely endangered/already *in situ* extinct. Then, large-scale urbanisation and deforestation in under-developed countries like India have destroyed the natural habitats of many species, including medicinal plants.

The present writers are fully convinced that collection of medicinal plants from natural habitats can never meet the required demands. Only *ex-situ* cultivation of practically all herbaceous species of medicinal plants is the only method for their conservation. One such species is *Chlorophytum borivilianum* which not very long ago was widely distributed in the hilly regions of the States of Maharashtra, Gujarat and Rajasthan.

However, there is no mention of this species in Cooke's *Flora of Bombay Presidency* (1958) or even in the recently published *Flora of Rajasthan* (Shetty and Singh, 1993). This species was reported for the first time by Santapau and Fernandes (1955) from Salsette Island near Mumbai. Kothari and Hajra (1983), Shah (1983) and Ahamedulla and Nayar (1987) have listed this as a rare and threatened species endemic to Maharashtra and Gujarat. Nayar and Sastry (1988) have entered it in the Red Data Book on Indian Plants. Purohit *et al* (1994) reported this species for the first time from several forests in Udaipur District. 'Safed moosli' as it is locally called, used to be collected as a minor forest product by the tribal people of the area. However, ever since its medicinal properties became popular, it has been almost completely uprooted by certain unscrupulous elements who are now cultivating it and making huge profits while the poor tribals have been deprived of this means of their livelihood which was also a matter of heritage.

It is only recently under a project funded by the Department of Science and Technology, Government of India, New Delhi, that the present writers provided seedling tubers to 100 rural/tribal women (one kg to each free of cost) to make additional income and which has proved very successful.

In the present work, the main object was to augment the production of tuberous roots as a result of pre-treatment by certain hormones.

MATERIAL AND METHOD

Prof. Y. D. Tiagi collected about one kg of tuberous roots of *Chlorophytum borivilianum* from the Aravalli forests in the year 1995 and cultivated them in big pots in his garden all these years. Ten kg of these tubers were provided to us for this experimental work in 1999. The cluster of tuberous roots remain attached to the under surface of a more or less discoid stem (or crown) which is cut vertically in such a manner so that 2-3 tubers each weighting about 2-3 gm remain attached to the under surface of the portion of the crown. Root tubers without a portion of the crown will not sprout. Such cut tubers are dried for a period of 15-20 days during the first fortnight of June so that the cut surfaces get suberised. Prior to sowing such seeding tubers were soaked in different concentrations of different growth regulants for a duration of 48 hours. After the pre-treatment, the seeding tubers were washed with tap water. Tuberous roots soaked in tap water constituted the controls.

OBSERVATIONS

These are recorded in Table 1 along with the statistical analyses of the data. It would be seen that pre-treatment of seeding tuberous, one or more concentration/duration augments the production of tuberous roots in a conspicuous manner and the results are statistically significant. Although some pre-treatments were superior to the control, another notable fact is that there is also a lot of variation among the experimental controls as also under natural conditions.

DISCUSSION

Any treatment which leads to increased production of roots and biomass may also lead to higher production of roots in *Chlorophytum borivilianum* is most welcome. Among the numerous chemical substances, natural and synthetic, which profoundly influence growth and differentiation of plant cells and organs in addition to seed germination, are a category designated by the term 'hormone' or growth regulants. It was the British physician, E. H. Starling (1905; see Hopkins, 1999) who coined the term 'hormone' to describe chemical substances which co-ordinated body functions among animals. The concept of hormones in plants may be traced back to the observations of Duha Mel-du-Monceau (1758; see Hopkins, 1999) who observed the formation of root on the swellings that occur above the girdle wound around the stem of woody plants. However, the real

TABLE 1: ***Chlorophytum borivilianum***
Effect of Certain Concentrations of Growth Regulants on Tuberous Root Production
(Values are Means of Three Replicates Each)

A: IAA

Concentration ppm	a: Numbers of Tubers/Plants	b: Fresh Weight of Tubers per Plant (g fresh weight)
Control	10.00	12.33
50 ppm	11.33	14.33
100 ppm	16.00	18.00
200 ppm	9.33	8.67

CRD ANOVA Table a

No.	Source	DF	SS	MS	F
1.	Treatment	3	81.333	27.11	9.295**
2.	Error	8	23.333	2.916	

CV = 14.64 SE = 0.986 CD(5%) = 3.216 CD(1%) = 4.679

CRD ANOVA Table b

No.	Source	DF	SS	MS	F
1.	Treatment	3	136.667	45.555	15.185**
2.	Error	8	24.000	3.000	

CV = 12.99 SE = 1.00 CD(5%) = 3.261 CD(1%) = 4.745

B: NAA

Concentration ppm	a: Numbers of Tubers/Plants	b: Fresh Weight of Tubers per Plant (g fresh weight)
Control	10.00	8.67
50 ppm	12.00	12.33
100 ppm	15.33	17.33
200 ppm	10.33	9.33

CRD ANOVA Table a

No.	Source	DF	SS	MS	F
1.	Treatment	3	53.583	17.861	4.560*
2.	Error	8	31.333	3.916	

CV = 16.61 SE = 1.14 CD(5%) = 3.726 CD(1%) = 5.422

CRD ANOVA Table b

No.	Source	DF	SS	MS	F
1.	Treatment	3	140.25	46.75	3.951
2.	Error	8	94.666	11.833	

CV = 28.87 SE = 1.99 CD(5%) = 6.477 CD(1%) = 9.424

Continued...

...Continued

C: GA_3

Treatment GA_3	a: Numbers of Tubers/Plants	b: Fresh Weight of Tubers per Plant (g fresh weight)
Control	10.67	6.00
100 ppm	16.67	10.33
200 ppm	12.67	12.00
300 ppm	13.00	10.67

CRD ANOVA Table a

No.	Source	DF	SS	MS	F
1.	Treatment	3	56.250	18.750	1.630
2.	Error	8	92.000	11.500	

CV = 25.59 SE = 1.96 CD(5%) = 6.385 CD(1%) = 9.291

CRD ANOVA Table b

1.	Treatment	3	60.916	20.305	2.936
2.	Error	8	55.333	6.916	

CV = 26.97 SE = 1.52 CD(5%) = 4.952 CD(1%) = 7.205

D: KINETIN

Concentration ppm	a: Numbers of Tubers/Plant	b: Fresh Weight of Tubers per Plant (g fresh weight)
Control	8.00	18.00
50 ppm	10.66	23.00
100 ppm	17.00	38.30
200 ppm	13.33	24.00

CRD ANOVA Table a

No.	Source	DF	SS	MS	F
1.	Treatment	3	121.795	40.589	24.464**
2.	Error	8	11.410	1.426	

CV = 9.7 SE = 0.69 CD(5%) = 2.249 CD(1%) = 3.272

CRD ANOVA Table b

1.	Treatment	3	524.250	174.75	46.600**
2.	Error	8	30.00	3.75	

CV = 7.67 SE = 1.126 CD(5%) = 3.646 CD(1%) = 5.305

beginning of plant hormone research is seen in a series of simple and clear experiments conducted by Charles Darwin (1881). It is these researches which ultimately led to the discovery of auxins by Went (1929, 1934, 1938, 1951). The term 'hormone' was introduced in plant physiology by H. Fitting (quoted by Hopkins, 1999).

According to current usage in plant physiology, hormones are naturally occurring organic substances which in low concentrations exert a profound influence on physiological processes. There are certain synthetic substances such as NAA, IBA, phenyl acetic acid (PPA), 2,4-D, etc. which too affect plant growth. So it is more appropriate to use the term 'growth regulants' for all such substances, natural or synthetic. IBA was originally thought to be synthetic but later its isolation from seeds and leaves of maize by Epstein *et al* (1980, 1989) showed that it is not so.

Plant hormones profoundly affect plant growth. In the present investigation, certain concentrations of kinetin pre-treatment of seeding tubers resulted in a spectacular increase in the production of tuberous roots but one or more concentration of all the above-mentioned hormones resulted in greater production of tuberous roots than the controls and in this connection kinetin was better than IAA, NAA and GA_3 (Table 1).

Thus, it can be seen that hormones which profoundly affect the various growth parameters also affect the production of tuberous roots in *Chlorophytum borivilianum*. A perusal of this vast literature shows that research on the effect of hormones *vis-a-vis* growth and development (and also seed germination) will never end because the effect they elicit from the treated plants vary from species to species and concentration/duration and also the mode of application. Therefore, the research work done on hormones *vis-a-vis* growth parameters is very diverse and extensive. One of the recent reviews on the subject is by Davies (1995). A terse review of the important findings including some historical milestones is given in the following lines.

A milestone in elucidating the importance of growth hormones was created by auxinologist Went way back in the 1920s (Thimann and Went, 1937). IAA as an endogenous hormone was identified, its biosynthetic pathway, its role in cell elongation, differentiation of secondary growth, mechanism of apical dominance, retardation of abscission and its role in development of root primordia have been well documented. Practical application of hormones was first discovered by horticulturists. Based on the formative effect of these hormones, several agricultural uses have been identified. Now a stage is set to judiciously and meaningfully use these growth substances to induce the desired pattern of growth in plants to achieve maximum productivity (Malik, 1995). In fact, application of growth regulators has become a necessary input for crop improvement. The widespread use of growth regulators by nursery men, florists and horticulturists indicates that they are valuable aids to rooting. There is usually a considerable saving of time, often amounting to well over one-third of the usual rooting period. Since rooting is more rapid, there is less opportunity for the cuttings to deteriorate and as a rule, the root systems produced are much more massive. As already mentioned, different species of plants respond variously to different growth regulators and no one hormone can be regarded as effective in all cases. Successful propagation of peach by stem cuttings with the aid of plant growth regulators and kept in mist chambers has been reported by Cochran (1945), Harrison (1958), Hartman and Hansen (1958), Hartmann and Kester (1976) and Sharpe(1956).

Since the discovery of auxins and their identification as a growth hormone, an enormous amount of literature has accumulated describing their effect on the growth of plants. In some cases auxin is stimulatory but inhibitory in others and in still other cases a necessary participant in growth activity of another plant hormone (namely, cytokinins and gibberellins). Application of IAA in lanolin paste to the severed end of a young stem stimulates the rate of formation and number of roots initiated. This discovery was not only of scientific interest but has also opened the door to commercial application of IAA to promote root formation in cuttings of economically useful plants (Went and Thimann, 1937). Cleland and Burstrom (1961) demonstrated that the amount of solute present in the cell sap increases in a cell treated with IAA. Auxin-induced cell wall extension strongly suggests that IAA exerts its influence at a point very close to the gene level. There appears to be an intimate relationship between the effects of auxin on nucleic acid and growth, a relationship first suggested by Skoog in 1954.

Since that time there have been numerous studies supporting Skoog's suggestion that the action of auxin in regulating growth is associated with nucleic acid metabolism (Coartney *et al,* 1967; Key and Shannon, 1964; Masuda *et al,* 1967; Nooden, 1968; Knypl, 1966). In view of the fact that exogenously applied IAA can induce the synthesis of new RNA and protein has been demonstrated in a variety of plant tissues. For example, applied IAA induced RNA and protein synthesis in *Rhoeo* leaves (Sacher, 1967), yeast cells (Shimoda *et al,* 1967), green pea stem sections (De Hertogh *et al,* 1965), bean endocarp (Sacher, 1967), and oat coleoptile sections (Masuda *et al,* 1967). Devlin and Jackson (1961) and Jackson (1960) emphasised that roots are much more sensitive to auxin than stems and real stimulation of root elongation may be achieved if low concentrations are used. The application of relatively high concentration of IAA to roots, not only retards root elongation but causes a noticeable increase in the number of branch roots.

Long ago, Thimann (1934, 1963) indicated that root formation is controlled by auxins in plants. Similar results were obtained by Thimann and Koepfli (1935), Cooper (1936) and Thakurta and Dutt (1941) with IAA. Ellott (1977) emphasised that in the maize plant the elongation of primary root and the geo-responses are regulated by interaction of growth promoting, acropetally moving IAA derived primarily from the fruit and shoot system with IBA moving in a basipetal direction from the root cap. The primary action of IAA in promotion of cell elongation may involve the stimulation of a proton pump in the cell membrane. Exogenously applied auxins affect rooting by stimulating cambial activity and differentiation of cambial derivatives into xylem (Nanda *et al,* 1967, 1968). According to Nanda (1970) and Nanda and Kochhar (1972, 1985) auxins play multifarious roles. These are concerned with the division and elongation of meristematic cells, differentiation of cambial initials into root primordia and in the mobilisation of reserve food materials by enhancing the activity of hydrolysing enzymes. Gregori and Somantarai (1950) and Nanda *et al* (1968) hypothesised that increased rooting in auxin treated cuttings has been considered to be partly due to enhanced hydrolysis of nutritional reserves under the influence of auxins. Biswas and Choudhuri (1977) applied foliar spray of IAA on rice and found increased grain yield.

Similar results were obtained by Chatterjee *et al* (1977) and Singh *et al* (1984). Singh and Dara (1971) reported that IAA increased the plant height and tillers in wheat. Chauhan and Maheshwari (1968) studied the effect of certain plant growth regulators, seasons and types of cuttings on root initiation and vegetative growth in stem cuttings of peach variety *sharbati* and concluded that IBA at 50 ppm concentration gave the highest rooting in all the three seasons tried. Nanda *et al* (1968) and Chauhan and Maheshwari (1968) have studied the effect of auxin on some tree species. It has been demonstrated that the response varied with the auxins, its concentration and the planting season. They found that 90 per cent stem cuttings of *Dalbergia sisoo* rooted in the month of August when treated with 100 ppm concentration of IAA while 2,4-D completely inhibited rooting. Sharma (1993) reported that IAA treatment at 500 ppm concentration initiated early flowering and fruiting in the cuttings of *Commiphora wightii* and *Commiphora agallocha.* One hundred per cent sprouting was observed in cuttings of *Commiphora agallocha* when treated with 100 to 1,000 ppm concentration IAA. Ahuja (2000) observed that *Tinospora cordifolia* exhibited 100 per cent sprouting at 200 and 500 ppm concentration of IAA and IBA.

Manohar (1966) could induce rooting in stem cuttings in certain plants by treatment with different concentrations of IBA. Blommaert (1959) recorded 80 per cent rooting in guava cuttings taken with an axillary bud and a portion of the stem in mist chambers after treatment with 4,000 ppm IBA. Similar results were obtained by Jolicoeur (1962) in two varieties of guava by Floor (1963) in some pear varieties by Tarasenko and Vesitev (1966), in softwood cuttings of plum and by Singh (1979) in *Ixora rosea.* Singh *et al* (1989) reported that pre-treatment of stem cuttings with 5,000 ppm concentration of IBA significantly enhanced the percentage of sprouting of 'guggal' cuttings. On the contrary, Sharma (1993) observed maximum sprouting in guggal only at 700 ppm and 1,000 ppm concentrations of IBA. Fuchs (1986) observed that IBA applied to root segments of *Rosa multiflora* var. '*Kanagawa*' showed increased number of regenerated roots, as well as root length and the best results were obtained with 1,000 ppm concentration of IBA. Shah *et al* (1983) reported similar results in guggal cuttings.

Gibberellic acid is known to cause cell elongation and mobilisation of food materials. During germination it activates the amylase enzymes which convert complex substances to simple substances required for the germinating seedlings. Kumar and Baijal (1978) reported that gibberellic acid mobilised the reserve food material stored in seed and tubers of potato by activating amylase enzyme and therefore helps in germination. Germination percentage, plant height, tillering and grain yield of wheat and barley seed improved after treating the seed with 10 ppm of gibberellic acid before sowing (Chippa and Lal, 1978; Verma and Singh, 1978). Improvement in germination percentage, ear bearing shoots, grains per ear, grain weight and yield of wheat was also observed after treating the wheat seed before sowing with 15 ppm of gibberellic acid (Shah, 1983).

Paul and Misra (1976) reported that soaking the rice seeds in certain concentrations of IAA, GA_3, CCC before sowing had more pronounced positive effect on shoot than root elongation. Singh *et al* (1984) observed very little effect on paddy yield and its attributes. Treatment of cotton seed with 100 ppm gibberellic acid increased the hypocotyl length and dry weight of roots. On the contrary, decrease in root length by treatment with gibberellic acid has also been reported (Brar and Singh, 1982, 1983).

Brian *et al* (1955, 1960) and Gundersen (1958) demonstrated that gibberellic acid in general inhibits root formation in many plants. However, they promote root as well as shoot formation on stem cutting of *Bryophyllum tubiflorum* (Nanda, Purohit and Bala, 1968), *Pisum sativum* (Erikson, 1972) and *Ipomoea fistulosa* (Nanda *et al,* 1972). The view has been expressed that root induction caused by gibberellic acid in these plants may be mediated through an increase in the auxin concentration and adequate supply/availability of nutrients, not only for stimulation of shoot but also for stimulation of roots as well.

Hansen (1976) observed that at low concentration gibberellins promoted root initiation in pea cuttings. But Brian *et al* (1960) concluded that gibberellins at high concentrations consistently inhibited adventitious root formation. This inhibition is a direct local effect that prevents the early cell division involved in transformation of mature stem tissues to a meristematic condition. Tomar and Ramgiry (1977a, 1977b) found that 50 ppm concentration of gibberellic acid showed maximum number of tubers per plant. Hormones at lower concentrations cause desirable change but at higher concentrations may cause various adverse effects as reported by Elebeltagy *et al* (1981). On the contrary, Sharma (1993) observed that higher concentrations of gibberellic acid (700 ppm and 1,000 ppm) were superior to the control for sprouting of stem cuttings in both the species of *Commiphora.* According to Ahuja (2000), higher concentrations of gibberellic acid (500 ppm and 1,000 ppm) were found to be slightly superior for sprouting as well as for production of both above and below-ground biomass in *Tinospora cordifolia.*

Bhadoria (1980) concluded that yield of potato could be increased by treatment with gibberellic acid and 2,4-D. According to Elebeltagy *et al* (1981) cycocel and gibberellic acid were superior for a desirable change in the yield of potato. Singh *et al* (1993) studied the radioprotective effect of gibberellic acid in black gram [*Vigna mungo* (L.) Hepper] and found that gibberellic acid at 100 ppm and 250 ppm concentrations showed a significant recovery in the radiation induced damage in plant growth. Godha and Kumar (1966) concluded that the combined application of gibberellic acid and nitrogen significantly increased the flower yield per plant of *Chrysanthemum.* Tomar and Ramgiry (1977a, 1977b) stated that gibberellic acid (50 ppm) treatment at the seedling stage seems to offer valuable scope for obtaining higher yield in commercial cultivation of tomato.

2,4-dichlorophenoxy acetic acid (2,4-D) is one of the most widely used synthetic auxins for the initiation of roots. Many phenoxy compounds such as 2, 4, 5-T, 2, 4, 5-TP, 2, 4 and 5-TB have also been found to be useful as root initiators. All of these have promontory effect at very low concentrations. Anbazagan (1978) observed that 25 ppm concentration of 2,4-D appreciably increased the bunch height, advanced the maturity of bunches and improved the quality of fruits in certain banana cultivars. Bhadoria (1980) found increased yield of potato when treated with 2,4-D. According to Grace (1939) 2, 4-D promotes rooting in low concentrations. Ahuja (2000) reported that 2,4-D at 500 ppm concentration resulted in a high percentage of rooting in *Tinospora cordifolia* and also improved the growth of the plant by increasing the biomass when compared with the control. However, Sharma (1993) observed inhibitory effect of 2,4-D on rooting in stem cuttings of *Commiphora wightii* and *Commiphora agallocha.*

Another phenoxy type growth promoting substance is NAA (Naphthalene acetic acid). It has been observed to affect the growth, development and yield of wheat, barely and rice (Choudhuri *et al,* 1980; Orsi and Tallarico, 1983; Singh and Gill, 1985; Grewal and Gill, 1986). Leaf area index and chlorophyll content of fresh leaves increased with NAA spray which helped the crop to trap more of photosynthetically active radiation and, in turn, significantly improved the ear bearing shoots/plant, number of filled up grains/panicle, grain weight and grain yield of paddy (Grewal and Gill, 1986). The beneficial effect of spray of NAA on the chlorophyll content, tillering, grain/ear and paddy yield was also observed by Choudhuri *et al* (1980). In groundnut, NAA application (40 ppm) twice, namely 40 and 80 days after sowing the groundnut markedly improved the pod yield of groundnut (Gopalkrishnan and Srinivasan, 1975). Subbireddy and Shah (1984) observed that NAA (25 or 50 ppm) improved the pod yield of groundnut by favourably influencing the pods/plant and 100 kernel weight. Grewal (1980) observed a significant increase in pod yield of groundnut with spray of NAA (60 ppm). Gowda *et al* (1976) and Singh *et al* (1978) emphasised that the beneficial effect of growth regulators on groundnut production was due to the favourable effect of these growth regulators on various plant physiological processes.

NAA spray at the optimum concentration and at the proper stage of the crop can also boost up the production of pulses. Foliar spray of NAA (25 ppm) at the flowering stage substantially increased the pod/plant, grain weight and thus the yield of blackgram (Mehrotra *et al,* 1968) and chickpea (Bengal *et al,* 1982). In mung bean, an increase in yield was observed with NAA 50 ppm by Kaul *et al* (1974). Singh (1984) observed no significant effect of 50 ppm spray of NAA on mung bean. Pigeon pea responded significantly to 100 ppm spray of NAA at the flowering stage (Vikhe *et al,* 1983).

The response of cotton to NAA spray is not consistent. Positive effect of NAA spray on the seed cotton yield was recorded by Dastur and Prakash (1954), Bhatt (1972), Rao *et al* (1976) and Brar and Singh (1983). NAA spray increased the setting percentage of bolls (Dastur and Prakash, 1954) and favourably affected the carbohydrate-nitrogen metabolism, resulting in increased dry matter production of cotton (Dastur and Bhatt, 1956). Muthoo and Chetan (1997) found that 30 ppm concentration of NAA improves the quality and yield of fruits in peach. Contrary to the results of above workers, no significant effect of NAA spray on seed cotton yield were observed by Singh (1967) and Sodhi (1979).

The above account clearly indicates that spray of NAA improves the production yield of various crops, namely, cotton, rice, wheat, barley, groundnut and pulses. According to Ahuja (2000) stem of *Tinospora cordifolia* with NAA responded positively to rooting and increased biomass. Sharma (1993) established successful rooting in *Commiphora wightii* at certain concentrations of NAA.

A number of naturally occurring compounds classed as cytokinins have been found in plants. These have a basic chemical structure of an N^6–substituted adenine. Synthetic cytokinins available for experimental use include benezyladenine, kinetin and others. Kinetin is also known as 6-furfurylaminopurine. It is used to break the dormancy, improve the germination, tillering/shoot and sink capacity of various crops. Kinetin has been reported to improve the growth of plants because it causes cell division apart from activation of various enzymes. Treatment of the wheat seed with 10 ppm of kinetin before sowing improved the emergence percentage, ear bearing shoots, number of grains/ear, grain weight, dry matter/plant and harvest index. Root length, coleoptile length and chlorophyll content of fresh leaves of wheat also increased with kinetin treatment (Kaur, 1980). Kinetin spray (10 ppm) at anthesis and again one week later increased the number of grains/panicle, percentage of filled up spikelets, grain weight and yield of rice (Singh *et al,* 1984). Meredith *et al* (1970) demonstrated that IAA improves rooting by stimulation, elongation and development of pre-formed root initials whereas kinetin possibly stimulates the formation of additional root initials. On the contrary, Humphries and Maciejewska–Potapczyk (1960) suggested that kinetin strongly inhibited formation of roots in the hypocotyls of *Phaseolus vulgaris* not by inhibiting cell division but by influencing the kind of cell produced. Cytokinins which stimulate cell division have been found to act as a promoter of rooting in certain cases (Allsopp and Szweykewska, 1960; Bachelard and Stowe, 1963; Meredith *et al,* 1970). The inhibitory effect of kinetin in *Commiphora wightii* but promontory in *Commiphora agallocha* was reported by Sharma (1993).

Ahuja (2000) found that in the non-bitter variety of *Tinospora cordifolia* certain concentrations of kinetin (up to 100 ppm) included rooting whereas in the bitter one it was at 200 ppm concentration. Certain concentrations of kinetin affected increase in fresh weight and dry weight in both the varieties. In the present work also, the effect of kinetin in augmenting fresh weight production of tuberous root has been found to be spectacular (Table 1).

In conclusion, it can be said that the endogenous levels of hormones play a vital role in the regulation of plant metabolism, growth and production. The same can be achieved by the exogenous application of hormones. However, the response of different species vary not only to different growth regulators and concentrations but at times, the results are conflicting and more comprehensive studies should continue on the subject.

REFERENCES

Ahmedulla, M. and Nayar, M. P. *Endemic Plants of the Indian Region*, Howrah, 1987.

Ahuja, K. (Miss). Studies on Phenotypic Variation, Clonal Propagation and Phytochemistry of *Tinospora cordifolia* (Willd.) Ex. Hoof. f. et Thomas. Ph.D. Thesis. University of Rajasthan, Jaipur, 2000.

Ahuja, P. Ecophysiological observations on the seeds of certain desert plants with special reference to germination, productivity and energetics. Ph.D. Thesis. University of Rajasthan, Jaipur, 1974.

Allsopp, A. and Szweykowska, A. 'Foliar abnormalities including repeated branching and root formation induced by kinetin in attached leaves of *Marsilea'*. *Nature* 186: 813-814, 1960.

Ambasta, S. P. (Ed.). *The Useful Plants of India*. New Delhi: Publications and Information Directorate, C.S.I.R., 1986.

*Anbazagam, A. Studies on the effect of ethrel and 2,4-D on certain banana cultivars. M.Sc. (Agr.) Thesis. Tamil Nadu Agricultural University, 1978.

Arber, A. *Herbals, Their Origin and Evolution*, 2nd edn., London, 1938.

Bachelard, E. P. and Stowe, B. B. 'Rooting of cuttings of *Acer rubrum* L. and *Eucalyptus camaldulensis* Deyn.' *Aust. J. Bio. Sci.* 16: 751-767, 1963.

Bengal, D. B., Desmukh, S. N. and Patil, V. A. 'Note on the effect of growth regulators and urea on yield attributes of gram (*Cicer arietinum*)' . *Legume Res.* 5: 54-56, 1982.

*Bhadoria, S. P. S. Effect of GA_3 and 2,4-D on growth and yield of potato. M.Sc. Thesis. J.N.K.V.V., Jabalpur, 1980.

Bhatia, A. K., Pandita, M. L. and Khurana, S. C. 'Effect of plant growth substances and sprouting conditions on sprout growth'. *J. Indian Potato Assn.* 18: 151-154, 1991.

Bhatt, J. G. 'Low concentration sprays of naphthalene acetic acid for more cotton'. *Indian Fmg.* 22: 36-37, 1972.

Biswas, A. K. and Chaudhuri, M. A. 'Regulation of leaf senescence in rice by hormones sprayed at different developmental stages and its effect on yield'. *Indian J. Agric. Sci.* 47: 38, 1977.

*Blommaert, K. L. J. 'Propagate guavas by means of leaf bud cuttings'. *Fmg. S. Afr.* 35: 29-32, 1959.

Brar, Z. S. and Singh, M. 'Effect of certain chemicals on the distribution of biomass and productivity of cotton'. *Indian J. Ecol.* 9: 277-280, 1982.

Brar, Z. S. and Singh, M. 'Effect of plant regulators on biomass and productivity of cotton (*Gossypium hirsutum*)'. *Indian J. Ecol.* 10: 254-259, 1983.

*Brian, P. W. and Hemming, H. G. 'The effect of gibberellic acid on shoot growth of pea seedling'. *Physiol. Plant.* 8: 669-681, 1955.

Brian, P. W., Hemming, H. G. and Lowe, D. 'Inhibition of rooting of cuttings by gibberellic acid'. *Ann. Bot.* 24: 407-409, 1960.

Chatterjee, A., Mandal, R. K. and Sircar, S. M. 'Effect of growth substances on productivity, photosynthesis and translocation of rice varieties'. *Indian J. Plant Physiol.* 19: 131, 1977.

*Chauhan, K. S. and Maheshwari, L. D. 'Effect of certain plant growth regulators, seasons and types of cuttings on root initiation and vegetative growth in stem cuttings of peach, variety *Sharbati*'. *Indian J. Hort.* 51: 136-140, 1968.

Chippa, B. R. and Lal, P. 'Effect of pre-soaking of seeds with salt and hormones and different quality of water on wheat'. '*J. Indian Soc. Soil. Sci.* 26: 350-356, 1978.

Cleland, R. E. and Burstrom, H. 'Theories of the auxin action on cellular elongation. A summary'. In: *Encyclopaedia of Plant Physiology.* (Ed.). Ruhland, W. Berlin: Springer, 14: 807, 1961.

Coartney, J. S., Morre, D. J. and Key, J. L. 'Inhibition of RNA synthesis and auxin-induced cell wall extensibility and growth by actinomycin D'. *Plant Physiol.* 42: 434, 1967.

Cochran, G. W. 'Propagation of peaches from softwood cuttings'. *Proc. Amer. Soc. Hort. Sci.* 46: 230-240, 1945.

Cooke, J. *The Flora of the Presidency of Bombay*, vol. 3, Kolkata: Botanical Survey of India, 1958.

Cooper, W. C. Transport of root forming hormones in woody cuttings' . *Plant Physiol.* 11: 779-793, 1936.

Core, E. W. *Plant Taxonomy*. Englewood Cliffs, N.J., U.S.A.: Prentice-Hall Inc., 1955.

*Darwin, C. *The Power of Movement in Plants.* New York: D. Appleton and Company, 1881.

Das, N. K., Patau, K. and Skoog, F. 'Initiation of mitosis and cell division by kinetin and indoleacetic acid in excised tobacco pith tissue'. *Physiol. Plant* 9: 640, 1956.

Dastur, R. H. and Bhatt, J. B. 'Effect of chemical hormones on carbohydrate and nitrogen content of cotton plant'. *Indian J. Agric. Sci.* 26: 39-42, 1956.

Dastur, R. H. and Prakash, Ved. 'Response of cotton plant to some growth regulating substances'. *Indian Cotton Grow. Rev.* 8: 1-6, 1954.

Davies, P. J. (Ed.). *Plant Hormones.* Dordrecht: Kluwer Academic Publishers, 1995.

*De Hertogh, A. A., McCune, D. C., Brown, J. and Antoine, D. 'The effect of antagonists of RNA and protein biosynthesis on IAA and 2,4-D induced growth of green pea stem sections'. *Contrib. Boyce Thompson Inst.* 23: 23, 1965.

Devlin, R. M. and Jackson, W. T. 'Effect of p-chlorophenoxyisobutyric acid on rate of elongation of root hair of *Agrostris alba* L.' *Physiol. Plant* 14: 40, 1961.

*Doak, B. W. 'The effect of various nitrogenous compounds on the rooting of *Rhododendron* cuttings treated with naphthalene acetic acid'. *New Zealand Jour. Sci. and Tech.* 21: 336-343, 1940.

*Elebeltagy, M. S., Abd, E. L., Hussain, S. O. and Mekesound, M. A. 'GA in relation to abnormal potato tuber formation'. *Egyptian J. Hort.* 8: 131-132, 1981.

Elliott, M. C. 'Auxin and the regulation of root growth'. In: *Plant Growth Regulation.* Berlin Heidelberg, New York: Springer-Verlag, 1977.

Epstein, E., Chen, K. H. and Cohen, J. D. 'Identification of Indole-3-butyric acid as an endogenous constituent of maize kernels and leaves'. *J. Pl. Growth Regul.* 8: 215-223, 1989.

Epstein, E., Cohen, J. D. and Bandurski, R. S. 'Concentration and metabolic turnover of indoles in germinating kernels of *Zea mays*'. *Plant Physiol.* 65: 415-421, 1980.

*Erikson, E. N. In: *Royal Vet. Agric. Year Book*. Copenhagen, 1972.

*Floor, J. 'The propagation of pear varieties by cuttings'. *Meded. Dir. Tuinb.* 26: 687-691 (*Hort. Abst.* 34: 2208), 1963.

Fuchs, H. W. M. 'Root regeneration of rose plants as influenced by applied auxins'. *Acta Horticulturae* 189: 101-107, 1986.

Godha, S. and Kumar, A. 'Studies on the effect of growth regulators on growth and flowering of *Chrysanthemum*'. Nat. Symp. on *Current Trends in Biotech. and Pl. Path: Prof. Uma Kant Felicitation Volume,* September. 20-21, Abst., p. 51, Jaipur, 1996.

*Gopalkrishnan, S. and Srinivasan, P. S. 'Effect of planofix on NAA formulation on groundnut'. *Pesticides*: 23-25, 1975.

Gowda, S. T., Ramachandra, T. V., Muniyappa, T. V. and Krishnamurthy, K. 'Response of groundnut to planofix (NAA)'. *Pesticides*: 31-33, 1976.

Grace, N. H. 'Vegetative propagation of conifers 1. Rooting of cuttings taken from upper and lower regions of Norway spruce tree'. *Can. J. Res.* 17: 178-180, 1939.

Gregory, F. G. and Somantarai, B. 'Factors concerned in the rooting response of isolated leaves'. *J. Exp. Bot.* 1: 153-169, 1950.

*Grewal, H. S. and Gill, H. S. 'Influence of NAA and nitrogen on the growth and yield of late-planted paddy (*Oryza sativa* L.)'. *J. Agric. Sci. Camb.* 106: 37-40, 1986.

*Gundersen, K. 'Some experiments with gibberellic acid'. *Acta Horti. Gotoburgensis* 22: 87-110, 1958.

Hansen, J. 'Adventitous root formation induced by gibberellic acid and regulated by irradiance to the stock plants'. *Physiol. Plant* 32: 170-173, 1976.

Harrison, T. B. 'Note on the vegetative reproduction of peach cuttings'. *Canad. J. Pl. Sci.* 38: 515-516, 1958.

*Hartmann, H. T. and Hansen, C. J. 'Effect of season of collecting, indolebutyric acid and pre-planting storage treatments on rooting of Marianna plum, peach and quince hardwood cuttings'. *Proc. Amer. Soc. Hort. Sci.* 71: 57-66, 1958.

Hartmann, H. T. and Kester, D. S. *Plant Propagation: Principles and Practices*. Englewood Cliffs, New Jersey, U.S.A.: Prentice Hall Inc., 1976.

Hopkins, W. G. *Introduction to Plant Physiology*. New York: John Wiley & Sons, Inc., 1999.

Humphries, E. C. and Maciejewska Potapezyk, W. 'Effect of indole acetic acid, naphthalene acetic acid and kinetin on phosphorus fraction in hypocotyls of dwarf bean (*Phaseolus vulgaris*)'. *Ann. Bot.* 24: 311-316, 1960.

Jackson, W. T. 'Effect of indole acetic acid on rate of elongation of root hair of *Agrostis alba* L.' *Physiol. Plant* 13: 36, 1960.

Jacobs, W. P. *Plant Hormones and Plant Development.* Cambridge, U.K.: Cambridge University Press, 1979.

*Jolicoeur, J. A. 'The rooting of guava cuttings treated with hormone under mist in Haiti'. *Proc. Caribb. Reg. Amer. Soc. Hort. Sci.* 57-59 (*Hort. Abst.* 34: 7704), 1962.

Jones, A. M. and Herman, E. M. 'KDEL-containing auxin-binding protein is secreted to the plasma membrane and cell wall'. *Plant Physiology* 101: 595-606, 1993.

Jones, A. M. and Prasad, P. 'Auxin-binding proteins and their possible roles in auxin mediated plant cell growth'. *Bioassays* 14: 43-48, 1992.

Kaul. J. N., Sekhon, H. S. and Singh, K. B. 'Preliminary studies on the effect of hormonal application on the yield of mung'. *J. Res. Punjab Agric. Univ.* 11: 359-361, 1974.

*Kaur, P. Effect of CCC and kinetin on the physiology of wheat under different salinity levels. M.Sc. Thesis. Punjab Agric. University, Ludhiana, 1980.

Key, J. L. and Shannon, J. C. 'Enhancement by auxin of ribonucleic acid synthesis in excised soybean hypocotyl tissue'. *Plant Physiol.* 39: 360, 1964.

Knypl, J. S. 'Specific inhibitors of RNA and protein synthesis as suppressors of the IAA and coumarin induced growth responses'. *Acta. Soc. Bot.*, Poland, 35: 357-373, 1966.

Kothari, M. I. and Hajra, P. K. 'Gujarat and Rajasthan region'. In: *Materials for a Catalogue of Threatened Plants of India.* (Eds.). Jain, S. K. and Sastry. A. R. K., Howrah, 1983.

Kshetrapal, A. and Sharma, M. K. 'Studies on the effect of certain growth regulators on the germination and seedling growth of *Boswellia serrata* Roxb.' *J. Environ. and Poll.* 3: 179-183, 1996.

Kumar, D. and Baijal, B. D. 'Changes in amylase activity and total sugar during storage in potatoes raised from growth regulators treated tubers'. *Indian J. Exp. Biol.* 16: 269-270, 1978.

Malik, C. P. 'Plant growth regulators: Software for plant development and crop productivity'. Presidential Address, 82nd Ind. Sci. Congr. Assoc., Botany Section, pp. 1-34, 1995.

Manohar, M. S. 'Influence of source of the performance of softwood cuttings of guava'. *Fmr.* 11: 191-194, 1966.

Masuda, Y., Tanimoto, E. and Wada, S. 'Auxin-stimulated RNA synthesis in oat coleoptile cells'. *Physiol. Plant* 20: 713, 1967.

Mehrotra, O. N., Saxena, H. K., Raya, H. M. and Nath, S. 'Effects of growth regulators on fruiting and yield of blackgram (*Vigna mungo*) in India'. *Exp. Agri.* 4: 339-344, 1968.

*Meredith, W. C., Joiner, J. N. and Biggs, R. H. 'Influence of indole-3-acetic acid and kinetin on rooting and indole metabolism of *Feijoa sellowiana*'. *J. Amer. Soc. Hort. Sci.* 95: 49-52, 1970.

Muthoo, A. K. and Chetan, T. 'Effect of different growth regulators and hand thinning of physio-chemical characteristics of peach Cv. Flordasun'. *Ad. Plant Sci.* 10: 61-64, 1997.

Nanda, K. K. 'Investigations on the use of auxin in vegetative reproduction of forest plants'. *Final Report P.L. 480 Project* A7-F, 5-11, 1970.

Nanda, K. K. and Kochhar, V. K. *Vegetative Propagation of Plants.* New Delhi, Ludhiana: Kalyani Publishers, 1985.

Nanda, K. K., Kochhar, V. K. and Gupta, S. 'Seasonal variation in morphactin effects in rooting hypocotyls of *Impatiens balsamina* and its relationship with auxin and nutrition'. *Proceedings of the All India Symposium on Biology of the Land Plants*, Meerut, 1972.

Nanda, K. K., Purohit, A. N. and Bala, A. 'Seasonal rooting response of stem cuttings of some forest tree species to auxins'. *Indian Forester* 154-162, 1968.

Nayar, M. P. and Sastry, A. R. K. *Red Data Book on Indian Plants* Howrah 2: 142, 1988.

Nooden, L. 'Studies on the role of RNA synthesis in auxin induction of cell enlargement'. *Plant Physiol.* 43: 140, 1968.

*Orsi, S. and Tallarico, R. 'Use of plant growth regulators and biostimulants in wheat and barley'. *Informators Agario* 39: 27539-27541, 1983.

Paul, S. C. and Mishra, D. 'Studies on early seedling growth of rice with IAA, GA and CC'. *Science and Culture* 42: 171, 1976.

Phinney, B. O. 'Gibberellin A1, dwarfism and shoot elongation in higher plants'. In: *The Biosynthesis and Metabolism of Plant Hormones.* (Eds.). Crozier, A. and Hillman, J. R. Cambridge, U.K.: Cambridge University Press, pp. 17-41, 1984.

Purohit, S. D., Dave, A. and Tiagi, Y. D. '*Chlorophytum borivilianum* Sant. & Fernand. (Liliaceae), an interesting species from the Aravallis in Rajasthan'. *Rheeded* 4: 113-115, 1994.

Rao, G. G. G., Koruddi, V. R. and Sridhara, H. 'Effect of planofix (NAA) spray on rainfed cotton'. *Cotton Res.* 5: 34-35, 1976.

Sacher, J. A. 'Senescence: Action of auxin and kinetin in control of RNA and protein synthesis in subcellular fractions of bean endocarp'. *Plant Physiol.* 42: 1334, 1967.

Sen, P. K. and Basu, R. N. 'Effect of growth substances on root formation in cuttings of *Justicia gendarussa* L. as influenced by varying levels of nitrogen nutrition of stock plants'. *Indian J. Pl. Physiol.* 3: 72, 1960.

Shah, G. L. 'Rare species with restricted distribution in Gujarat'. In: *An Assessment of Threatened Plants of India.* (Eds.). Jain, S. K. and Rao, R.R. Howrah, pp. 50-54, 1983.

Shah, P. R., Patel, D. B., Patel, D. H. and Dalal, K. C. 'Hormonal effect on germination of guggal cuttings'. *India Drugs*: 435-437, 1983.

Sharma, M. K. Studies on the ecophysiology and reproductive biology of *Boswellia serrata* Roxb. Ph.D. Thesis. University of Rajasthan, Jaipur, 1998.

Sharma, R. Reproductive biology of guggal plant, *Commiphora wightii* (Arnott.) Bhandari and *Commiphora agallocha*. Ph.D. Thesis. University of Rajasthan, Jaipur, 1993.

Sharpe, R. H. 'Softwood cuttings of peach under mist'. *Proc. Amer. Soc., Hort. Sci*: 67: 102-106,1956.

Shetty, B. V. and Singh, V. *Flora of Rajasthan* (3 vols.). Kolkata: Botanical Survey of India, 1993.

Shimoda, C., Masuda, Y. and Yanagishima, N. 'Nucleic acid metabolism involved in auxin-induced elongation of yeast cells'. *Physiol. Plant* 20: 299, 1967.

*Singh, G. Effect of dates of sowing and growth regulators on growth and yield of mung. M.Sc. Thesis. Punjab Agric. University, Ludhiana, 1984.

Singh, G., Sekhon, N. and Kaur, M. 'Effect of growth regulators on some yield contributing parameters in groundnut (*Arachis hypogea*)'. *J. Res. Punjab Agric. Univ.* 15: 106-111, 1978.

Singh, G., Singh, S. and Gurung, S. B. 'Effect of growth regulators on rice productivity'. *Tropical Agric.* 61: 106-108, 1984.

Singh, H. and Dara, B. L. 'Influence of pre-soaking of seeds with gibberellins and auxins on growth and yield attributes of wheat under high salinity sodium adsorption ratio and boron levels'. *Indian J. Agric. Sci.* 41: 998-1003, 1971.

Singh, H. and Gill, H. S. 'Effect of foliar spray of NAA on the growth and yield of late sown wheat and barley'. *Indian J. Ecol.* 12: 267-272, 1985.

Singh, P., Sharma, M. L. and Mukherjee, S. 'Effect of indole butyric acid on sprouting in plant cuttings of *Commiphora wightii* (Arnott) Bhandari'. *Indian Drugs* 26: 575, 1989.

Singh, S. P. 'Note on auxins on root formation in *Ixora rosea* Sims. cuttings during winter under intermittent mist'. *Curr. Agri.* 3: 225-227, 1979.

Sivagami, S., Vijayan, K. P. and Natarajaratnam, N. 'Effect of nutrients and growth regulating chemicals on biochemical aspects and hormonal balance with reference to apical dominance in mango'. *Acta. Horticulture* 231: 476-482, 1988.

*Skoog, F. Substances involved in normal growth and differentiation of plants'. *Brookhaven Symp. Biol.* 6 (BNL 258): 1-21, 1954.

Skoog, F. and Miller, C. O. 'Chemical regulation of growth and organ formation in plant tissues cultured *in vitro*'. *Symp. Soc. Expt. Biol.* 11: 118-131, 1957.

*Sodhi, K. S. Effect of growth regulators, defoliants and nitrogen levels on *Hirsutum* cotton. M.Sc. Thesis. Punjab Agric. University, Ludhiana, 1979.

*Spiegel, P. Auxins inhibitors in canes of *Vitis*'. *Bull. Res. Coun., Israel* 4: 176-183, 1954.

Subbireddy, C. and Shah, C. B. 'Effect of growth regulators in Spanish bunch and Virginia runner groundnut cultivars'. *Indian J. Agron.* 29: 516-521, 1984.

*Tarasenko, M. T. and Vesitev, B. S. 'The rooting of cuttings under artificial mist'. *Vestn. Sel.-Hoz. Nauki.* 11:112-115 (*Hort. Abst.* 37: 2557), 1966

Thakurta, A. G. and Dutt, B. K. 'Vegetative propagation of mango from *gootes* (Marcotte) and cuttings by treatments with high concentration of auxin. *Curr. Sci.* 10: 297, 1941.

Thimann, K. V. 'On an analysis of activity of two growth-promoting substances on plant tissues'.. *Proc. Kon. Acad. Wet.*, Amsterdam 38: 896,1935.

Thimann, K. V. 'On the nature of inhibition caused by auxin'. *American J. Bot.* 24: 407, 1937.

Thimann, K. V. 'Plant growth substances: past, present and future'. *Ann. Rev. Plant Physiol.* 14: 1-18, 1963.

Thimann, K. V. 'The synthetic auxins: relation between structure and activity'. In: *Plant Growth Substances.* (Ed.). Skoog, F. Madison, Wisconsin, U.S.A.: University Wisconsin Press, 1951.

Thimann, K. V. *Hormones in Action in the Whole Life of Plants.* Amherst,, U.S.A.: University Massachusetts Press, 1977.

*Thimann, K. V. Studies on the growth hormone of plants. VI. The distribution of the growth substance in plant tissues'. *J. Gen. Physiol.* 18: 23, 1934.

*Thimann, K. V. and Koepfli, J. B. 'Identity of the growth promoting and root forming substances of plants'. *Nature* 135: 101-102, 1935.

Tomar, I. S. and Ramgiry, S. R. 'Effect of growth regulators on growth and yield of potato (*Solanum tuberosum* L.)'. *Adv. Plant Sci.* 10: 51-54, 1997a.

Tomar, I. S. and Ramgiry, S. R. 'Effect of growth regulators on yield and yield attributes in tomato (*Lycopersicon esculentum* Mill)'. *Adv. Plant Sci.* 10: 29-31, 1997b.

Trewavas, A. 'How do plant growth substances act?' *Plant Cell Environment* 4: 203-228, 1981.

Trewavas, A. 'How do plant growth substances act?' *Plant Cell Environment* 14: 1-12, 1991.

Trivedi, A. P. Ecological observations on *Utricularia stellaria* L.F. with special emphasis on biological productivity, ecological energetics and seed germination. Ph.D. Thesis. University of Rajasthan, Jaipur, 1974.

*Uhrstrom, I. 'The time effect of auxin and calcium on growth and elastic modules in hypocotyls'. *Physiol. Plantarum* 22: 271-287, 1969.

Verma, A. N. and Tandon, P. 'Effect of growth regulators on germination and seedling growth of *Pinus kesiya* Royle ex Gord and *Schima khasiana* Dyer'. *India J. For.* 11: 32-36, 1988.

Verma, H. S. and Singh, P. 'Effect of seed treatments with IAA, IBA and GA on growth and yield of barley'. *Indian J. Agri. Res.* 12: 59-60, 1978.

*Vikhe, S. V., Bengal, D. B. and Patil, V. A. 'Effect of growth regulators and urea on the pod number of pigeon pea cv. 148'. *International Pigeon Pea News Letter* 2: 39-40, 1983.

Went, F. W. 'On a substance causing root formation'. *K. Akad. van Wetensch, te Amsterdam Proc.* 32: 35-39; 1929.

Went, F. W. 'On the growth-accelerating substances in the coleoptile of *Avena sativa*'. *Proc. Kon. Acad. Weten.* Amsterdam 35: 723, 1926.

Went, F. W. 'On the pea test method for auxin, the plant growth hormone'. *Kon. Acad. Weten. Amsterdam, Proc. Sect. Sci.* 37: 547, 1934.

Went, F. W. 'Specific factors other than auxin affecting growth and root formation'. *Plant Physiol.* 13: 55, 1938.

Went, F. W. 'The development of stems and leaves'. In: *Plant Growth Substances.* (Ed.). Skoog, F. Madison, Wisc., U.S.A.: University Wisconsin Press, 1951.

Went, F. W. and Thimann, K. V. *Phytohormones.* New York: The Macmillan Company, 1937.

Yomo, H. and Jinoma, H. 'Production of gibberellin-like substances in the embryo of barley during germination'. *Planta* 71: 113-118, 1996.

*Not seen in original.

—oo(O)oo—

17

Current Advances in Herbal Based Contraceptive Research: A Worldwide Scenario

A. S. Ansari and S. C. Joshi

Population explosion is the major planetary crisis and the World Health Organisation has put great attention on the search for a safe, cheap and socially accepted form of contraception (Waites, 1999). Many indigenous plants were used by Ayurvedic physicians in India from time immemorial for prevention of conception. A number of plant species have been tested for fertility regulation beginning from the last five decades by national and international agencies (van de Walle, 1997; Sharma, 2001; Cocks and Moller, 2002). They exert their effects equally on both female and male reproductive systems. On females, the plants have been evaluated for spermicidal, anti-implantational or post-coital and abortifacient activities, while in males their effects are seen as an anti-spermatogenic, post-testicular effects on sperm motility and viability and anti-gonadotropic properties (Kamboj and Dhawan, 1989; Lohiya and Ansari, 1999). In the present chapter, recent trends on the plant-based contraceptive research is reviewed with the hope that further research will take place to solve the population explosion problem.

Alangium salviifolium

Alangium salviifolium (Linn. F) Wang (Family: Alangiaceae) is a medicinal plant used in India, China and the Philippines (Kirtikar and Basu, 1987). It possesses many medicinal properties like acrid, astringent, emollient, anthelmintic, diuretic and purgative properties and is used in rheumatism, leprosy, inflammation and dog bite. Root bark is an antidote for several poisons. Fruit are used as a poultice for treating burning sensation and haemorrhage. The leaves are used for treatment of rheumatism (Warrier and Nambiar, 1964).

Daily administration of petroleum ether, ethyl acetate, chloroform, methanol and aqueous extracts at the dose of 100 mg/kg of *Alangium salviifolium* stem bark in female rats for eight days starting from the first day of pregnancy showed significant abortifacient activity. In addition to this observation, petroleum ether and ethyl acetate extracts also exhibited anti-implantation property. The treatment also led to resorption of fertilised ovum. A comparison of different extracts used in the present study was also made. Chloroform extract was found to be least effective followed by petroleum ether extract. Methanol extract showed total resorption sites in two animals. Aqueous and ethyl acetate extracts have also exhibited good activity. It has been concluded from these studies that *Alangium salviifolium* exhibited mainly abortifacient activity and less anti-implantation activity (Murugan *et al*, 2000).

Andrographis paniculata

Andrographis paniculata (Acanthaceae), commonly known as 'King of Bitters' (kalmegh in Hindi) is an annual herb, common in hedgerows throughout the plains of India, cultivated in gardens from Lucknow to Assam, specially in Bengal. Common medicinal properties of this plant are as follows. The roots and leaves of this plant are said to be stomachic, tonic, antipyretic, alterative, anthelmintic, febrifuge and cholagogue (Nadkarni and Nadkarni, 1954).

Burgos and associates (1997) found no subchronic testicular tôxicity of standardised dried extract of *Andrographis paniculata* in male Sprague Dawley rats when treated at 20, 200 and 1,000 mg/kg for 60 days. No alteration in the reproductive organ weight, testicular histology, ultrastructural analysis of Leydig cells and testosterone levels was observed after 60 days of treatment, whereas *Andrographis paniculata* leaves, when fed to male albino rats, causes the arrest of spermatogenesis. The active compound isolated was andrographolide found to be one of the major constituents of this plant. The compound was administered to three-month-old male Wistar albino rats at two dose levels for 48 days. The results showed that sperm count decreased, the spermatozoa were not motile, and several of them possessed abnormalities. The seminiferous epithelium was-thoroughly disrupted and in the seminiferous tubules, fully differentiated spermatozoa were far too limited; cells in the divisional stages were prevalent; multinucleate giant cells were abundant and Leydig cells appeared intact. It is inferred that andrographolide could affect spermatogenesis by preventing cytokinesis of the dividing spermatogenic cell lines. The multinucleate giant cells are comparable to the.symplasts generated by cytochalasin-D and ursolic acid due to action at stages V-VII of the spermatogenic cycle. Sertoli cell damage and spermatotoxic effects are also apparent. Thus, the study points to a male reproductive toxic effect of this compound when used as a therapeutic; the study also confirms the possible prospective use of andrographolide in male contraception (Akbarsha and Murugaian, 2000).

Azadirachta indica

The neem tree (*Azadirachta indica* Juss.) originated in the Indian subcontinent, where its medical and insecticidal properties are well known (Schmutterer, 1981; Anonymous, 1982). Kaushic and Upadhyay (1995) examined the mode of anti-fertility action of intrauterine neem treatment (IUNT) on ovarian functions and uterine responsiveness to ovarian hormones in adult Wistar rats. The treated animals had normal reproductive cycles. Unilateral IUNT followed by mating resulted in degeneration of embryos on the treated side as noted between days 3-5 post coitum. The study shows that the mode of anti-fertility action of IUNT is not because of uterine unresponsiveness to the ovarian hormones but is due to impairment of embryo development.

Praneem (a purified extract of neem, *Azadirachta indica*) at a dose of 0.6 ml was given orally from day 8 to 10 of pregnancy caused complete resorption of embryos in female Wistar rats.

Cytokines of Th1 type, that is, gamma interferon and TNF, were raised on administration of Praneem, which may be the probable cause of pregnancy termination (Mukherjee and Talwar, 1996). For the purpose of using neem as a long-term contraceptive, an activity guided fractionation and biologically active fraction from neem seeds was carried out. Sequentially extracted fractions of neem seeds were tested orally at an early post implantation stage in rats. The hexane extract of the neem seeds was found to be biologically active and was the precursor for the final active fraction. The active fraction, identified as a mixture of six components, could completely abrogate pregnancy in rodents up to a concentration of 10 per cent. No apparent toxic effects could be seen following treatment with the fraction. The treatment with the active fraction caused a specific activation of T lymphocyte cells of CD8+ subtype as well as phagocytic cells followed by elevation in cytokines gamma-interferon and TNF. Mukherjee *et al* (1999) concluded from this study that a pure active fraction of neem seeds may be used for early post implantation contraception.

Calotropis procera

Calotropis procera or madar belongs to the family Asclepiadaceae and is found in north, western and central India from Sind, and in Punjab, Bengal, Bihar and Maharashtra, and in drier climate of the Deccan. The alcoholic extracts of root and leaves of this plant were found to have anti-cancer activity against human epidermal carcinoma of the nasopharynx in tissue culture (Dhar *et al*, 1968; Bhakuni *et al*, 1969).

Effects of ethanol and aqueous extracts of *Calotropis procera* (Ait.) R.Br. root have been studied on oestrous cycle and on some parameters of oestrogenic functionality in rats. Both extracts have been shown to interrupt the normal oestrous cycle in 60 and 80 per cent, respectively, of rats treated. The rats exhibited prolonged dioestrous stage of the oestrous cycle with consequent temporary inhibition of ovulation (Circosta *et al*, 2001). Recently, Kamath and Rana (2002) studied the effect of ethanolic extract of the roots of *Calotropis procera* in albino rats to explore its anti-fertility and hormonal activities. A strong anti-implantation (inhibition 100 per cent) and uterotropic activity was observed at the dose level of 250 mg/kg (1/4 of LD_{50})). No anti-estrogenic activity could be detected.

Carica papaya

The papaya (*Carica papaya* L., Family: Caricaceae) is a large herbaceous plant cultivated throughout the tropical world and in the warmest parts of the subtropics. The genus includes about 40 species, of which *Carica papaya* is the most important and widely cultivated in India. Papain extracted from pulp of papaya fruit is reported to possess embryotoxic activity (Satyavati *et al*, 1987). Oral administration of aqueous suspension of ripe papaya seed powder (20 mg/animal/day) for eight weeks produced sterility in 40 per cent of male rats without affecting genital organs (Das, 1980).

After publication of the findings of Das (1980), several experiments were conducted by Chinoy and associates (Chinoy and Geetha Ranga, 1984; Chinoy and George, 1983; Chinoy *et al*, 1985, 1994; Verma and Chinoy, 2002) using aqueous extracts. Marked inhibition of fertility in male rodents was observed following either oral or intramuscular administration of crude aqueous extract at varying dose regimens ranging between 0.5 and 20 mg/kg/day and concluded that it caused functional sterility in treated animals (Chinoy and Geetha Ranga, 1984; Chinoy and George,

1983; Chinoy *et al*, 1985, 1994). Vyas and Jacob (1984) have also reported sterile mating in rabbits when normal females were mated with males treated with (100 and 200 mg/animal/day; oral for 10 and 20 days) aqueous suspensions of papaya seed powder.

Udoh and Kehinde (1999) also conducted preliminary studies on the anti-fertility effect of *Carica papaya* seeds on the gonads of male albino (Wistar) rats. Crude ripe papaya seeds at 50 and 100 mg/kg body weight dose regimens were administered orally for eight weeks. Histological observations at both doses showed dose dependent degenerative changes of the germinal epithelium and germ cells, a reduction in the number of Leydig cells and the presence of vacuoles in the tubules. At a high dose, many empty tubules containing degenerated spermatozoa and cell debris in the lumen was observed in epididymis. The epididymidal epithelium appeared normal. At a low dose, a milder effect was observed. The epithelial tissue appeared to be normal.

Lohiya and co-workers conducted several experiments with various extracts, their chromatographic fractions and isolated compounds from the sub-fractions in rats, rabbits and langur monkeys. For instance, administration of crude ethanolic (Lohiya *et al*, 1992), aqueous (Lohiya *et al*, 1994a) (10 and 50 mg/animal/day for 30, 60 and 90 days) and chloroform (5 mg/animal/day) extracts (Lohiya and Goyal, 1992), chromatographic fractions of crude chloroform extract, that is, chloroform, ethyl acetate and methanol fractions (Lohiya *et al*, 1994b) at 2 and 5 mg/animal/day dose regimens curtailed fertility of male rats to a varying degree. Prime effects were observed on cauda epididymal sperm motility associated with morphological defects and reduced sperm count. Chloroform extract also showed severe oligozoospermia following 90 days and uniform azoospermia following 120 days of treatment in male rabbits (Lohiya *et al*, 1999a). Total sperm motility inhibitory activity within 60 days in rats and uniform azoospermia within 15 days in rabbits was achieved with benzene chromatographic fraction (Lohiya *et al*, 1999b; Pathak *et al*, 2000). Similar results were obtained with sub-fractions and isolated compounds in both rats and rabbits and with aqueous extract in rabbits (Lohiya *et al*, 2000a). No toxicity sign was evident up to 180 days of study period. The treatment was completely reversible following withdrawal of treatment. Uniform reversible azoospermia after 90 days of treatment and total sperm motility inhibitory activity after 60-90 days of treatment with chloroform extract (50 mg/kg/day, oral for 360 days) with no toxicity was noticed in langur monkeys (Lohiya *et al*, 2002).

Lohiya and associates (2000b) also examined anti-spermatogenic/sperm immobilisation properties of the seed extracts of *Carica papaya* with the aim that it could cause human sperm immobilisation *in vitro*. In this study, chloroform extract, benzene chromatographic fraction of the chloroform extract, its methanol and ethyl acetate sub-fractions and the isolated compounds from the sub-fractions of the seeds of *Carica papaya* were used at concentrations ranging from 0.1 to 2 per cent. A dose-dependent spermicidal effect showing an instant fall in the sperm motility to less than 20 per cent at 2 per cent concentration was observed. Isolated compounds ECP 1 and ECP 2 were more effective inducing a motility of less than 10 per cent. Many of the spermatozoa became vibratory on the spot. Total inhibition of motility was observed within 20-25 minutes at all concentrations of all products. Scanning and transmission electron microscopy showed deleterious changes in the plasma membrane of the head and mid-piece of spermatozoa.

Carica papaya seeds have not only been evaluated for inhibition of male fertility, but study has also been carried out for abortifacient properties. Oderinde *et al,* (2002) conducted an experiment to investigate the abortifacient potential of aqueous extract of *Carica papaya* (Linn.) seeds in female

Sprague-Dawley rats. Daily oral doses of 100 and 800 mg/kg body weight were administered from day 1-10 post-coitum. No significant differences in total body weight were found in foetuses exposed to these regimes. However, in the group treated with 100 mg/kg body weight, there was a significant increase ($p < 0.05$) in the implantation sites and foetal weight was significantly decreased ($p < 0.05$) compared to the controls. No dead or malformed foetuses were found. However, in the group treated with 800 mg/kg body weight, there was obvious vaginal bleeding but no treatment-related increase in implantation sites compared with control. There was however, complete resorption of about 30 per cent of the foetuses was noticed. The surviving foetuses were stunted when compared with the control but were without any external malformations.

Cimicifuga racemosa

The rhizome of black cohosh (*Cimicifuga racemosa*) is used widely for the treatment of menopausal complaints. Zierau *et al* (2002) evaluated this plant for estrogenic and anti-estrogenic effects of ethanolic and iso-propanolic extracts on proliferation of MCF-7 cells and on gene expression. Estrogenic properties of plant extracts could neither be detected in proliferation assays, nor on gene expression using an estradiol-inducible yeast assay or the oestrogen-inducible MVLN cells. In contrast, in all three experimental systems *Cimicifuga racemosa* antagonised estradiol-induced activities. Estradiol-induced stimulation of proliferation was inhibited by a dosage of >1 microg/ml of extract concentration, gene expression was suppressed by doses of 100-1,000 microg/ml of *Cimicifuga racemosa* extracts. From these results, the authors concluded that extracts from the rhizome of *Cimicifuga racemosa* contain compounds with anti-estrogenic properties (Zierau *et al*, 2002).

Ferula hormonis

Khleifat *et al* (2001) investigated the effects of an aqueous extract of *Ferula hormonis* on social aggression, fertility and some physiological and biochemical parameters in male mice. Daily ingestion of 3 mg/kg b. wt. of aqueous extract of *Ferula hormonis* for six weeks inhibited social aggression and reduction of body wet weight and other accessory reproductive organs. The ingestion of this extract by male mice resulted in a significant reduction of their fertility. This treatment caused a significant decrease in the number of pregnant females, number of implantations and viable foetuses in females impregnated by males that ingested this extract. The numbers of epididymal sperm and their motility were dramatically reduced. Concomitant increases in sperm abnormalities were also observed. The authors concluded that *Ferula hormonis* exposure during pre-puberty period puts the exposed animals at significant risk for reduced reproductive capacity in adulthood.

The anti-fertility, anti-implantation and ovarian histological alterations of the ethanolic extract of *Ferula hormonis* have been investigated in female mice (Homady *et al*, 2002). The intragastric application of 3 mg/kg per day of such extract for six weeks resulted in a significant reduction in female mice fertility. Furthermore, it caused a decrease in the number of mated females, the total number of implantations and the number of viable foetuses. These changes were also associated with ovarian atrophy and a concomitant increase in the connective tissue. The ova showed degeneration while most of the ovarian follicles suffered follicular atresia.

Globularia Species

Two species of *Globularia* (Family: Globulariaceae) namely, *Globularia alypum* and *Zygophyllum gaetulum* possess hypoglycaemic activity (Skim et al, 1999). Methanol and dichloromethane extracts (1, 10 and 100 microg/ml) obtained from the leaves and stems of *Globularia alypum* L *in vitro* produced a dose dependent abolition of the contractile effects of histamine and serotonin in the guinea-pig ileum and rat uterus, respectively (Bello *et al*, 2002).

The effect of the ethanolic extracts of *Globularia arabica* and *Globularia alypum* dried leaves was monitored on fertility. The intragastric ingestion by female Sprague-Dawley rats at 800 mg/kg dose of ethanolic extracts of *Globularia arabica* and *Globularia alypum*, from day one to day six of pregnancy, did not cause pregnancy failure. However, the ingestion of ethanolic extracts of *Globularia alypum* significantly reduced the number of viable foetuses. The number of resorptions was significantly increased in pregnant females administered ethanolic extracts of both *Globularia* arabica and *Globularia alypum*. The ingestion of 800 mg/kg of ethnologic extracts of both plants for 30 consecutive days by adult female rats had no significant effect on the occurrence of pregnancy. However, the ingestion of extracts of both species increased the number of resorptions and only *Globularia alypum* extract caused a significant reduction in the number of viable foetuses. These results indicate that ingestion of *Globularia arabica* and *Globularia alypum* could have some reproductive toxicity in female rats (Elbetieha *et al*, 2000).

***Gossypium* Species**

The seed, stem and root of three species of *Gossypium* (Family: Malvaceae; cotton plant), that is, *Gossypium herbaceum, Gossypium hirsutum* and *Gossypium arboreum* generally contain gossypol which is a yellow pigment, insoluble in water, soluble in 5 per cent NaOH (pH 7.4) or alcohol. It is reported to possess anti-spermatogenic effect in a number of animal species like rat, mice, hamster, dog, monkey and in human beings (Chang *et al*, 1978; Lohiya *et al*, 1990). Gossypol acetic acid is the most potent derivative of gossypol (Wang *et al*, 1979; Sonenberg *et al*, 1988). Gossypol exerts its contraceptive effect during spermatogenesis including the post-testicular development and maturation of spermatozoa in the epididymis. Desquamation of the germinal epithelium occurred in the form of the multinucleated giant cells derived from spermatids (Hoffer, 1985; Sonenberg *et al*, 1988). The onset of gossypol induced infertility seems to be dose and duration dependent. Distinct species specificity in its effects was evident; the rabbit was extremely resistant with no effects on fertility following the administration of 10 mg/kg/day for 14 weeks (Chang, 1978). Administration of gossypol in rhesus monkeys at 4 mg and 20 mg dose regimens for a period of three months did not induce any change in sperm count (Bardin *et al*, 1981). Progressive motility, however, was significantly reduced along with morphological alterations in the spermatozoa.

Clinical trials have been carried out at a number of centres in the People's Republic of China. The first trial was reported by Qian *et al* (1972) using the higher doses ranged from 60 to 70 mg/day for a period of five to six weeks. Reversible anti-fertility effects along with no serious side effects were observed. After the conduction of this study, several experiments were carried out with low dose level. For instance, in a study, Liu and co-workers (1981) gave 20 mg/day gossypol orally for 60-75 days during loading phase and 50 mg/week during maintenance phase. The contraceptive efficacy estimated was 99.07 per cent. Brazilian volunteers were also treated with 20 mg gossypol acetic acid/day for four months which was followed by 60 mg/week during maintenance phase. A significant reduction in sperm motility, increase in number of immature cells in ejaculate and severe oligospermia/azoospermia developed in all subjects at the end of the loading phase (Coutinho and Melo, 1988). Xu *et al* (1988) studied long-term administration of gossypol in Chinese subjects for 6 to 12 years. The dose of loading phase was 20 mg/day and 40 mg/week during maintenance phase. When 15 subjects stopped drug intake for 6-12 months, 12 subjects exhibited sperm count more than 4×10^6/ml, whereas three taking the drug for 7-8 years did not recover.

Fatigue (12.6 per cent); gastro-intestinal symptoms (7.4 per cent), decreased libido and potency (5.0 per cent), dizziness (3.8 per cent) and dryness of mouth (3.1 per cent) were main untoward side effects noticed during these studies (Bajaj and Madan, 1983). Some individuals also suffered from somnolence, palpitation, puffiness of eyelids, decreased sweating, skin rash and changes in the ECG and SGPT. Though it was not confirmed that these side effects were due to gossypol treatment and most of the side effects were observed during loading phase of the study. These effects were transient and disappeared during the recovery phase. The circulatory levels of testosterone and LH remained unaltered by gossypol administration (Xue, 1981; Coutinho and Melo, 1988; Yu and Chan, 1998). While, in some subjects, FSH levels were increased (Gu and Wang, 1984; Zhang *et al*, 1989). The most serious side effect of gossypol administration was hypokalemia. It was reported in 66 cases out of 8,806 treated men (Qian *et al*, 1980; Liu and Lyle, 1987; Waites *et al*, 1998) that hypokalemia caused due to potassium deficiency in the body led to muscular paralysis and other physiological complications.

To overcome the hypokalemic symptoms, supplementation of potassium salt was advised by some scientists (Qian *et al*, 1980), while others did not agree with this view (Liu *et al*, 1988). Toxicological screening has shown that rats, guinea pigs and hamsters are unsuitable as models for studies on hypokalemic paralysis (Qian, 1981). Therefore, expressing serious concern about hypokalemia and other related side effects, the World Health Organisation (WHO, 1984) advised scientists to defer clinical trials and carry out toxicological investigations in suitable animal model with the possibility of extrapolation of findings in the human situation.

Studies have been planned in langur monkeys to overcome the drawbacks of gossypol by Lohiya and associates (1990). In a study, highly purified gossypol acetic acid was orally administered at 5, 7.5 and 10 mg/animal/day alone and also in combination with potassium chloride at 0.25, 0.50 and 0.75 mg/animal/day/dose regimens, respectively. The treatment caused a dose and duration dependent suppression in sperm motility along with increased abnormality and gradual decrease in the sperm count leading to oligo, severe oligo/azoospermia at the end of medication, respectively. Serum potassium concentration decreased significantly in gossypol alone groups, while values were comparable to pre-treatment in combination groups except at 5 mg/day dose regimen where serum potassium levels were below normal. Serum GOT and GPT values were elevated significantly in both the groups. No other untoward side effects were observed. All the gossypol induced effects returned to normalcy. Experiments with langur monkey suggested that the gossypol induced hypokalemic could be counteracted with supplementation of potassium salt (Kumar *et al*, 1997; Sharma *et al*, 1999).

A multicentre, international and dose finding study has been carried out to remove the controversies existing with gossypol with the aim to evaluate gossypol as a contraceptive pill for men at doses lower than those previously prescribed and in men from various ethnic origin. A total of 151 men from Brazil, Nigeria, Kenya and China were divided into two groups. Both groups received 15 mg gossypol/day for 12 or 16 weeks to reach spermatogenesis suppression. Subjects were then randomised to either 7.5 or 10 mg/day for 40 weeks. In addition, 51 men were enrolled as a control group. In all, 81 subjects attained spermatogenesis suppression. Only one man discontinued treatment because of tiredness. Potassium levels fluctuated within the normal range. FSH increased consistently. Testicular volume decreased, but after discontinuation, values returned to levels not statistically different from admission. Of 19 subjects in the 7.5 mg/day dose group, 12 recovered sperm counts higher than 20 million/ml within 12 months of discontinuing gossypol. In the 10 mg/day group, sperm counts recovered in only 10 of 24 subjects. 8 of the 43 patients remained azoospermic one year after stopping gossypol. All men diagnosed with varicocele failed to reverse spermatogenesis suppression. Gossypol blood levels indicated that sperm suppression occurs independently of concentration, whereas spermatogenesis recovery appears to be concentration-dependent. When taken for one year, gossypol causes no reduction in sexual desire or frequency of intercourse. The reported hypokalemia of early studies has not confirmed in the latest trials (Coutinho *et al*, 2000). The only concern at present appears to be lack of reversibility in over 20 per cent of subjects. Gossypol should be prescribed preferably to men who have completed their families or for those who would accept permanent infertility after a few years of use (Coutinho, 2002).

Hibiscus rosa-sinensis

Hibiscus rosa-sinensis (Linn.) (Family: Malvaceae; gudhal in Hindi) is an evergreen glabrous shrub 1.5-2.4 metres high. It is cultivated as an ornamental plant throughout India and Myanmar. Its leaves are considered emollient, aperient, anodyne and laxative. Mixed with the juice of *Vernomia cineria*, it is used to stimulate expulsion of remnant after child birth. Roots are demulcent and used for cough. The flowers are attributed to possess contraceptive properties in Ayurvedic literature, Materia Medica and folklore (Satyavati *et al*, 1987).

Hibiscus rosa-sinensis has been investigated extensively for its anti-fertility effect. Different parts of the plant have been screened for their effect on the reproductive system. For instance, the benzene extract of flowers of this plant at the dose of 100 mg/kg revealed post-coital anti-fertility effect in female albino rats, leading to 80 per cent reduction in the implantation site on the tenth day of pregnancy. The foetal loss in the rats was within the normal range, indicating the absence of any early abortifacient. The petroleum ether extract was devoid of anti-fertility effect, whereas the solvent ether and ethanolic extracts of the flowers did not show any significant activity. However, in the rats treated with ethanolic extract of the flower petals, a change in the sex ratio of the pups born was observed. There was a higher incidence of male:female pups born in the extract-treated rats (Batta and Santhakumari, 1971).

The leaves, flowers, bark, stem and roots of *Hibiscus rosa-sinensis* in the form of their aqueous, alcoholic (90 per cent) and petroleum ether extracts were also assessed, but only the alcoholic extracts of flowers and roots showed some resorptive activity (Prakash and Mathur, 1976). The administration of benzene extract of flowers at a dose of 250 mg/kg from day one to 10 of pregnancy in rats was found to be most active for prevention of pregnancy when compared with the petroleum ether and aqueous extract. However, the alcoholic extract exhibited 50-70 per cent activity in female rats in a dose 250 mg/kg (Kholkute and Udupa, 1974; Kholkute *et al*, 1976a).

The total benzene extract of *Hibiscus rosa-sinensis* showed anti-estrogenic activity in bilaterally ovariectomised immature albino rats (Kholkute and Udupa, 1976a). The extract led to a reversible disruption of the oestrus cycle of rats which largely depend on the dose and duration of treatment (Kholkute *et al*, 1976b). The mechanism of action of its anti-fertility activity is mediated via inhibition of implantation and absorption of foetuses (Kholkute and Udupa, 1976b, 1978).

Prakash (1979a) studied the effect of the 50 per cent ethanolic and benzene extracts of *Hibiscus rosa-sinensis* flowers on the acid and alkaline phosphatase activity rate on uterus. A dose-related and remarkable increase in the acid phosphatase and decrease in alkaline phosphatase was noticed. Both extracts were found with an anti-estrogenic property (Prakash, 1979, 1979b, 1979c) which was further confirmed in another experiment on guinea pigs (Prakash, 1980).

To find the active principle responsible for anti-fertility activity, quercetin, cyaniding and hentriacontane were isolated from the benzene extract of the flowers of *Hibiscus rosa-sinensis*. However, none had shown any anti-fertility potential. Moreover, the mother liquor prevented pregnancies in 60 per cent of treated rats (Kholkute *et al*, 1976c).

The benzene extract of *Hibiscus rosa-sinensis* flowers was also assessed for its contraceptive effects in male rats (Kholkute *et al*, 1972; Kholkute and Udupa, 1974; Kholkute, 1977). Oral administration of the benzene extract at the dose of 250 mg/kg for a period of 30, 45 and 60 days led to a duration dependent varying damage in germinal epithelium. There was a significant reduction in the weight of the reproductive organs and pituitary gland after 60 days of treatment. The concentrations of alkaline phosphatase in the ventral prostate, citric acid in seminal vesicle and fructose in dorsolateral prostate were declined. Histological observation of the testes revealed marked degenerative changes in various seminiferous tubule elements along with disappearance of spermatocytes. Leydig cells appeared atrophic. Loss of secretory activity was observed in accessory reproductive organs and pituitary showed degranulation of gonadotrophs. All altered parameters restored to normalcy within 30 days of treatment. Bioassay in immature castrated rats revealed the absence of androgenic or anti-androgenic property in the extract suggesting that the anti-spermatogenic effect was possibly mediated via the pituitary (Kholkute and Udupa, 1974; Kholkute, 1977).

The flower extract of *Hibiscus rosa-sinensis* has also been reported for its anti-spermatogenic property in bat (*Rhinopoma kinneari* Wroughton). Spermatogenically active testes showed cytotoxic and cytostatic effects. Marked depletion was observed in germ cells and spermatozoa (Singhwi and Lall, 1980). An attempt to study the effect of the flower extract histochemically on the testicular lactate dehydrogenase on bat did not produce any conclusive results mainly due to considerable variation in the results in the treated and normal animals (Singhwi and Lall, 1981). Extracts of the flower of *Hibiscus rosa-sinensis* administration to albino male mice resulted in the decrease of spermatogenic elements of testis and epididymal sperm count. The drug also showed androgenic action in immature mice (Reddy *et al*, 1997).

Though this plant possesses anti-fertility activity in both male and female animals, it is receiving attention as a potential post-coital anti-fertility agent. Several investigations have been undertaken with the benzene extract of flowers of *Hibiscus rosa-sinensis* for anti-fertility activity in female albino rats (Singh *et al*, 1982), as a potential source of contragestative agent (Kabir *et al*, 1984; Pal *et al*, 1985; Pakrashi *et al*, 1986), electrolyte concentration in uterine flushing during various stages of reproduction (Prakash *et al*, 1990) and effects of oestrus cycle and ovarian activity (Murthy *et al*, 1997). A preliminary clinical trial with benzene and water insoluble portion of the benzene extract of red petals of *Hibiscus rosa-sinensis* when administered orally at 750 mg/day from day 7-22 day of menstrual cycle in women showed cent per cent pregnancy intercepting effects.

Piper betle

Piper betle (Family: Piperaceae) commonly known as paan or tambuli is a twining plant cultivated all over India except the dry north-western parts. The leaves and roots of *Piper betle* were reported to be of any anti-fertility action in rats and mice (Bhaduri *et al*, 1968). Khosa and Singh (1972), however, investigated a mild anti-fertility effect in rats, with regard to an amorphous compound obtained from benzene extract of roots.

Sarkar and associates (2000) conducted a set of experiments with two different doses in Swiss male albino mice using alcoholic extract of the leaf-stalk of *Piper betle* Linn. for anti-fertility activity. Initially, 500 mg of the leaf-stalk extract for 30 days and then 1,000 mg for the next 30 days/animal/day/kg body weight were administered orally. The extract reduced fertility to zero per cent within 60 days. A significant suppression of cauda epididymal sperm count and motility was observed. Biochemical parameters did not show any marked alterations in testosterone content in serum nor 17β-hydroxysteriod dehydrogenase (17β-HSD) activity in testes although fructose content in seminal vesicles was reduced as are the weights of reproductive organs. A non-appreciable increment on cholesterol content in testes was observed. Absolute recovery of the altered parameters was noticed. It was concluded that the contraceptive effect of the extract of leaf-stalk of *Piper betle* Linn. is mainly on the maturation process of spermatozoa in epididymides without influencing hystemic hormonal profiles.

Striga orobanchoides

Four successive solvent extracts of the whole plant *Striga orobanchoides* have been screened for anti-fertility activity in albino rats. Of these, the ethanolic extract was found to be most effective in causing significant anti-implantation activity. The anti-fertility activity was reversible on withdrawal of treatment with the extract. It was concluded that the ethanolic extract at 200 mg/kg showed estrogenic activity (Hiremath *et al*, 1994).

The two flavones, apigenin and luteolin, isolated from *Striga orobanchoides*, were investigated for endocrine and contraceptive properties. Doses ranging from 5 to 25 mg/kg body weight/day of these compounds when administered from day one to day four of pregnancy showed dose-dependent and significant anti-implantation activity. The mean effective dose for both compounds was found to be 25 mg/kg body weight. Oral administration of these compounds caused a significant increase in uterine weight, uterine diameter, thickness of the endometrium and epithelial cell height in immature ovariectomised rats. The uterotrophic potency was less than that of ethinyl estradiol. Simultaneous administration of these compounds with ethinyl estradiol caused a significant increase in uterine weight, uterine diameter, thickening of the endometrium and height of endometrial epithelium. The extent of these changes was also less than that in only ethinyl estradiol-treated rats. The compounds exhibited estrogenic properties at their contraceptive dose level when given alone. However, in combination with ethinyl estradiol, both compounds exhibited slight anti-estrogenic activity (Hiremath *et al*, 2000).

Tripterygium wilfordii

Tripterygium wilfordii Hoof f., a perennial twining vine belonging to the family Celastraceae, is cultivated and grown widely in Southern China and usually found growing densely on the shaded hill slopes. The herb, commonly called Lei Gong Teng (Thunder God Vine) or Mang Cao (rank grass) in China, has been used as a medicinal herb in Chinese traditional medicine in the treatment of rheumatoid arthritis, chronic nephritis, tuberculosis and other pulmonary diseases without serious side effects. Long-term medication of this plant leads to a decrease in testicular weight or menstrual disturbance in some patients (Anonymous, 1978). In the late 1970s, the active constituents, that is, the multiglycosides of *Tripterygium wilfordii* (GTW) were extracted from the root xylem (Qian, 1987).

Many preliminary experiments were conducted in mice, rats and human beings. In a study, when both male and female hybrid rats were fed simultaneously, a laboratory chow containing GTW for 4.5 months, the body weight growth, birth rate and litter size were decreased (Zheng *et al,* 1983). The feeding of GTW with laboratory diet to Wistar rats at the dose level of 30 mg/kg body wt./day for 35 or 80 days leads to marked seminiferous tubule damages together with a decrease in the serum testosterone level in the 80-day group (Zheng *et al*, 1985). Qian *et al* (1988, 1995) carried out further studies on the effect of GTW on fertility. In an experiment with Wistar rats, GTW was given through gastric gavage at a dose of 10 mg/kg/day, 6 times a week, the fertility of the rats began to decrease by the end of four weeks of medication and at the end of the eighth week all animals were infertile with a significant decrease in the density and vitality of cauda epididymal sperms. The fertility recovered following four weeks of the withdrawal of the treatment. Chan and Ng (1995) demonstrated adverse effect of extracts of the plant on cultured mice embryo development.

In the clinical practice with the crude extract of the plant for the treatment of various diseases, clinicians have observed the fact that a decrease in the testicular volume may take place in a few patients after a long-term treatment with the drug. Yu (1983) reported that in rheumatoid arthritis patients, taking only the crude extract or the crude extract plus GTW for a period of 2-56 months, necrospermia or azoospermia occurred. Only in the case taking the crude extract plus GTW for 56 months, the testicular size decreased significantly. Libido and potency were normal in all the cases. In patients taking only the crude extract, seminological indices were found to be essentially within the normal range after three months of cessation of treatment. Qian *et al* (1995) also carried out a comparative retrospective study on the seminal indices and the blood hormonal profiles in rheumatoid arthritis patients with or without GTW therapy. Treatment group was administered 20-30 mg GTW/day for 1.5-5 months. The sperm density of the ejaculated spermatozoa was far lower in the treated that in the control group. Sperm motility of the treated subjects was zero, indicating that they were infertile at the time of semen analysis. No significant side effects were seen, the libido and potency and the serum levels of testosterone and LH were normal. The serum FSH levels, however, were significantly high in the treated group. All the parameters restored to normalcy within 2 to 4 months after cessation of drug intake.

The WHO Task Force initiated the Bioassay directed compound isolation studies (WHO, 1995). To date, a series of six male anti-fertility diterpene epoxide have been isolated. Their chemical structures have been identified and found to be triptolide, tripdiolide, triptolideno, tripchlorolide, 16-hydroxytriptolide and T7/19. At the ED95 dosage levels, all compounds act mainly on metamorphosing spermatids, testicular and epididymal spermatozoa with exfoliation and inhibition of basic nuclear protein turnover of late spermatids, delayed spermiation, sperm head-tail separation and microtubule, microfilaments and membrane damages. Preliminary toxic evaluation suggested that all compounds are immunosuppressive at dose level 5-12 times their anti-fertility doses (Qian *et al,* 1995).

OTHER PLANTS

Acalypha indica L. (Family: Euphorbiaceae) extracts were tested for post-coital anti-fertility activity in female albino rats. The petroleum ether and ethanol extracts were found to be most effective in causing significant anti-implantation activity. The anti-fertility activity was reversible on withdrawal of the treatment of the extracts. Both the extracts at 600 mg/kg body weight showed estrogenic activity. Histological studies of the uterus confirmed estrogenic activity (Hiremath *et al*, 1999).

The effect of an ethanolic extract (200 mg/kg/day, intraperitoneally, for 20 days) and a hydroalcoholic extract (300 mg/kg/day, orally for 30 days) of *Achillea millefolium* L.(yarrow) flowers caused exfoliation of immature germ cells, germ cell necrosis, and seminiferous tubule vacuolisation in Swiss male mice (Montanri *et al*, 1998b).

Different doses of aqueous extracts from the leaves of *Aloe buettneri, Justicia insularis, Hibiscus macranthus* and *Dicliptera verticillata*, locally used to regulate the menstrual cycle and to treat dysmenorrhea or infertility in women, were given daily to 22 day old rats for 5, 10, 15, 20 and 25 days by gastric intubation. The results showed a decrease in growth rate of animals treated with 94 mg/kg per day at the end of the experimental period. The ovarian and uterine weights were high in all treated groups especially within the pubertal period (36-41 days old) when compared to the respective controls. Ovarian and uterine protein levels, as well as serum oestradiol level was significantly high in the groups given 49 or 94 mg/kg per day of the plant extracts (52 and 42 per cent, respectively). A concomitant decrease in ovarian cholesterol was observed in the same treated groups (Telefo *et al*, 1998).

The methanolic extract of *Asparagus pubescens* Bak root dose-dependently (0.5-1.5 g/kg) protected the animals from conception for 4-14 gestational periods in rabbits, rats and mice (Nwafor *et al,* 1998).

The effects of a hexanic extract of *Austroplenckia populnea* leaves were studied at a range of doses during 7 and 14 days male rats. At the dose of 1 g/kg/day caused reduction in cauda epididymal sperm number (Mazaro *et al*, 2000).

Bursera species are commonly used in religious services due to their sweet smell after burning the whole plant, known as 'copal' in many Central American countries. Serrano and Garcia-Suarez (2001) evaluated the sperm agglutinating activity of two species on human and boar sperm. Aqueous extracts from stem and leaves were prepared. Capacitated sperm samples were used in all cases. Different agglutinating capacities were observed. The most frequent sperm agglutination response was that involving the heads. Agglutinating activity was higher from stem than leaf extracts.

Cassia fistula (Family; Leguminosae) commonly known as sonhali or amultas is a common plant throughout India and Myanmar. Pulp, root-bark, seeds and leaves have purgative properties and are also used as tonic and febrifuge. Fruit is also cathartic (Nadkarni and Nadkarni, 1954; Iyengar *et al*, 1966; Satyavati *et al,* 1976). Aqueous extract of seeds of *Cassia fistula* administration to mated female rats from day 1-5 of pregnancy at the doses of 100 and 200 mg/kg body weight (oral) resulted in 57.14 per cent and 71.43 per cent prevention of pregnancy, respectively, whereas 100 per cent pregnancy inhibition was noted at 500 mg/kg b. w. In the uterine bioassay test carried out in immature bilaterally ovariectomised female rats, aqueous extract of seeds of *Cassia fistula* (100 mg/kg b. w.) increased the uterine wet weight ($p < 0.05$) and luminal epithelial cell height ($p < 0.001$) but did not induce premature opening of the vagina suggesting a mild estrogenic activity. However, it significantly ($p < 0.001$) prevented the oestrogen-induced uterotrophic effect when administered in combination with estradiol valerate (EDV, 0.1 mg/kg b. w.). It was concluded that the extract possesses an anti-estrogenic nature in the presence of a strong oestrogen (Yadav and Jain, 1999).

Crude ethanolic extract of seeds of *Cichorium intybus* and aerial parts of *Guetterda andamonica, Memcylon lushingtonii* and *Solanum crassypetalum* and their fractions (chloroform- or butanol-insoluble fractions) exhibited post-coital contraceptive efficacy in adult female Sprague-Dawley rats (Keshri *et al*, 1998).

An ethanolic leaf extract of *Colebrookia oppositifolia* was orally fed to male rats at dose levels of 100 and 200 mg/kg for 8-10 weeks caused weight loss of testes and epididymides, while, seminal vesicles and ventral prostate showed a significant loss in their respective weights at the higher dose only. Reduced sperm count and motility resulted in 100 per cent negative fertility at 200 mg/kg dose level. Treated animals showed a notable depression of spermatogenesis. Following the treatment at 100 and 200 mg/kg, the preleptotene spermatocytes were decreased by 46.5 and 39.8 per cent, the secondary spermatocytes by 13.4 and 12.7 per cent, the step-19 spermatids by 36.6 and 35.2 per cent, and the mature Leyding cells by 31.2 and 39.5 per cent, respectively. At both dose levels, the seminiferous tubule diameter, Leydig cells nuclear area and cytoplasmic area, as well as the cross-sectional surface area of Sertoli cells, were highly significantly reduced when compared to controls. A significant fall in the total protein and sialic acid content and acid phosphatase enzyme activity of the testes, epididymides, seminal vesicle and ventral prostate, as well as in the glycogen content of testes, was also observed at both dose levels in comparison with controls (Gupta *et al*, 2001).

Traditional reputation of the plant *Inula viscosa* indicates that it is used as an abortifacient. To prove this, recently Al-Dissi and co-workers (2001) conducted an experiment on the effects of *Inula viscosa* leaf extracts in rats. The aqueous extract administered i.p. on day 1-6 of gestation, totally diminished foetal implantation and caused a significant ($P < 0.05$) reduction in the number of corpora lutea and blood progesterone levels. Meanwhile, administration on day 13-15 of gestation exhibited mid-term abortion. Furthermore, petroleum ether and dichloromethane, but not methanol, extracts exhibited pronounced abortifacient effects. It was concluded that the plant possesses anti-implantational and luteolytic activity.

Maytenus ilicifolia Mart. is being used for stomach disorders and fertility control in South America. Montanari and Bevilacqua (2002) verified its potential as an abortifacient. The lyophilised hydroalcoholic extract of its leaves was administered orally at a dose of 1,000 mg/kg/day to mice between the first and third day of pregnancy (DOP), between the fourth and sixth DOP, or between the seventh and ninth DOP. The extract caused a pre-implantation embryonic loss, but it did not have an effect on implantation or organogenesis. Morphological alterations of the reproductive system, not an embryotoxic effect, were not found. Montanari *et al* (1998a) also evaluated the effects of this plant on spermatogenesis.

The petroleum ether extract of the leaves of *Mentha arvensis* L., at the oral doses 10 and 20 mg/mouse per day for 20, 40 and 60 days in male albino mice showed a dose and duration dependent reduction in the number of offspring of the treated male mated with normal females. The results suggest that the petroleum ether extract of the leaves of *Mentha arvensis* possess reversible anti-fertility property without adverse toxicity in male mice (Sharma and Jacob, 2001, 2002).

Chronic administration of *Mondia whitei* L. root bark extract (400 mg/kg/day) for 55 days caused testicular lesions resulting in the cessation of spermatogenesis, degenerative changes in the seminiferous tubules and epididymides. The wet weight of the seminal vesicle increased, whereas the weights of testes, epididymides and ventral prostate were unchanged. The treatment also resulted in a partial anti-fertility effect, and an increase in the protein content of the testes and epididymides. The cholesterol contents of the testes were significantly elevated after 55 days, whereas testosterone and 17β-oestradiol contents of the testes were unchanged. Serum protein was elevated but serum testosterone was unchanged. A recovery period resulted in normal spermatogenesis and fertility, suggesting reversible anti-spermatogenic and anti-fertility effects of the plant (Watcho *et al,* 2001).

Anti-fertility effects of an alcohol extract of the whole plant, *Phyllanthus amarus* at a dose of 100 mg/kg body weight for 30 days orally was investigated in cyclic adult female mice (Rao and Alice, 2001). The results revealed that the cohabited females with normal male mice were unable to become pregnant as their cyclicity was affected. Upon withdrawal of feeding for 45 days, these effects were reversible.

The *Ricinus communis* seed extract was found to possess anti-implantation and abortifacient effect. It was also observed that the seed extract prolonged the oestrus cycle of guinea pigs. The dioestrus phase was significantly prolonged as well. After stopping administering the extract, however, the normal dioestrus phase and oestrus cycle started to resume. The seed extract also reduced the weight of the uterus without affecting that of the ovaries significantly (Makonnen *et al,* 1999).

Petroleum ether, chloroform, ethanol and aqueous extracts of the aerial parts of the plant *Rivea hypocrateriformis* (Convolvulaceae) were tested for anti-implantation and pregnancy interruption properties in female albino rats. Among these, the ethanol extract was found to be most effective in causing significant anti-implantation and interruption of early pregnancy. The anti-fertility activity of ethanol extract was reversible on exogenous administration of hydroxy progesterone. However, the same ethanol extract was found to be ineffective in interruption of late pregnancy. Among the four extracts subjected to preliminary phytochemical screening, the active ethanol extract showed positive tests for alkaloids, glycosides, saponins, tannins and phenolic compounds (Shivalingappa *et al;* 2001).

Salvia fruiticosa belongs to the family Labiatae. The anti-implantation, anti-fertility and reproductive toxicity potentials of aqueous and ethanolic extracts of *Salvia fruiticosa* leaves have been investigated in male and female rats. The ingestion of 200, 400 and 800 mg/kg of aqueous or 400 mg/kg of ethanolic extracts of *Salvia fruiticosa* from day one to day six of pregnancy by female rats did not cause pregnancy failure whilst the ingestion of an ethanolic extract reduced the number of viable foetuses and increased the number of resorptions in the pregnant rats. The ingestion of aqueous extract (800 mg/kg) or ethanolic extract (400 mg/kg) of *Salvia fruiticosa* for 30 consecutive days by adult female rats had no effect on the occurrence of pregnancy. However, the ingestion of these extracts reduced both the number of implantations and viable foetuses and increased the number of resorptions in the pregnant females. The ingestion of aqueous extract (800 mg/kg) or ethanolic extract (400 mg/kg) or *Salvia fruiticosa* for 30 consecutive days by adult male rats had no effect on the number of females impregnated by these males. However, the number of implantations and viable foetuses were reduced in females impregnated by males which ingested either aqueous or ethanolic extracts of *Salvia fruiticosa*, whereas the number of resorptions was increased in females impregnated by males administered either aqueous or ethanolic extracts of *Salvia fruiticosa*. On the other hand, the pre-natal exposure of male and female rat offspring to 400 mg/kg ethanolic extract of *Salvia fruiticosa* had no effects on the timing of testicular descent and vaginal opening, respectively. The ingestion of *Salvia fruiticosa* may produce adverse effects on the fertility of male and female rats (Al-Hamood *et al,* 1998).

Verma *et al* (2002) evaluated anti-fertility activity of *Sarcostemma acidum* (Roxb.) Voigt. stem extract in male rats. Animals were treated with 70 per cent methanol extract of *Sarcostemma acidum* stem orally at two dose levels (50 and 100 mg/kg/day) for 60 days. The treatment resulted in an arrest of spermatogenesis without any systemic side effects. Sperm motility as well as sperm density was reduced significantly. Treatment caused a 80 per cent reduction in fertility at the 50 mg dose and complete suppression of fertility at the 100 mg dose. The protein and glycogen content of the testes, fructose in the seminal vesicle and protein in epididymides were significantly decreased. Cholesterol in the testes was elevated. Treatment at both of the doses caused a marked reduction in the number of primary spermatocytes (preleptotene and pachytene), secondary spermatocytes and spermatids. The number of mature Leydig cells was decreased, and degenerating Leydig cells was increased proportionately. No noticeable side effects were observed.

CONCLUSION

A large number of plants have been screened during the last five-year period. Looking into the trends there are only a few plants on which extensive studies have been undertaken. On other plants, hardly one or two publications have appeared so far. There may be the following reasons for non-development of herbal-based male contraceptive. The first reason may be the requirement of extensive financial and technical inputs. The lack of systematic study, namely, inadequate numbers of vehicle-treated controls, poor experimental design, problems related to insolubility of crude plant extracts, variation in routes of administration, diversity in reproductive function and control among various laboratory species and problems in identifying plant names appears to be the second reason. Finally, the herbal contraceptives being used by humans as a traditional medicine may be ineffective in animal models. Therefore, the need for proper recording of time and place of collection, proper authentication of plants, formulation of uniform protocol for extraction and clinical trials may help in identifying plant products for fertility regulation.

REFERENCES

Akbarsha, M. A. and Murugaian, P. 'Aspects of the male reproductive toxicity/male anti-fertility property of andrographolide in albino rats: Effects on the tests and cauda epididymidal spermatozoa'. *Phytother. Res.* 14: 432-435, 2000.

Al-Dissi, N. M., Salhab, A. S. and Al-Hajj, H. A. 'Effects of Inula viscosa leaf extracts on abortion and implantation in rats'. *J. Ethnopharmacol.* 77: 117-121, 2001.

Al-Hamood, M. H., Elbetieha, A., Alkofahi, A. and Bataineh, H. 'Reproductive toxicity potentials of *Salvia fruiticosa* (Labiatae) in rats'. *J. Ethnopharmacol.* 61: 67-74, 1998.

Anonymous. 'Neem may be source of safe insecticides'. *IRRI Reporter* 82: 2, 1982.

Anonymous. *Encyclopaedia of Chinese Medicines*. vol. 2. Hong Kong and Shanghai: Commercial Press. Jiang Su Medical School, pp. 2460-2470, 1978.

Bajaj, J. S. and Madan, R. 'Regulation of male fertility'. In: *Research on the Regulation of Human Fertility: Needs of Developing Countries and Priorities for the Future*. vol. 2. Background Documents. Scriptor, Copenhagen, Denmark, pp. 729-767, 1983.

Bardin, C. W., Sundaram, K. S. and Chang, C. S. Paper presented at the workshop on Gossypol, Programme for Applied Research on Fertility Regulation, Chicago, 1981.

Batta, S. K. and Santhakumari, G. 'The anti-fertility effect of *Ocimum sanctum* and *Hibiscus rosa-sinensis*'. *Indian J. Med. Res.* 59:777-778, 1971.

Bello, R., Moreno, L., Primo-Yufera, E. and Esplugues, J. '*Globularia alypum* L. extracts reduced histamine and serotonin contraction *in vitro*'. *Phytother. Res.* 16: 389-392, 2002.

Bhaduri, B., Ghose, C. R., Bose, A. W., Moze, B. K. and Basu, U. P. 'Anti-fertility activity of some medicinal plants'. *Indian J. Exp. Biol.* 6: 252-253, 1968.

Bhakuni, D. S., Dhar, M. L., Dhar, M. M., Dhawan, B. N. and Mehrotra, B. N. 'Screening of Indian plants for biological activity'. Part II. *Indian J. Exp. Biol.* 7: 250-252, 1969.

Burgos, R. A., Caballero, E. E., Sanchez, N. S., Schroeder, R. A., Wikman, G. K. and Hancke, J. L. 'Testicular toxicity assessment of *Andrographis paniculata* dried extract in rats'. *J. Ethnopharmacol.* 58:219-224, 1997.

Chan, W. Y. and Ng, T. B. 'Adverse effect of *Tripterygium wilfordii* extract on mouse embryonic development'. *Contraception* 51: 65-71, 1995.

Chang, M. C. 'Development of the oral contraceptives'. *American J. Obstet. Gynecol.* 132: 217-219, 1978.

Chinoy, J. J., D'Souza, J. M. and Padman, P. 'Effects of crude aqueous extract of *Carica papaya* seeds in male albino mice'. *Reprod. Toxicol.* 8: 75-79, 1994.

Chinoy, N. J. and Geetha Ranga, M. 'Effects of *Carica papaya* seed extracts on the physiology of the vas deferens of albino rats'. *Acta Eur. Fertil.* 15: 59-64, 1984.

Chinoy, N. J. and George, S. M. 'Induction of functional sterility in male rats by low dose *Carica papaya* seed extract treatment'. *Acta Eur. Fertil.* 14: 425-432, 1983.

Chinoy, N. J., Geetha Ranga, M., Rao, M. V., Verma, R. J., George, S. M., Patel, K. G. and D'Souza, J. M. 'The reversible anti-fertility effects of extracts of *Carica papaya* seeds on male rats'. In: *Methods for the Regulation of Male Fertility.* (Eds.).Anand Kumar, T. C. and Waites, G. M. H. New Delhi: Indian Council of Medical Research, pp 95-106, 1985.

Circosta, C., Sanogo, R. and Occhiuto, F. 'Effects of *Calotropis procera* on oestrous cycle and on estrogenic functionality in rats'. *Farmaco.* 56: 373-378, 2001.

Cocks, M. and Moller, V. 'Use of indigenous and indigenised medicines to enhance personal well-being: A South African case study'. *Social Sci. Med.* 54: 387-397, 2002.

Coutinho, E. M. 'Gossypol: a contraceptive for men'. *Contraception* 65: 259-263, 2002.

Coutinho, E. M. and Melo, J. F. 'Clinical experience with gossypol in non-Chinese men: a follow up'. *Contraception* 37: 137-152, 1988.

Coutinho, E. M., Athayde, C., Atta. G., Gu, Z. P., Chen, Z. W., Sang, G. W., Emuveyan, E., Adekunle, A. O., Mati, J. and Otubu, J. 'Gossypol blood levels and inhibition of spermatogenesis in men taking gossypol as a contraceptive. A multicentre, international, dose-finding study'. *Contraception* 61: 61-67, 2000.

Das, R. P. 'Effect of papaya seed on the genital organs and fertility of male rats'. *Indian J. Exp. Biol.* 18: 408-409, 1980.

Dhar, M. L., Dhar, M. M., Dhawan, B. N., Mehrotra, B. N. and Ray, C. 'Screening of Indian plants for biological activity'. Part I. *Indian J. Exp. Biol.* 6: 232-247, 1968.

Elbetieha, A., Oran, S. A., Alkofahi, A., Darmani, H. and Raies, A. M. 'Fetotoxic potentials of *Globularia arabica* and *Globularia alypum* (Globulariaceae) in rats'. *J. Ethnopharmacol.* 72:215_219, 2000.

Gu, Z. P. and Wang, W. C. 'The effect of gossypol on reproductive endocrine function in man (abstract)'. In: Symposium of Fertility Regulation in Male. Nanjing, 14-16 December, 1984. Organised by the Ministry of Public Health of the People's Republic of China and the World Health Organisation's Special Programme of Research Development and Research Training in Human Reproduction. Abstracts. (Nanjing, China, Jiangsu Family Planning Institute, 1984), 1984

Gupta, R. S., Yadav, R. K., Dixit, V. P. and Dohhal, M. P. 'Anti-fertility studies of *Colebrookia oppositifolia* leaf extract in male rats with special reference to testicular cell population dynamics'. *Fitoterapia* 72: 236-245.

Hiremath, S. P., Badami, S., Hunasagatta, S. K. and Patil, S. B. 'Anti-fertility and hormonal properties of flavones of *Striga orobanchoides*'. *Pharmacology* 391: 193-197, 2000.

Hiremath, S. P., Badami, S., Swamy, H. K., Patil, S. B. and Londonkar, R. L. 'Anti-fertility activity of *Striga orobanchoides*'. *Biol. Pharm. Bull.* 17: 1029-1031, 1994.

Hiremath, S. P., Rudresh, K., Badami. S., Patil, S. B. and Patil, S. R. 'Post-coital anti-fertility activity of *Acalypha indica* L.' *J. Ethnopharmacol.* 67: 253-258, 1999.

Hoffer, A. P. 'Ultrastructural, biochemical, and endocrine studies on the effects of gossypol and its isomeric derivatives in the male reproductive tract'. In: *Gossypol: a Potential Contraceptive for Men* (Ed.). Segal, S. J. New York: Plenum Press, pp. 143-186, 1985.

Homady, M. H., Khleifat, K. M., Tarawneh, K. A. and Al-Raheil, I. A. 'Reproductive toxicity and infertility effect of *Ferula hormonis* extracts in mice'. *Theriogenology* 57: 2247-2256, 2002.

Iyengar, M. A., Pendse, G. S. and Narayana, N. 'Bioassay of *Cassia fistula* L. (Argavadha)'. *Planta Medica* 14: 289, 1966.

Kabir, S. N., Bhattacharya, K., Pal, A. K. and Pakrashi, A. 'Flowers of *Hibiscus rosa-sinensis*, a potential source of contragestive agent. I. Effect of benzene extract on implantation of mouse'. *Contraception* 29: 385-397, 1984.

Kamath, J. V. and Rana, A. C. 'Preliminary study on anti-fertility activity of *Calotropis procera* roots in female rats'. *Fitoterapia* 73: 111-115, 2002.

Kamboj, A. P. and Dhawan, B. N. 'Fertility regulating plants on Indian scene—an update'. In: *Contraceptive Research Today and Tomorrow*. (Eds.). Toteja, G. S., Mokkapati, S., Singh, B. K., Sharma, R. S. and Saxena, B. N. New Delhi: Indian Council of Medical Research, pp. 115-125, 1989.

Kaushic, C. and Upadhyay, S. 'Mode of long-term anti-fertility effect of intrauterine neem treatment (IUNT)'. *Contraception* 51: 203-207, 1995.

Keshri, G., Lakshmi, V. and Singh, M. M. 'Post-coital contraceptive activity of some indigenous plants in rats'. *Contraception* 57: 357-360, 1998.

Khleifat, K., Homady, M. H., Tarawneh, K. A. and Shakhanbeh, J. 'Effect of *Ferula hormonis* extract on social aggression, fertility and some physiological parameters in pre-pubertal male mice'. *Endocr. J.* 48: 473-482, 2001.

Kholkute, S. D. and Udupa, K. N. 'Antiestrogenic activity of *Hibiscus rosa-sinensis* Linn. flowers'. *Indian J. Exp. Biol*: 14: 175-176, 1976a

Kholkute, S. D. and Udupa, K. N. 'Anti-fertility properties of *Hibiscus rosa-sinensis* Linn.' *J. Res. Indian Med.* 9: 99-102, 1974.

Kholkute, S. D. and Udupa, K. N. 'Biological profile of total benzene extract of *Hibiscus rosa-sinensis* flowers'. *J. Res. Indian Med. Yoga Homoeop.* 13: 107-112, 1978.

Kholkute, S. D. and Udupa, K. N. 'Effects of *Hibiscus rosa-sinensis* on pregnancy of rats'. *Plants Med.* 29: 321-329, 1976b.

Kholkute, S. D., Chatterjee, S. and Udupa, K. N. 'Effect of *Hibiscus rosa-sinensis* Linn. on oestrous cycle and reproductive organs in rats'. *Indian J. Ex. Biol.* 14: 703-704, 1976b.

Kholkute, S. D., Chatterjee, S., Srivastava, D. N. and Udupa, K. N. 'Anti-fertility effect of the alcoholic extract of Japa (*Hibiscus rosa-sinensis*)'. *J. Res. Indian Med.* 7: 72-75, 1972.

Kholkute, S. D., Mudgal, V. and Deshpande, P. J. 'Screening of indigenous medicinal plants for anti-fertility potentiality'. *Planta Med.* 29: 151-155, 1976a.

Kholkute, S. D., Srivastava, D. N., Chatterjee, S. and Udupa, K. N. 'Effects of some compounds isolated from *Hibiscus rosa-sinensis* flowers on pregnancy in rats'. *J. Res. Indian Med. Yoga Homoeop.* 11: 106-112, 1976c.

Kholkute. S. D. 'Effect of *Hibiscus rosa-sinensis* on spermatogenesis and accessory reproductive organs in rats'. *Planta Med.* 31: 127-135, 1977.

Khosa, R. L. and Singh, R. H. 'Betel root—an anti-fertility agent'. *J. Res. Indian Med.* 7: 65-66, 1972.

Kirtikar, K. R. and Basu, B. P. *Indian Medicinal Plants*, vol. II. Dehradun: International Book Distributor, 1987.

Kumar, M., Sharma, S. and Lohiya, N. K. 'Gossypol-induced hypokalemia and role of exogenous potassium salt supplementation when used as an antispermatogenic agent in male langur monkey'. *Contraception* 56: 251-256, 1997.

Liu, G. Z. and Lyle, K. C. 'Clinical trial of gossypol as a male contraceptive drug. Part II. Hypokalemia study'. *Fertil. Steril.* 48: 462-465, 1987.

Liu, G. Z., Ch'iu-Hinton, K., Cao, J., Zhu, C. and Li, B. 'Effect of K salt or a potassium blocker on gossypol-related hypokalemia'. *Contraception* 37: 111-117, 1988.

Liu, Z. Q., Liu, G. Z., Hei, L. S., Zhang, R. A. and Yu, C. Z. 'Clinical trial of gossypol as a male anti-fertility agent'. In: *Recent Advances in Fertility Regulation* (Eds.). Chang, C. F., Griffin, D. and Woolman, A. Geneva: S. A. Atar Press, pp. 160-163, 1981.

Lohiya, N. K. and Ansari, A. S. 'Male contraceptive agents'. In: *Comparative Endocrinology and Reproduction.* (Eds.). Roy, K. P., Krishna, A. and Haldar, C. New Delhi: Narora Publishing House, pp. 260-277, 1999.

Lohiya, N. K. and Goyal, R. B. 'Anti-fertility investigations on the crude chloroform extract of *Carica papaya* Linn. seed in male albino rats'. *Indian J. Exp. Biol.* 30: 1051-1055, 1992.

Lohiya, N. K., Goyal, R. B., Jayaprakash, D., Ansari, A. S. and Sharma, S. 'Anti-fertility effects of aqueous extract of *Carica papaya* seeds in male rats'. *Planta Med.* 60: 400-404, 1994a.

Lohiya, N. K., Goyal, R. B., Jayaprakash, D., Ansari, A. S., Srivastava, S. and Singh, P. 'Anti-fertility effects of *Carica papaya* seeds in male rats'. In: *Current Concepts in Fertility Regulation and Reproduction* (Eds.). Puri, C. P. and Van Look, P. F. A. New Delhi: Wiley Eastern Limited, pp. 177-192, 1994b.

Lohiya, N. K., Goyal, R. B., Jayaprakash, D., Sharma, S., Kumar, M. and Ansari, A. S. 'Induction of reversible anti-fertility with a crude ethanol extract of *Carica papaya* seeds in albino male rats'. *Int. J. Pharmacog.* 30: 308-320, 1992.

Lohiya, N. K., Kothari, L. K., Manivannam, B., Mishra. P. K. and Pathak, N. 'Human sperm immobilisation effect of *Carica papaya* seed extracts: an *in vitro* study'. *Asian J. Androl.* 2: 103-109, 2000b.

Lohiya, N. K., Manivannan, B., Mishra, P. K., Pathak, N., Sriram, S., Bhande, S. S. and Panneerdoss, S. 'Chloroform extract of *Carica papaya* seeds induces long-term reversible azoospermia in langur monkey'. *Asian J. Androl.* 4: 17-26, 2002.

Lohiya, N. K., Mishra, P. K., Pathak, N., Manivannan, B. and Jain, S. C. 'Reversible azoospermia by oral administration of the benzene chromatographic fraction of the chloroform extract of the seeds of *Carica papaya* in rabbits'. *Adv. Contracept.* 15: 141-161, 1999b.

Lohiya, N. K., Pathak, N., Mishra, P. K. and Manivannam, B. 'Contraceptive evaluation and toxicological study of aqueous extract of the seeds of *Carica papaya* in male rabbits'. *J. Ethnopharmacol.* 70: 17-27, 2000a.

Lohiya, N. K., Pathak, N., Mishra. P. K. and Manivannan, B. 'Reversible contraception with chloroform extract of *Carica papaya* Linn. seeds in male rabbits'. *Reprod. Toxicol.* 13: 59-66, 1999a.

Lohiya, N. K., Sharma, K., Kumar, M. and Sharma, S. 'Limitations in developing gossypol acetic acid as a male contraceptive'. *Contraception* 41: 519-532, 1990.

Makonnen, E., Zerihun, L., Assefa, G. and Rostom, A. A. 'Anti-fertility activity of *Ricinus communis* seed in female guinea pigs'. *East Afr. Med. J.* 76: 335-337, 1999.

Mazaro, R., Di Stasi, L. C., Filho, S. A. and De Grava Kempinas, W. 'Decrease in sperm number after treatment of rats with *Austroplenckia populnea*'. *Contraception* 62: 45-50, 2000.

Montanari, T. and Bevilacqua, E. 'Effect of *Maytenus ilicifolia* Mart. on pregnant mice'. *Contraception* 65: 171-175, 2002.

Montanari, T., de Carvalho, J. E. and Dolder, H. 'Antispermatogenic effect of *Achillea millefolium* L. in mice'. *Contraception* 58: 309-313, 1998b.

Montanari, T., de Carvalho, J. E. and Dolder, H. Effect of *Maytenus ilicifolia* Mart. ex. Reiss on spermatogenesis'. *Contraception* 57: 335-339, 1998a.

Mukherjee, S. and Talwar, G. P. 'Termination of pregnancy in rodents by oral administration of praneem, a purified neem seed extract'. *Am. J. Reprod. Immunol.* 35: 51-56, 1996.

Mukherjee, S., Garg, S. and Talwar, G. P. 'Early post-implantation contraceptive effects of a purified fraction of neem (*Azadirachta indica*) seeds, given orally in rats: possible mechanisms involved'. *J. Ethnopharmacol.* 67: 287-296, 1999.

Murthy, D. R., Reddy, C. M. and Patil, S. B. 'Effect of benzene extract of *Hibiscus rosa sinensis* on the estrous cycle and ovarian activity in albino mice'. *Biol. Pharm. Bull.* 20: 756-758, 1997.

Murugan, V., Shareef, H., Rama Sarma, G. V. S., Ramanathan, M. and Suresh, B. 'Anti-fertility activity of the stem bark of *Alangium salviifolium* (Linn. F) Wang in Wistar female rats'. *Indian J. Pharmacol.* 32: 388-389, 2000.

Nadkarni, A. K. and Nadkarni, K. M. *Nadkarni's Materia Medica,* edn. 3, vol. I. Bombay: Popular Book Depot, 1954.

Nwafor, P. A., Okwuasaba, F. K. and Onoruvwe, O. O. 'Contraceptive and non estrogenic effects of methanolic extract of *Asparagus pubescens* root in experimental animals'. *J. Ethnopharmacol.* 62:117-122, 1998.

Oderinde, O., Noronha, C., Oremosu, A., Kusemiju, T. and Okanlawon, O. A. 'Abortifacient properties of aqueous extract of *Carica papaya* (Linn.) seeds on female Sprague-Dawley rats'. *Niger. Postgrad. Med. J.* 9: 95-98, 2002.

Pakrashi, A., Bhattacharya, K., Kabir, S. N. and Pal, A. K. 'Flowers of *Hibiscus rosa-sinensis*, a potential source of contragestive agent. III. Interceptive efficacy of benzene extract in mouse'. *Contraception* 34: 523-536, 1986.

Pal, A. K., Bhattacharya, K., Kabir. S. N. and Pakrashi, A. 'Flowers of *Hibiscus rosa- sinensis*, a potential source of contraceptive agent. II: Possible mode of action with reference to anti-implantation effect of the benzene extract'. *Contraception* 32: 517-529, 1985.

Pathak, N., Mishra., P. K., Manivannan, B. and Lohiya, N. K. 'Sterility due to inhibition of sperm motility by oral administration of benzene chromatographic fraction of the chloroform extract of the seeds of *Carica papaya* in rats'. *Phytomedicine* 7: 325-333, 2000.

Prakash, A. O. and Mathur, R. 'Screening of Indian plants for anti-fertility activity'. *Indian J. Exp. Biol.* 14: 623-626, 1976.

Prakash, A. O. 'Acid and alkaline phosphatase activity in the uterus of rat treated with *Hibiscus rosa-sinensis* Linn. extracts'. *Curr. Sci.* 48: 501-506, 1979a.

Prakash, A. O. 'Effect of *Hibiscus rosa-sinensis* Linn. extracts on corpora lutea of cyclic guinea pigs'. *Sci. Cult.* 46: 330-335, 1980.

Prakash, A. O. 'Protein concentration in rat uterus under the influence of *Hibiscus rosa-sinensis* Linn. extracts'. *Proc. Indian Natl. Sci. Acad.* 45B: 327-335, 1979b.

Prakash, A. O. 'Protein concentration in the rat uterus. Response to *Hibiscus rosa-sinensis* extracts'. *Experientia* 35: 1122-1125, 1979c.

Prakash, A. O., Mathur, A., Mehta, H. and Mathur, R. 'Concentrations of Na^+ and K^+ in serum and uterine flushing of ovariectomised, pregnant and cyclic rats when treated with extracts of *Hibiscus rosa-sinensis* flowers'. *J. Ethnopharmacol.* 28: 337-347, 1990.

Qian, S. Z. 'Effect of gossypol on potassium and prostaglandin metabolism and mechanism of action of gossypol'. In: *Recent Advances in Fertility Regulation.* (Eds.). Chang, C. F., Griffin, D. and Woolman, A. Geneva: S. A. Atar Press, pp. 151-159, 1981.

Qian, S. Z. '*Tripterygium wilfordii*, a Chinese herb effective in male fertility regulation'. *Contraception* 36: 335-345, 1987.

Qian, S. Z., Hu, J. H, Ho, L. X., Sun, M. X., Huang, Y. Z. and Fang, J. H. Cited In: Qian, S. Z. and Wang, Z. G. (1984). 'Gossypol: a potential anti-fertility agent for males'. *Annual. Rev. Pharmacol. Toxicol.* 24: 329-360, 1972.

Qian, S. Z., Jiang, G. W., Wu, X. Y., Xu, Y., Li, Y. Q. and Zhou, Z. H. 'Gossypol related hypokalemia: clinicopharmacologic studies'. *Chin. Med. J.* 93: 477-482, 1980.

Qian, S. Z., Xu, Y. and Zhang, J. W. 'Recent progress in research of *Tripterygium*: a male anti-fertility plant'. *Contraception* 51: 121-129, 1995.

Qian. S. Z., Hu, Y. Z., Wang, S. M., Luo, Y., Tang, A. S., Shu, S. Y., Zhou, J. W. and Rao, T. Y. 'Effects of *Tripterygium hypoglaucum* (Levl.) Hutch on male fertility'. *Adv. Contracept.* 4: 307-310, 1988.

Rao, M. V. and Alice, K. M. 'Contraceptive effects of *Phyllanthus amarus* in female mice'. *Phytother. Res.* 15: 265-267, 2001.

Reddy, C. M. Cited In: Lohiya, N. K. (2000). 'Plant products for contraception: how to make it a reality?' *ISSRF Newsletter* 2000 July (5): 9-12, 1997.

Sarkar, M., Gangopadhyay, P., Basak, B., Chakrabarty, K., Banerji, K., Adhikary, P. and Chatterjee, A. 'The reversible anti-fertility effect of *Piper betle* Linn. on Swiss albino male mice'. *Contraception* 62: 271-274, 2000.

Satyavati, G, V., Raina, M. K. and Sharma, M. '*Medicinal Plants of India*. vol. I. New Delhi: Indian Council of Medical Research, 1976.

Satyavati, G. V., Gupta, A. K. and Tondon, N. '*Medicinal Plants of India*. vol. 2. New Delhi: Indian Council of Medical Research, 1987.

Schmutterer, H. 'Some properties of components of the neem tree and their use in pest control in developing countries'. *Med. Fac. Landbouww. Rijksuniv. Gent*, 46/1, 1981.

Serrano, H. and Garcia-Suarez, M. D. 'Effect of water extracts of Bursera species on sperm aggregation: contraceptive potential'. *Adv. Reprod.* 5: 51, 2001.

Sharma, D. C. 'India to regulate indigenous medicine sector'. *Lancet* 358: 1249, 2001.

Sharma, N. and Jacob, D. 'Anti-fertility investigation and toxicological screening of the petroleum ether extract of the leaves of *Mentha arvensis* L. in male albino mice'. *J. Ethnopharmacol.* 75: 5-12, 2001.

Sharma, N. and Jacob, D. 'Assessment of reversible contraceptive efficacy of methanol extract of *Mentha arvensis* L. leaves in male albino mice'. *J. Ethnopharmacol.* 80: 9-13, 2002.

Sharma, S., Kumar, M., Goyal, R. B., Manivannan, B. and Lohiya, N. K. 'Reversible antispermatogenic effect of gossypol in langur monkeys (*Presbytis entellus entellus*)'. *Adv. Contracept.* 15: 15-27, 1999.

Shivalingappa, H., Satyanarayan, N. D. and Purohit, M. G. 'Anti-implantation and pregnancy interruption efficacy of *Rivea hypocrateriformis* in the rat'. *J. Ethnopharmacol.* 74: 245-249, 2001.

Singh, M. P., Singh, R. H. and Udupa, K. N. Anti-fertility activity of a benzene extract of *Hibiscus rosa-sinensis* flowers on female albino rats'. *Planta. Med.* 44: 171-174, 1982.

Singhwi, M. S. and Lall, S. B. 'Cytostatic and cytotoxic effects of flower extract of *Hibiscus rosa-sinensis* on spermatogenically and androgenically active testes of a non-scrotal bat *Rhinopoma kinneari* Wroughton'. *Indian J. Exp. Biol.* 18: 1405-1406, 1980.

Singhwi, M. S. and Lall, S. B. 'Effect of flower extract of *Hibiscus rosa-sinensis* on testicular lactate dehydrogenases of a non-scrotal bat *Rhinopoma kinneari* Wroughton'. *India J. Exp. Biol.* 19: 359-361, 1981.

Skim, F., Lazrek, H. B., Kaaya, A., el Amri, H. and Jana, M. 'Pharmacological studies of two anti-diabetic plants: *Globularia alypum* and *Zygophyllum gaetulum*.' *Therapie* 54: 711-715, 1999.

Sonenberg, M., Huang, J. T., Ren, Y. F., Su, T. L., Watanabe, K. A., Haspel, H. C., Corin, R. E. and Hoffer, A. P. 'Anti-fertility and other actions of gossypol analogues'. *Contraception* 37: 247-255, 1988.

Telefo, P. B., Moundipa, P. F., Tchana, A. N., Tchouanguep, D. C. and Mbiapo, F. T. 'Effects of an aqueous extract of *Aloe buettneri, Justicia insularis. Hibiscus macranthus, Dicliptera verticillata* on some physiological and biochemical parameters of reproduction in immature female rats'. *J. Ethnopharmacol.* 63: 193-200, 1998.

Udoh, P. and Kehinde, A. 'Studies on anti-fertility effect of pawpaw seeds (*Carica papaya*) on the gonads of male albino rats'. *Phytother. Res.* 13: 226-228, 1999.

Van de Walle, E. 'Flowers and fruits: two thousand years of menstrual regulation'. *J. Interdisciplin. Hist.* 28: 183-203, 1997.

Verma, P. K., Sharma, A., Mathur, A., Sharma, P., Gupta, R. S. and Joshi, S. C. 'Effect of *Sarcostemma acidum* stem extract on spermatogenesis in male albino rats'. *Asian J. Androl.* 4: 43-47, 2002.

Verma, R. J. and Chinoy, N. J. 'Effect of papaya seed extract on contractile response of cauda epididymal tubules'. *Asian J. Androl.* 4: 77-78, 2002.

Vyas, D. K. and Jacob, D. 'Effect of papaya (*Carica papaya*) seeds on the reproductive structures and fertility of the male rabbit'. *Indian Zoologist* 8: 105-108, 1984.

Waites, G. M. 'The contribution of Asian scientists to global research in andrology'. *Asian J. Androl.* 1: 7-12, 1999.

Waites, G. M., Wang, C. and Griffin, P. D. 'Gossypol: reasons for its failure to be accepted as a safe, reversible male anti-fertility drug'. *Int. J. Androl.* 21: 8-12, 1998.

Wang, Y. E., Luo, Y. G. and Tang, X. C. 'Gossypol: reasons for its failure to be accepted as a safe, reversible male anti-fertility drug'. *Acta Pharm. Sinica.* 14: 662-669, 1979.

Warrier, P. K. and Nambiar, R. *Indian Medicinal Plants—A Compendium of 500 Species*. Vol. I. Madras: Orient Longmans Ltd., 1964.

Watcho, P., Kamtchouing, P., Sokeng, S., Moundipa, P. F., Tantchou, J., Essame, J. L. and Koueta. N. 'Reversible anti-spermatogenic and anti-fertility activities of *Mondia whitei* L. in male albino rat. *Phytother. Res.* 15: 26-29, 2001.

WHO. 'Annual Technical Report 1994, Special Programme of Research, Development and Research Training in Human Reproduction. Geneva: World Health Organisation, 1995.

WHO. Annual Report, Special Programme of Research, Development and Research Training in Human Reproduction. Geneva: World Health Organisation, 1984.

Xu, D., Cai, W. J., Zhu, B. H., Dong, C. J., Zheng, Z. C. and Gao, Z. Q. 'Clinical safety of long-term administration of gossypol in 32 cases'. *Contraception* 37: 129-135, 1988.

Xue, S. P. 'Studies on the anti-fertility effect of gossypol, a new contraceptive for males'. In: *Recent Advances in Fertility Regulation* (Eds.). Chang, C. F., Griffin, D. and Woolman, A. Geneva: S. A. Atar Press, pp. 122-146, 1981.

Yadav, R. and Jain, G. C. 'Anti-fertility effect of aqueous extract of seeds of *Cassia fistula* in female rats'. *Adv. Contracept.* 15: 293-301, 1999.

Yu, D. Y. Cited in: Xiao, P. G. and Wang, N. G. 'Can ethnopharmacology contribute to the development of anti-fertility drugs?' *J. Ethnopharmacol.* 32: 167-177, 1991.

Yu, Z. H. and Chan, H. C. 'Gossypol as a male anti-fertility agent—why studies should have been continued'. *Int. J. Androl.* 21: 2-7, 1998.

Zhang, G. Y., Meng-Chun, J., Jin-Lai, C. and Wen-Qing, Y. 'The effect of long-term treatment with crude cotton seed oil on pituitary and testicular function in men'. *Int. J. Androl.* 12:404-410, 1989.

Zheng, J. R., Fang, J. L., Xu, L. F., Gao, J. W., Guo, H. Z., Li, Z. R. and Sun, H. Z. Cited In: Wu, F. C. (1988). 'Male contraception: current status and future prospects'. *Clin. Endocrinol.* 9: 43-65, 1985.

Zierau, O., Bodinet, C., Kolba, S., Wolf, M. and Vollmer, G. 'Anti-estrogenic activities of *Cimicifuga racemosa* extracts'. *J. Steroid Biochem. Mol. Bio.* 80:125-130, 2002.

—oo(O)oo—

18

PLANTS WITH ANTIOXIDATIVE PROPERTIES IN RADIOPROTECTION WITH REFERENCE TO *AMARANTHUS* AND *SPINACIA*

A. L. BHATIA AND MANISH JAIN

OXYGEN is a double-edged sword. We cannot live without oxygen but at same time we are continuously exposed to oxygen toxicity. However molecular oxygen is neither very reactive nor very toxic. The apparent toxicity of oxygen is actually due to free oxygen radicals formed by partial reduction of molecular oxygen. Moreover, a free radical of any species is capable of independent existence (hence the term 'free'). Generally enhanced reactivity of free radicals over more stable molecules results from the fact that more energy is required, for example, to maintain two separate species with an unpaired electron than to allow them to come together and share electrons such that a filled molecular orbital is formed, eventually with formation of a covalent bond. Moreover, the reactivity of free radical is inversely related to stability.

Free radicals are produced in the body as by-products of normal cellular metabolic activities such as prostaglandin synthesis, mitochondrial electron transport, endoplasmic reticulum enzyme activity, oxyhaemoglobin, auto-oxidation and phagocytosis as well as when exposed to environmental pollutants, drugs, pesticides and ionising radiation producing severe damaging effects on body tissues. Normally a balance is maintained between the oxidative attack of free radicals and the anti-oxidative defence system prevailing in the cells and tissues of our body, but when the balance is tilted more towards generation of free radicals then degenerative changes set in causing many degenerative diseases. The most important reduction of free radicals in aerobic cells involve molecular oxygen and its radical derivatives (superoxide radical O_2).

Moreover, the rate of univalent pathway and the consequent formation of free radical is significantly increased by uncoupled oxidative phosphorylation, hyperbaric oxygen treatment and in various pathophysiological conditions such as inflammatory immunologic disorders, metabolism of drugs and alcohol, exposure to UV and therapeutic radiation, cancer, myocardial infraction, cataract, rheumatoid arthritis, ischemia repurfusion, ageing, signal transduction mechanisms, auto-oxidation of molecules (such as catecholamines) and deficiency of antioxidants.

RADIATION AND GENERATION OF FREE RADICALS

Exposure to living organisms to gamma radiation also causes homalytic fission of O-H bonds in water (living organisms contain more than 70 per cent water) to give $H^{\cdot}$ and $OH^{\cdot}$ radical that reacts at a diffusion controlled rate with almost all molecules in living cells. Hence, when OH^{-} is formed *in vivo*, it damages whatever is next to it, it cannot migrate significant distance within the cell. Further, the harmful effects of excess exposure to gamma radiation on living organisms are thought to be initiated by an attack of OH^{-} on protein, DNA and lipids. Hydroxyl radical attack DNA in a multiplicity of ways. One of the main products of attack on the DNA bases is δ–hydroxyguanine, a miscoding lesion often leading to G → T transversions. An excessive rise in intracellular free Ca^{2+} can also activate endonucleases and cause DNA fragmentation. Other oxyradicals include singlet oxygen ($O^{\cdot -}$), peroxyl and alkoxyl radicals and oxides of nitrogen. However, oxyradicals such as H_2O_2 and HOCl cannot be classified as free radicals as they still contain a pair of electrons in the outer orbit. Therefore, the term 'reactive oxygen species' (ROS) is preferentially used to cover all these chemical species. Radiation causes free radical formation and results in cumulative damage on irreplaceable vital molecules as those of nuclear DNA, membrane lipid and collagen, a basic component of connective tissue and causes lipid peroxidation (Fitechett, 1985; Yagi, 1988; Halliwell *et al,* 1992). Lipid peroxidation has been implicated in diseases such as cancer (Cerutti, 1985) and ageing (Harman, 1981).

Biological materials particularly membranes contain higher concentration of polyunsaturated fatty acid (PUFA). In the presence of a free radical initiator (such as O_2^{-} or OH^{-}) and O_2, they may be oxidised to alkanes, aldehydes and hydroperoxide. This process is known as lipid peroxidation and occurs in both plant and animal cells. It is a complex process and peroxidation of linoleic acid alone results in the formation of at least 20 degradation products. The loss of PUFA leads to extensive damage to the fine structure, permeability and other functions of cellular membrane and concomitant release of destructive lysosomal enzymes. If these hydroperoxides or secondary products are not removed, they may react with inactive essential proteins, enzymes and nucleic acids and ultimately lead to irreversible damage to the cell. Lipid peroxidation (LPO) is oxidative deterioration of polyunsaturated lipids and it involves ROS and transition metal ions. It is a molecular mechanism of cell injury leading to generation of peroxides and lipid hydroperoxides which can decompose to yield a wide range of cytotoxic products most of which are aldehydes, such as malondialdehyde (MDA), 4 hydroxynonenal, etc. The stimulation of LPO as a consequence of tissue injury can sometimes make significant contribution to worsening of injury. LPO is a highly destructive process and cellular organelles/whole organism lose biochemical function and/or structural architecture, which may lead to damage or death of cell.

WIDESPREAD USE OF RADIATION

Today we are living in the era of nuclear energy. With the widespread and increasing use of nuclear energy and radiation, it has become imperative to understand the basic mechanisms of interaction of radiation with living matter. There is need for the precise evaluation of biological risks involved and optimisation of gainful uses of radiation in research, medicine, industry, military and agriculture. At present, ionising radiation and radioisotopes have become very useful in medical sciences both for diagnostic and therapeutic purposes including cancer. Similarly with the use of radiation in industrial and technological areas, the chances of natural or unpredictable accidental exposure to radiation become unavoidable. This is significant for persons working in the area of radiation and nuclear energy.

Unfortunately, most of the technology has failed to address the harmful effects of radiation. The nuclear weapon is the most destructive creation of humankind in history. The gruesome destructive effects of the nuclear bomb were demonstrated with unforgettable pain at Hiroshima and Nagasaki during World War II on 6 and 9 August, 1945. According to reports published by the U. S. National Academy of Sciences and the U. S. Environmental Protection Agency, exposure to radiation doses will continue due to continuous nuclear weapon testing, and it is estimated that hundreds of additional cancers will result from atmospheric nuclear testing. Nuclear tests, including those performed underground are likely to cause damage to natural resources that will last for centuries. There are two kinds of environmental factors associated with radioactivity from underground tests: (i). radioactivity contamination may escape into the atmosphere, or (ii). the radioactivity may be released into ground water or to the surface or both the two factors may have a combined effect. The major sources of radiation exposure are of two types, natural and man-made. Of all exposures, more than 80 per cent is contributed by natural sources, of which the radon gases and their decay products account for almost 70 per cent. Some parts of coastal Kerala and Tamil Nadu in South India have radioactivity levels 5-10 times higher than in other parts of the country. This is due to the presence of thorium deposits in the sand containing the monazite minerals. More than 20 per cent of the population working in the high background areas in Kerala receives an annual dose of approximately 5mSv/y, while a smaller population receives about 10-20 mSv/y. Medical uses of radiation and radio-isotopes constitute the major sources (more than 95 per cent) of man-made exposures.

World scientific organisations like United Nations Scientific Committee on the Effects of Atomic Radiation (UNSCEAR), International Commission on Radiological Protection (ICRP), Committee on the Biological Effects of Ionising Radiation (BEIR), National Radiological Protection Board (NRPB), etc. have been concerned for a long time with evaluating the risk from radiation exposure to man and environment. ICRP has recommended exposure limits for radiation workers and the public, with an aim to control and reduce unwanted exposures. Under these guidelines every country has to set its own limits to keep the exposures as low as reasonable and achievable (ALARA). ICRP in its recommendations (1991) has suggested an annual limit of 20 mSv (2 rems) for occupational exposure and 1 mSv (0.1 rem) for members of the public.

With the advancement and use of radiation for diagnostic and therapeutic purposes in medical sciences, it has been demonstrated that there is no threshold dose of radiation for the human body. Although, nuclear accidents are spectacular, frightening and can cause immediate death because of the incredible amount of energy involved, the long-term problems resulting from the exposure to radiation are even worrisome.

Radiation is converted to other forms of energy when it is absorbed by matter. This energy conversion results in damage at the cellular, tissue, organ or organism level when individuals are irradiated. The degree and kind of damage vary with the kind of radiation, the amount of radiation, the duration of the exposure and the particular type of cells irradiated and other factors like age, sex and species of the animal. In contrast to other forms of radiation, ionising radiation has the capacity to break chemical bonds. It imparts energy to living cells through random interactions with atoms, giving rise to ions and reactive radicals; these in turn cause molecular changes that may lead ultimately to biological injury. The effects of large doses are easily seen and can be quantified because there is high incidence of death at these levels. However, harmful biological effects from low doses are much more difficult to demonstrate and analyse. Moderate doses of radiation are known to increase the likelihood of cancer and birth defects. The higher the dose, the more incidence of abnormality. Lower doses may cause temporary cellular changes, but it is difficult to demonstrate long-term effects.

Thus, there is a need to evolve means to protect radiation workers and the common man from radiation exposure. This holds true also in the medical field especially during treatment of cancer, where the cancer cells have to be killed and the normal cells need protection.

Experimental and clinical studies on radiation protection and recovery have been concerned primarily with:

1. The need for information on protection of human populations who may have to be or have been exposed to external radiation, for example, the military and civilians during nuclear warfare, occupational exposure to personnel in nuclear power reactors and in medicine and research.
2. The protection against damage produced by internally administered isotopes and techniques of radio-element removal.
3. The elucidation of mechanisms by which protective agents act.

ANTIOXIDATIVE DEFENCE SYSTEM

To meet the challenges of free radicals/ROS, aerobic organisms have been equipped with powerful batteries of mechanisms that protect them from the adverse effects of lipid peroxidation and other manifestations of oxygen toxicity. These are commonly known as 'antioxidant defence system'. The term 'system' is used deliberately, since it is believed that many different antioxidants work together in concert for the homeostatic regulation of redox state of the body. Antioxidant defence systems can be classified into two major groups:

1. **Enzymatic Antioxidants:** This category includes superoxide-dismutase, catalase, glutathione peroxidase, glutathione reductase, glutathione S-transferase and glutamyl transpeptidase and function by direct or sequential removal of ROS thereby terminating their activities
2. **Non-Enzymatic Antioxidants:** It includes metal binding proteins and low molecular weight non-enzymatic antioxidants consisting of scavenging molecules that are either endogenously produced (glutathione, ubiquinols cytochrome–c and uric acid or those derived from the diet (carotenoids, ascorbic acid, α–tocopherol, riboflavin, lipoic acid, selenium and zinc).

Conclusively, the aerobic life is challenged by partially reduced oxygen species (O_2^-, OH^-, H_2O_2) which are transiently formed during the biological processes. Due to their higher reactivity, as compared to molecular dioxygen, they are considered to be potentially toxic to cells, especially because of their lesions in germline DNA that increase the incidence of genetic diseases and cancer progeny. Simultaneously, these free radicals or ROS can attack lipids, proteins and carbohydrates to induce oxidation, cleavage, cross-linking and modification that eventually cause damage. Moreover, the influence of free radicals mediated oxidation is amplified because it proceeds by a chain mechanism and only one radical can initiate chain reaction that may propagate over and over again. Further, oxidative stress can result from or can be enhanced by a large variety of conditions, including nutritional imbalance, exposure to chemicals and physical agents in the environment, strenuous physical activities, injuries and hereditary disorders. A normal cell may control or prevent such adverse reactions by physically separating oxygen from susceptible molecules by providing molecules that effectively compete for oxygen by lysing, inactivating or removing damaged molecules or by rapidly repairing damaged molecules. For this, aerobic organisms are provided with an array of defence systems. The preventive antioxidants decompose peroxides or sequester metal ions to reduce the generation of free radicals whereas the chain-breaking antioxidants scavenge the free radicals to inhibit the radical attack and/or break the chain reaction. Thus, a decline balance exists between oxidants and antioxidants or the susceptibility of a given tissue to oxidative stress is a function of overall balance between the degrees of oxidative damage, which may be attributed to insufficient antioxidant potentials.

ROLE OF ANTIOXIDANTS/RADIOPROTECTIVE AGENTS

In the past few years, the role of dietary antioxidants (such as vitamin C, E, β-carotene and biological trace elements, zinc and selenium) in health and diseases has attracted increasing attention and numerous trials are in progress to ascertain the potential benefits of antioxidant supplements to patients with a variety of diseases.

Antioxidants are molecules which can safely *interact* with free radicals and terminate the chain reaction before vital molecules are damaged. Although there are several enzyme systems within the body that scavenge free radicals, the principal micronutrient (vitamin) antioxidants are vitamin E, β-carotene and vitamin C. A potent radioprotector neutralises free radicals and mitigates oxidative stress and may also stimulate inherent oxidant defence systems.

Modification of radiation response can be achieved by means of chemical substances that can significantly decrease the magnitude of the response when present in a biologic system during irradiation. This type of modification may be classified as chemical protection and substances responsible for it may be termed 'chemical protectors' or chemical radioprotectors. In recent years there has been a growing interest in the research concerned with the modification of radiation injury in biological systems.

Ever since the discovery of radiation protection by several synthetic compounds such as cysteine (Patt *et al*, 1949), 2-mercaptopropionylglycine (MPG) (Sugahara *et al*, 1970), WR-2721 (Yuhas *et al*, 1980), lipoic acid (Ramakrishnan *et al*, 1992), deoxyspergualin (Nemoto *et al*, 1995), dipyridamole and adenine monophosphate (Pospisil *et al*, 1995) have been tested to find out their protective action on the biological system. However, the application of these radioprotective drugs in clinical radiotherapy is limited due to their inherent toxicity at the effective doses required to obtain significant therapeutic gains.

Knowing the threat from radiation to human health and life, scientists make an endeavour to look for an antidote since such pollutants are unavoidable from our environment. This has necessitated search for the non-toxic radioprotective agents. It seems that certain natural and synthetic compounds quench the reactive energy of free radicals generated due to such miscreants. The herbal extracts contain large number of compounds, many of which offer protection against reactive oxygen species on the contrary to synthetic ones which cause toxicity. Herbal preparations are being exploited in Indian the system of medicine, Ayurveda, since ancient times. Hence, the present study is an attempt to investigate the role of two important hitherto ignored herbs against free radicals generated by gamma irradiation.

NATURAL ANTIOXIDANTS IN HERBS

The body of knowledge about plants, herbs and spices and their respective and collective roles in promoting human health is modest. Dietary compounds, their role in maintaining human health and their interactions with established nutrients need to be determined to be research priorities. A number of fruits and vegetables have been shown to actually combat the deleterious effects of metabolic oxidation generated naturally or by increasing pollutants in the environment.

Recently, interest has been generated to develop the potential drugs of plant origin for the modification of radiation effects. The plants that show good antioxidant activity include *Allium cepa* (Onion), *Allium sativum* (Garlic), *Aloe camells* (Sinensis) (Green tea), *Curcuma longa* (Turmeric), *Emblica officinalis* (Amla), *Glycyrrhiza glabra* (Liquorice), *Hemidesmus indicus* (Anantamul), *Mangifera indica* (Mango), *Ocimum sanctum* (Tulsi), *Picrorrhiza kurroa* (Katuka), *Tinospora cordifolia* (Guduchi), *Withania somnifera* (Ashwagandha) and *Zingiber officinale* (Ginger).The Indian system of medicine offers a large number of plants in the treatment of different diseases including cancer. Plant foods such as cereals, vegetables, fruits, pulses, nuts, spices and beverages contain many biologically active micronutrients other than vitamins and minerals. These are known as phytochemicals. Plant products appear to have an advantage over the synthetic compounds because of low/no toxicity at the effective dose with minimum/no side effects. Several plant extracts like garlic (Gupta, 1988), ginseng (Pande *et al,* 1998a), *Aloe vera* (Pande *et al,* 1998b), *Podophyllum* (Goel *et al,* 1999), *Ocimum* (Uma Devi *et al,* 2000), *Rubia cordifolia* (Pande *et al,* 1994); *Withania* (Bhattacharya *et al,* 1996; Panda and Kar, 1997); caffeine from coffee (Hebbar *et al,* 2001) have been investigated for their anti-oxidative efficacy. Rich source of non nutrient antioxidants are beans, cloves, turmeric and mustard (Fruta *et al,* 1997) and herbal drug preparations such as Liv.52 (Saini *et al,* 1985; Daga *et al,* 1995) and Rasayanas (Kumar *et al,* 1999) have been used for radioprotection. There are still a large number of plants and Ayurvedic formulations whose antioxidant activities need to be examined in relation to their potential therapeutic and related beneficial properties.

According to recent studies, antioxidant vitamins in various products and other foods may actually represent a modern day 'Fountain of Youth'. In an effort to beef up bodily defences to combat free radical activity, scientists are studying the effects of increasing the individual's antioxidant levels through diet and dietary supplements. A large number of compounds from various plant sources have been shown to possess antioxidant properties (Bhattacharya *et al,* 1996; Lee *et al,* 1996; Yen *et al,* 1996). Antioxidants of plant origin are vitamin E and C, selenium, phenolic compounds, carotenoids, flavonoids, etc. (Chanda, 1997). Vitamin C or L-ascorbic acid is considered to be the most important antioxidant in extracellular fluids (Stocker and Frei, 1991), and has many cellular activities of an antioxidant nature (Moser and Bendich, 1991). So ascorbic acid can protect biomembranes against peroxidation damage. Ascorbic acid can also act to protect membranes against peroxidation by enhancing the activity of a tocopherol, the chief lipid-soluble, chain-breaking antioxidant (Packer *et al,* 1979). Ascorbic acid reduces the tocopheroxyl radical and thereby restores the radical-scavenging activity of α-tocopherol (Lambelet *et al,* 1985).It has been assumed that nutritional intervention to increase intake of phyto-antioxidants may reduce threat of free radicals.

SPINACIA AND *AMARANTHUS*

Spinacia oleracea L. (Eng.–*Spinach*, Hindi–Palak) is a common herb, native of S. W. Asia. Leaves are eaten as vegetable. *Spinacia* is reported to be a good source of minerals, vitamin B-complex, vitamin K, ascorbic acid and β-carotene. Besides these, *Spinacia* also contains two important carotenoids, lutein and zeaxanthin. In plants, zeaxanthin has a well-accepted photoprotective role. When plants are exposed to excess light, zeaxanthin is synthesised and it helps to dissipate energy that cannot be used for photosynthesis so that the plant is protected from light damage. The observations have led to the conclusion that zeaxanthin is the carotenoid that protects the photosynthetic apparatus when photon flux density is high (Demmig 1990; Schubert *et al,* 1994). Lutein and zeaxanthin are structural isomers, differing only by the placement of one double bond. From *Spinacia* leaves, five new naturally occurring flavonoids have been isolated (Ferreres *et al,* 1997).

Researchers at the University of Utah Medical School found that people who eat plenty of lutein rich foods have a low risk of developing colon cancer. Zeaxanthin rich diets have been linked to lower risk of oesophageal cancer. According to a recent study, examining antioxidant levels in 40 common fruits and vegetables, wild blueberries, straw berries and *Spinacia* were top-rated. Interestingly the chemical structure of haemoglobin and chlorophyll are quite similar, therefore, in addition to being a good source of iron, *Spinacia* helps combat anaemia too. *Spinacia* and *Amaranthus* have high concentration of β-carotene and are easily available and therefore may prove efficient antioxidants.

In pre-Columban times *Amaranthus* grain was one of the basic foods of the New World nearly as important as corn and beans. Thousands of hectares of Aztec, Inca and other farmland were planted with the tall, leafy, reddish plants. Some 20,000 tons of *Amaranthus* grain were sent from 17 provinces to Tenochtitlan (present day Mexico City) in annual tribute to the Aztec emperor Montezuma (*Modern Prospects for an Ancient Crop*, 1984). With the passage of time, corn and beans became two of the leading crops that feed the world while grain *Amaranthus* faded into obscurity and today is largely forgotten.

To diversify the food base, we should not overlook lesser known indigenous crops such as *Amaranthus* which began attracting increased research attention in 1972 when Australian plant physiologist John Downton found that the seed also contains a protein of unusual quality. *Amaranthus* are broad brilliantly coloured leafy plants, one of the few non-grasses that produce significant amount of edible 'cereal' grain. They grow vigorously, resist drought, heat and pests and adapt readily to new environments, as weeds also that are inhospitable to conventional cereal crops. In the tropics, *Amaranthus* can be produced the year round with little effort. They afford a nutritious dish which contains abundant provitamin-A, the vitamin particularly necessary in the tropics for eye health. *Amaranthus* also produces protein efficiently. It is high in the amino acid lysine. Cereals are considered 'unbalanced' in terms of amino acid composition because generally they lack sufficient amounts of lysine for optimum health. *Amaranthus* protein, however, has nearly twice the lysine content of wheat protein, three times that of maize and, in fact, as much as is found in milk, the standard of nutritional excellence. It is, therefore, a nutritional complement to conventional cereals. *Amaranth* protein itself is low in leucine, but this amino acid is found in excess in conventional plant protein sources.

Amaranthus is gaining popularity also in the north-western plains of India as well as in the hills of southern India under the common names 'rajgira' (king seed), 'ramdana' (seed sent by god) and 'keerai'. In India, the family is represented by 17 genera and about 50 species. Familiar plants of this family are *Amaranthus blitum, Amaranthus paniculatus, Amaranthus gangeticus, Celosia argentea, Comphrena globosa, Achyranthes aspera* (Puthkanda).

The leaves are rich in protein as well as in vitamins and minerals; most *Amaranthus* species have edible leaves and several species are already widely used as potherbs (boiled greens). Over the years, growers have selected types with leaves and stems of high palatability. In recent taste tests at the U. S. Department of Agriculture in Beltsville, Maryland, most of 60 participants said that cooked *Amaranthus* leaves tasted at least as good as *Spinacia.* Their mild *Spinacia* like flavour, high yield, ability to grow in hot weather and high nutritive value have made *Amaranthus* a popular vegetable crop.

A future promise of vegetable *Amaranth* is the development of leaf protein concentrates. Compared with most other species, *Amaranth* leaf protein is highly extractable. In one trial, *Amaranthus* had the highest level of extractable protein among 24 plant species studied. During the extraction of leaf protein, most other nutrients are extracted as well; for example, provitamin-A (β-carotene), polyunsaturated lipids (linoleic acid) and iron. Harmful compounds are eliminated, as they remain in the soluble phase. The resulting leaf nutrient concentrate is especially useful for young children and other persons with particularly high protein, vitamin A and iron needs. The protein quality of the *Amaranthus* leaf nutrient concentrate (determined by amino acid composition, digestibility and nutritional effectiveness) is excellent. It has been assumed that nutritional intervention to increase intake of phyto-antioxidants may reduce threat of free radicals. Out of these, β-carotene has excellent antioxidant property. *Amaranthus* has 14,190 mg/100 gm of carotene and *Spinacia* has 5,580 mg/100 gm of carotene present (Gopalan *et al*, 1996).

The carotenoids are brightly yellow to red pigments occurring in plants and are introduced into humans and animals through dietary intake of vegetables and fruits. These are synthesised by higher plants and belong to the group of 'fat soluble' antioxidant vitamins (electron donors). Carotenoids are important micronutrients for human health (Casten Miller and West, 1998). So far, almost 600 carotenoids have been identified and described. In addition to their provitamin-A activity, carotenoids may have several other important biological functions in animals and man (Van-vliet, 1996). Of the two major carotenoid families, the hydrocarbon and the xanthophylls carotenoids (oxygenated carotenoids), the hydrocarbon carotenoids are more likely to have provitamin-A activity with b-carotene being the most active. Evidence is available that b-carotene can indeed function as an effective radical trapping antioxidant (Burton and Ingold, 1984; Gerster, 1993; Bhatia, 1996, 1998; Sisodia *et al,* 1999). The role of vitamin A and β-carotene in protection against radiomimetic drugs was indicated by Seifter and collaborators (1984). Antioxidant capacity of β-carotene is linked to the length of its polyene chain as indicated in Figure 1.

Non-beta carotene carotenoids possessing also at least seven to nine conjugated bonds became candidates as singlet oxygen quenchers and free radical scavengers. The quenching efficiency of carotenoids increases with increasing numbers of conjugated bonds (Conn *et al,* 1991).

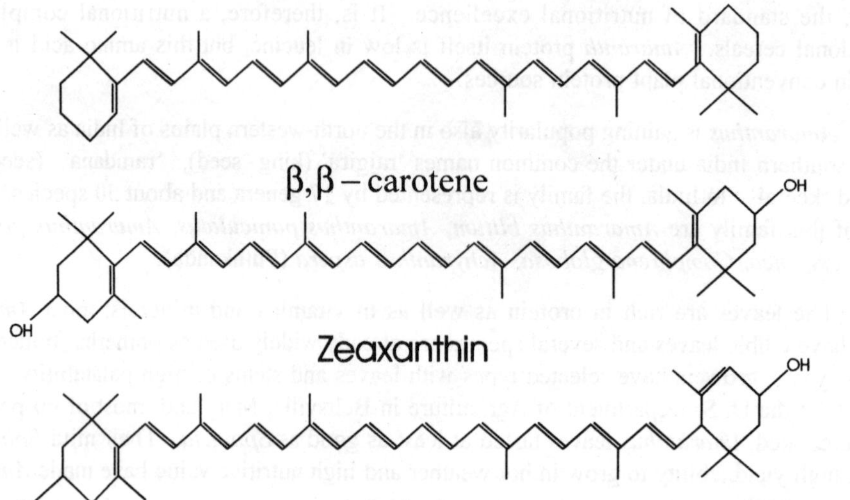

Figure 1. Chemical structures of carotene family members.

Flavonoids are known to display a broad array of pharmacological and biochemical actions (Middleton and Kandaswami, 1992, 1993). The flavonoids are typical phenolic compounds and powerful chain-breaking antioxidants (Torel *et al,* 1986; Pratt, 1992) occurring widely in the plant kingdom and are especially common in leaves, flowering tissues and woody parts such as stems and barks (Mc Clure *et al,* 1975).

Mentha extract has shown to have antioxidant and anti-peroxidant properties due to the presence of eugenol, caffeic acid, rosmarinic acid and α-tocopherol (Rastogi and Mehrotra, 1991; Krishnaswamy and Raghuramulu, 1998; Al-Sereiti *et al,* 1999). The aqueous extract has also been screened for antibacterial activity against *Pseudomonas solanacearum* (Lirio *et al,* 1998). Recently, Aqil *et al* (2001) evaluated anti-fungal activity peppermint oil against *Aspergillus niger*, *Alternaria alternata* and *Fusarium chlamydosporum*.

Cucurmin, containing a double bond in conjugation with phenyl ring is a powerful radical scavenger (Elizabeth and Rao, 1990). Graf (1992) has showed that the feluric acid present in plants, due to its phenolic nucleus and an extended side chain conjugation, readily forms a resonance stabilised phenoxyl radical which accounts for its potent antioxidant potential. Rajakumar and Rao (1993) have demonstrated that isoeugenol, which has a conjugated double bond, is a good radical scavenger. They suggested that the double bond in conjugation with the phenyl ring plays an important role in the antioxidant activity of this compound. Cotelle *et al* (1993) opined that polyphenolic flavonoids inhibit lipid peroxidation by forming less reactive aryloxyl radicals with free radicals.

Besides being an antioxidant and precursor to vitamin A, β-carotene may be more important in our diet than vitamin A for the following reason. People with low tissue levels of β-carotene were found to be usually prone towards getting a number of different types of cancer (Peto *et al,*

1981). It has therefore been recommended that β-carotene be used for protection against different types of human cancers and photosynthesised oxidative damage because free radicals and related reactive species may be some part in these pathology. As radiation damage also occurs due to the attack of free radicals on cell membranes, decrease or removal of free radicals might lead to a decrease in the extent of damage.

RADIOPROTECTORS OF PLANT ORIGIN

A major concern regarding synthetic chemical radioprotectors is their inherent toxicity. Research on the chemical radioprotectors needs to be expanded to include studies on the drugs which could prevent radiation induced behavioural disruption and performance decrement as well as studies on the agents that could modify the behavioural toxicity of radioprotectors (Bogo, 1988). The most effective protectors have the greatest behavioural side effects, as measured by alterations in locomotor activity (Landauer *et al*, 1989).

Recently, interest has been generated to develop the potential drugs of plant origin for modification of radiation effects. Plant products appear to have an advantage over the synthetic compounds in terms of low/no toxicity at the effective dose and have minimum/no side effects.

Radioprotection by various plant products has been studied by several workers (Bhargava and Singh, 1981; Singh *et al*, 1991; Tshyb and Yarmonenko, 1991; Sen *et al*, 1992; Uma Devi and Ganasoundri, 1995; Singh *et al*, 1995; Arora and Goel, 2000). Singh *et al* (1995) observed LD50/30 for *Chlorella vulgaris* E-25 (algae mutant) in pre- and post- treated mice to 8.66 and 9.0 Gy, respectively, compared to control value of 7.80 Gy and the dose reduction factor (DRF) as 1.11 and 1.15 for pre- and post- treated mice, respectively. Uma Devi *et al.* (1999) observed that two flavonoids, orientin and vicenin, isolated from the leaves of the Indian plant *Ocimum sanctum* provided protection against death from gastrointestinal syndrome as well as bone marrow syndrome when injected intraperitoneally before whole-body exposure to 11 Gy gamma radiation.

Saini *et al* (1978) showed radioprotection in Swiss albino mice after treating the animals with herbal formulation Liv.52. Daga *et al* (1995) found Liv.52 to be effective against radiation induced haematological alterations in Swiss albino mice and reported that pre-administration of Liv.52 significantly protects the erythrocyte counts in peripheral blood. Gupta (1988) showed hypolipidemic action of garlic unsaturated oils in irradiated mice. Farooqui and Kesavan (1992) observed caffeine as a radioprotector against radiation induced damage in mice after whole-body gamma irradiation. Hebbar *et al* (2001) also advocated the potent radioprotective action of caffeine in terms of survival of lethally whole-body irradiated mice.

Ginseng is one of those plants which has shown to be effective on radiation caused bone marrow death (Takeda *et al*, 1982). Pande *et al* (1998a) reported the radioprotective effect of ginseng and *Aloe vera* in Swiss albino mice (Pande *et al*, 1998b). Radioprotective effect of *Ocimum sanctum* extract has also been reported in mice (Ganasoundari *et al*, 1997; Uma Devi *et al*, 1999; Uma Devi *et al*, 2000). Radiomodifying effects of root extract of *Withania somnifera* and *Plumbago rosea* have been reported by Ganasoundari *et al* (1997) and Uma Devi *et al* (1999). Goel *et al* (1999) showed protective effects of an aqueous extract of roots of *Podophyllum hexandrum* against radiation damage in Swiss albino mice.

Rutin was capable of modifying membrane dependent processes such as free radical induced membrane lipid peroxidation (Saija *et al*, 1995). Shimoi *et al* (1996) conclude that plant flavonoids

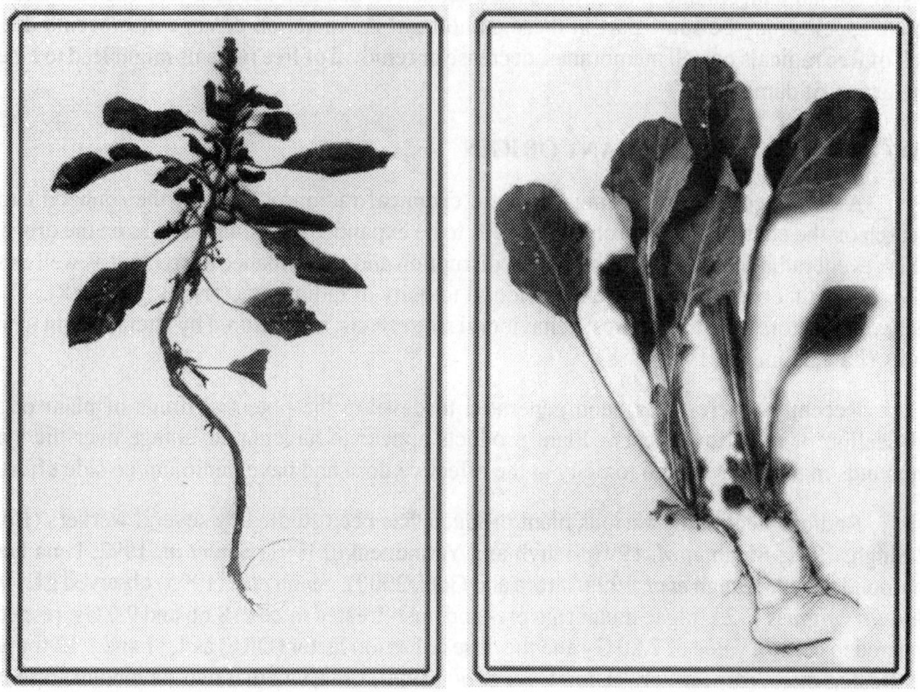

***Amaranthus paniculatus* Linn.**
Family—Amaranthaceae
RUBHL No. 19866

***Spinacia oleracea* L.**
Family—Chenopodiaceae
RUBHL No. 19867

Figure 2. Amaranthus and Spinach.

which show antioxidant activity *in vitro* also function as antioxidants *in vivo*, and their radioprotective effect may be attributed to their radical scavenging activity. The aqueous extract of the *Ocimum* leaves, containing orientin and vicenin flavonoids, has also been claimed to have radioprotective effects *in vivo* and antioxidant activity *in vitro* (Uma Devi and Ganasoundari, 1995; Ganasoundari *et al*, 1997; Uma Devi *et al*, 2000). The cellular radiation damage is markedly modified by natural free radical scavengers like α-tocopherol and carotenoids or by membrane structural agent cholesterol (Pandey and Mishra, 1999).

Rasayans is a group of drug preparations used in Ayurvedic system of medicine to improve the health of the body (Singh, 1990). Kumar *et al* (1996) observed that the oral administration of Rasayans protected mice from radiation induced leucopenia and reduced the formation of lipid peroxidase in liver as compared to controls. Pre-treatment of some antioxidants like curcumin, bixin, ellagic acid and α-tocopherol before exposure to gamma rays, significantly declined the serum and lipid peroxidase enzymes (Thresiamma *et al*, 1996).

Liv.52 (a non-toxic herbal preparation) has been reported to be clinically effective in treating hepato-toxicity and a wide range of hepatic disorders of different etiology (Sule *et al*, 1968). More recently, Saxena (1997) observed its hepato-protective role against irradiation and/or methylmercuric chloride (MMC) intoxication.

SPECIAL STUDIES WITH REFERENCE TO *AMARANTHUS* AND *SPINACIA*

Fruits and vegetables are key sources of antioxidants, nutrients that disarm harmful molecules (free radicals), the undesirable by-products of various metabolic functions. Free radicals damage over a time is called oxidative stress. It is believed to play a leading role in certain diseases and age-related changes. Although the body also produces antioxidants, over time, its production declines. Nutritional intervention with fruits and vegetables may play an important role in protecting against and possibly reversing the cognitive declines seen from ageing. To determine whether an increase in antioxidant rich fruit and vegetable consumption might offset these age-related declines in antioxidant production, and their consequences, the present study has been undertaken.

Twenty five foods cultivated and consumed by the tribals of Andhra Pradesh, India, comprising cereals/millets, legumes, tubers and miscellaneous foods collected seasonally from 20 tribal villages were analysed by Rajyalakshmi and Geervani (1994) for proximate composition, vitamins and minerals. Among the miscellaneous foods analysed, rajgeera seed (*Amaranthus paniculatus*) had protein content of 22 g per 100 g.

In this context, recently work has been started on antioxidant rich fruits and vegetables. *Amaranthus* and spinach have been top-rated as they are rich in antioxidant properties which may be due to presence of large quantity of β-carotene and other constituents known to possess antioxidant properties.

It has been reported that *Amaranthus paniculatus* (Linn.) contains good natural sources of carotenoids (14,190 μg/100 gm of edible portion), vitamin C, folate, folic acid, high level of nutritional critical lysine and methionine amino acid, protein content (22 gm/100 gm of edible portion) and promising oil composition with regard to polyunsaturated fatty acid [Prakash *et al,* 1995, 2000; Guil *et al,* 1997, Special Series No. 42 ICMR; Rajyalakshmi and Geervani, 1994). *Amaranthus* contains provitamin-A (β-carotene), vitamin C, E and riboflavin (Vietmeyer, 1983; Krishnaswamy and Raghuramulu, 1998). Bergman *et al* (2001) studied the chemical identity of several of these antioxidant components in water extract of spinach leaves. The study demonstrated for the first time the presence of both flavonoids and P-coumaric acid derivatives as antioxidant components in the aqueous extract of spinach leaves.

The foliage of 62 specimens of *Amaranthus* belonging to 10 species of grain and four of vegetable type were analysed by Prakash *et al* (1995) for vitamin C content. Most of the specimens had promising oil composition with regard to unsaturated fatty acids. Devadas Rajammal *et al* (1996) studied the consumption pattern of β-carotene rich foods from 500 households of Coimbatore district. The total β-carotene contents of five commonly consumed β-carotene rich food, both in raw and cooked states were determined. Results indicated that amaranth tender (*Amaranthus gangeticus*) and ponnanganni (*Alternanthera sessilis*) were one of the carotene-rich foods available round the year.

Amaranthus has been found to affect absorption of cholesterol and bile acids, cholesterol lipoprotein distribution, hepatic cholesterol content and cholesterol biosynthesis whereas *amaranth* grain and oil did not affect these pathways identically (Berger *et al*, 2003). Lowering of non-HDL cholesterol and raising HDL cholesterol by *Amaranthus* grain or oil (5 per cent); it decreased total and non-high-density lipoprotein (HDL) cholesterol by 15 and 22 per cent, respectively. *Amaranth* grain (20 per cent; providing 1.4 per cent *Amaranthus* oil) was found to decrease very low-density lipoprotein (VLDL) cholesterol by 21-50 per cent; and increased fecal excretion of particular neutral sterols and the bile acid ursodeoxycholate. *Amaranthus* oil (5 per cent) additionally increased the cholesterol synthesis rate, possibly due to compensatory mechanisms; and decreased hepatic cholesterol ester, indicating reduced cholesterol ester availability for VLDL secretion and consistency with reduced VLDL cholesterol.

The fish fed on diets containing *Amaranthus* seeds at different levels showed better growth than the control, because of the good-quality proteins available in *Amaranthus* seeds (Virk and Saxena, 2003). Growth in terms of body weight gain was maximum in fish fed on diets containing 20 per cent *Amaranthus* seeds, that replaced rice bran and groundnut oil cake in the feed. In the two species used, *Labino rohita* showed better growth performance than *Cyprinus carpio*. *Amaranthus* seeds were used at three different levels (20 per cent, 35 per cent, 50 per cent) in fish diets under a semi-intensive fish culture system and their impact on the growth of common carp, *Cyprinus carpio*, and rohu, *Labeo rohita*, was studied.

Klimczak *et al* (2002) reported the antioxidant activity of ethanolic extracts of *Amaranthus* seeds. Antioxidant activity of ethanolic extracts obtained from two *Amaranthus* species was evaluated in a beta-carotene-linoleic acid model system. Addition of *Amaranthus* extracts in the range of 0.01-0.1 per cent inhibited degradation of a beta-carotene in a model emulsion during incubation at 60 degrees C; 0.05 per cent addition of *Amaranthus* seeds extract was proposed as practically applicable. The total content of phenolic compounds was estimated by the Folin-Ciocalteu method and ranged from 39.17 mg/100 g of *Amaranthus caudatus* to 56.22 mg/100 g of *Amaranthus paniculatus* seeds. Free phenolic acids contained in ethanolic extracts of *Amaranthus*seeds were purified and isolated by solid-phase extraction (SPE) and identified by reversed-phase high-performance liquid chromatography (RP-HPLC). The technique involved gave a good separation of the free phenolic acids in the *Amaranthus* seeds. Significant differences in phenolic acid profiles of both *amaranth* species were observed. Lipid peroxidation and anti-oxidative defence system in blood, liver and heart tissues, nitric oxide metabolites content in brain tissue of rats under binary action of small-doses of ionising radiation and fluoride intoxication treated by *amaranth* oil and interval hypoxic training have been studied by Konyk *et al,* (2002). Complex using of *amaranth* oil and interval hypoxic training results in increase of both enzymatic, as non-enzymatic links of antioxidant defence in all investigated tissues. This complex can be used for binary action of ionising radiation and fluoride intoxication correction. It was revealed that it also enhanced NO system metabolites content in brain gomogenate. In these conditions, lipid peroxidation processes in liver and heart tissues normalise in comparison to essential increase level LPO under binary action influence. It is supposed that complex using of *amaranth* oil and interval hypoxic training results in increase of organism adaptive possibility.

Amaranthus paniculatus (Linn.) proves efficient antioxidants (Bhatia and Jain, 2003). To evaluate its anti-oxidative efficacy, healthy Swiss albino mice from an inbred colony were selected and divided into three groups having equal number of males and females in each group. All of these animals were initially trained in Hebb William's Maze, model D[1]. After initial training of 10 days, two groups were supplemented with methanolic extract of *Amaranthus paniculatus* (Linn.) at a dose of 600 and 800 mg/kg bw per day, respectively for 15 days. One group without any treatment served as normal. It has been observed that mice, supplemented with extract took lesser time to reach the goal (Figure 3) than normal (without any treatment). Furthermore, after supplementation of *Amaranthus*, followed by exposure to 9 Gy of gamma radiation by 60Co beam therapy unit, the survived mice took lesser time to reach their goal than those without plant extract. Control mice (not supplemented with AE extract) showed continuous decline in their learning performance. Mice of control group died within 12 days after exposure. Irradiated males try to recover from the tenth day onwards but they died up to day 12. But in experimental mice (AE treated), after initial decline in learning ability after exposure, recovery was noticed and not only this 70 per cent of them survived beyond the observation period (Figures 4, 5). Male mice showed faster learning ability as compared to females in all groups. After irradiation too, the males took lesser time to reach their goals. Learning in all the groups before exposure has been much faster between nine and 15 days. After radiation, however, it was followed by a sudden spurt and delayed learning response up to 12 days. Recovery was greater in males than females in treated groups. Recovery was greater in males of 600 mg/kg bw per day than other groups. Learning has been almost at the same level from the 14th day onwards, which indicates that both the dose levels have been found equally effective.

Amaranthus gangeticus Linn., widely considered as a weed, has been found to protect brain biochemical activity in mouse and may prove beneficial for clinical use as a radioprotector (Verma *et al*, 2002). To evaluate the anti-oxidative efficacy of *Amaranthus*, healthy Swiss albino mice from an inbred colony were treated with alcoholic extract of *Amaranthus gangeticus* leaves (AE) for two weeks, at 800 mg/kg body weight, before radiation exposure. Irradiated mice were examined and autopsied at intervals of 1, 3, 7, 15 and 30 days after exposure. Brain was removed by skull dissection, and various biochemical changes were sought. Radiation caused a maximum increase of 27 per cent in LPO and a maximum decrease of 27.96 per cent in protein content at day seven in controls. However, in the experimental group, the increase in LPO was 9.98 per cent and the increase in protein content was 18.78 per cent at day seven. By day 30 after irradiation, AE brought these values to near-normal levels.

The cholesterol content of eggs got reduced by diet manipulation, using two naturally available and already proved hypocholesteromic agents, red palm oil (RPO) and grain *Amarantus* (Punita and Chaturvedi, 2000). Thirteen experimental rations using raw and popped grain *Amarantus* and RPO were fed to 24 week-old hens for a period of six weeks, singularly and in combination. Total lipids, cholesterol and PUFA contents were analysed in the experimental and control eggs. The results showed that RPO and RPO+ popped *Amarantus* feeding resulted in a maximum reduction in total lipids and cholesterol contents. Significant increase was observed in linoleic acid content in RPO+ popped *Amarantus*; raw *Amarantus* and RPO-fed groups.

Yadav and Sehgal (1995) studied the concentration of ascorbic acid and beta-carotene in spinach and *Amarantus* leaves as affected by various domestic processing and cooking methods which included storage of leaves in polythene bags or without packing for 24 and 48 hours in refrigerator at 5°C; at 30°C in polythene bags; drying (sun and oven); blanching (5, 10, 15 minutes); open pan and pressure cooking. Ascorbic acid content of fresh leaves was 624.1 to 629.0 mg and beta-carotene content was 35.3 to 53.1 mg/100 g dry weight. The per cent loss of ascorbic acid ranged from 1.1 to 6.3 and 55.3 to 65.9 while lower losses (0.0 to 1.3 and 1.5 to 2.1) of beta-carotene were observed in leaves stored in refrigerator and at 30°C, respectively. A markedly greater reduction in ascorbic acid and beta-carotene was observed in dried, blanched and cooked

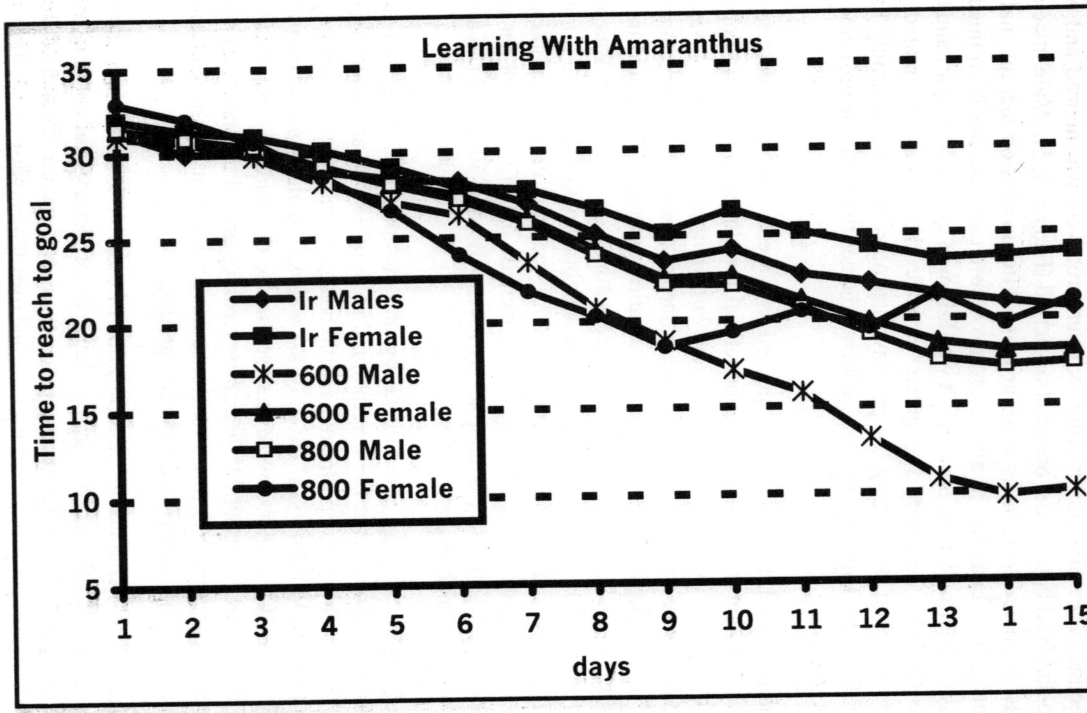

Figure 3. Protection by *Amaranthus* against irradiation: Linear trends of time (sec.) taken by 15-day *Amaranthus paniculatus* L. pre-treated and trained male and female mice after gamma radiation exposure to 9Gy on day 0. Note that the regression coefficients are best for irradiated males and females which died by 15th day of observation. However, the *Amaranthus*-fed animals survived against radiation-induced damage and the value of 'y' shows greater consistency in relation to their learning in terms of time to reach the goal.

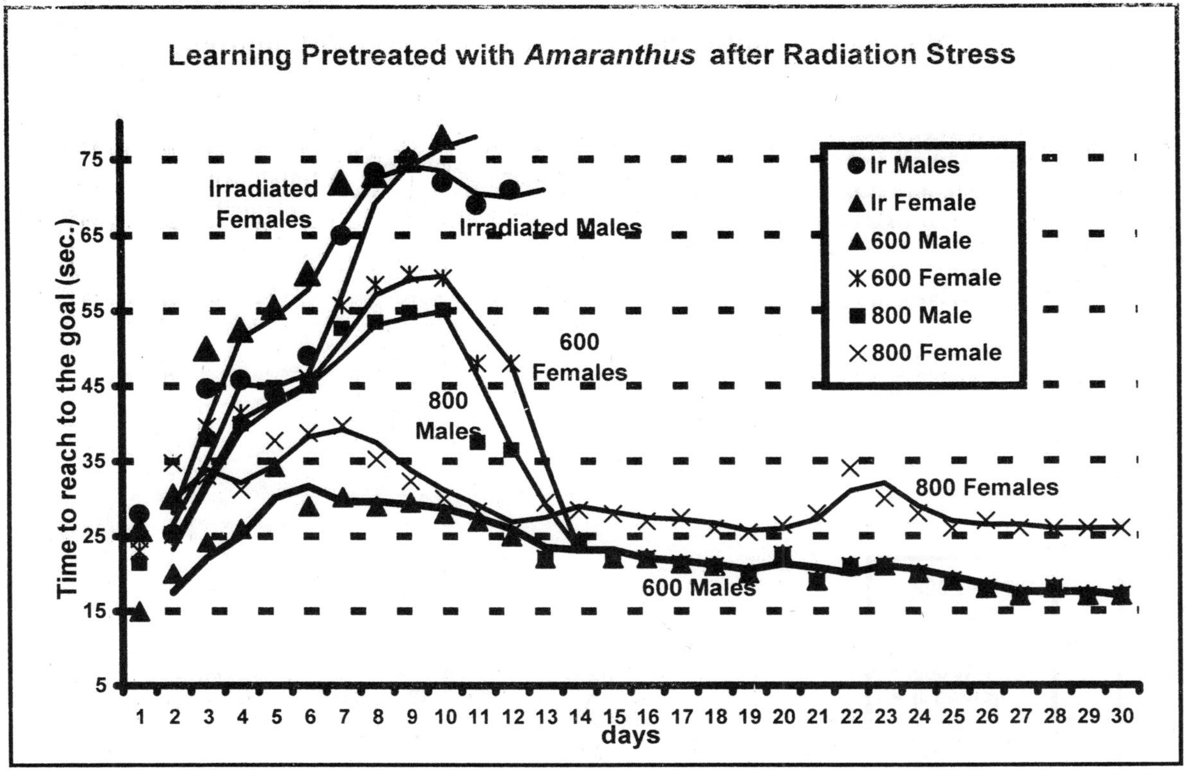

Figure 4. Protection by *Amaranthus* against irradiation: Time (sec.) taken by 15 days *Amaranthus paniculatus* L. pretreated and trained male and female mice to reach the goal after gamma radiation exposure in 9Gy on day 0. Note that 600 mg/day resulted in the best learning in males against radiation induced changes.

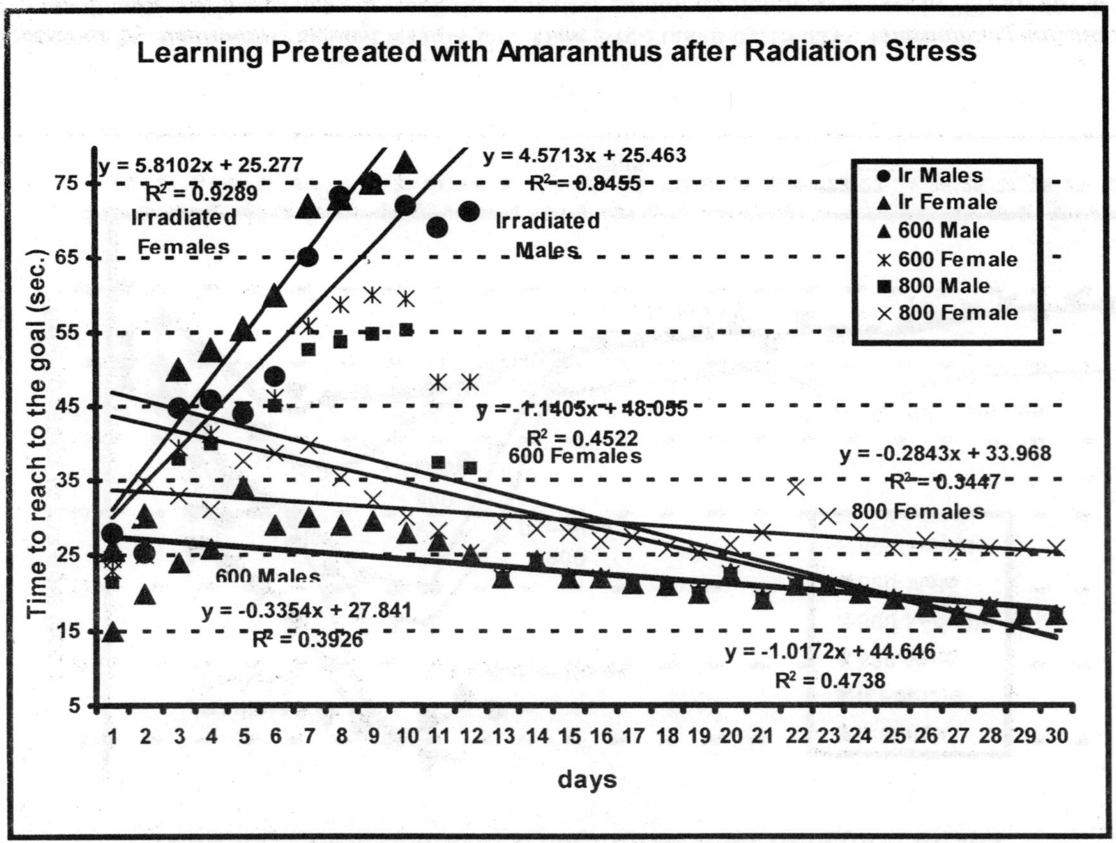

Figure 5. Learning in mice with different doses of *Amaranthus*: Time (sec.) taken by 10 days trained miced and female mice before irradiation to reach the goal during daily administration of *Amaranthus paniculatus* L. extract orally. Note the dose 600 mg/day resulted in better learning in male mice in 15 days period.

leaves. The study recommended the storage of leaves in refrigerator, drying in oven, blanching for shorter time and cooking in pressure cooker for better retention of these two vitamins.

Spinacia oleracea L. (English–Spinach; Hindi-Punjabi–Palak) belonging to family Chenopodiaceae is a commonly occurring herb and is reported to be good source of minerals, vitamin B complex, ascorbic acid, carotenoids (β-carotene, lutein, zeaxanthine), flavonoids, apocyanin and p-coumaric acid (Bergman *et al*, 2001; Gerster, 1993; Zennie and Dwayne, 1977; Burton and Ingold, 1989). Whole plant is used for remedy of urinary calculi and leaves are used for bowel and lung inflammations, fibrile affliction, cooling (Jain and Fillips, 1991).

Raw spinach is a healthy addition to salads, but to get the full benefit from this leafy green it should be cooked at least some of the time. Cooking makes the antioxidant carotenoids responsible for much of spinach's nutritional potency easier for the body to absorb. Spinach was shown to be effective in preventing age-related dopamine decrease, and maintaining the ability to remove calcium ions from the cell. Spinach helped with water maze performance, possibly because this task requires visual input, and spinach is known to preserve vision.

Spinach contains a very effective natural antioxidant system (NAO) which is claimed to be capable of preventing lipid peroxidation both in plant and animal systems (Grossman *et al*, 1994). The potential physiological role of NAO as an antioxidant was shown in several *in vitro* and *in vivo* systems (Grossman *et al*, 1994; Lomnitski *et al*, 2000a, 2000b, 2000c; Zurovsky *et al*, 1994). Its efficacy in preventing lipid-peroxidation in the skin of mice, rats and humans has been reported (Grossman *et al*, 1994). Recently, the efficacy of NAO in preventing LPS-induced hepatic injury both in rats and rabbits was demonstrated (Ben-Shaul *et al*, 1999; Lomnitski *et al*, 2000).

Presence of flavonoid-like compounds in spinach was first reported by Weatherky and Cheng (1943). Zane and Wender (1961) established the structure of isolated flavonoid from spinach leaves as patuletin and also described the presence of spinacetin in this extract. Aritomi *et al* (1986) reported the presence of seven flavonol glycosides in the methanolic extract of spinach leaves. Ferreres *et al* (1997) isolated and identified five novel naturally occurring flavonoids from alcoholic extracts of spinach leaves. Studies of Bergman *et al* (2001) indicate that several of the flavonoids and new naturally occurring compounds are present in the water extract of spinach leaves and contribute to its anti-oxidant activity.

Flavonoids (as also present in spinach) are known to display a broad array of pharmacological and biochemical actions (Middleton and Kandaswami, 1992). The flavonoids are typical phenolic compounds and powerful chain-breaking antioxidants (Torel *et al*, 1986). It was reported that lipid peroxidation can be inhibited by flavonoids possibly through their activity as strong 0_2^- Scavengers (Baumann *et al*, 1980) and singlet oxygen quenchers (Sorata *et al*, 1984). The ability of some phenolic compounds to act as antioxidant has been shown (Velioglu *et al*, 1998). Flavonoids are reported to possess anti-tumour promoter (Fujiki *et al*, 1986), anti-metastatic (Bracke *et al*, 1988) and anti-proliferative (Kandaswami *et al*, 1991) properties. Shimoi *et al* (1994) demonstrated that some plant flavonoids protect against radiation-induced micronucleus formation. Several naturally-occurring flavonoids have been reported to have antioxidant properties and to scavenge free radicals (Husain *et al*, 1987; Robak and Gryglewski, 1988; Hu *et al*, 1995). Shimoi *et al* (1996) attributed the radioprotective effect of antioxidant plant flavonoids to their ability to scavenge free radicals. Copper, manganese and zinc contents are present in maximum amounts in *Spinacia* (Singh *et al*, 2001). Adequate zinc supplementation inhibits lipid peroxidation and has been described as an antioxidant. Increased availability of Zn, Cu, Mn results in increased/ proper activity of Cu Zn SOD and Mn/Fe SOD.

In addition to the flavonoids, the spinach extract was found to contain derivatives of the isomers of p-coumaric acid. P-coumaric derivatives are very strong antioxidants. The presence of p-coumaroyl-meso-tartric acid detected in spinach leaves in large amounts was reported by Winter and Herrmann (1986).

Molnar *et al* (1995) determined selenium concentrations via hydride generation atomic absorption spectrometry in more than 100 convenience fast foods including 34 vegetarian dishes. The foods were purchased mainly in Ayrshire, Scotland, but few of them came from other parts of the U. K. The results indicate a considerable amount of selenium in certain mushrooms, spinach, fish, offal and chicken-based products. The selenium content of beef and pork-based products was generally somewhat lower. Vegetarians having a sufficient intake of mushrooms (in particular button and closed cap mushrooms) and spinach do not seem to be at risk of selenium deficiency provided of course that the selenium in mushrooms, in particular, is bioavailable.

Observed beneficial effects of increased vegetable intake may be contributed by carotenoids, folate and vitamin C. Currently, knowledge on the bioavailability of these compounds from vegetables is limited. Van het Hof KH *et al* (2000) compared the efficacy of different vegetables at the same level of intake (that is, 300 g/d), in increasing plasma levels of carotenoids, folate and vitamin C and they investigated that disruption of the vegetable matrix would enhance the bioavailability of these micronutrients. Bioavailability of lutein and folate from spinach can be improved by disruption of the vegetable matrix.

Guil *et al* (1997) studied the nutritional (ascorbic acid, dehydroascorbic acid and carotenes), anti-nutritional and toxic components (oxalic acid, nitrate and nitric acid) determined in 16 popular species of wild edible plants, which were collected for human consumption in South East Spain. Carotenoid content was 15.4 mg/100 g and nitrate contents were 597 mg/100 g in *Amaranthus viridis* L.

Perring *et al* (1997) reported that people aged of 65 and older, having higher ascorbic acid and beta carotene plasma level showed better memory performance. Castenmiller *et al* (2000) studied the effect of the food matrix and dietary fibre on the bioavailability of folate. In a controlled, three-week dietary intervention study, two men and 42 women were divided into six groups to receive either a control diet (n = 10), or the control diet plus 20 g/MJ per day (n = 12 per group) of whole-leaf spinach, minced spinach or liquefied spinach to which dietary fibre (10 g/kg wet weight) was added. The sixth group received the control diet plus a synthetic carotenoid supplement with similar amounts of β-carotene and lutein as found in spinach. A significantly higher plasma folate response was found for the pooled spinach groups than for the control group. Among the spinach groups no significant differences were detected. However, the plasma folate response of the pooled minced and liquefied spinach groups was greater than that of the whole-leaf spinach group ($p = 0.03$). Re-addition of dietary fibre to the liquefied spinach to compensate for the fibre broke down during liquefaction did not reduce the plasma folate response. The consumption of the carotenoid supplement did not have an effect on plasma folate concentrations compared with the control group. The food matrix in which the folate is entrapped plays a role in folate bioavailability.

Spinach portions augmented satiety and reduced the post-prandial glucose response. The total satiety scores seemed to be correlated positively to both the dietary fibre and the water content in the vegetable (Gustafsson *et al*, 1995).

Bickford *et al* (2000) reported that diets supplemented with either spinach, strawberries, blue berries, nutritional sources of antioxidants, reverse age induced decline in beta-adrenergic receptor function in cerebellar purkinje neurons measured using electrophysiological techniques. The spinach diet improved learning on a run way motor task, previously shown to be modulated by cerebellar nor-epinephrine.

Increased vulnerability to oxidative stress may be the major factor involved in CNS functional declines in ageing and age-related neurodegenerative diseases, and that antioxidants, for example, vitamin E, may ameliorate or prevent these declines. Joseph *et al* (1998) examined whether long-term feeding of Fischer 344 rats, beginning when the rats were six months of age and continuing for eight months, with diets supplemented with a fruit or vegetable extract identified as being high in antioxidant activity, could prevent the age-related induction of receptor-mediated signal transduction deficits that might have a behavioural component. Thus, the following parameters were examined: (1). oxotremorine-enhanced striatal dopamine release (OX-K+-ERDA), (2). cerebellar beta receptor augmentation of GABA responding, (3). striatal synaptosomal 45Ca2+ clearance, (4). carbachol-stimulated GTPase activity, and (5). Morris water maze performance. The rats were given control diets or those supplemented with strawberry extracts (SE), 9.5 gm/kg dried aqueous extract (DAE), spinach (SPN 6.4 gm/kg DAE), or vitamin E (500 IU/kg). Results indicated that SPN-fed rats demonstrated the greatest retardation of age-effects on all parameters except GTPase activity, on which SE had the greatest effect, whereas SE and vitamin E showed significant but equal protection against these age-induced deficits on the other parameters. For example, OX-K+-ERDA enhancement was four times greater in the SPN group than in controls. Thus, phytochemicals present in antioxidant-rich foods such as spinach may be beneficial in retarding functional age-related CNS and cognitive behavioural deficits and, perhaps, may have some benefit in neuro-degenerative disease.

Cytochrome b (6) f complex with stoichiometrically bound β-carotene molecule was purified from spinach chloroplasts by Yan *et al* (2001). The configuration of this beta-carotene was studied by reversed-phase HPLC and resonance Raman spectroscopy. Both the absorption spectrum of this β-carotene in dissociated state and the Raman spectrum in native state could be unambiguously assigned top a 9-cis configuration. This finding was in contrast to the predominantly all-trans isomers commonly found in that the 9-cis β-carotene is an authentic component and may have a unique structural and functional role in cytochrome b(6) f complex.

Singh *et al* (2001) analysed six green leafy vegetables and herbs—spinach, amaranth, Bengal gram, cauliflower, mint, coriander and carrots for moisture, protein, ascorbic acid, beta-carotene, total iron, ionisable iron (as percentage of total iron) *in vitro* iron (percentage of total iron), copper, manganese and zinc. Moisture content of the leaves and carrots varied from 75.1 per cent (Bengal gram) to 95.4 per cent (carrot) and protein from 9.83 per cent (carrots) to 30.9 (mint) per cent. Ascorbic acid, beta-carotene, total iron and ionisable iron contents were at a maximum in case of Bengal gram leaves whereas level of ionisable iron and *in vitro* iron as a per cent of total iron was highest in carrots. Copper, manganese and zinc contents were maximum in spinach.

Antioxidant-rich fruits and vegetables are plentiful in the summer when sweet peaches, juicy tomatoes and just-picked corn are easily available. Fortunately, some of the best sources of antioxidants are at their peak during the autumn and winter months. According to laboratory tests by researchers at the Human Nutrition Research Centre on Ageing at Tufts University, the vegetables kale, beets, spinach and Brussels sprouts, as well as oranges, were ranked among the most potent weapons against free radicals—the cell-damaging compounds believed to accelerate ageing and contribute to heart disease, cancer and other diseases. The test, called oxygen radical absorbance capacity, or ORAC, measures the total antioxidant potency of foods or supplements. It is a more precise way of determining the free radical-destroying power of a food than just focusing on individual nutrients, because ORAC takes into consideration the effect of all of the plant's compounds—including many phytochemicals that are not traditionally considered nutrients—and the impact they have when they work in concert. Very simply, a sample of a food or a chemical substance (such as vitamin E) is put in a test tube to measure how well and for how long it disarms free radicals. The test substance is then given an ORAC score that reflects its power. The researchers estimate that the average person's daily ORAC intake from diet alone is about 1,200 units. In a study of 36 older people, boosting fruit and vegetable intake to reach 3,200 ORAC units a day increased the antioxidant potential of the blood by 10 to 15 per cent—enough to have an impact on disease prevention. The researchers think most people should strive to consume 1,000 to 2,500 ORAC units above what they currently get.

Regularly consumed fruits and vegetables of mixed varieties available on the U. K. market were analysed by Proteggente *et al* (2002) for the composition of the major individual phenolic components. The total phenolic content (applying the Folin assay) and the vitamin C levels were also determined. The antioxidant capacities of aqueous/methanolic extracts were comparatively assessed. The results were calculated in terms of 100 g fresh weight (FW) uncooked portion sizes. Fruit and vegetables rich in anthocyanins (for example, strawberry, raspberry and red plum) demonstrated the highest antioxidant activities, followed by those rich in flavanones (for example, orange and grapefruit) and flavonols (for example, onion, leek, spinach and green cabbage), while the hydroxycinnamate-rich fruit (for example, apple, tomato, pear and peach) consistently elicited the lower antioxidant activities. The antioxidant activities (TEAC) in terms of 100 g FW uncooked portion size were in the order: strawberry >> raspberry = red plum >> red cabbage >>> grapefruit = orange > spinach > broccoli > green grape approximately/= onion > green cabbage > pea > apple > cauliflower, tomato approximately/= peach = leek > banana approximately/= lettuce.

Castenmiller *et al* (1999) examined the effect of variously processed spinach products and of dietary fibre on serum carotenoid concentrations, subjects received, over a three-week period, a control diet (n = 10) or a control diet supplemented with carotenoids or one of four spinach products (n = 12 per group): whole leaf spinach with an almost intact food matrix, minced spinach with the matrix partially disrupted, enzymatically liquefied spinach in which the matrix was further disrupted and the liquefied spinach to which dietary fibre (10 g/kg wet weight) was added. Consumption of spinach significantly increased serum concentrations of all-trans-beta-carotene, cis-beta-carotene (and consequently total beta-carotene), lutein, alpha-carotene and retinol and decreased the serum concentration of lycopene. Serum total beta-carotene responses (changes in serum concentrations from the start to the end of the intervention period) differed significantly between the whole leaf and liquefied spinach groups and between the minced and liquefied spinach groups. The lutein response did not differ among spinach groups. Addition of dietary fibre to the liquefied spinach had no effect on serum carotenoid responses. The relative bioavailability as compared to bioavailability of the carotenoid supplement for whole leaf, minced, liquefied and liquefied spinach plus added dietary fibre for beta-carotene was 5.1, 6.4, 9.5 and 9.3 per cent, respectively, and for lutein 45, 52, 55 and 54 per cent, respectively. Bioavailability of lutein from spinach was higher than that of beta-carotene and that enzymatic disruption of the matrix (cell wall structure) enhanced the bioavailability of beta-carotene from whole leaf and minced spinach, but had no effect on lutein bioavailability.

Sommerburg *et al* (1998) reported that substantial amounts of lutein and zeaxanthin (30-50 per cent) are present in kiwi fruit, grapes, spinach, orange juice, zucchini (or vegetable marrow), and different kinds of squash that can be consumed to increase dietary intake of lutein and zeaxanthin. Lutein and zeaxanthin, xanthophylls found in corn and in leafy greens such as kale and spinach, are believed to function as protective antioxidants in the macular region of the human retina (Snodderly, 1995). The retinal carotenoids lutein (L) and zeaxanthin (Z) that form the macular pigment (MP) may help to prevent neovascular age-related macular degeneration. A study was done by Hammond Jr. (1997) to determine whether MP density in the retina could be raised by increasing dietary intake of L and Z from foods. Serum concentrations of L, Z and beta-carotene were measured by high-performance liquid chromatography. It was found that spinach diet increased the MP density and it remained elevated for at least several months after resuming an unmodified diet.

Lutein and zeaxanthin are the only carotenoids in the macular region of the retina [referred to as macular pigment (MP)]. Foods that are rich in lutein and zeaxanthin can increase MP density. Response to dietary lutein and zeaxanthin in other tissues has not been studied. A study was done by Johnson *et al* (2000) to examine tissue responses to dietary lutein and zeaxanthin and relations among tissues in lutein and zeaxanthin concentrations. Seven subjects consumed spinach and corn, which contain lutein and zeaxanthin, with their daily diets for 15 weeks. At 0, 4, 8 and 15 weeks and two months after the study, serum, buccal mucosa cells, and adipose tissue were analysed for carotenoids, and MP density was measured. It was found that serum and buccal cell concentrations of lutein increased significantly from baseline during dietary modification. Serum zeaxanthin concentrations were greater than at baseline only at four weeks, whereas buccal cell and adipose tissue concentrations of zeaxanthin did not change. Adipose tissue lutein concentrations peaked at eight weeks. Changes in adipose tissue lutein concentration were inversely related to the changes in MP density, suggesting an interaction between adipose tissue and retina in lutein metabolism. To investigate the possibility of tissue interactions, they examined cross-sectional relations among serum, tissue and dietary lutein concentrations, anthropometric measures and MP density in healthy adults. Significant negative correlation was found between adipose tissue lutein concentrations and MP for women, but a significant positive relation was found for men. Sex differences in lutein metabolism may be an important factor in tissue interactions and in determining MP density.

Slattery *et al* (2000) evaluated association between dietary alpha-carotene, beta-carotene, lycopene, lutein, zeaxanthin and beta-cryptoxanthin and the risk of colon cancer in the U. S. population. The major dietary sources of lutein in subjects with colon cancer and in control subjects were spinach, broccoli, lettuce, tomatoes, oranges and orange juice, carrots, celery and greens. The data suggest that incorporating these foods into the diet may help reduce the risk of developing colon cancer. Lutein was inversely associated with colon cancer in both men and women. The greatest inverse association was observed among subjects in whom colon cancer was diagnosed when they were young and among those with tumours located in the proximal segment of the colon. The associations with other carotenoids were unremarkable.

Yin *et al* (2000) analysed that serum level of carotenoid, including all-trans-beta-carotene, cis-beta-carotene, cryptoxanthin and lutein were significantly higher after intervention in yellow-green vegetable group, as compared to their baseline levels. However, in the light-coloured vegetable group, all those components, including all-trans-beta-carotene, 13-cis-beta-carotene and lutein, decreased significantly after intervention, as compared with those at their baseline levels. Serum carotene level correlated significantly with that of retinol, and their coefficient of correlation was greater in the winter than in the autumn. They concluded that carotenoid nutrition status can be improved by supplementation of green and yellow vegetables.

Noakes *et al* (2002) investigated that consuming an additional daily serving of a high-carotenoid vegetable (carrots, sweet potatoes, pumpkins, tomatoes, apricots, spinach or broccoli.) or fruit when consuming spreads containing sterol or stanol esters maintains plasma carotenoid concentrations while lowering LDL-cholesterol concentrations significantly.

The effects of spinach leaf protein concentrate (SPPC) on serum and liver lipid concentrations and on serum free amino acid concentrations were examined in rats fed a cholesterol-free diet containing two and 10 per cent fats. The serum total cholesterol, triacylglycerol and phospholipid concentrations in the rats fed on SPPC diet containing two per cent corn oil were significantly lower than those of the rats fed a corresponding casein diet. When 10 per cent corn oil or lard was used, the serum cholesterol-lowering effect of the SPPC became insignificant, but the serum and liver triacylglycerol concentrations were kept at significantly lower levels. Both the amounts of fecal neutral steroids and bile acids were significantly higher in the rats fed the SPPC than those of the casein-fed rats. The concentrations of serum threonine, serine, glutamine, glycine, cystine and isoleucine were significantly higher in the rats fed the SPPC diet containing two per cent corn oil compared with those of the control rats, but when the dietary fat was raised to 10 per cent, only glycine showed a higher serum concentration. These results indicate that the SPPC has a stronger cholesterol-lowering effect at a lower dietary fat level, two per cent, and the activity is partly due to the inhibition of intestinal absorption of cholesterol and bile acid, and partly due to an increase in the concentration of some of the serum amino acids (Satoh, *et al,* 1995).

Pre-treatment with both antioxidants for eight days reduced, in some organs, the necrotic and inflammatory changes associated with the LPS challenge. Endotoxin lipopolysaccaride (LPS) enhances the formation of reactive oxygen species such as superoxide anion radicals, peroxides and their secondary product, malondialdehyde, especially in the liver. Lomnitski *et al* (2000a) studied the histopathological changes in several organs and compared among groups of male Wistar rats that had been injected with LPS following prophylactic pre-treatment with either of two antioxidants, a group that had been injected with LPS without pre-treatment with antioxidants, an untreated control group, and groups that had been injected with either of the two antioxidants only. The antioxidants used were a water-soluble natural antioxidant from spinach (NAO) and the NADPH oxidase inhibitor apocynin. Exposure to LPS alone was associated with multifocal hepatocellular necrosis and acute inflammation, thymic and splenic lymphoid necrosis, ocular retinal haemorrhage and acute endophthalmitis, adrenal medullary vacuolation and necrosis and acute inflammation, and decreased adrenal cortical cytoplasmic vacuolation (consistent with depletion of steroidal hormone contents). These findings suggest a potential therapeutic application for these antioxidants in clinical sepsis The possible therapeutic efficacy of NAO has been claimed in the treatment of clinical endotoxemia associated with gram-negative bacterial species that is known to be associated with oxidative stress. Lomnitski *et al* (2000b) demonstrated that endotoxin lipopolysaccharide

(LPS) promotes oxidative stress and associated pathological changes in a rat model and that use of selected antioxidants was effective in reducing LPS-related lipid peroxidation product formation in the liver, as well as LPS-related pathological changes in different organs. In this study, several toxicological parameters (that is, clinical signs, blood chemistry and histopathological changes) were compared among groups of male New Zealand rabbits injected with LPS following prophylactic pre-treatment with either of two antioxidants, a group injected with LPS without pre-treatment with antioxidants, groups injected with either of the two antioxidants only, and an untreated control group. The antioxidants used were a water-soluble natural antioxidant (NAO) from spinach and the NADPH oxidase inhibitor, apocynin. Exposure to LPS alone was associated clinically with depression, tachypnea, outer ear vasodilation and iris congestion; biochemically with a significant increase in blood total bilirubin, transaminase activity and glucose, total cholesterol and triglyceride levels; macroscopically with multiple whitish areas in the liver; and histologically with hepatocellular focal necrosis and acute inflammation, thymic and splenic lymphoid necrosis and depletion, acute uveitis and haemorrhages in the ciliary processes, and decreased adrenal cortical cytoplasmic vacuolation considered consistent with depletion of steroidal hormone contents. The NAO had more effective prophylactic capacities than the apocynin. The protective effects were obvious in all investigated parameters. The possible therapeutic efficacy of NAO and apocynin in the prevention of liver damage related to clinical endotoxemia known to be associated with oxidative stress (Lomnitski *et al*, 2000c). The immunoreactivity of inducible nitric oxide synthase and cyclo-oxygenase-2 was compared among groups of male Wistar rats comprising those injected with lipopolysaccharide following pre-treatment with either natural antioxidant from spinach or the antioxidant apocynin, with lipopolysaccharide without pre-treatment with antioxidants, with each of the two antioxidants alone, and untreated controls. The negative nitrotyrosine immunoreactivity of the lipopolysaccharide-related hepatic lesions may indicate that there was relatively low interaction between superoxide anions and nitric oxide to form peroxynitrite or that the expression levels of the nitrotyrosine were below the limit of detection. In all treatment groups a positive correlation ($P < 0.05$, $r = 0.86$) found between the inducible nitric oxide synthase and cyclo-oxygenase-2 scores suggests a strong relationship between these two parameters.

He *et al* (1999) studied the effect of a fat-soluble extract of spinach powder (SPFE) on the proliferation of human gastric adenocarcinoma cell line (SGC-7901) *in vitro* by using four kinds of assays (cell growth assay, colony forming assay, MTT colorimetric assay and 3H-TdR incorporation assay). The results indicated that SPFE inhibited the proliferation and colony forming ability of SGC-7901 cells. And in MTT assay, SPFE inhibited the viability of SGC-7901 cells, but no inhibitory effect of SPFE was observed on the viability of lymphocytes in peripheral blood of healthy people. Finally, in the 3H-TdR incorporation test, both SPFE and beta-carotene showed significant inhibitory effects on DNA synthesis in SGC-7901 cells, but SPFE was more effective than beta-carotene.

Broccoli and spinach possessed the highest total phenolic content (Chu *et al*, 2002). Anti-proliferative activities were also studied *in vitro* using HepG(2) human liver cancer cells. Spinach showed the highest inhibitory effect, followed by cabbage, red pepper, onion and broccoli. Kayashima and Katayama (2002) reported that oxalic acid present in spinach suppressed *in vitro* lipid peroxidation in a concentration-dependent manner. Howard *et al* (2002) reported that growing conditions, as well as biotic and abiotic stresses, influenced phenolic metabolism because over-winter spinach, which was planted in late fall and harvested in the spring, had much higher levels of total phenolics and antioxidant capacity than spinach planted in early fall and harvested in late fall. Lee *et al* (2002) reported that spinach in the dough decreased accumulation of the polar compounds in soybean oil during frying but had little effect on the fried dough. It also reduced conjugated diene and aldehyde formation in the lipid of fried dough during storage. Improvement in lipid oxidative stability, presumably due to pigments in spinach, was more noticeable in the fried products during storage than in the frying oil. In the same manner, the effect of spinach products on lipid oxidation is affected by processing (Castenmiller *et al,* 2002). The consumption of carotenoid-rich foods like spinach, even for a short period of time, gives protection against oxidative stress. The results obtained seem to suggest that this protective role is not specifically related to carotenoids. However, they may contribute together with other substances present in vegetables to lymphocyte resistance to oxidative damage.

β-CAROTENE AND OTHER CAROTENOIDS

Radioprotective, Antioxidative and Other Effects

Carotenoids are a class of natural fat-soluble pigments found principally in plants, algae and photosynthetic bacteria, where they play a critical role in the photosynthetic process. They also occur in some non-photosynthetic bacteria, yeasts and moulds, where they may carry out a protective function against damage by light and oxygen. Although animals appear to be incapable of synthesising carotenoids, many animals incorporate carotenoids from their diet. Within animals, carotenoids provide bright coloration, serve as anti-oxidants, and can be a source for vitamin A activity (Ong and Tee, 1992; Britton *et al* 1995).

Carotenoids are natural compounds with lipophilic properties; more than 500 different compounds have been identified. Most carotenoid content and extended system of conjugated double bond, is responsible for their antioxidant activity. Carotenoids are thought to act as antioxidants, which scavenge free radicals and other oxidants involved in disease processes (Ames, 1987; Krinsky, 1989; Liebler, 1996).

β-carotene is the most potent form of available carotene. It is present in dark green leafy vegetables, carrots and yellow, red fruits such as peaches and apricots. β-carotene is defined as provitamin-A because it is converted to vitamin A once in the body. This is different than pre-formed vitamin A (retinol) which is normally found in fish liver oils. In addition to providing with a safe source of vitamin A, β-carotene works with other natural protectors to defend anti-oxidant cells from harmful free radical damage.

Carotenoids are substances synthesised only in plants which serve to protect the plants from the free radicals generated during photosynthesis (Moore, 1957). Antioxidant functions are associated with lowering DNA damage, malignant transformation and other parameters of cell damage *in vitro* as well as epidemiologically with lowered incidence of certain types of cancer and degenerative disease, such as ischemic heart disease and cataract. People with low tissue levels of β-carotene are found to be usually prone towards getting a number of different types of cancer (Peto *et al,* 1981). It has therefore been recommended that β-carotene be used for protection against certain types of human cancers and photosensitised oxidative damage (Bertram and Bortkiewioz, 1995; Albanes *et al,* 1995) because free radicals and related reactive species may play some part in their pathology. β-carotene has been extensively used in cancer chemopreventive studies in which it displayed suppressing activity against oral and colon tumours (Tanaka *et al,* 1994; Alabaster *et al,* 1995). Most convincing reports support a direct connection between a high intake of fruits and vegetables and a low incidence of cancer and cardiovascular disease. The literature lacks specific information on the possible medical contribution of natural carotenoids, isomers of carotenoids and carotenoids fatty acid esters. Experimental nutritional and medical studies with natural carotenoids originating from different plants, fruits, vegetables and algae have been very limited and research is in its infancy. ß-carotene is present in most plants and algae.

β-carotene has been thought to be of value to human and other species not only as a precursor to vitamin A but also for having excellent antioxidant properties (Krinsky and Deneke, 1982; Krinsky, 1989). Although it is not easy to define a compound as an anticarcinogen, β-carotene, a well known antioxidant, is a provitamin that plays an important role in reducing the mutagenecity of many chemicals (Stich *et al,* 1988; Renner, 1990; Mukherjee *et al,* 1991; Salvadori *et al,* 1992a, 1992b, 1993,1994) and its mechanism of action is under active study. Few studies evaluating its ability as radioprotector have been conducted.

The role of β-carotene and vitamin A in radiation protection with their antioxidant properties has been indicated by Siefter and collaborators (1983, 1984). β-carotene supplementation produced a greater residual antitumour action than vitamin A supplementation, after the supplement was discontinued which may have been due to greater tissues storage of β-carotene. Seifter *et al* (1988) carried out experiments to determine low supplemental vitamin A and β-carotene influences the course of radiation sickness in C^3 H mice after partial body irradiation (30 Gy) and total body irradiation (450-750 rad). They observed that supplemental vitamin A prevented the radiation induced adrenal hypertrophy and weight loss and lesioned lymphocytopenia due to irradiation in partial body irradiation. In total body irradiation, the supplemental vitamin A and β-carotene decreased mortality as evidenced by increases in the radiation dose required to kill 15 per cent of mice within 30 days.

Vitamin A and β-carotene are unique radio-protective agents of broad applicability. Total body irradiation caused gastric and intestinal bleeding in CBA mice and Sprague-Dawley rats, supplemental vitamin A and β-carotene reduced ulceration and bleeding (Levenson *et al,* 1984). Weitberg *et al* (1985) demonstrated that β-carotene gave protection against oxygen radical induced chromosome damage which were measured by frequencies of sister chromatid exchanges. β-carotene and vitamin A also offer good protection against some radiomimetic drug like cyclophosphamide and streptozotocin. Vitamin A and β-carotene were found to obviate lympnocytopenia, decreased growth rate and impaired wound healing due to either streptzotocin or cyclophosphamide (Stratford *et al,* 1980; Weinzweig *et al,* 1987). A beneficial influence of b-carotene on the condition of patients under radiotherapy was also observed by Mill (1988).

There is a growing body of evidence regarding the beneficial properties of β-carotene in human and animal diets (Mathews-Roth, 1991; Gerster, 1993). Feeding studies in the rat showed that β-carotene was as effective in protecting red blood cells against oxidative damage with vitamin E (Zamora *et al,* 1991). β-carotene inhibits the oxidative modification of low-density lipoproteins when added in near-physiological concentration to both cell-free and cellular *in vitro* systems (Jialal *et al,* 1993).

Reactive oxygen species occur in tissues and cells and can damage DNA, proteins, carbohydrates and lipids. These potentially deleterious reactions are controlled in part by antioxidants that eliminate pro-oxidants and scavenge free radicals. Their ability as antioxidants to quench radicals may explain some anti-cancerous properties of the carotenoids independent of their provitamin-A activity, but other functions may play a role as well (Sies *et al,* 1992).

Beliaev *et al* (1992) reported the radiomodifying efficiency of short term and chronic medicinal and treatment prophylactic enrichment of rations with artificial β-carotene, administered at single doses of 0.1-10.0 mg, after acute external gamma irradiation of adult non-linear and Wistar rats (0.029 Gy/s) or female SBA mice (0.0037 Gy/s), where the absorbed dose was equal to 8.3 Gy or 9.9-9.5 Gy, respectively. Suspension of β-carotene paste in olive oil accelerated death of rats irradiated at doses of 8 and 7 Gy (P = 0.04), and shortened their life span. At a dose of 6 Gy single and long-term enrichment of rations with β-carotene decreased the rate of death within 30 days from 33.3 per cent to 16.7 per cent (P = 0.14) and 3.3 per cent (P = 0.01), while their life time was increased from 48 days to 67 days (P = 0.05) and 508 days (P = 0.01). β-carotene was found to affect favourably the radiation induced (5 Gy) leukocytopenia, and decreased thymus mass (6 Gy) and body weight (8 Gy). In treatment-prophylactic enrichment with β-carotene of mice (9.9 Gy) ration their survival was increased from 15 per cent to 30 per cent and life span from 14.4 days to 28.9 days (P = 0.05). During medicinal or treatment-prophylactic courses of β-carotene death of mice (9.7 Gy) was decreased from 75 per cent to 35 per cent (P = 0.01) or 60 per cent and life time was increased from 16.7 days to 22.17 days and 39.9 days (P = 0.05). Sies *et al* (1992) reported that carotenoids, notably β-carotene and lycopene as well as oxycarotenoids (for example, zeaxanthin and lutein), exert antioxidant functions in lipid phases by O_2 or free radicals quenching. There were pronounced differences in tissue carotenoid patterns, extending also to the distribution between the all trans and various cis isomers of the respective carotenoids. Ei Nahas *et al* (1993) evaluated the radioprotective effect of vitamin C and E in the groups of whole body irradiated rats and observed that only vitamin C and not E was able to decrease frequency of chromosome damage induced by irradiation.

Abraham *et al* (1993) used mouse bone marrow micronucleus test to evaluate the possible role of β-carotene and other dietary constituents in modulating chromosomal damage induced by gamma-radiation. They noticed reduction of micronuclei due to the radioprotective effect of β-carotene. Umegaki *et al* (1994) also showed that β-carotene given *in vivo* prevents induction of micronuclei by X-rays in human lymphocytes. Bitterman *et al* (1994) tested the efficacy of dietary supplementation by natural β-carotene on the ability of rats to cope with a CNS oxidative insult induced by exposure high pressure of oxygen using freely moving rat model with exposure to HBO and continuous monitoring of EEG. They demonstrated the protective effect of β-carotene rich *Dunaliella baradawil* against hyperoxia induced CNS seizures on exposure to high oxygen pressure.

When the dietary intake of different carotenoids was analysed, the sum of lutein and zeaxanthin, the retinal carotenoids forming the macular pigment had the strongest protective effects against neovascular age-related mascular degeneration (AMD) (Seddon *et al,* 1994). An especially beneficial effect was assigned to intake of spinach, which is rich in lutein but not zeaxanthin (Krinsky *et al,* 1990).

β-carotene, apart from the main source of retinol, has been reported to be potent free-radical quenchers, singlet oxygen scavengers and lipid antioxidants (Gey, 1994; Blot *et al,* 1995). The observational epidemiological studies continue to accumulate impressive evidence that food rich in the antioxidant vitamins (Gey, 1994) and β-carotene (Kohlmier and Hastings, 1995) have an important role in the prevention of cardiovascular disease, as well as in cancer prevention (Byers and Guerrero, 1995; Van Popple and Goldbohm, 1995). Bertram *et al* (1995) also concluded that carotenoids can inhibit neoplastic transformation and modulate the expression of gene products in both human and mouse cells.

The possibility of β-carotene as an anti-ageing and anti-radiation drug has also been discussed by Bhatia, (1996). Salvadori *et al* (1996) evaluated the protective effect of β-carotene after whole body exposure of mice to 2 Gy of X-rays. spleenocyte, reticulocytes, bone marrow cells and spermatids were evaluated for the frequency of micronuclei induced by X-rays. Mice were treated with β-carotene (10, 25 and 50 mg/kg body weight) for five consecutive days and four hours after last treatment, the animals were irradiated. The radioprotective effect of β-carotene was observed in spleenocytes, reticulocytes and spermatids but not in bone marrow cells. Low dose response relationship for β-carotene was detected. Ben-Amotz *et al* (1996) observed the possible anti-oxidative effect against whole-body irradiation of a natural β-carotene, composed of equal amounts of the all-trans and 9-cis isomers, obtained from the unicellular alga *Dunaliella Baradawil.* They found a normal increase in body weight and no ill effects were noted in the groups of rats whose diet was supplemented by β-carotene before and after irradiation, compared with the reduction in the specific growth rate in the group of rats irradiated without β-carotene. Liver β-carotene and retinol decreased significantly after irradiation compared with the rats, which were not irradiated. This decrease was not shown in rats fed β-carotene prior to irradiation, and the effect of irradiation was partially cured by supplementation with β-carotene after irradiation. These results suggested that 9-cis β-carotene and retinol protect *in vivo* against the cellular damage by free radicals induced after whole-body irradiation. Iyama *et al* (1996) reported that the amount of thiobarbutaric acid reactive substance (TBARS) in mice's kidney, liver and lung, decreased with increasing amounts of β-carotene accumulated in these tissues, that is, inverse correlation was obtained. These results indicated that β-carotene can suppress lipid peroxidation in mouse tissue.

Cozzi *et al* (1997) suggested that ascorbic acid and β-carotene are effective in reducing $H_2O_2^-$ induced cister chromatid exchange. They concluded that both vitamins act as scavengers of endogenous and H_2O_2 induced reactive oxygen species. Knopacka *et al* (1998) studied the modifying effect of treatment with vitamins C and E and β-carotene on clastogenic activity of gamma rays in mice. Vitamins were administered orally, either for five consecutive days before or immediately after irradiation with 2 Gy of gamma rays. The result showed that pre-treatment with vitamin E (100-200 mg/kg/day) and β-carotene (3-12 mg/kg/day) were effective in protecting against micronucleus induction by gamma rays.

Chen *et al* (1988) investigated the effect of dietary carotenoid-rich extracts of carrots, tomatoes and orange juice on rat liver-y-glutamyl transpeptidase-positive preneoplastic foci induced by aflatoxin B. They concluded that carotenoid-rich extracts of these three foods substantially inhibited biochemical and cellular events thought to play a role in the early stages of hepatocarcinogenesis.

It was also reported in our laboratory that β-carotene protects radiation-induced lipid peroxidation in mice liver and spleen (Ramesh *et al*, 1997). Knopacka *et al* (1998) studied the modifying effect of treatment with vitamin C, E, and β-carotene on clastogenic activity of gamma rays in mice. Vitamins were administered orally, either for five consecutive days before or immediately after irradiation with 2 Gy of gamma rays. The result showed that pre-treatment with vitamin E (100-200 mg/kg/day) and β-carotene (3-12 mg/kg/day) were effective in protecting against micronucleus induction by gamma rays.

Vitamins (rhodopsin, ascorbic acid, tocopherol, riboflavin and folate) function as antioxidants and prevent xenobiotic induced LPO and generation of oxygen-free radicals. Vitamin C reduces chemical toxicity by decreasing the covalent binding of reactive intermediate reducing quinones, eliminating free radical metabolites, (Correa, 1992).

Kanazawa *et al* (1992) reported that ascorbic acid deficiency in guinea pigs led to decrease in CYPIAI and CYPIIE isoforms of cytochrome P450, responsible for activation of aflatoxin. Recently, vitamins C and E have shown to reduce the extent and severity of gastric ulcers resulting from immobilisation stress and also to enhance the immunity in rats (Ray *et al,* 1989).

Ben-Amotz *et al* (1998) observed the protective effect of natural β-carotene supplementation in children exposed to radiation from the Chernobyl accident. Attempts were made to evaluate 709 children (324 boys and 385 girls) who had been exposed long-term to different doses of radiation during and after the Chernobyl accident and had moved to Israel between 1990 and 1994. Upon arrival, all of them underwent a check-up for most common clinical disorders and were then divided into various groups according to their residences (distance from the reactor) and the level of irradiation exposure. The results obtained from this study indicated that irradiation increased the susceptibility of lipids to oxidation in the Chernobyl children and that natural beta-carotene may act as an *in vivo* lipophilic or radioprotector.

Slyshenkov *et al* (1999) exposed rats to a total dose of 0.75 Gy of gamma radiation receiving 3 doses of 0.25 Gy at weekly intervals. During two days before each irradiation, the animals received daily doses of 26 mg pantothenol or 15 mg β-carotene/kg body mass. Animals were killed after third irradiation, and their blood and livers were analysed. In livers of animals not supplied with either pantothyenol or β-carotene and killed one hour after irradiation, a large accumulation of lipid peroxidation products was observed. The contents of CoA, pantothenic acid, total phospholipids, total glutathione decreased considerably. All these effects were alleviated in animals supplied with β-carotene and were completely abolished with pantothenol; seven days after irradiation most of these changes disappeared spontaneously, whereas supplementation with β-carotene shortened the time required for normalisation of biochemical parameters.

El-Habit *et al* (2000) studied the modifying effect of β-carotene on gamma-induced elevation of oxidative reactions and genotoxicity in male rats. β-carotene was gavaged at a dose of 5 mg/kg.b.wt for seven consecutive days before whole body gamma irradiation with 7 Gy (single dose). The biochemical and cytogenetic determinations were carried out 1, 24 and 72 hours after radiation exposure. The results revealed that administration of β-carotene pre-irradiation significantly inhibited the decrease in plasma β-carotene, significantly reduced the levels of TBARS in plasma and liver. Significant protection of the radiation induced changes in the activities of SOD and catalase were also recorded in the blood and liver of β-carotene treated and irradiated rats. β-carotene significantly inhibited frequency of radiation induced MN. These results suggest that β-carotene could play a modulatory role against the cellular damage affected by free radicals induced by whole body irradiation.

Zhang and Omaye (2000) studied the effect of β-carotene on protein oxidation under different oxygen tensions and with other antioxidants in human serum albumin. High concentration of β-carotene produced more protein oxidation in the presence of high O_2 tensions by a peroxidant mechanism. Mixture of β-carotene, alpha tocopherol and ascorbic acid provided better protective effects of protein oxidation than any single compound.

An anthology of the works of our laboratory with β-carotene started since 1991 with financial assistance from the University Grants Commission in collaboration with Prof. A. S. Kapoor, Prof. Emeritus and Ex-Vice Chancellor, University of Rajasthan, Jaipur. β-carotene was found to offer good protection against external gamma radiation on different tissues. however, at an optimum dose of 30 mg/kg body weight given orally for certain length of period. The protective action of β-carotene against gamma radiation showed its effect was dependent on the dose as well as on the mode of administration. The protective effect of β-carotene after whole body exposure of mice was observed in developing brain, testis, liver and hemopoietic tissues like spleen. A dose response relationship for β-carotene was detected. β-carotene prevents the radiation induced lipid peroxidation in mice liver and spleen of Swiss albino mice after oral administration. It was also reported in our laboratory that β-carotene protects radiation-induced lipid peroxidation in mice liver and spleen (Ramesh *et al*, 1997).

Ramesh *et al* (1997) indicated that β-carotene prevents the radiation induced lipid–peroxidation in mice liver and spleen when Swiss albino mice were administered oral dose of β-carotene 50 mg/kg body weight for two weeks and exposing to 3 Gy of gamma radiation. With the same plan of radiation doses and β-carotene treatment, a significant decrease in the cholesterol and glycogen level was seen. β-carotene in irradiated animals supplemented with β-carotene. However, β-carotene does not produce any significant difference in the sham-irradiated animals. Besides, all the studies show an inverse relationship in the effect of protein and lipid peroxidation. After irradiation, the amount of TBARS n mol/mg tissue increases with the passage of time whereas the protein after initial raise decreases on latter intervals. The initial increase in protein may be due to an unscheduled DNA synthesis or repair mechanism (Manda and Bhatia, 2000).

A study on Swiss albino mice, taking β-carotene along with a cocktail of vitamins (The vitamin mixture contains β-carotene 42 mg/kg body weight, vitamin A 1600 IU/kg body weight, vitamin C 48 mg/kg body weight, vitamin E 0.2 IU/kg body weight and Zinc 0.1 mg/kg body weight) were found to have prolonged survival by 40 per cent and animals survived up to 10 days more after 11 Gy exposure. There was a sudden decrease in body weight of radiation exposed group whereas in the vitamin treated group the weight loss was gradual (Ramesh *et al,* 1997).

Manda (1999) studied effects of β-carotene on the sensitivity of mouse spermatogonia to radiation. He found that an appreciable protective potential of β-carotene against radiation damage in the stem spermatogenic cells and hence, possibly with plausible mutational changes. Bhatia *et al* (1999), Sisodia *et al* (1999) and Manda *et al* (2000) studied the role of β-carotene against radiation induced lipid peroxidation in mice testis and other organs, namely, brain, liver, etc. They reported that β-carotene ameliorates radiation induced lipid peroxidation in mouse brain and testis. They found that the radiation induced lipid peroxidation as reflected by the thiobarbutiric acid reactive substance (TBARS) or malondialdehyde (MDA) content could be prevented to an extent by β-carotene in mouse brain and testis.

Bhatia *et al* (2001) investigated the most effective and optimum dose level of β-carotene against gamma irradiation. Swiss albino mice were administered different oral doses of β-carotene (20, 30, 50 and 70 mg/kg of their body weight) for two weeks and then exposed to 9 Gy of gamma radiation. A correlation between doses of β-carotene after irradiation and recovery interval in the body weight indicated the longer time interval at lower doses of β-carotene. Both mortality data and body weight recovery show 30 mg/kg body weight as an optimal dose level of β-carotene.

Sharma (2001) studied radioprotective efficacy of β-carotene in relation to ageing of mice and found that anti-oxidative property of b-carotene offered more significant protection in young mice as compared to old age group of animals. Sharma (2001) evaluated the effect the β-carotene vs radiation on mice cerebellum of different age groups, namely, 1, 2, 3 and 6 weeks of age. He concluded that severity of damage diminishes gradually as age advances; maximum damage is noticed in mice when the treatment is initiated from one week of age. Granular layer is more affected compared to the molecular layer. The overall picture shows the protection rendered by β-carotene ranges up to 40 per cent in the case of young mice, whereas it hardly crosses 20 per cent in the case of adult mice. One or two doses of β-carotene are not adequate to exert protective effect on the cerebellum of mice against gamma radiation.

Sisodia *et al* (2002) studied the possible radioprotective role of β-carotene on mice cerebellum with relation to age. They found that highest efficacy of β-carotene is noticed when the treatment initiates from one week of age and anti-oxidative property of β-carotene seems to afford significant protection against radiation induced neuromorpho-metrical changes in young developing mice.

Even though the β-carotene studies in mouse, rat and hamster may not reflect the human situation because of species-specific differences in β-carotene metabolism and kinetics, the uniformity of the findings in animal models does lend support to a potential chemopreventive and radioprotective effect of β-carotene. This potential effect needs to be further explored in humans.

DOSE RELATIONSHIP AND TOXICITY OF β-CAROTENE AND OTHER CAROTENOIDS

β-carotene has found wide use as a colorant in food, cosmetic and drug industries and it was therefore essential to conduct reliable toxicity studies of this substance through use of an accepted range of techniques. When this was done, no mutagenecity was found with the Ames test nor in the mouse bone marrow micronuclei test (Bagdon *et al*, 1960; Heywood *et al*, 1985). Detailed toxicity trials led to β-carotene being placed in the U. S. Food and Drug Administration (FDA) category of food generally recognised as safe (GRAS), both for use as a colorant in the food, drug and cosmetic industries and as a dietary supplement and nutrient (*Life Science*, 1979). β-carotene has been used for at least 20 years to treat patients with genetically inherited photosensitivities, and it has been reported in this context that ingestion of large amount of pure β-carotene does not produce toxic side effects (Mathews-Roth, 1986).

A large body of evidence is available from treatment of patients with erythropoietic protoporphyria (EPP) showing that β-carotene causes no unwanted side effects even when used in very high doses of up to 180 mg daily for many years (Mathews-Roth *et al*, 1977). Brubacher *et al* (1985) suggested that β-carotene bioavailabity is dose-dependent, high and low β-carotene doses may lead to different tissue distribution.

Occasionally there is reversible yellowing of the skin at doses above 30 mg/day (Bendich, 1988; Mathews-Roth, 1991). This again indicates that in a person with an adequate vitamin A status, β-carotene is not converted to retinol or retinoic acid in undesirable amounts. In extensive animal studies, β-carotene was shown to be equally non-toxic. It was neither cytotoxic nor mutagenic. In contrast to retinoic acid it does not produce any teratogenic effects (Mathews-Roth, 1989).

In a short-term (Phase I) toxicity trial of supplemental β-carotene in a small number of human volunteers, a progressive decrease in serum vitamin E concentration was reported during a nine-month supplementation with 15, 30, 45 and 60 mg β-carotene/day (Xu *et al,* 1992). This study raised a question that had been thought to be settled in the particular case of β-carotene interaction with tocopherol, because earlier studies had not shown any such interaction. However, Goodman *et al* (1994) showed no evidence of lowered vitamin E concentration in a study of 2,319 participants supplemented with 30 mg β-carotene/day and 25,000 IU retinol/day for up to six years. In some other comprehensive studies regarding the β-carotene and α tocopherol interaction, Albanes *et al* (1992), Mclarty (1992) and Nierenberg *et al* (1994) found no effect of β-carotene on serum α-tocopherol concentration.

Abraham *et al* (1993) evaluating the protective action of β-carotene (0.5 and 2.5 mg/kg) against gamma-radiation in mouse bone marrow observed that its effect was dependent on the dose and time/frequency of administration. However, no dose-response relationship was observed by Salvadori *et al* (1996) since 10 mg of β-carotene had almost the same effect of 50 mg and 25 mg/kg.

Questions to the safety of the ingestion of high doses of β-carotene have been raised by the Alpha-tocopherol b-carotene cancer prevention study in Finland (ATBC, 1994) and another study by Heinonen and Albanes (1994). In both the studies, a higher incidence of lung cancer amongst smoking men that receive β-carotene was observed in comparison with smokers that did not receive β-carotene. However, there are so many epidemiological evidences suggesting the decreased cancer risks with increased consumption of β-carotene (Temple and Basu, 1987; Alam and Alam, 1987; Suda *et al,* 1986; Van Popple, 1993). Despite these, β-carotene remains a major candidate for the prevention of disease *de novo*, and Finland's ATBC (1994) cancer prevention study illustrates the pitfalls of relying on clinical trials to answer questions about the benefits of nutrients in disease prevention (Block, 1995). Evidence from human toxicity trials is not available but there is much circumstantial evidence that 15.50 mg/day is without side effect except for hypercarotenemia in some subject at high intakes (Diplock, 1995).

Even though β-carotene studies in mouse, rat and hamster may not reflect the human situation because of species-specific differences in β-carotene metabolism and kinetics, the uniformity of the findings in animal models does lend support to a potential chemopreventive effect of β-carotene. This potential effect needs to be further explored in humans.

A dose-dependent relationship of β-carotene was also observed by Ni and Pei (1997), when studying the effect of β-carotene on radiation induced mutation at T-lymphocyte hypoxanthine-guanine phosphoribosyl transferase (HGPRT) locus in rat. Mutant frequency at the HGPRT locus was elevated by 60 Co-gamma 3.75 Gy, and was reduced by β-carotene 20 and 10 mg/kg ($P > 0.05$), but not by β-carotene 5 mg/kg. It showed a dose-dependent relationship. MDA was significantly reduced in plasma of rats given β-carotene after 60 Co-gamma radiation. There was positive correlation between MDA and mutant frequency at the HGPRT locus $r = 0.9978$, $P < 0.05$). They concluded that radiation induced mutation is inhibited by β-carotene, associated with antioxidant action. The non-beta carotene carotenoids have not yet been submitted to detailed toxicity studies, but given their structures they are likely to be as safe as beta carotene.

COMBINATION OF DRUGS

Radioprotective efficacy of the protectors can be enhanced by using them in a combination. These radioprotections are chosen in such a manner that they enable to reduce the doses of individual compounds to provide various mechanisms of radioprotective action and to achieve a higher total radioprotection. Therefore, in the past years, interest has been developed for the use of a combination of various protective compounds because it seemed very unlikely that a single compound would possess all the required properties to protect a cellular system in mammals. Therefore, combination of agents has been chosen either to complement each other in protective activity or to reduce toxicity and side effects.

No adverse effects were observed in the animals treated with different concentrations of *Amaranthus paniculatus* (Linn.) (Amaranthus) and *Spinacia oleracea* L. (spinach) in terms of sickness and mortality. Also, there was no significant change in the body weight, urination and defecation pattern. After the preliminary observations with different doses of Amaranthus (AE) and Spinach (SE) extracts against radiation, it was inferred that 600 mg/kg b.wt. of AE and 1,100 mg/kg b.wt of SE are the most effective concentrations for radioprotection. Therefore, a detailed investigation was performed at the optimum dose of AE (600 mg/ kg b.wt./day) and SE (1,100 mg/ kg b.wt./day). For this purpose, mice were treated with AE and SE for 15 consecutive days prior to irradiation (9 Gy) to get maximum protection against radiation injury. The protective effect of the above plant extracts against radiation injury was assessed by the survival assay. DRF was calculated to see the radioprotective efficacy of drug by treating the animals with different doses of gamma radiation (6, 9, 12 Gy) and DRF was calculated as 1.43 for AE and 1.65 for SE. In another experiment, both the drugs were given in combination at their effective dose level calculated according to 1 kg b. wt./day. DRF in combination treatment of both the plant extracts was calculated as 1.72. The radioprotective effect of AE, SE and AE + SE on the liver of mice was also studied one day to 30 day post-irradiation. A significant increase in the normal hepatic cells, glutathione, cholesterol as well as a significant decrease in abnormal cells, binucleated cells, glycogen, protein, lipidperoxidation, alkaline and acid phosphatases were observed in animals pre-treated with AE, SE, AE + SE as compared to control (irradiated) animals.

Hepatic cells can be protected against radiation damage which was evident in increased survivability in plants extract (single and in combination) pre-treated irradiated animals and a subsequent increase (decrease was less in comparison to control) in glutathione and decrease in lipid peroxidation have been observed. The possible mechanism of radioprotection by the studied plants extract may be mediated through the hepatic cells which are protected against the radiation induced free radical damage by lowering the lipid peroxidation level. The protection rendered by *amaranthus* and spinach in the whole body irradiated mouse is of significant degree at 5 Gy dose level of gamma radiation (Jain, 2002).

CONCLUSION

Amaranthus paniculatus (Linn.) (English name–Amaranth; Hindi name–Lal Choulai), has good quantity of carotenoid content, vitamin C, high level of nutritionally critical lysine and methionine amino acids (Guil *et al*, 1997; Prakash *et al,* 1995; Koch *et al*, 1965). Whole plant is used as emollient, astringent, diuretic, blood purifier, haemorrhagic diathesis and biliousness (Jain *et al*, 1998). Amaranthus contains provitamin-A (β-carotene), vitamins C and E and riboflavin (Vietmeyer, 1983; Krishnaswamy and Raghuramulu, 1998).

Spinacia oleracea L. (English–Spinach; Hindi, Punjabi–Palak) belonging to family Chenopodiaceae is a commonly occurring herb and is reported to be good source of minerals, vitamin B complex, ascorbic acid, carotenoids (β-carotene, lutein, zeaxanthine), flavonoids, quercetin, apocyanin and p-coumaric acid (Bergman et al, 2001; Gerster, 1993; Zennie and Dwayne, 1977; Burton and Ingold, 1989). Whole plant is used for remedy of urinary calculi and leaves are used for bowel and lung inflammations, fibrile affliction, cooling (Jain and Fillips, 1991).

The protection afforded by plant extracts might be due to their rich antioxidant constituents like β-carotene, lutein, zeaxanthin, flavonoids, p-coumaric acid, ascorbic acid, quercetin, selenium, zinc and folate present in them. Of the common carotenoids present in food, beta carotene, alpha carotene, lycopene, lutein and zeaxanthin can be considered potential prophylactic agents against oxidative stress. They are absorbed by humans in reasonable amounts and they have antioxidant properties (Gerster, 1993). Many epidemiological and oncological studies suggest that humans on a diet high in carotenoid-rich fruits and vegetables, who maintain higher than average levels of serum carotenoids, have a lower incidence of several types of cancer (Chan 1995). The higher β-carotene content of these plants along with other carotenoids seems to emerge as potent radioprotector which seems to be acting through one or more anti-oxidative mechanisms against free radicals generation. Free radicals have been implicated in the pathogenesis of a variety of diseases, resulting usually from defective natural antioxidant defences. Potential antioxidant therapy should therefore, include either natural antioxidant enzymes or agents which are capable of augmenting the function of these oxidative free radical scavenging enzymes (Bast *et al,* 1991).

The studies in our laboratories have shown that the extract of these plants exerts its radioprotective effect in two ways: (i). it is able to curb the initial damage caused due to radiation (by antioxidant activity), and (ii). it stimulates the cellular regeneration in the post-irradiation period (particularly hematopoietic regeneration, liver recovery, gastrointestinal system recovery).

Our experimental findings and review of literature thus conclusively suggest that the extract of *Amarantus* and spinach may offer radioprotection by the following mechanisms:

1. By decreasing radiation induced lipid peroxidation level

It was observed that plant extract treatment (in our laboratory) significantly alters the MDA (Malondialdehyde) level in unirradiated animals and it significantly lowers the generation of the radiation induced lipid peroxidation in terms of MDA. Inhibition of lipid peroxidation in biomembranes can be caused by antioxidants (Konings and Drijver, 1979; Konings and Orsterloo, 1980). The basic effect of radiation on cellular membrane is believed to be the peroxidation of membrane lipids. Lipid peroxidation can be initiated by lipid radiolytic products, including hydroxyl and hydroperoxyl radicals (Raleigh, 1987).

2. By inhibiting the radiation induced depletion of endogenous glutathione

Oral administration of these plant extracts to Swiss albino mice did not significantly influence the endogenous GSH level in liver, by its mere presence while radiation exposure protects the endogenous GSH depletion due to irradiation. The increased GSH level suggests that protection by these plants may be mediated through the modulation of cellular antioxidant levels.

GSH is a versatile protector and executes its radioprotective function through free radical scavenging, restoration of the damaged molecule by hydrogen donation, reduction of peroxides and maintenance of protein thiols in the reduced state (Bump and Brown, 1990). The thiol hypothesis describes the mechanism of the effect of radioprotectors. Revesz and Modig (1965) for the first time put forward a hypothesis that the radioprotective action of aminothiols is mediated through their capacity to release glutathione. Graevsky *et al* (1966) assumes the participation of -SH groups in the process of protection against ionising radiation. It believes that the administered radioprotective substance by itself has no protective effect, but its administration stimulates the release of endogenous -SH substances and these substances are the genuine radioprotectors. Reduced glutathione (GSH) offers protection against oxygen derived free radicals and cellular lethality following exposure to ionising radiation (Biaglow *et al*, 1987). It has been observed that the chemicals, which modify the radiation damage (radiosensitisers) are electron acceptors (Quintiliani, 1970). If electron acceptors are able to enhance radiation effect then electron donors ought to be radioprotective substances (Lohman *et al*, 1967). Thus, it is possible that -SH compounds which are electron donors might act by transferring an electron to biomolecules and hence afford protection.

3. By decreasing acid phosphatases activity

Acid phosphatase activity in plants pre-treated irradiated animals was measured significantly lower than control. This suggests that plant extract may help in causing early recovery by helping in the rapid removal of cellular debris from the tissues, collected due to radiation damage. Acid phosphatase is a lysosomal enzyme which hydrolyses the ester linkage of phosphate ester and helps in the autolysis of the degenerated cells. Acid phosphatase helps in early recovery from radiation damage by removing debris.

The anti-radiation effects shown by the plants may be due to presence of phytoantioxidants such as carotenoids (β-carotene, lutein and zeaxanthine), folic acid, ascorbic acid, vitamin E, p-coumaric acid, quercetin and flavonoids whose anti-oxidative mechanism has been already explained.

REFERENCES

Abraham, S. K., Sharma, L. and Kesavan, P. C. 'Protective effects of chlorogenic acid, curcumin and b-carotene against gamma radiation-induced *in vivo* chromosomal damage. *Mutation Res.* 303: 109-112, 1993.

Alabaster, O., Tang, Z. C., Frost, A. and Shivapurkar, N. 'Effect of β-carotene and wheat bran fibre on colonic aberrant crypt and tumour formation in rats exposed to azoxymethane and high dietary fat'. *Carcinogenesis* 16: 127-132, 1995.

Alam, B. S. and Alam, S. Q. 'The effect of different levels of dietary β-carotene on DMBA induced salivary gland tumours. *Nutr. Cancer*. 9: 93-101, 1987.

Albanes, D., Heinonen, O. P. and Huttunen, J. K. 'The effect of α-tocopherol and β-carotene supplementation on cancer incidence in the alpha-tocopherol b-carotene cancer prevention study'. *Am. J. Clin. Nutr.* 62: (Suppl.) 1423s-1430s, 1995.

Albanes, D., Virtamo, J. and Rautalahti, M. 'Serum β-carotene before and after β-carotene supplementation'. *Eur. J. Clin. Nutr.* 46: 15-24, 1992.

Alpha Tocopherol Beta-Carotene Cancer Prevention Study Group 'The effect of vitamin E and beta-carotene on the incidence of lung cancer and other cancers in male smokers'. *N. Engl. J. Med.* 330: 1029-1035, 1994.

Al-Sereiti, M. R., Abu-Amer, K. M. and Sen, P. 'Pharmacology of rosemary (*Rosmarinus officinalis* Linn.) and its therapeutic potential'. *Ind. J. Exp. Biol.* 37: 124-128, 1999.

Ames, B. N. 'Dietary carcinogens and anticarcinogens oxygen radicals and degenerative diseases'. *Science.* 221: 1256-1264, 1987.

Aqil, F., Beg, A. Z. and Ahmad, I. '*In vitro* toxicity of plant essential oils against soil fungi'. *J. Med. Aro. Plant Sci.* (JMAPS), 22/4A & 23/1A: 177 –182, 2001.

Aritomi, M,, Kokori, T. and Kawasaki, T. 'Flavonol glycosides in leaves of *Spinacia oleracea*'. *Phytochemistry.* 25: 231-234, 1986.

Arora, R. and Goel, H. C. 'Herbal radioprotectors'. Abstract *Proceedings of International Conference on Radiation Biology.* 17-19 February, 2000, Thiruvanthapuram, India. p. 87, 2000.

Bagdon, R. E., Zbinder, G. and Studer, A. 'Chronic toxicity studies of β-carotene'. *Toxicol. Appl. Pharmacol.* 2: 225-236, 1960.

Bast, A., Haenen, G. R. M. M. and Doelman, C. G. A. 'Oxidants and antioxidants: State of the art'. *Am. J. Med.* 91: (Suppl. 3C): 2-9, 1991.

Baumann, J., Wurm, J. and von Bruchhausen, F. 'Prostaglandin synthetase inhibition by flavonoids and phenolic compounds in relation to their O_2^- scavenging properties'. *Arch. Pharm.* (Weinheim) 313: 330-337, 1980.

Beliaev, I. K., Zaraiskii, A. V. Limberg, V. K. and Vakulova, L. A. 'Modification of the body's resistance to acute ionising radiation by synthetic beta-carotene'. *Vopr Med. Khim.* 38(6): 39-42, 1992.

Ben-Amotz, A., Rachmilevich, B., Greenberg, S., Sela, M. and Weshler, Z. 'Natural beta-carotene and whole body irradiation in rats'. *Radiat. Environ. Biophys.* 35(4): 285-288, 1996.

Ben-Amotz, A., Yatziv, S., Sela, M., Greenberg, S., Rachmilevich, B., Shwarzman, M. and Weshler, Z. 'Effect of natural beta-carotene supplementation in children exposed to radiation from the Chernobyl accident'. *Radiat. Environ. Biophys.* 37(3): 187-193, 1998.

Bendich, A. 'The safety of β-carotene'. *Nutr. Cancer* 11: 207-214, 1988.

Ben-Shaul, V., Sofer, Y., Bergman, M., Zurovsky, Y. and Grossman, S. 'Lipopolysaccharide-induced oxidative stress in the liver: comparison between rat and rabbit'. *Shock.* 12: 288-293, 1999.

Berger, A., Gremaud, G., Baumgartner, M., Rein, D., Monnard, I., Kratky, E., Geiger, W., Burri, J., Dionisi, F., Allan, M. and Lambelet, P. 'Cholesterol-lowering properties of amaranth grain and oil in hamsters'. *Int J. Vitam. Nutr. Res.* 73(1): 39-47, 2003.

Bergman, M., Varshavsky, L., Gottlieb Hugo, E. and Grossman, S. 'The antioxidant activity of aqueous Spinach extract: Chemical identification of active fractions'. *Phytochemistry* 58:143-152, 2001.

Bertram, J. S. and Bortkiewioz, H. 'Dietary carotenoids inhibit neoplastic transformation and modulate gene expression in mouse and human cells'. *Am. J. Clin. Nutr.* 62 (Suppl.): 1327s-1336s, 1995.

Bhargava, K. P. and Singh, N. 'Anti-stress activity of *Ocimum sanctum* (Linn.)'. *Ind. J. Med. Res.* 73: 443-447, 1981.

Bhatia, A L. and Jain, M. '*Amaranthus paniculatus* (Linn.) improves learning after radiation stress'. *J. Ethnopharmacol.* 85(1):73-79, 2003.

Bhatia, A. L. 'The anti-ageing role of vitamin A and β-carotene'. *Ind. J. Gerontol.* 12(3-4): 70-79. 1998.

Bhatia, A. L. β-carotene as a function of age: The possibility of its anti-ageing property'. In: *Ageing: Indian Perspective and Global Scenario* (Ed). Kumar, Vinod, pp. 445-447, 1996.

Bhatia, A. L. and Manda, K. 'Role of β-carotene against radiation induced lipid-peroxidation in mice testes'. *Res. J. Chem. Environ.* 4(1): 59-61, 2000.

Bhatia, A. L., Sisodia, R., Manda, K. and Sharma, M. 'Dose dependent study on the effectiveness of β-carotene on the survivability of mice against lethal gamma irradiation'. *Rad. Prot. Env.* 24 (1 & 2): 96-101, 2001.

Bhattacharya, S. K., Satyam, K. and Ghosal, S. 'Antioxidant activity of glycowithanolides from *Withania somnifera*'. *Ind. J. of Expl. Biol.* 35: 236-239, 1996.

Biaglow, J. E., Varnes, M. E., Epp, E. R. and Clark, E. P. In: *Anticarcinogenesis and Radiation Protection*". (Eds). Cerrutti, P. A., Nygaard, O. F. and Simic, M. G. New York: Plenum Press, pp. 387-391, 1987.

Bickford, P. C., Gould, T., Briederiok, L., Chadman, K., Pollock, A., Youn, D., Shukitt- Hale, B. and Joseph, J. 'Antioxidant rich diets improve cerebellar physiology and motor learning in aged rats'. *Brain Res.* 866 (1-2): 211-217, 2000.

Bitterman, N., Melamed, Y. and Ben-Amotz, A. 'β-carotene and CNS oxygen toxicity in rats'. *American Physiological Society,* pp. 1073-1076, 1994.

Block, G. 'Are clinical trials really the answer'. *Am. J. Clin. Nutr.* 62: 1517-1520, 1995.

Blot, W. J., Li, J. Y., Taylor, P. R., Guo, W., Dawsey, S. M. and Li, B. 'The linxial trials: mortality rates by vitamin-mineral intervention group'. *Am. J. Clin. Nutr.* 62 (Suppl.): 1424S-1426S, 1995.

Bogo, V. 'Behavioural radioprotection'. *Pharmacol. Ther.* 39: 73, 1988.

Bracke, M. L., Depestel, G., Castronovo, V., Vijneke, B., Foidart, J. M., Vakaet, L. C. A. and Marcel, M. M. 'Flavonoids inhibit malignant tumours invasion *in vitro*'. In: *Plant Flavonoids in Biology and Medicine.* II. *Biochemical, Cellular and Medicinal Properties* (Eds.). Cody, V., Middleton, E., Harborne, J. B. and Beretz, A., pp. 219-233. New York: Alan R. Liss, 1988.

Britton, G., Liaaen-Jensen, S. and Pfander, H. 'Carotenoids today and challenges for the future'. In: *Carotenoids.* vol. 1A: *Isolation and Analysis.* (Eds.). Britton, G., Liaaen-Jensen, S. and Pfander, H. Basel: Birkhäuser, pp. 162-166, 1995.

Brubacher, G. B. and Weiser, H. 'The vitamin A activity of beta-carotene'. *Internatl. J. Vit. Nutr. Res.* 55: 5-15, 1985.

Bump, E. A and Brown, M. 'Role of glutathione in the radiation response of mammalian cells *in vitro* and *in vivo*'. *Pharmacol. Ther.* 47: 17-22, 1990.

Burton, G. W. and Ingold, K. U. 'β-carotene: an unusual type of lipid antioxidant'. *Science* 224: 569-573, 1984.

Byers, T. and Guerrero, N. 'Epidemiologic evidence for vitamin C and vitamin E in cancer prevention'. *Am. J. Clin. Nutr.* 62: (Suppl.): 1385s-1392s, 1995.

Castenmiller, J. J. and West, C. E. 'Bioavailability and bioconversion of carotenoids'. *Ann. Rev. Nutr.* 18: 19-38, 1998.

Castenmiller, J. J., Linssen, J. P., Heinonen, I. M., Hopia, A. I., Schwarz, K., Hollmann, P. C. and West, C. E. 'Antioxidant properties of differently processed spinach products' *Nahrung* 46(4): 290-293, 2002.

Castenmiller, J. J., van de Poll, C. J., West, C. E., Brouwer, I. A., Thomas, C. M. and van Dusseldorp, M. 'Bioavailability of folate from processed spinach in humans. Effect of food matrix and interaction with carotenoids'. *Ann Nutr Metab.* 44(4):163-169, 2000.

Castenmiller, J. J., West, C. E., Linssen, J. P., van het Hof, K. H. and Voragen, A. G. 'The food matrix of spinach is a limiting factor in determining the bioavailability of beta-carotene and to a lesser extent of lutein in humans'. *J Nutr.* 129(2): 349-355, 1999.

Cerutti, P. A. 'Peroxidant status and tumour production'. *Science.* 227: 331-381, 1985.

Chan, T. Y. 'Shellfish-borne illness. A Hong Kong perspective'. *Trop. Geogr. Med.* 47(6): 305-307, 1995.

Chandha, S. L. 'Natural source of antioxidants and their adequacy in diet to prevent atheroscelerosis. *Mediquest.* 14(3): 337-351, 1997.

Chen, L. H., Boissonneault, G. A. and Glavert, H. P. 'Vitamin C, vitamin E and cancer'. *Anticancer Res.* 8: 739-748, 1988.

Chu, Y. F., Sun, J., Wu, X. and Liu, R. H. 'Antioxidant and antiproliferative activities of common vegetables'. *J. Agric. Food Chem.* 50(23): 6910-6916, 2002.

Conn, P. F., Schalch, W. and Truscott, T. G. 'The singlet oxygen and carotenoid interaction'. *J. Photochem. Photobiol. B. Biol.* 11: 41-47, 1991.

Correa, P. *Cancer Res.* 52: 6735, 1992.*

Cotelle, N., Bernier, J. L., Cattaeu, J. P., Henichart, J. P. and Pasandon, D. 'Inhibition of macrophage superoxide production by two phenylated flavonones from *Erythrina sigmoidea*'. *Natural Prod. Lett.* 3: 79-83, 1993.

Cozzi, R., Ricordy, R., Aglitti, T., Gatta, V., Perticone, P. and Salvia, R. 'Ascorbic acid and β-carotene as modulators of oxidative damage'. *Carcinogenesis* 18(1): 223-228, 1997.

Daga, S. S., Jain, V. K. and Goyal, P. K. 'Radioprotective role of Liv.52 on circulating erythrocytes against sub-lethal doses of gamma radiations'. *Proceedings of International Symposium on Radiomodifiers in Human Health.* Manipal, India. 1995.

Demmig-Adams, B. 'Carotenoids and photoprotection in plants: a role for the xanthophyll zeaxanthin'. *Biochim. Biophys. Acta.* 1020:1-24, 1990.

Devadas Rajammal, P., Chandrasekhar, U., Premakumari, S. and Saishree, R. 'Consumption pattern of carotene rich foods and development of a year calendar'. *Biomed. Environ. Sci.* 9(2-3): 213-222, 1996.

Diplock, A. T. 'Safety of antioxidant vitamins and β-carotene'. *Am. J. Clin. Nutr.* 62 (Suppl): 1510S-1516S, 1995.

Ei-Nahas, S. M., Mattar, F. E. and Mohamed, A. A. 'Radioprotective effect of vitamin C and E'. *Mutation Research* 301: 143-147.

Elizabeth, K. and Rao, M. N. A. 'Oxygen radical scavenging activity of Cucurmin'. *Int. J. Pharm.* 58: 237-242, 1990.

Farooqi, Z. and Kesavan, P. C. 'Radioprotection by caffeine pre-treatment in the bone marrow chromosomes of mice given whole body gamma irradiation'. *Mutat. Res.* 269(2): 225-229, 1992.

Ferreres, F., Castaner, M. and Tomas-Barbern, A. 'Acylated flavonol glycosides from spinach leaves *(Spinacia oleracea)*'. *Phytochemistry* 45: 1701-1705, 1997.

Fitechett, M., Gilbert, B. C. and Jeffy, M. *Phil. Trans. R. Soc.*, London, B31, 517-529, 1985.

Fruta, S. Y., Nishiba and Suda. J. 'Flourometric assay for screening antioxidative activity of vegetables'. *J. of Food Sci.* 62: 526-528, 1997.

Fuziki, H., Horiuchi, T., Yamashita, K., Hakii, H., Iwashima, A., Hirata, Y. and Sugimura, T. 'Inhibition of tumour promotion by flavonoids'. In: *Plant Flavonoids in Biology and Medicine: Biochemical, Pharmacological and Structure Activity Relationships.* (Eds.). Cody, V., Middleton, E. and Harborne, J. B.) New York: Alan R. Liss, pp. 429-440, 1986.

Ganasoundari, A., Zare, S. M. and Uma Devi, P. 'Modification of bone marrow radiosensitivity by medicinal plant extracts'. *Brit. J. Radiol.* 70: 599, 1997.

Gerster, H. 'Anticarcinogenic effect of common carotenoids'. *Int. J. Vit. Nutr. Res.* 63: 93-121, 1993.

Gey, K. F. 'The relationship of antioxidant status and the risk of cancer and cardiovascular disease: A critical evaluation of observational data. In: *Free Radicals in the Environment, Medicine and Toxicology.* (Eds.). Nohl, H., Esterbauer, H. and Rice-Evans, C. London: Richelieu Press, pp. 181-219, 1994.

Goel, H. C., Prasad, J. and Sharma, A. K. 'Protective effect of *Podophyllum* against radiation damage'. *Adv. Radiat. Biol. & Peace* (2): 27-33, 1999.

Goodman, G. E., Metch, B. J. and Omenn, G. S. 'The effect of long-term β-carotene and vitamin A administration on serum concentrations of alpha-tocopherol'. *Cancer. Epidemiol. Biomarkers,* Prev. 3: 429-432, 1994.

Gopalan. C., Sastri, R. B. V. and Balasubramanian, S. C. *Nutritive Value of Indian Foods.* Hyderabad: National Institute of Nutrition, I. C. M. R., pp. 1-156, 1996.

Graevsky, E. Y., Konstantinova, M. A., Nekrasova, I. V., Sokolova, O. M. and Toresenko, A. E. 'Increase in the content of endogenous sulphydryl compounds as the mechanism of radioprotective action'. *Nature.* 212: 475, 1966.

Graf, E. 'Antioxidant potential of feluric acid'. *Free Radic. Biol. Med.* 13: 435-439, 1992.

Guil, J. L., Rodriguez–Garcia, I. and Torija, E. 'Nutritional and toxic factors in selected wild edible plants'. *Plant Foods Hum. Nutr.* 51(2): 99-107, 1997.

Gupta, N. K. 'Hypolipidemic action of garlic unsaturated oils in irradiated mice'. *Nat. Acad. Sci. Lett.* 11(12): 401, 1988.

Gustafsson, K., Asp, N. G., Hagander, B. and Nyman, M. 'Satiety effects of spinach in mixed meals: Comparison with other vegetables'. *Int. J. Food Sci. Nutr.* 46(4): 327-334, 1995.

Halliwell, B., Gutteridge, J. M. C. and Cross, C. E. *J. Lab. Clin. Med.* 119: 398-620, 1992.

Hammond, B. R. Jr., Johnson, E. J., Russell, R. M., Krinsky, N. I., Yeum, K. J., Edwards, R. B. and Snodderly, D. M. 'Dietary modification of human macular pigment density'. *Invest Ophthalmol. Vis Sci.* 38(9):1795-1801, 1997.

Harman, D. 'The ageing process'. *Proc. Natl. Acad. Sci.*, U.S.A., 78: 7124-7128, 1981.

He, T., Huang, C. Y., Chen, H. and Hou, Y. H. 'Effects of spinach powder fat-soluble extract on proliferation of human gastric adenocarcinoma cells'. *Biomed Environ Sci.* 12(4): 247-252, 1999.

Hebbar, S. A., Mitra, A. K., Satav, J. G., George K. G. and Verma, N. C. 'Radioprotection by caffeine'. Satellite meeting, International Conference IARP-IC-2KI, Jaipur, 2001.

Heinonen, O. P. and Albanes, D. 'The effects of vitamin E and β-carotene on the incidence of lung cancer and other cancers in male smokers'. *N. Engl. J. Med.* 330: 1029-1035. 1994.

Heywood, R., Palmer, A. K., Gregson, R. L. and Hummlev, H. 'The toxicity of β-carotene'. *Toxicology* 36: 91-100, 1985.

Howard, L. R., Pandjaitan, N., Morelock, T. and Gil, M. I. 'Antioxidant capacity and phenolic content of spinach as affected by genetics and growing season'. *J. Agric. Food Chem.* 50(21): 5891-5896, 2002.

Hu, J. D., Calomine, M., Lasure, A., Debruyne, T., Pieters, A., Vlientinck, A., Vanden, D. A. and Berghe 'Structure-activity relationship of flavonoids with superoxide scavenging activity'. *Biol. Trace Element Res.*: 47: 327-331, 1995.

Husain, S. R., Cillarat, J. and Cillard, P. 'Hydroxyl radical scavenging activity of flavonoids'. *Phytochemistry* 26: 2489-2492. 1987.

Iyama, T., Takasuga, A. and Azuma, M. 'β-carotene accumulation in mouse tissues and a protective role against lipid peroxidation'. *Int. J. Vitam. Vit. Nutr. Res.* 66(4): 301-305, 1996.

Jain, M. Evaluation of antioxidative efficacy of certain plants extract: A study on mice liver. Ph.D. Thesis. University of Rajasthan, Jaipur, 2002.

Jain, S. K. and De Fillipps, R. A. *Medicinal Plants of India.* Michigan, U.S.A.: Reference Publication, Inc., pp. 18-24, 1991.

Jain, S., Shukla, S. D., Sharma, K. and Bhatnagar, M. 'Phytoantioxidants: Therapute implication of antioxidants in neuro degenerative changes in brain'. *Ind. J. Gerontol.* 12(3-4): 60-69, 1998.

Jialal, I., Norkus, E. P., Cristol, L. and Grundy, S. M. 'β-carotene inhibits oxidative modification of low-density lipoprotein'. *Biochem. Biophys. Acta.* Cited by Gerster, H. (1993). 'Anticarcinogenic effect of common carotenoids'. *Int. J. Vit. Nutr. Res.* 63: 93-122. 1993.

Johnson, E. J., Hammond, B. R., Yeum, K. J., Qin, J., Wang, X. D., Castaneda, C., Snodderly, D. M. and Russell, R. M. 'Relation among serum and tissue concentrations of lutein and zeaxanthin and macular pigment density'. *Am. J. Clin. Nutr.* 71(6):1555-1562, 2000.

Joseph, J. A., Shukitt-Hale, B., Denisova, N. A., Prior, R. L., Cao, G., Martin, A., Taglialatela, G. and Bickford, P. C. 'Long-term dietary strawberry, spinach, or vitamin E supplementation retards the onset of age-related neuronal signal-transduction and cognitive behavioural deficits'. *J. Neurosci.* 18(19): 8047-8055, 1998.

Kandaswami, C., Perkins, E., Solonink, D. S., Drzewiecki and Middleton, E. Jr. 'Antiproliferative effects of citrus flavonoids on a human squamous cell carcinoma *in vitro*'. *Cancer Lett.* 56: 147-152, 1991.

Kayashima, T. and Katayama, T. 'Oxalic acid is available as a natural antioxidant in some systems'. *Biochim. Biophys. Acta.* 1573(1):1-3, 2002.

Klimczak, I., Malecka, M. and Pacholek, B. 'Antioxidant activity of ethanolic extracts of amaranth seeds'. *Nahrung.* 46(3):184-186, 2002.

Knopacka, M., Widel, M. and Rzeszowska-Wolny, J. 'Modifying effect of vitamin C, E and beta-carotene against gamma-ray-induced DNA damage in mouse cells'. *Mutat. Res.* 417(2-3): 85-94, 1998.

Koch, B., Kota Mand and Howafn, I. M. 'Fodder crops as leaf protein. *Agrobotanika* 7: 19-28, 1965.

Kohlmier, L. and Hastings, S. B. 'Epidemiologic evidence of a role of carotenoids in cardiovascular disease prevention'. *Am. J. Clin. Nutr.* 62(Suppl.): 1370S-1376S, 1995.

Konings, A. W. T. and Drijver, E. B. 'Radiation effects on membranes. I. Vitamin E deficiency and lipid peroxidation'. *Radiat. Res.* 80: 494-497, 1979

Konings, A. W. T. and Oosterloo, S. K. 'Radiation effects on membranes. II. A comparison of the effects of X-irradiation and ozone exposure with respect to the relation of antioxidant concentration and the capacity for lipid peroxidation'. *Radiat. Res.* 81: 200, 1980.

Konyk, U. V., Hzhehots'kyi, M. P. and Koval'chuk, S. M. 'Metabolic effect of amaranth oil and impulse hypoxic training under chronic fluoride intoxication and small doses of ionising radiation'. *Fiziol. Zh..* 48(6):80-85, 2002.

Krinsky, N. I. 'Antioxidant functions of carotenoids'. *Free Rad. Biol. Med.* 7: 617-635. 1989.

Krinsky, N. I. and Deneke, S. M. 'Interaction of oxygen and oxy-radicals with carotenoids'. *J. Nat. Cancer Inst.* 69: 205-210, 1982.

Krinsky, N. I., Russett, M. D., Handelman, G. J. and Snodderly, D. M. 'Structural and geometrical isomers of carotenoids in human plasma. *J. Nutr.* 120: 1654-1662, 1990.

Krishnaswamy, K. and Raghuramulu, N. 'Bioactive phyto-chemicals with emphasis on dietary practices'. *Ind. J. Med. Res.* 108: 167, 1998.

Kumar, P., Kuttan, R. and Kuttan, G. 'Effect of 'Rasayanas', a herbal drug preparation on immune response and its significance to cancer treatment'. *Ind. J. Exp. Biol.* 37: 27-32, 1999.

Kumar, P., Kuttan, V. R. and Kuttan, G. 'Radioprotective effects of rasayans'. *Ind. J. Exp. Biol.* 34: 848-850, 1996.

Lambelet, P., Saucy, F. and Loliger, J. 'Chemical evidence for interaction between vitamin E and C'. *Experientia.* 41: 1384-1388, 1985.

Landauer, M. R., Walden, T. L. and Davis, H. D. 'Behavioural effects of radioprotective agents in mice. Combination of WR-2721 and 16,16 dimethyl prostaglandin E2. Frontiers of Radiation Biology'. Proceedings of the 21st Annual Meeting of the European Society for Radiation Biology. (Eds.). Riklis, E., Weinheim, V. C. H., Deerfield Beach, F. L. and Balaban, Rehovot. Philadelphia, 1989.

Lee, J., Lee, S., Lee, H., Park, K. and Choe, E. 'Spinach (*Spinacia oleracea*) powder as a natural food-grade antioxidant in deep-fat-fried products'. *J. Agric. Food Chem.* 50(20): 5664-5669, 2002.

Lee, Ji-hylon; Jong-Cheol, P. and Jae-Sue, C. 'Antioxidant activity of *Ecklonia stolonifera*'. *Archives of Pharmacol. Res.* 3: 223-227, 1996.

Levenson, S. M., Gruber, C. A., Rettura, G., Gruber, D. K., Demetriou, A. A. and Seifter, E. 'Supplemental Vit. A prevents the acute radiation induced defect in wound healing'. *Ann. Surg.* 200: 494-512, 1984.

Liebler, D. C. and McClure, T. D. 'Antioxidant reactions of beta-carotene: Identification of carotenoid-radical adducts'. *Chem. Res. Toxicol.* 9(1): 8-11, 1996.

Lirio, L. G., Hermano, M. L. and Fontanilla, M. Q. 'Antibacterial activity of medicinal plants from the Philippines'. *Pharmaceut. Biol.* 36: 357, 1998.

Lohmann, W., Momeni, M. and Nette, P. 'On the possible involvement of charge transfer complexes (redox systems) in radioprotection'. *Strahlentherapie.* 134: 590, 1967.

Lomnitski, L., Carbonatto, M., Ben-Shaul, V., Peano, S., Conz, A., Corradin, L., Maronpot, R. R., Grossman, S. and Nyska, A. 'The prophylactic effects of natural water-soluble antioxidant from spinach and apocynin in a rabbit model of lipopolysaccharide-induced endotoxemia'. *Toxicol. Pathol.* 28(4): 588-600, 2000b.

Lomnitski, L., Foley, J. E., Grossman, S., Shaul, V. B., Maronpot, R. R., Moomaw, C. R., Carbonatto, M. and Nyska, A. 'Effects of apocynin and natural antioxidant from spinach on inducible nitric oxide synthase and cyclooxygenase-2 induction in lipopolysaccharide-induced hepatic injury in rat'. *Pharmacol. Toxicol.* 87(1): 18-25, 2000c.

Lomnitski, L., Nyska, A., Ben-Shaul, V., Maronpot, R. R., Haseman, J. K., Harrus, T. L., Bergman, M. and Grossman, S. 'Effects of antioxidants apocynin and the natural water-soluble antioxidant from spinach on cellular damage induced by lipopolysaccaride in the rat'. *Toxicol. Pathol.* 28(4): 580-587, 2000a.

Manda, K. Investigation on the possible radioprotective effect of β-carotene on mice testis. Ph.D. Thesis, University of Rajasthan, Jaipur, India, 1999.

Manda, K. and Bhatia, A. L. 'Effect of spermatogonia to radiation'. *Natl. Acad. Sci Ind.*, 1999.

Manda, K., Sharma, M., Sisodia, R. and Bhatia, A. L. 'β-carotene deplets radiation induced lipid peroxidation in mouse brain and testes'. *Ind. J. Gerntol.* 12(1-4): 10-14, 2000.

Mathews-Roth, M. M. 'Beta-carotene therapy for erythropoietic protoporphyria and other photosensitivity diseases'. *Biochemic.* 68: 875-884, 1986.

Mathews-Roth, M. M. 'Beta-carotene: clinical aspects'. In: *New Protective Roles for Selected Nutrients.* (Eds.). Spiller, A. and Scale, J. *Curr. Top. Nutr. Dis.* 22: 17-38, 1989.

Mathews-Roth, M. M. 'Recent progress in the medical application of carotenoids'. *Pure Appl. Chem.* 63: 147-156, 1991.

Mathews-Roth, M. M., Pathak, M. A., Fitzpatrick, T. B., Harber, L. H. and Kass, E. H. 'Beta carotene therapy for erythropoietic protoporphyria and other photosensitivity diseases'. *Arch. Dermatol.* 113: 1229-1232, 1977.

Mc Clure, J. W. '*In the Flavonoids*, vol. 2. (Eds.). Harborne, J. B., Mabry, T. J. and Mabry. H. New York: Academic Press, p. 970, 1975.

McLarty, J. W. 'An intervention trial in high-risk asbestos-exposed persons'. In: *The Biology and Prevention of Aerodigestive Tract Cancer.* (Eds.). Newell, G. R. and Hongs, W. K. New York: Plenum, pp. 141-149, 1992.

Middleton, Jr. E. and Kandaswami, C. 'Effects of flavonoids on immune and inflammatory cell functions'. *Biochem. Pharmacol.* 43: 1167-1179, 1992.

Middleton, Jr. E. and Kandaswami, C. 'The impact of plantvonoids on mammalian biology; implication for immunity, inflammation and cancer. In: *The Flavonoids: Advances in Research Since 1986.* (Ed.). Harborne. J. B. London: Chapman & Hall, pp. 619-652, 1993.

Mills, E. E. D. 'The modifying effect of beta-carotene on radiation and chemotherapy induced oral mucositis'. *Br. J. Cancer.* 57: 416-417, 1988.

Molnar, J., MacPherson, A., Barclay, I. and Molnar, P. 'Selenium content of convenience and fast foods in Ayrshire, Scotland'. *Int. J. Food Sci. Nutr.* 46(4): 343-352, 1995.

Moore, T. *Vitamin A.* Amsterdam: Elsevier Publication Co., 1957.*

Moser, U. and Bendich, A. 'Vitamin C'. In: *Handbook of Vitamins.* (Ed.). Machlin, L. J. New York: Marcel Dekker, pp. 195-232, 1991.

Mukherjee, A. K., Agarwal, M. A., Aguilar and Sharma, A. 'Anticlastogenic activity of β-carotene against cyclophosphamide in mice *in vivo*'. *Mutation Res.* 263: 41-46, 1991.

Nemoto, K., Horiuchi, K. and Miyamoto, T. 'Deoxyspergualin is a new radioprotector in mice'. *Radiat. Res.* 141: 223, 1995.

Ni, Q. G. and Pei, Y. 'Effect of beta-carotene on ^{60}Co-gamma-induced mutation at T-lymphocyte hypoxanthine-guanine phosphoribosyl transferase locus in rats'. *Zhongguo Yao Li xue Bao.* 18(6): 535-536, 1997.

Nierenberg, D. W., Stukel, T. A., Mott, L. A. and Greenberg, E. R. 'Steady-state serum concentration of alpha tocopherol not-altered by supplementation with oral beta carotene'. The Polyp Prevention Study Group. *J. Natl. Cancer Inst.* 86: 117-120, 1994.

Noakes, M., Clifton, P., Ntanios, F., Shrapnel, W., Record, I. and McInerney, J. 'An increase in dietary carotenoids when consuming plant sterols or stanols is effective in maintaining plasma carotenoid concentrations'. *Am. J. Clin. Nutr.* 75(1): 79-86, 2002.

Ong, A. S. H. and Tee, E. S. 'Natural sources of carotenoids from plants and oils'. *Meth. Enzymol..* 213: 142-167, 1992.

Packer, J. E., Slater, T. E. and Wilson, R. L. 'Direct observation of a free radical interaction between vitamin E and vitamin C'. *Nature.* 278: 737-738, 1979.

Panda, S. and Kar, A. 'Evidence for free radical scavenging activity of Ashwagandha root powder in mice'. *Ind. J. Phys. Pharm.* 41: 424-426, 1997.

Pande, S., Kumar, M. and Kumar, A. 'Evaluation of radio-modifying effect of root extract of *Panax ginseng*'. *Phytother. Res.* 12: 13-18, 1998a.

Pande, S., Kumar, M. and Kumar, A. 'Investigation of radio-protective efficacy of *Aloe vera* leaf extract'. *Pharmaceut. Biol.* 36: 1, 1998b.

Pandey, B. N. and Mishra, K. P. 'Radiation induced oxidative damage: Modification by cholesterol in liposomal membrane'. *Radiat. Phys. Chem.* 54: 481, 1999.

Pandey, S., Sharma, M. and Chaturvedi, P. 'Protective effect of *Rubia cordifolia* on lipid peroxide formation in isolated rat liver homogenate'. *Ind. J. Exp. Biol.* 32: 180-183, 1994.

Patt, H. M., Tyree, E. B., Straub, R. L. and Smith, D. E. 'Cystein protection against X-irradiation'. *Science* 110: 213-215, 1949.

Perrig, W. J., Perrig, P. and Stahelin, H. B. 'The relation between antioxidants and memory performance in the old and very old'. *Journal of the American Geriatrics Society.* 45(6): 718-724, 1997.

Peto, R., Doll, R., Buckley, J. D. and Sporn, M. B. 'Can dietary β-carotene materially reduce human cancer rates'. *Nature.* 290: 201-208, 1981.

Pospisil, M., Hofer, M., Znojil, V., Vacha, J., Netikova, J. and Hola, H. 'Radioprotection of mouse hemopoiesis by dipyridamole and adenine monophosphate in fractional treatment'. *Radiat. Res.* 142: 16-21, 1995.

Prakash, D., Joshi, B. D. and Pal, M. 'Vitamin C in leaves and seed oil composition of the *Amaranthus* species'. *Int. J. Food Sci. Nutr.* 46(1): 47-51, 1995.

Prakash, Niranjen, A. and Tewari, S. K. 'Nutritional composition of weed flora of sodic soil'. *JMAPS*; 22/4A, 23/1A, 450-454, 2000.

Pratt, D. E. In: *Phenolic Compounds in Food and Their Effect on Health* II. (Eds.). Hvang, M. T., HOC-H. and Lee C. Y. *American Chemical Society.*, Washington, 1992.

Proteggente, A. R., Pannala, A. S., Paganga, G., Van Buren, L., Wagner, E., Wiseman, S., Van De Put, F., Dacombe, C. and Rice-Evans, C. A. 'The antioxidant activity of regularly consumed fruit and vegetables reflects their phenolic and vitamin C composition'. *Free Radic. Res.* 36(2): 217-233, 2002.

Punita, A. and Chaturvedi, A. 'Effect of feeding crude red palm oil (*Elaeis guineensis*) and grain amaranth (*Amaranthus paniculatus*) to hens on total lipids, cholesterol, PUFA levels and acceptability of eggs'. *Plant Foods Hum. Nutr.* 55(2):147-157, 2000.

Quintiliani, M. 'Radiation sensitisation at the molecular level'. Abstract in IV. Int. Cong. Radait. Res., Evian, France, 1970.

Rajakumar, D. V. and Rao, M. N. A. 'Dehydrozyngerone and isoeugonol as inhibitors of lipid peroxidation and as free radical scavengers'. *Biochem. Pharmacol.* 46: 2067, 1993.

Rajyalakshmi, P. and Geervani, P. 'Nutritive value of the foods cultivated and consumed by the tribals of south India'. *Plant Foods for Human Nutrition* 46 (1): 53-61, 1994.

Raleigh, J. A. 'Radiation protection in model membranes'. In: *Protaglandins and Lipid Metabolism in Radiation Injury* (Eds.). Walden, Jr., T. L. and Hughes, H. N. New York: Plenum Press, pp. 3-28, 1987.

Ramakrishnan, N., Wolfe, W. W. and Catravas, G. N. 'Radioprotection of hemopoietic tissues in mice by lipoic acid'. *Radiat. Res.* 130: 360, 1992.

Ramesh, S., Manda, K. and Bhatia, A. L. 'Protective effect of β-carotene on radiation induced lipid peroxidation'. *Current Science* 73(5): 470-471, 1997.

Rastogi, R. P. and Mehrotra, B. N. *Compendium of Indian Medicinal Plants.* vol. 3, (1980-81) New Delhi: CDRI and PID, 1991.

Renner, H. W. '*In vivo* effects of single or combined dietary antimutagens on mutagens induced chromosomal aberrations'. *Mutation Res.* 244: 185-188, 1990.

Revesz, L. and Modig, H. 'Cysteamine induced increase of cellular glutathione level: A new hypothesis of the radioprotective mechanism'. *Nature.* 207: 430, 1965.

Robak, J. and Gryglewski, R. J. 'Flavonoids are scavengers of superoxide anion'. *Biochem. Pharmacol.* 37: 837-841, 1988.

Saija, A., Scalese, M., Lanza, M., Morzullo, D., Bonina, F. and Castelli, F. 'Flavonoids as antioxidant agents: Importance of their interaction with biomembranes'. *Free Radic. Biol. Med.* 19: 481, 1995.

Saini, M. R., Kumar, S., Uma Devi, P. and Saini, N. 'Late effects of whole-body irradiation on the peripheral blood of mice and its modification by Liv.52'. *Radiobiol. Radiother.* 26-28: 487, 1985.

Saini, M. R., Uma Devi, P. and Yadav, S. S. 'Radiation protection of bone marrow lymphocytes by 2-merctaptopropionyl-glycine (MPG)'. *Experientia.* 34: 16-27, 32, 1978.

Salvadori, D. M. F., Ribeiro, L. R. and Natrajan, A. T. 'Effect of β-carotene on clastogenic effects of mitomycin C, methyl methanesulfonate and bleomycin in Chinese hamster ovary cells'. *Mutagenesis* 9: 53-57, 1994.

Salvadori, D. M. F., Ribeiro, L. R. and Natrajan, A. T. 'The anticlastogenicity of β-carotene evaluated on human hepatoma cells'. *Mutat. Res.* 303: 151-156, 1993.

Salvadori, D. M. F., Ribeiro, L. R., Oliveira, M. D. M., Pereira, C. A. B. and Becak, W. 'β-carotene as a modulator of chromosomal aberrations induced in mouse bone marrow cells'. *Environ. Mol. Mutagen.* 20: 206-210, 1992b.

Salvadori, D. M. F., Ribeiro, L. R., Oliveira, M. D. M., Pereira, C. A. B. and Becak, W. 'The protective effect of β-carotene on genotoxicity induced by cyclophosphamide'. *Mutation Res.* 265: 237-244, 1992a.

Salvadori, D. M. F., Ribeiro, L., Yiao, Y., Boei, J. J. and Natrajan, A. T. 'Radioprotection of β-carotene evaluated on mouse somatic and germ cells'. *Mutat. Res.* 356: 163-170, 1996.

Satoh, A., Hitomi, M. and Igarashi, K. 'Effects of spinach leaf protein concentrate on the serum cholesterol and amino acid concentrations in rats fed a cholesterol-free diet'. *J. Nutr. Sci. Vitaminol* (Tokyo) 41(5): 563-573, 1995.

Saxena, A. Entero-hepatic response against the combined effect of mercury and radiation in mice and its modification by Liv.52. Ph.D. Thesis, University of Rajasthan, Jaipur, India, 1997.

Schubert, H., Kroon, B. M. A. and Mathijs, H. C. P. '*In vivo* manipulation in the green algae *Chlorella pyrenoidosa*'. *J. Biol. Chem.* 269: 7267-7272, 1994.

Seddon, J. M., Ajani, U. A. and Sperduto, R. D. 'Dietary carotenoids, vitamins A, C, and E, and advanced age-related macular degeneration'. *JAMA.* 272: 1413-1420, 1994.

Seifter, E., Mendecki, J., Holtzman, S., Jacob, D., Friedenthal, F., Davis, L. and Weizweig, J. 'Role of Vitamin A and ß-carotene in radiation protection relation to antioxidant properties'. *Pharmac. Ther.* 39: 357-365, 1988.

Seifter, E., Rettira, G., Padwer, J., Stratford, F., Goodwin, P. and Levenson, S. M. 'Regression of C3HBA mouse tumour due to X-ray therapy combined with supplemented β-carotene or vitamin A'. *J. Natl. Cancer Inst.* 71: 409-417, 1983.

Seifter, E., Rettira, G., Padwer, J., Stratford, F., Weinzweig, J., Demetration, A. A. and Levenson, S. M. *J. Natl. Cancer. Inst.* 73: 1167-1177, 1984.*

Sen, P., Malti, P. C., Puri, S., Audulav, N. A. and Voldman, A. V. 'Mechanism of anti-stress activity of *Ocimum sanctum* Linn.: *Eugenol* and *Tinospora malabarica* in experimental animals'. *Ind. J. Exp. Biol.* 30: 592, 1992.

Sharma, M. Investigation on the beta-carotene vs radiation effects on mice cerebellum. Ph.D Thesis. Submitted to University of Rajasthan, Jaipur, 2001.

Shimoi, K., Masuda, S., Shen, B., Furugori, B. and Kinae, N. 'Radioprotective effect of antioxidative plant flavonoids in mice'. *Mutat. Res.* 350: 153, 1996.

Shimoi, K., Mishida, S., Furogori, M., Osaki, S. and Kinae, N. 'Radioprotective effects of antioxidative flavonoids in γ-ray irradiated mice'. *Carcinogenesis* 15: 2669-2672, 1994.

Sies, H., Sthal, W. and Sundquist, A. R. 'Antioxidant functions of vitamins, vitamin E and C, beta-carotene and other carotenoids'. *Ann. N.Y. Acad. Sci.*, September 30. 669: 7-20, 1992.

Singh, G., Kawatra, A. and Sehgal, S. 'Nutritional composition of selected green leafy vegetables, herbs and carrots'. 56(4): 359-64, 2001.

Singh, K. *Proceedings of Ayurveda Seminar on Cancer,* Thrissum, 15-21, 1990.

Singh, N., Mishra, N., Srivastava, A. K. and Dixit, K. S. 'Mechanism of anti-stress activity of *Ocimum sanctum* Linn., *Eugenol* and *Tinospora malabarica* in experimental animals'. *Ind. J. Exp. Biol.* 30: 592-596, 1991.

Singh, S. P., Ashu, B. T. and Kesavan, P. C. 'Post exposure radioprotection by *Chlorella vulgaris* (E-25) in mice'. *Ind. J. Exp. Biol.* 33: 612-615, 1995.

Sisodia, R., Manda, K. and Bhatia, A. L. 'The possible radioprotective role of beta-carotene and vitamin A'. *Adv. Radiation Biol. and Peace.* 2: 211-218, 1999.

Sisodia, R., Sharma, M. and Bhatia, A. L. 'Qualitative and quantitative study on the radioprotective role of β-carotene on mice cerebellum'. *J. Enviro. Sci.,* 2002.

Slattery, M. L., Benson, J., Curtin, K., Ma, K. N., Schaeffer, D. and Potter, J. D. 'Carotenoids and colon cancer'. *Am. J. Clin. Nutr.* 71(2): 575-582, 2000.

Slyshenkov, V. S., Omelyanchik, S. N., Moiseenok, A. G., Petushok, N. E. and Wojtczak, L. 'Protection by pantothenol and beta-carotene against liver damage produced by low dose gamma irradiation'. *Acta. Biochem. Pol.* 46(2): 239-248, 1999.

Snodderly, D. M. 'Evidence for protection against age-related macular degeneration by carotenoids and antioxidant vitamins'. *Am. J. Clin. Nutr.* 62(Suppl): 1448S-1461S, 1995.

Sommerburg, O., Keunen, J. E., Bird, A. C. and van Kuijk, F. J. 'Fruits and vegetables that are sources for lutein and zeaxanthin: The macular pigment in human eyes'. *Br. J. Ophthalmol.* 82(8): 907-910, 1998.

Sorata, Y., Takahama, U. and Kimura, M. 'Protective effect of quercetin and rutin on photosensitised lysis of human erythrocyte in the presence of hematoporphyrin'. *Biochem. Biophys. Acta.* 799: 313-317, 1984.

Stich, H. F., Rosin, M. P., Horny, A. P., Mathew, B., Sankaranarayan, R. and Nair, M. K. 'Remission of oral leukoplaskias and micronuclei in tobacco/betel quid chewers treated with ?-carotene and with β-carotene plus vitamin A'. *Int. J. Cancer.* 42: 195-199, 1988.

Stocker, R. and Frei, B. 'Endogenous antioxidant defences in human blood plasma'. In: *Oxidative Stress: Oxidants and Antioxidants.* (Ed.). Sies, H. London: Academic Press, pp. 213-243, 1991.

Stratford, F., Seifter, E., Rettura, G. and Levenson, S. M. 'Impaired wound healing due to cyclophosphamide: Alleviation by supplemental Vit. A'. *Surg. Forum.* 31: 224-225, 1980.

Suda, D., Schwartz, J. and Shklar, G. 'Inhibition of experimental oral carcinogenesis by topical beta-carotene'. *Carcinogenesis.* 7: 711-715, 1986.

Sugahara, T., Tanaka, Y, Nagata, W. and Kano, E. 'Radiation protection by MPG'. Proc. Int. Symp., Thiola, Osaka, Japan: 267, 1970.

Sule, C. R., Pai, V. R., Damania, R. F. *et al.* 'Studies with Liv.52 therapy in infective hepatitis'. *J. Ind. Med. Prof.* 14: 6391-6395, 1968.

Takeda, A., Katoh, N. and Yonezawa, M. 'Restoration of radiation injury by ginseng. III. Radioprotective effect of thermostable fraction of ginseng extract on mice, rats and guinea pig'. *J. Radiat. Res.* 23:150, 1982.

Tanaka, T., Makita, H., Ohnishi, M., Hirose, Y., Wang, A., Mori, H., Satoh, K., Hara, A. and Ogawa, H. 'Chemoprevention of 4-nitroquinoline I-oxide-induced oral carcinogenesis by dietary curcumin and hesperidin: Comparison with the protective effect of β-carotene'. *Cancer Res.* 54: 4653-4659, 1994.

Temple, N. J. and Basu, T. K. 'Protective effects of β-carotene against colon tumours in mice'. *J. Natl. Cancer Inst.* 78: 1211-1214, 1987.

Thresiamma, K. C., George, J. and Kuttan. R. 'Protective effect of curcumin, ellagic acid and bixin on radiation induced toxicity'. *Ind. J. Exp. Biol.* 34: 845-847, 1996.

Torel, J., Cillard, J. and Cillard, P. 'Antioxidant activity of flavonoids and reactivity with peroxyradical'. *Phytochemistry.* 25: 383-386, 1986.

Tshyb, A. F., Yarmonenko, S. P. and Ogaki, M. 'Clinical evaluation of *Chlorella vulgaris* strain E-25 as a nutrition additive (preliminary results)'. Summary of the Japan, May 11-12, 1991.

Uma Devi, P. and Ganasoundari, A. 'Radioprotective effect of leaf extract of Indian medical plant *Ocimum sanctum'*. *Ind. J. Exp. Biol.* 33: 205-208, 1995.

Uma Devi, P. and Ganasoundri, A. 'Modulation of glutathione and antioxidant enzymes by *Ocimum sanctum* and it role in protection against radiation injury'. *Ind. J. Exp. Biol.* 37: 262-268, 1999.

Uma Devi, P. and Hossain, M. 'Risk from low dose foetal irradiation. *Proceedings of International Conference on Radiation Biology.* 17-19 February, Thiruvananthapuram, India, 2000.

Umegaki, K., Ikegami, S., Inoue, K., Ichikawa, T., Kobayashi, S., Soeno, N. and Tomabechi, K. 'Beta-carotene prevents X-ray induction of micronuclei in human lymphocytes'. *Am. J. Clin. Nutr.* 59: 409-412, 1994.

Van het Hof, K. H., Tijburg, L. B., Pietrzek, K. and Weststrate, J. A. 'Influence of feeding different vegetables on plasma level of carotenoids, folate and vitamin C. Effect of disruption of the vegetable matrix'. *B. R. J. Nutr.* 82(3): 203-212, 2000.

Van Poppel, G. 'Carotenoids and cancer: An update with emphasis on human intervention studies'. *Eur. J. Cancer* 29A/9: 1335-1344, 1993.

Van Poppel, G. and Goldbohm, R. A. 'Epidemiologic evidence for β-carotene and cancer prevention'. *Am. J. Clin. Nutr.* 62(Suppl.): 1393(S)-1402(S), 1995.

Van Vliet, T. 'Absorption of beta-carotene and other carotenoids in humans and animal models'. *Eur. J. Clin. Nutr.* 50 (Suppl 3): S32-S37, 1996.

Velioglu, Y. S., Mazza, G., Gao, Y. L. and Oomah, B. D. 'Antioxidant activity and total phenolics in selected fruits, vegetables and grain products'. *J. Agric. Food Chem.* 46: 4113-4117, 1988.

Verma, R. K., Sisodia, R. and Bhatia, A. L. 'Radioprotective role of *Amaranthus gangeticus* Linn.: A biochemical study on mouse brain'. *J. Med. Food* 5(4):189-195, 2002.

Vietmeyer, N. D. 'Amaranth: Return of the Aztec mystery crop'. *Sci Future* 186-195, 1983.

Virk, P. and Saxena, P. K. 'Potential of *Amaranthus* seeds in supplementary feed and its impact on growth in some carps'. *Bioresour. Technol.* 86(1): 25-27, 2003.

Weatherby, L. and Cheng, L. 'Determination of flavons or quercetin-like substances in certain naturally occurring products'. *J. Biochem.* 48: 707, 1943.

Weinzweig, J., Weinzweig, N., Levenson, S. M., Mendecki, J., Goodwin, P. and Seifter, E. 'Prevention of the tumour induced wound healing defect by supplemental vitamin A'. *Fed. Proc.* 46(4): 5087, 1987.

Weitberg, A. B., Weitzman, S. A., Clark, E. R. and Stossel, T. P. 'Effects of antioxidants on oxidant-induced sister chromatid exchanges formation'. *J. Clin. Invest.* 75: 1835-1841, 1985.

Winter, M. and Hermann, K. 'Esters and glucosides of hydroxycinnamic acids in vegetables'. *J. Agric. Food Chem.* 34: 616-620, 1986.

Xu, M. J., Plezia, P. M. and Albers, D. S. *et al.* 'Reduction in plasma or skin alpha-tocopherol concentration with long-term oral administration of beta-carotene in humans and mice'. *J. Natl. Cancer Inst.* 84: 1559-1565, 1992.

Yadav, S. K. and Sehgal, S. 'Effect of home processing on ascorbic acid and beta-carotene content of spinach (*Spinacia oleracea*) and amaranth (*Amaranthus tricolor*) leaves'. *Plant Foods Hum. Nutr.* 47(2): 125-131, 1995.

Yagi, K. In: *The Biological Rate of Reactive Oxygen Species in Skin* (Eds.). Hyasi, O., Imamure, S. and Miyachi, Y. Tokyo Press, pp. 109-116, 1998.

Yan, J., Liu, Y., Mao, D., Lil, L. and Kuang, T. 'The presence of 9-cis-beta-carotene in cytochrome b (6) f complex from spinach'. *Biochim. Biophys. Acta.* 1506(3): 182-188, 2001.

Yen, Grow-Chin; She, Chig, W. and Pin-der D. 'Extraction and identification of components from the levels of mulberry'. *J. of Agri. and Food Chem.* 44: 1687-1690, 1996.

Yin, S., Gu, X. and Xu, Q. *et al.* 'Effect of green and yellow vegetables on serum carotenoid in children'. *Zhonghua Yu Fang Yi Xue Za Zhi.* 34(2): 89-91, 2000.

Yuhas, J. M., Spellman, J. M. and Culo, F. 'The role of WR-2721 in radiotherapy and/or chemotherapy'. *Cancer Clin. Trials.* 3: 221, 1980.

Zamora, R., Hidalgo, F. J. and Tappel, A. L. 'Comparative antioxidant effectiveness of dietary β-carotene, vitamin E, selenium and colnzyme Q 10 in rat erythrocytes and plasma'. *J. Nutr.* 121: 50-56, 1991.

Zane, A. and Wender, S. H. 'Flavanols in spinach leaves'. *J. O. Chem.* 26: 4718, 1961.

Zennie, M., Thomas and Dwayne Ogzewalk, C. 'Ascorbic acid and vitamin A content of edible wild plants of Ohio and Kentucky'. *J. Eco Botany* 31:76-79, 1977.

Zhang, P. and Omaye, S. T. 'Beta-carotene and protein oxidation: Effect of ascorbic acid and alpha-tocopherol'. *Toxicology* 146(1): 37-47, 2000.

Zurovsky, Y., Eligal, Z., Grossman, S., Bergman, M. and Gafter, U. 'Glycerol-induced augmentation of sensitivity to endotoxin in rats'. *Toxicon.* 32: 17-26, 1994.

*Not seen in original.

—oo(O)oo—

19

Medicinal Plants: Need for Protection

Tapan Mukherjee

NEARLY all cultures, from ancient times, have used plants as a source of medicine. In many developing countries, traditional medicine is still the mainstay of health care, and most of the drugs and cures used come from plants. In developed countries, many people are turning to herbal remedies, especially for minor ailments, and modern scientific medicine still depends on plants, and the knowledge gained from plants, for some essential drugs. Among human beings, seeking relief from sickness is as natural as eating. The use of plants for alleviation of human suffering is, perhaps, as old as humans themselves. People in India and China are known to have used plants in organised health care regimes for over 5,000 years. Medicinal plants originate from almost every part of the globe. They range from small perennial herbs adapted to high elevation mountain areas, to the enormous baobab, one of Africa's most renowned trees. Plants are harvested for local use on virtually every continent.

INDIAN SCENARIO

India is one of the world's 12 regions having the largest biodiversity. India has 16 agroclimatic zones. It has 45,000 plant species of which 15,000-20,000 possess proven medicinal value. It is estimated that worldwide about 24 hectares of rain forest disappear every minute. This destruction also reduces the supply of medicinal plants many of which grow in forests. India's forests are the home of extremely rich biodiversity and two hot spots have been identified—the Eastern Himalayan region and the Western Ghats. Over 45,000 plant species, several of them endemic, are found in the country. Indian plant varieties have provided the germplasm to a great number of crops. But now the forest area accounts only for about 23 per cent of the total land area in the country.

According to the World Health Organisation (WHO) more than one billion people rely on herbal medicines to some extent. The WHO has listed 21,000 plants, which have been reported having medicinal uses around the world. India has a rich medicinal plant flora of some 2,500 species; of these; at least 150 species are used commercially for pharmaceutical purposes on a fairly large scale. The World Health Organisation estimates that as many as 80 per cent of the world's population depends on plants for their primary healthcare (Farnsworth *et al*, 1995). The Indian systems of medicine have identified 1,500 medicinal plants, of which 500 species are mostly used in the preparation of drugs. India with its diversified biodiversity has a tremendous potential and advantage in this emerging area.

The industrial uses of medicinal plants are many. These range from traditional medicines, herbal teas and health food such as neutraceutical to galenicals, phytopharmaceuticals and industrially produced pharmaceuticals. Furthermore, medicinal plants constitute a source of valuable foreign exchange for most developing countries.

Today's healthcare systems rely largely on plant material. Much of the world's population depends on traditional medicine to meet daily health requirements, especially within developing countries. Use of plant-based remedies is also widespread in many industrialised countries and numerous pharmaceuticals are based on or derived from plant compounds. Similarly, cosmetics and other household products may contain plants of medicinal or therapeutic value.

THREAT OF EXTINCTION

The widespread use of plants has generated the assumption that plants identified as having medicinal properties will be available on a continuing basis. However, till date, no dedicated effort has been made to ensure this. In the face of the threats of increasing demand, a vastly increasing human population and extensive destruction of plant-rich habitats, there can be no guarantee that we will continue to benefit indefinitely from this valuable resource provided by medicinal plants. Unfortunately, the products of biological and cultural diversity are undervalued. The forests have a high level of endemism, and contain many medicinal plants with potential value in new natural products development.

Today, many medicinal plant species face extinction or severe genetic loss but detailed information is lacking. For most of the endangered species, no conservation action has been taken, and for most countries there is not even a complete inventory of medicinal plants. Traditional people, whose very existence is now under threat, hold much of the knowledge on their use. Herbalists now report having to walk increasingly greater distances for herbs that once grew almost outside their door. As habitats for plants disappear and over harvesting for commercial uses reduces stocks of wild medicinal plant material, there is a corresponding drop in the availability of the plants used as the first and last resort for health care by many rural populations.

The herbal medicine trade is booming business worldwide. In India, for example, there are 46,000 licensed pharmacies manufacturing traditional remedies, 80 per cent of which come from plants (Alok, 1991). Another example is Hong Kong, which is claimed to be the largest market in the world, importing over US$ 190 million annually (Kong, 1982). In Durban (South Africa), in 1929, there were only two herbal traders; by 1987, there were over 70 herbal trader shops registered. The species-specific nature of the demand for medicinal plants is responsible for generating long distance trade across international boundaries. According to Malla (1982), 60-70 per cent of the medicinal herbs collected in Nepal are exported to India, with 85-200 tons exported annually between 1972 and 1980. Similarly the Hong Kong market imports *Aquilaria* heartwood for incense manufacture from the rain forests in Thailand and Malaysia.

Despite the increasing use of medicinal plants, their future seemingly, is being threatened by complacency concerning their conservation. Reserves of herbs and stocks of medicinal plants in developing countries are diminishing and in danger of extinction as a result of growing trade demands for cheaper healthcare products and new plant-based therapeutic markets in preference to more expensive target-specific drugs and biopharmaceuticals.

With few exceptions, prices paid to gatherers are very low, and bear no relation to annual sustainable off-take. In many cases, the wild plants are also treated as resources available to anybody without control. To make a living, commercial medicinal plant gatherers are forced to exhaust rather than manage these resources.

CONSERVATION

Conservation is the planned management of natural resources, to retain the natural balance, diversity and evolutionary change in the environment. It is a protective measure taken

(i). to prevent the loss of genetic diversity of a species; (ii). to save a species from becoming extinct; and

(iii). to protect an ecosystem from damage so as to promote its sustained utilisation.

Myers (1988, 1990) has recognised 18 hotspots. These have now been increased to 25 (Myers *et al*, 2000), which harbour 44 per cent of all endemic plant species (300,000). Among the 25 hotspots of the world, the Western Ghats, the Eastern Himalayas and the Andaman-Nicobar Islands, have been recognised as the two-mega diversity hotspots of India. These two areas also figure in the list of eight hottest hotspots (Myers *et al*, 2000).

The following 24 areas, often termed as micro-hotspots, have also been identified in India: Andamans, Nicobars, Agasthyar Hills, Annamalai Hills, Nilgiri-Silent Valley, Palni Hills, Shimoga-Kanara, Mahabaleshwar, Konkan, Satpura Range, Tirupathi Hills, Visakhapatnam Hills, Deccan Hills, Chotanagpur Plateau, Kutch, Aravalli Hills, Khasia-Jaintia Hills, Patkoi-Lushai Hills, Cachar-Mikir Hills, Arunachal Pradesh, Sikkim Himalayas, Garhwal Himalayas, Lahaul Himalayas and Kashmir Himalayas. Some of these areas are a part of the two Indian hotspots recognised by Myers *et al*, (2000).

Little attention has been paid to the socio-economic and conservation aspects of medicinal plant resources, probably due to the relatively small volumes involved and the specialist nature of the informal trade in them. However, the management of traditional medicinal plant resources is probably the most complex Indian resource management issue facing conservation agencies, healthcare professionals and resource users. As pressure is increasing on diminishing medicinal plant supplies, constructive resource management and conservation actions must be identified, based upon a clear understanding of the surrounding medicinal plant use.

Traditional medical practitioners constitute the most abundant and in many cases, valuable health resources present in the community. They are important and influential members of their communities who should be associated with any move to develop health services at a local level. The populations of developing countries worldwide continue to rely heavily on the use of traditional medicines as their primary source of healthcare. Ethnobotanical studies carried out throughout the country confirm that native plants are the main constituents of traditional medicines.

Medicinal plants are now being given serious attention, as is evidenced by the recommendation given by the World Health Organisation in 1970 (Wondergem *et al*, 1989) that proven traditional remedies should be incorporated within national drug policies. The World Health Organisation (WHO), IUCN–The World Conservation Union and the World Wide Fund (WWF) for Nature convened an International Consultation on the conservation of medicinal plants in March 1988 in Chiang Mai, Thailand. For the first time, the Consultation brought together in the same forum, policy-makers and scientists from the two key areas of health care and nature conservation.

Nearly all cultures, from ancient times to today, have used plants as a source of medicine. In many developing countries, traditional medicine is still the mainstay of health care, and most of the drugs and cures used come from plants. In developed countries, many people are turning to herbal remedies, especially for minor ailments, and modern scientific medicine still depends on plants, and the knowledge gained from plants, for some essential drugs. With this widespread use has come the assumption that plants identified as having medicinal properties will be available on a continuing basis. However, no concerted effort has been made to ensure this, and in the face of the threats of increasing demand, a vastly increasing human population and extensive destruction of plant-rich habitats such as the tropical forests, there can be no guarantee that we will continue to benefit indefinitely from this valuable resource provided by medicinal plants.

Today, many medicinal plant species face extinction or severe genetic loss but detailed information is lacking. For most of the endangered species no conservation action has been taken, and for most countries there is not even a complete inventory of medicinal plants. Much of the knowledge on their use is held by traditional societies, whose very existence is now under threat. Maintaining medicinal plant harvest and trade within sustainable levels presents a major challenge today and for the foreseeable future. A combined effort by those concerned with the conservation of medicinal plant species and/or the healthcare systems dependent on them will be crucial to ensuring the long-term viability of biodiversity.

The forests of India are estimated to harbour 90 per cent of India's medicinal plants diversity in the wide range of forest types that occur across the country. Probably only 10 per cent of the known medicinal plants of India are restricted to non-forest habitats. Hence, there is a strong case for incorporating "*in-situ* conservation of medicinal plants". About 10 per cent of India's plant species are currently endangered, underlying the urgency for conservation action. To protect medicinal plant biodiversity, species have been reintroduced to their natural habitats and *ex-situ* medicinal plant gardens have been created. These activities not only conserve medicinal plant resources, but also ensure the long-term provision of both quality plant seedlings for cultivation and rare plant products.

Plant collectors for screening take three basic approaches for obtaining samples. First, with random sampling, material is collected from the largest possible number of identifiable plant species within a habitat, with the emphasis on plants that are flowering or fruiting, so that good voucher specimens are obtained. A second approach is to focus collection of certain plant families that are known to be rich sources of interesting, biologically active compounds such as the *Apocynaceae*, *Euphorbiaceae*, *Asclepiadaceae*, *Menispermaceae* and Solanaceae. Third, collecting is guided by knowledge of traditional uses of plants.

Indiscriminate use of medicinal plants without ensuring sustainability through conservation has led to massive endangering of valuable plant bio-resources. There is an urgent need to conserve the medicinal plants, both *in situ* and *ex situ*. Attention paid to medicinal plants is minimal. *In situ* conservation is an ideal method of conservation, because it not only conserves a given species in its natural habitat but also carries all its associated elements.

Information relating to medicinal plants and traditional medicine can be found in documents and databases in a wide range of disciplines including botany, chemistry, ecology, medicine, etc. Access to relevant information by the public, decision makers and local communities is still very limited.

The Convention on Biological Diversity (CBD), signed by more than 160 member states of the United Nations provides an international legal framework for the conservation of biological diversity including access to and exchange of genetic materials. The issue of benefit sharing has received considerable attention during the last decade. Many developing countries are behind the rest of the world in the development of national policies with respect to genetic resources and trade in medicinal plants. There is an urgent need to adopt appropriate strategies to increase awareness of policy makers and donors about the need for sustainable use and conservation of medicinal plants and traditional medicine.

Biodiversity in both developing and developed countries has been accessed for long time, for various purposes, by outside researchers, private companies as well as local communities, with little or no returns to conservation activities. Bioprospecting has been practised for many years in different forms but in more recent times, the issue of sharing of benefits arising from bioprospecting has attained significance.

Conservation of alternative sources of supply of medicinal plants is crucial. However, it is important that plants are made available in large quantities and at low prices to take the pressure off wild stocks. The results of over-exploitation of medicinal plants is felt by those involved with traditional healing, either as collectors, traders, traditional practitioners, herbalists and researchers. Traditional medicines also have the potential to form the basis of pharmaceutical drugs for the treatment of a range of diseases. Thus, the loss of these potentially valuable genetic resources ultimately affects the whole society.

The conservation of biological resources is essential for basic human need, such as food security, health, shelter and clothing. A major part of these resources are located in the developing countries whose inhabitants have been innovating, selecting, conserving and protecting local species for ages. Erosion of resources mainly occurs because of the replacement of local varieties by improved varieties and species.

Medicinal plant gatherers are familiar with species that are becoming difficult to find, either because of limited geographical distribution, habitat destruction or over-exploitation. Their insight, coupled with botanical and ecological knowledge of the plant species involved, provide an essential source of information for a survey of this type. The emergence of commercial medicinal plant gatherers in response to urban demand for medicines and rural unemployment has resulted in indigenous medicinal plants being considered as an open access or common property resource instead of a resource only used by specialists.

Despite limited information on the population biology of medicinal plants, it is possible to classify target plant species according to demand, plant life form, part used, distribution and abundance (Cunningham, 1990). The large categories of traditional medicinal plants, which are under no threat at all, are the cause of little concern to TMPs or to conservation biologists.

The sustainable use of the medicinal plants was facilitated in the past by several inadvertent or indirect controls and some intentional management practices. Taboos, seasonal and social restrictions on gathering medicinal plants and the nature of plant gathering equipment all served to limit medicinal plant harvesting. A medicinal plants conservation and sustainable utilisation programme, if designed appropriately, can ensure increased access to health resources to the rural poor and create jobs and sustainable livelihoods. It has a special scope to advance the education of women and thus promote gender equity.

In spite of increasing urbanisation, a large proportion of the Indian population has retained their reliance upon this traditional approach to healthcare and continues to consult TMPs for medical treatment. Even where Western medicine is available, it is unlikely that it will be adopted without first establishing a framework for national economic growth which would allow for socio-economic and cultural changes to take place, and give access to formal education.

HERBAL MEDICINE

Herbal medicine has been virtually rediscovered in recent years. The renewed interest in herbal medicine is likely to continue due to increasing population and better affordability. Fresh market demands have not only brought in newer opportunities for the herbal drug industry, but are also posing threats to the phytoresources, especially in the developing economies. There is, therefore an urgent need to conserve the genetic diversity of medicinal plant resources. Together with it the ancient knowledge systems of traditional practitioners needs to be protected. With so much of herbal raw materials and finished products being consumed across the world in recent years, there is a greater need today than even before in ensuring that they are safe, efficacious and non-toxic.

The global sales of herbal medicines in the U. S. A. reached US $ 14 billion in 1996. Of this, 26 per cent was generated by Germany, 19 per cent in Asia, 17 per cent in Japan, 13 per cent in France, 12 per cent in the rest of Europe and 1 per cent in North America (Zhang, 1998). The international market of medicinal plant-related trade is US $ 60 billion with annual growth of 7 per cent (Anonymous, 1997). The volume of Germany's exports is second only to that of China (Lange, 1997). The largest imports are from India, followed by Bulgaria, Poland, Chile, Hungary, Argentina and Albania (Lange, 1996). The current value of trade in Indian systems of medicine and Homoeopathy is around Rs. 4,205 crores, roughly close to US $ 1 billion.

As many as 35,000-70,000 species of plants have been used at one time or another for medicinal purposes (Farnsworth *et al.*, 1991). By far the greater number of species is employed in herbal medicine and is used in unrefined or semi-processed form, often in mixtures, which sometimes also contain non-botanical ingredients. A few species are the sources of defined compounds used in the pharmaceutical industry. The overall quantities of plants used medically, in one way or another, are large. Approximately one-quarter of all prescriptions dispensed from community pharmacies in the U. S. A. contain one or more ingredients derived from higher plants. In many tropical and sub-tropical countries, as in Africa and South and East Asia, the majority of people resort to herbal medicine for the majority of their primary healthcare needs. There are also strong traditions of herbal medicine in parts of Europe such as Germany, France and Eastern Europe. The herbal sector is growing fast, increasing by 12-15 pr cent by value per year in the U. K., the U. S. A. and Italy (Abrahams, 1992). There are more than 2,000 herbal medical companies in Europe and more than 220 in the U. S. A.; Germany is the largest market in the world for herbal medicines, with annual sales of $ 1.2 billion representing nearly 25 per cent of the national pharmaceutical market. The U. S. A. is the next largest market with sales of $ 480 million (Thorpe and Warrier, 1992).

Today the availability of medicinal plants is under serious threat. Over 95 per cent of the medicinal plants used by Indian industry are collected from the wild. It is important to develop scientific harvesting technologies so that medicinal plants are harvested in the proper season, at the proper stage of their physiological growth, from the proper habitats and in a non-destructive and sustainable fashion. Agro-technologies urgently need to be developed for such prioritised species that are in high demand but in short supply and which cannot be sustainably collected from the wild. Market links also need to be developed between the collectors and growers of medicinal plants and the end users. The agro-technology developed in experimental fields needs to be transferred from the lab to the land and ultimately to the market place.

Medicinal plants are an accessible, affordable and culturally appropriate source of primary health care for more than 80 per cent of Asia's population. Marginalised people, who cannot afford or have access to formal health care systems, are especially dependent on these culturally familiar, technically simple, financially affordable and generally effective traditional medicines. As such, there is widespread interest in promoting traditional health systems to meet primary health care needs.

In the large majority of cases, companies investigating natural products work with small quantities of plant material. They look for the specific active compounds that may lead to new drugs, which are likely to be synthesised chemically. Sometimes, however, large quantities are required from wild collections or from cultivation. This is the case when synthesis poses a problem, as with the anti-cancer agent taxol, derived from the bark of the Pacific yew, *Taxus brevifolia*. It is also the case when treatments use herbal extracts, as in herbal and traditional medicines, or where whole extracts are required. Finally, it is the case when, although synthesis or cultivation is possible, harvesting material from the wild is cheaper.

Medicinal plants contain a wide variety of alkaloids, essential oils, carotenoids, bioflavonoids, etc. Traditional medicine in India and China has been practised for more than 5,000 years. Recent interest in the West and in America is more on a holistic approach, which has seen a tremendous resurgence. There is large-scale international trade in medicinal plants, used both for herbal medicine and for the manufacture of pharmaceutical drugs. There is also growing interest in obtaining samples of plant material, or traditional knowledge about plant uses, to explore for new commercial medical products.

INDIGENOUS OR TRADITIONAL MEDICINE

Indigenous medical systems have been and still are playing a major role in healthcare. However, traditional healthcare presently receives only about five per cent of the national budget in India. The knowledge base of indigenous peoples is now facing the threat of alienation through us outsiders. Local communities in the Asian, African and Latin American countries have a long history of dependence on traditional remedies, largely based on plants, for immediate access to relatively safe, cost-effective, efficacious and culturally acceptable solutions to primary health care.

In India, out of 4,752 communities, as many as 3,226, that is, around 70 per cent of the population are dependent on tradition plant-based medicine (Gadgil and Rao, 1998). These plant-based medicines are used for primary health care needs. Between 25-505 of modern drugs are derived from plants. Demand for medicinal plants is increasing in both developing and developed countries. There has been a recent growth of interest in traditional medicine from the international pharmaceutical industry, as well as from the national product industry in Asia, Europe and America. The practice of traditional medicine is widespread in China, India, Japan, Pakistan, Sri Lanka and Thailand. In China, about 40 pet cent of the total medicinal consumption is attributed to traditional tribal medicines.

Developed countries, in recent times, are turning to the use of traditional medicinal systems that involve the use of herbal drugs and remedies. About 1,400 herbal preparations are used widely, according to a recent survey in member-states of the European Union. Herbal preparations are popular and are of significance in primary health care in Belgium, France, Germany and The Netherlands. Such popularity of health care plant-derived products has been traced to their increasing acceptance and use in the cosmetic industry as well as to increasing public costs in the daily maintenance of personal health and well being. Since the vast majority of plants that are used to treat many of the diseases are collected from the wild, sound management of medicinal plant resources is critical, especially where traditional medicine prevails. Within traditional systems, reliance on natural medicinal resources can be attributed to cultural preferences, as well as to the high cost and inaccessibility of Western medicine.

Strategies for choosing which plants to investigate in the search for new medical products include the random selection of plants based on taxonomic affinity, or the pursuit of leads based on ethnobotanical knowledge. The use of plants in folk medicine has led to the discovery of the majority of major drugs used in Western medicine with an origin in plants (Hollman, 1991). Traditional knowledge, accumulated through years of experience, can be regarded as the product of a natural screening process. The search for new medical products based on plants often involves the movement of plant samples or information about plants between countries.

Indigenous medicinal systems are relying on crude herbal drug preparations. We have to adopt modern analytical methods and subject the drugs to enhanced quality control. This does not mean that traditional drugs should strictly adhere to the standardisation at par with chemical drugs. It is not possible to compare herbal drugs with chemical ones because most of the herbal medicines are mixtures of numerous chemical molecules. But it is necessary to develop standard specifications for herbal medicines by indicating the ingredients, the amount and range of the active principles, their therapeutic properties, etc. Traditional medicines can be prepared under enhanced quality control without sacrificing the therapeutic quality.

The most common medical treatments administered by traditional healers are hot and cold infusions, powders that are rubbed into the body where incisions have been made, poultices, lotions, ointments, vapour baths, emetics and enemas. Each year, thousands of indigenous plants are gathered from the forests and grasslands, putting severe pressure on the species collected. In addition, the habitat in which these species occur is shrinking as more and more natural vegetation is destroyed for agriculture, timber, industry and urban settlement. Research has shown that the massive demand for bark, roots and whole plants from wild populations is causing a critical decline in population of some plant species, and may lead to extinction of numerous species. Concern about this problem has brought conservationists and resource users together to investigate possible solutions.

Multinational companies have realised the potential of the plant-based remedies in drug development. In recent years, overseas firms have rushed to patent chemicals from natural sources that have been used locally for hundreds of years. This is *Biopiracy*, which is nothing less than the theft of indigenous resources and know-how.

A large portion of the population in a number of developing countries still relies mainly on traditional practitioners, including traditional birth attendants, herbalists and bonesetters, and local medicinal plants to satisfy greatly from country to country and from region to region. Despite its existence over many centuries and its expansive use during the last decade, in most countries, traditional medicine has not yet been officially recognised. Furthermore, research and training activities for traditional medicine has not received due support and attention. As a result, the quantity and quality of safety and efficacy data are far from sufficient to meet the demands for the use of traditional medicine in the world. Safety and efficacy data exist only in respect of much smaller number of plants, their extracts and active ingredients, as well as preparations containing them. There is need for validation and standardisation of phytomedicines and traditional medical practices so that this sector can be accorded its rightful place in the health care system.

The absence of an internationally agreed methodology for sharing economic benefits from the commercial exploitation of biodiversity with the primary conservers and holders of traditional knowledge and information is leading to a growing number of accusations of biopiracy committed by business and industry in developing countries. Biodiversity in both developing and developed countries has been accessed for a long time, for various purposes, by outside researchers, private companies as well as local communities, with little or no return to conservation activities. Bioprospecting has been practised for many years in different forms but in more recent times in particular with the development of CBD, the issue of sharing of benefits arising from bio prospecting has attained significance. There has been a recent growth of interest in traditional medicine from the international pharmaceutical industry, as well as from the national product industry. Traditional medicine has come to be viewed by the pharmaceutical industry as a source of 'qualified leads' in the identification of bioactive agents for use in the production of synthetic modern drugs. There is a need for validation and standardisation of phytomedicines and traditional medical practices so that this sector can be accorded its rightful place in the health care system.

Hundreds of medicinal plant species in the wild are threatened with extinction due to over harvesting, destructive collection techniques and conversion of habitats for single crop use. The relative high price of synthetic medicines in developing countries makes traditional medicines the only viable choice for the very poor. Relieving pressures on these wild plant populations is further complicated by the fact that many poor rely on the collection of these plants as their primary source of income. In order to ensure the viability of these plants, nurseries must be created to research plant species and encourage the cultivation of commonly used medicinal plants at home. Farming medicinal plants will help manage supply problems, regularise the trade, provide certifiable products of uniform quality and offer a new source of income to the rural poor. The challenge of documenting the vast data on medicinal plants lies primarily with the rural communities, which collect and harvest them. Medical practitioners represent an indigenous knowledge base, which is being lost at an alarming rate. Systematic collection of the traditional knowledge is vital to preserve the heritage and provide financial rewards for discoveries to those communities.

INTELLECTUAL PROPERTY RIGHTS (IPR) AND PROTECTION OF TRADITIONAL KNOWLEDGE

Intellectual Property Rights (IPR) are mechanisms to protect individual and industrial 'inventions' and are usually in effect for a specified period. To be eligible for a patent, inventions should be novel, non-obvious and useful. The World Trade Organisation controls international trade relations. For intellectual property rights, a patent war is emerging and there is the need that the developing countries like India should take up the challenge.

As the specialised U. N. agency responsible for the promotion of intellectual property world wide, WIPO was mandated in 1998 to undertake exploratory groundwork in order to provide an informal and realistic analysis of traditional knowledge and folklore protection. The sustained efforts towards modernisation of traditional knowledge system of the developing world will help create higher awareness about this vast knowledge base at national and international levels, and establish a scientific approach that will ensure higher acceptability of the system by practitioners of the modern system and public at large.

Today, there is a growing appreciation of the value of traditional knowledge even in the industrialised society of the West, as reflected by the interest shown in Ayurveda and tribal medicine. Many widely used products such as plant-based medicines and cosmetics are based on traditional knowledge. Traditional knowledge, innovations and creativity, including folklore, have received increasing attention in numerous policy areas, ranging from food and agriculture, environment, health, human rights and cultural policy, trade and economic development. The role of intellectual property rights in the protection of traditional knowledge and folklore is being considered in several of these policy contexts.

Some of the traditional knowledge systems are well-organised and documented. Indian systems of medicine (Ayurveda, Siddha, Unani, Tibetan or Amchi) and the Chinese system of medicine are about 5,000 years old. These traditional systems are reported to make use of about 1,000 plant genera and 2,500 species. In addition to these traditional systems, there exists a parallel stream of tribal and folk medicine all over the world. The role of indigenous people as protectors of biodiversity and as custodians of ancient knowledge systems, including the medicinal uses of plants, is well recognised.

An appropriate mechanism for co-ordination and implementation of policies relating to medicinal plants both at national and State levels are urgently needed. To accomplish the task, the Government of India through a notification of November 24, 2000, set up a Medicinal Plants Board. This board has identified 28 medicinal plant species which accounts for 62 per cent of the total value in the global market. These plants have been identified for cultivation, conservation and development. Drug development and patenting has taken place without the knowledge of the people in the country of origin, with no recompense for use of regional natural resources.

The developing countries, which are the major repositories of traditional knowledge (TK), are concerned about its progressive erosion and unsustainable commercialisation without adequate rewards for the owners of such knowledge. TK needs to be protected by appropriate legislative systems that will be acceptable to the international community. The present systems for protection of intellectual property and bio-resources, such as those under the TRIPS agreement of the WTO or the CBD are not adequate or appropriate for protection of community rights on TK and indigenous systems and practices.

Due to lack of documentation and poor dissemination of knowledge, much of indigenous knowledge is getting irretrievably lost. In the absence of searchable databases, disclosing that such knowledge exists as *prior art*, patent offices grant patents on the use of this knowledge to produce useful products. The patents on turmeric for wound healing activity, *karela, brinjal* and *jamun* for diabetes, neem formulations as insecticides and fungicides, *Phyllanthus amarus* as antiviral activity, etc. point out compulsions that their knowledge base is protected from unauthorised exploitation with no benefits accruing to them. India fought successfully revocation of turmeric and *basmati* patents granted by the United States Patent and Trademark Office (US PTO) and *neem* patent granted by the European Patent Office (EPO).

TRADITIONAL KNOWLEDGE DIGITAL LIBRARY (TKDL)

The Department of Indian Systems of Medicine and Homoeopathy (ISM & M) and National Institute of Science Communication (NISCOM), a constituent of the Council of Scientific and Industrial Research (CSIR), have initiated an effort to document TK available in all systems of indigenous medicine available in the public domain by creating Traditional Knowledge Digital Library (TKDL).

There are two distinct and potentially conflicting knowledge systems. The knowledge systems of the formal sector are recorded, well-documented and defended through national and international laws, whereas the knowledge systems of the informal sector are often oral, not documented and thus non-defendable. TKDL is the only viable route on patent grant prevention for non-original inventions in our traditional knowledge systems where pre-grant opposition facilities are not available, as post-grant opposition is complex and extremely expensive.

Following the grant of the controversial patents, an exercise has been initiated to prepare easily navigable computerised database of documented traditional knowledge relating to the use of medicinal plants, which are already in the public domain through the Traditional Knowledge Digital Library (TKDL). The database is being created in English, German, Spanish, French and Japanese, which would enable patent offices globally to search and examine the prevalent use/*prior art*, and thereby deny grant of patents of knowledge which is already in the public domain and help prevent biopiracy.

TKDL in its first phase, targets Ayurveda, which will be followed by Unani, Siddha, Naturopathy, Yoga and Folklore. The knowledge of Ayurveda available in the public domain is being documented by shifting and collating information on traditional knowledge from the existing literature covering Ayurveda, in digitised format, which will be available nationally and internationally in several Indian and international languages. The information is being structured as per the International Patent Classification (IPC) for the convenience of its use by the international patent examiners. Information from about 35,000 formulations and *shlokas* (verses and prose) will be put on the portal for realising the first stage objective of TKDL. TKDL will have the objective of preservation, protection and wealth creation. TKDL will ensure ease of retrieval of TK-related information by patent examiners thus ensuring avoidance on misappropriation of Indian TK. This will also clearly identify a large number of patents already granted on our traditional knowledge for non-original inventions, which may require cancellation.

CONCLUSION

Medicinal plants are now recognised throughout the world as an important component of natural resources of the respective countries. For all practical purposes, medicinal plants are no different from the other economically important species, whether occurring in the wild or cultivated. They are subject to the same risks and need the same degree of protection as other plant resources. There has been a rapid decline in the biodiversity of the world, more particularly during the past two decades or so. Biodiversity losses have been alarming in the developing countries in the tropics.

Biodiversity losses occur due to habitat destruction, over-harvesting, pollution, inappropriate and often accidental introduction of exotic plants and animals, etc. Habitat destruction is often related to development projects like land conversion, construction of dams, etc. Biodiversity is also lost due to sudden natural calamities like floods, cyclones, hurricanes, earthquakes, etc. Conservation of biodiversity is one of the paramount concerns the world over.

Action should be taken now to conserve the medicinal plant base of traditional medicine in, as well as safeguarding its potential for modern medicines in other parts of the world. A shift to a cash economy and the emergence of commercial harvesters into what was largely a specialist activity restricted to traditional medical practitioners have resulted in medicinal plants becoming a common property resource with few incentives for resource management or traditional conservation practice. In the context of major threats posed to natural habitats and the survival of particular species by agricultural expansion, deforestation and so on, over-exploitation of traditional medicines is occurring. Subject to uncertainties in demographic and urbanisation trends, the demand for traditional medicines is set to rise, putting increasing pressures on remaining areas of natural vegetation. Neither formal conservation legislation nor conservation practices are able to control the situation.

Traditional medical practitioners (TMPs) are aware of the conservation status of local medicinal plant resources and can be influential in changing local opinion so as to limit over-exploitation. There is a need that support is given to the formation of rural TMP associations and the self-sufficiency of TMPs, particularly in buffer ones. This might possibly be through local health services with the support of the WHO Traditional Medicine Programme. In particular, information should be disseminated to rural communities on appropriate cultivation methods for medicinal plants, which are in local demand. Very little goes unnoticed in communally owned areas so that if problems arise regarding the depletion of valued local resources, TMP associations or community leaders are likely to be at least as effective as forest guards and could draw on conservation or forest guard support where necessary.

The following species of medicinal plants from India have been considered to be 'endangered and threatened' for over a decade (Ayensu, 1986): *Acorus calamus, Alpinia galanga, Commiphora wightii, Dendrobium nobile, Dendrobium pauciflorum, Dioscorea deltoidea, Diplomeris hirsuta, Gentiana kurroo, Nelumbo nucifera, Paphiopedilum druryi, Podophyllum hexandrum, Rauvolfia serpentina, Santalum album* and *Saussurea lappa*. A very large number of other species of medicinal plants may include, for example, *Saraca asoca, Picrorrhiza kurroa, Costus speciosus, Berberis aristata, Gloriosa superba*, etc.

It is recommended that there should be rapid development of alternative supply sources through cultivation in large enough quantities and at a low enough price to compete with prices obtained by gatherers of wild stocks. This will satisfy market demands, result in more secure jobs and provide fewer incentives to gather from the wild. If this does not occur, key species will disappear from the wild, thereby undermining the local medicinal resource base.

However, the practical difficulties associated with the cultivation of medicinal plants should to be underestimated. The most vulnerable category of species, by their very nature, cannot be grown profitably due to their slow growth rates, especially as the land, which is most likely to be available for medicinal plant cultivation, is likely to be less productive agricultural land.

It is very important for the gene bank to collect information on uses and efficacy of medicinal plants than collect material for *ex-situ* conservation. Some popular and effective medicinal plants are threatened and need to be established in field gene banks until technology is available for storage of recalcitrant seeds. The ultimate goal of the conservation process is certainly to preserve the natural habitats of vulnerable medicinal plant species and to achieve sustainable exploitation in less vulnerable areas. However, seed and gene banks of vulnerable medicinal plant species should be maintained as a precaution and backup against extinction. The plants most likely to be collected for this purpose are the slow-growing species where commercial cultivation in unlikely and wild populations are jeopardised.

The conservation of medicinal plants is by necessity a long-term project requiring the development of trained staff supported by organisations and a general public that is aware of the issues at stake. Improvement in national education standards is a key factor in the conservation issue, which will come about only as a result of economic development.

REFERENCES

Abrahams, P. 'Herbal sales set to grow'. *Financial Times,* London, U. K., 2 October 1992.

Alok, S. K. 'Medicinal plants in India: Approaches to exploitation and conservation'. In: *Conservation of Medicinal Plants.* (Eds.). Akerele, O., Heywood, V. and Synge, H. Cambridge University Press, pp. 295-304, 1991.

Anonymous. 'Indian medicinal plants: A sector study'. *Occasional Paper*, No. 54. Mumbai: Export Import Bank of India, 1997.

Ayensu, S. E. 'World medicinal plant resources'. In: *Conservation for Productive Agriculture.* (Eds.). Chopra, V. L. and Khoshoo, T. N. New Delhi: ICAR, pp. 11-49, 1986.

Cunningham, A. B. *Man and Medicines: The Exploitation and Conservation of Traditional Zulu Medicinal Plants.* Hamburg: Mitheilungen aus dem Institut fur Allegemeine Botanik, 1990.

Farnsworth, N. R., Akerele, O., Bingel, A. S., Soejarta, D. D. and Eno, Z. 'Medicinal plants in therapy'. *Bulletin of the World Health Organisation* 63(6): 965-981, 1995.

Farnsworth, N. R., Akerele, O., Heywood, V. and Soejarto, D. D. 'Global importance of medicinal plants'. In: *Conservation of Medicinal Plants.* (Eds.). Akerele, O., Heywood, V. and Synge, H. Cambridge University Press, pp. 25-51, 1991.

Gadgil, M. and Rao, P. R. S. '*Nurturing Biodiversity: An Indian Agenda.* Ahmedabad: Centre for Environment Education, 1998.

Hollman, A. *Plants in Medicine*. London: U. K.: Chelsea Physic Garden, 1991.

Kong, Y. C. 'The control of Chinese medicines—A scientific overview'. In: *Yearbook Pharm. Soc.*, Hongkong, pp. 47-51; cited by Farnsworth, N. R., *Screening Plants for New Medicines*, pp. 83-97. In: *Biodiversity*. (Ed.). Wilson, E. O. Washington, DC, U. S. A.: National Academy Press, 1982.

Lange, D. 'Medicinal Plant Market Study in Germany—Germany, state of project'. *Medicinal Plants Conservation Newsletter* of the IUCN Species Survival Commission, Medicinal Plants Specialist Group 2:9-10, 1996.

Lange, D. 'Trade in plant material for medicinal and other purposes—A German case study'. *TRAFFIC Bull.* 17: 20-32, 1997.

Malla, S. B. *Medicinal Plants of Nepal*. FAO Regional Office for Asia and the Pacific, Report No. 64, Bangkok, FAO., 1982.

Myers, N. 'The biodiversity challenge: Expanded hotspot analysis'. *Environmentalist* 10: 243-256, 1990.

Myers, N. 'Threatened Biotas: Hotspots in tropical forests'. *Environmentalist* 8: 187-208, 1988.

Myers, N., Mittermeler, R. A., Mittermeler, C. G., da Fonseca, G. A. B. and Kent, J. 'Biodiversity hotspots for conservation priorities'. *Nature* 403: 853-858, 2000.

Thorpe and Warrier. 'Competitive positioning: Who's doing what in the herbal medical industry'. *Consultancy Report*, Private publication, U. K., 1992.

Wondergem, P., Senah, K. A. and Glover, E. K. 'Herbal drugs in primary healthcare: Ghana: An assessment of the relevance of herbal drugs in PHC and some suggestions for strengthening PHC. Amsterdam: Royal Tropical Institute, *Zimbabwe Science News*, 1989.

Zhang, X. 'Significance of traditional medicine in human health care'. WIPO Asian Regional Seminar on Intellectual Property Issues in the Field of Traditional Medicines, New Delhi, October 7-9, 1998, p. 6, 1998.

—oo(O)oo—

20

POTENTIAL MEDICINAL PLANTS: BOTANY, MEDICINAL USES AND CHEMICAL CONSTITUENTS

P. C. TRIVEDI AND SAMPAT NEHRA

THE use of plants for curing various human ailments figured in ancient manuscripts such as the Bible, the *Rig Veda*, the *Iliad* and the *Odyssey* and the *History of Herodotus*. Over 6,000 years ago, the ancient Chinese were using drug plants. The Egyptians, Babylonians, Sumerians, Greeks and Romans, all developed their respective characteristic *Materia Medica.* On the other side of the world, the Aztecs, Mayans and Incas had all developed primitive medicine. Some of the ancient Egyptian textbooks 'Papyri' written as early as 1600 BC indicate that the Egyptians had an amazingly complex *Materia Medica.* Apart from the names of many medicinal plants then known, the papyri also included several hundred recipes or prescriptions for various diseases.

The Greeks and Romans were familiar with many of the present-day drugs as is evident from the work of Hippocrates (460-370 BC), Aristotle (384-322 BC), Theophrastus (370-287 BC), Pliny the Elder (AD 23-79), Dioscorides (AD 50-100) and Galan (AD 131-201). They wrote extensively about medicinal herbs, giving their names along with a description of each plant, illustrations, their putative healing properties and also complex descriptions for the preparation of medicines. Hippocrates, the 'Father of Medicine' was the first to attempt a scientific explanation for diseases. His influence remains today in the Hippocratic Oath taken by young doctors upon their graduation from medical school. Dioscorides' treatise on medicinal plants *De Materia Medica* remained the supreme authority for over 16 centuries, during which the manuscript was laboriously copied and recopied with few additions.

About the beginning of the sixteenth century, several herbals of considerable merit were published, such as those of Brunfels (1530), Bock (1539), Fuchs (1542), Cordus (1561) and L'obel (1576). Although these works were a great improvement over earlier ones, they still propagated many myths and superstitions such as the 'Doctrine of Signatures' advocated by an eccentric genius Paracelsus (1493-1541) according to which all plants possessed certain signs given by God, which indicated their usefulness in treating diseases of similarly shaped organs in the human body.

THE INDIAN SYSTEM OF MEDICINE

The traditional system of medicine in India prescribing plant extractives in therapy dates back to the early age of the *Rig Veda* (4500-1600 BC). There is ample proof of the application of various recipes of Indian herbs in curing many maladies. The therapeutic efficacy of herbal medicines led to the evolution (2500-600 BC) of Ayurveda, which literally means 'Science of Life'. According to Ayurveda, health is an indication of normal biological processes, which would help to maintain mental and physical alertness and happiness.

Charaka Samhita, the first recorded treatise on Ayurveda, was followed by *Sushruta Samhita*, both compiled a century apart, believed to be not later than 900 BC. *The Encyclopaedia Britannica* (Macro 23, 886, 1988) however, recorded the period between 800 BC to the first century AD when *Charaka Samhita* appeared in its present form.

Charaka Samhita dealt primarily with medicine, *Sushruta Samhita*, on the other hand, was concerned with the advanced state of knowledge on the general principles and details of treatment. It was more systematic in its arrangement. Though mainly concerned with anatomy and surgery, it incorporated a comprehensive chapter on therapeutic (*Uttara Tantra*) dealing with general diseases such as fever, diarrhoea, lung diseases, etc.

The most important treatise, *Astanga Hridaya Samhita*, unrivalled for principles and practice of medicine, was written by Vagbhata, an Ayurvedic practitioner in the seventh century AD.

The period between 800 BC and 1000 AD could be considered as the golden age of the Indian system of medicine, particularly because of the availability of these three treatises which collectively became known as *Vridha Trayi* (Senior Triad) of Ayurveda. Of course, the place of *Kashyapa Samhita* in Ayurveda cannot be ignored since it embodied invaluable information about *Kaumarabhritya Tantra*, that is, maternity and child care (Chatterjee and Pakrashi, 1991).

The details of the definite properties of drugs prepared from indigenous plants and their uses, the extensive Materia Medica which was further enriched by addition of a large number of newer drugs during the Buddhist period, and the methods of administration of drugs akin to the present-day practice clearly showed the extent of advancement of the Indian indigenous system of medicine as well as the depth of knowledge of the then practitioners with regard to drug therapy and toxicology.

It is amazing to find how even in the ancient times the Indian *Materia Medica* could classify drugs based on their physiological actions and specify the details of the habitat of different plants, the parts to be used and the proper time for their collection, method of storage, etc. It is, thus abundantly clear that the users of the Ayurvedic system were fully aware of the important factors regulating the yield of active principles and as such the efficacy of the drug preparation.

DEVELOPMENT OF SYNTHETIC DRUGS

With the development of synthetic drugs, plant products lost their significance. From the crude beginning of the earlier physician-botanists, the study of drugs and drug plants has developed into modern pharmacognosy which deals with the knowledge of history, botany, preservation and commerce of crude drugs. Pharmacology is the study of the action of drugs on an organ or organism. Nature has provided a rich storehouse of herbal remedies to cure all mankind's ills. Throughout the world, primitive peoples have utilised several thousands of different plants and plant products as cures for human ailments.

The information on drugs and drug plants whose efficacy in medicine has been established is available in various authentic books known as 'Pharmacopoeia' and the drugs included therein are described as 'official'. The most important of these pharmacopoeia are the 'United States Pharmacopoeia', 'British Pharmaceutical Codex', 'Indian Pharmaceutical Codex' and 'National Formulary'.

In the present article, 26 plant species whose efficacy in medicine has now been tested and recognised have been included. Information regarding vernacular names in important languages, occurrence and distribution, botany of the plant, useful parts and medicinal uses and important chemical constituents has been given for these plants.

ACONITUM HETEROPHYLLUM WALL EX ROYLE

Vernacular Names: Sanskrit and Bengali: Ativisha; Hindi: Atish; Tamil: Ativadayam; English: Indian Atis.

Occurrence and Distribution: :Common in the alpine and sub-alpine belts of the Himalayan northwestern region at altitudes between 1,800 and 4,500 metres.

Botany of Plant: Family Rununculaceae. A perennial, erect, showy herb, stem 30.5-91.4 cm long, simple or branched from base, glabrous and puberulous above, broad, ovate or orbicular or somewhat five-lobed and toothed, upper three bid or entire. Flowers 2.5 cm long, helmet-shaped, bright, blue or greenish-blue with purple veins.

Useful Parts: Underground stem and root.

Medicinal Uses: Powdered root mixed with honey is effective for children suffering from cough, coryza, fever and vomiting. Root is considered to be aphrodisiac, digestive, valuable febrifuge, bitter tonic and useful in throat infections, abdominal pain and gastralagia.

Chemical Constituents: Diterpenoid alkaloid, alisine is the main constituent (0.4 per cent) of the root. Other includes atidine, histisine, helisine, hetidine, helerophyllisine, heterophylline, heterophyllidine, heteratisine, isoatisine, dihydroatisine, hestisinone and benzoyl heteratisine.

ACONITUM FEROX WALL. EX SER.

Vernacular Names: :Sanskrit: Vatsanava; Hindi: Bish; Bengali: Katbish; Tamil: Vashanabi; English: Indian aconite.

Occurrence and Distribution: Grass grows wild in the alpine Himalayas, Kashmir at an altitude of 3,600 metres.

Botany of Plant: Family: Ranunculaceae. A perennial herb. Roots tuberous, paired, daughter tuber ellipsoid to ovoid-oblong, 2.5-4.0 cm in length, with filiform root fibres. Leaves scattered, orbicular cordate to reniform, palmately five-lobed, resembling those of melon leaves; blade and petiole pubescent. Peduncle straight, bearing flowers on both sides. Flowers pale dirty blue, borne in a dense terminal raceme, 10-25 cm long, helmet-vaulted with a short sharp beak, resembling a pea flower. Follicle oblong; seeds long, obpyramidal to obovoid, winged along the raphe.

Useful Parts: Underground stem and root.

Medicinal Uses: The root and underground stems are highly toxic; but the toxicity may be reduced by suitable processing in small doses (0.023 to 0.018 g) they are beneficial in nasal catarrh, uvula hypertrophy, sore throat, gibbous, paralysis and chronic fever; in large doses it acts as narcotic poison and powerful sedative. Internally, the tincture of root (1 in 8 of alcohol in doses of 2 to 5 drops) is used in combination with other drugs for the treatment of fever and rheumatism. The root is considered to be a cardiac stimulant, hypoglycaemic, diaphoretic and antiphlogestic. Powdered roots in the form of liniment or paste is spread over the skin in cases of arthritis and scabies. *Aconitum ferox* finds application in the formulation of many useful Ayurvedic and Unani medicines.

Chemical Constituents: The roots contain toxic alkaloids, pseudoconitine along with chasmaconitine, indaconitine, bikhaconitine, veratroyl pseudoconitine and diacetyl pseudoaconitine.

AEGLE MARMELOS CORR. EX ROXB.

Vernacular Names: Sanskrit: Bilva; Hindi and Bengali: Bel; Tamil: Bilvam; English: Bael tree.

Occurrence and Distribution: Common throughout India in dry hilly areas, gardens and roadsides; also cultivated in various places in India.

Botany of Plant: Family Rutaceae. A spinous deciduous, aromatic tree, about 12 metres high; spines straight, strong, axillary. Leaves usually three-foliate, sometimes five foliolate; leaflets ovate-lanceolate, lateral sessile, terminal long-petiolded, acuminate, cuneate to obtuse at base. Flowers borne in few flowered, axillary panicles, greenish-white, sweet-scented. Fruits large, up to 15 cm diam.; globose, ovoid or pyriform, 8-15 celled; rind grey or greyish-yellow, woody pulp orange, sweet. Seeds numerous in aromatic pulp, oblong, compressed; testa woolly and mucilaginous. Flowers during April-May and fruits ripen during March-April.

Useful Parts: Fruits, seeds, leaves, bark and root.

Medicinal Uses: Fruits (ripe): alterative, cooling, laxative and nutritive; useful in habitual constipation, chronic dysentery and dyspepsia; tonic. (Unripe): antidiarroheal, astringent, demulcent, digestive and stomachic. Seeds: Laxative. Flowers: antidiarrohoel and antiemetic. Leaves: expectorant, febrifuge; fresh ones used in dropsy, efficacious in bronchial asthma. Bark (stem and root): beneficial in intermittent fever, melancholia and palpitation of heart. Root: One of the ingredients of Dashamulg, a common Ayurvedic formulation, particularly useful in loss of appetite and puerperal diseases.

Chemical Constituents: B-sitosterol (all parts); amino acids (fruits, leaves); dictamnine (pericarp, wood); marmesin (pericarp, bark, wood); marmin, umbelliferone (pericarp, bark); Skimmianine (leaves, bark); carbohydrate, carotene, fat, tannins and vitamins; imperatorin (marmelosin) and its isomers, alloimperatorin and marmelide, psoralen and tannic acid (fruits; a-d-phellandrene (rind, leaf, oil); N-2-methoxy-2-(4-methoxyphenyl-)-ethylcinnamamide, auraplen, isoimperatorim, isopimpinellin, marmelin and its methyl ether, osthol, scoparone, xanthotoxol and xanthotoxin (pericarp); arabinose, galactose D-galacturonic acid and rhaminose (fruit-gum-hydrolysate); linoleic, linolenic, oleic, palmitic and stearic acids (seeds, oil); caryophyllene, cineol, citral, citronellal, cuminaldehyde, cuminyl alcohol, p-cymene, ethyl-n-amylketone, methyl-n-heptylketone, eugeol, methleugeol, d-limonene and linalool (essential oil); N-2-ethoxy- and N-2 methoxy-2 (4-methoxyphenyl)-ethylcinnamamides, N-2-methoxy-2-[4-(3'3'-dimethylallyoxy) phenyl]- ethlycinnamamide, O-(3,3-dimethylallyl)- halbordivial, aegeline, aegelenine, anthocyanins and leucoanthocyanins, flavan-3-ols and flavone glycosides (leaves) γ-fagarine from the bark.

ANDROGRAPHIS PANICULATA (BURM.F.) WALL EX NEES.

Vernacular Names: Sanskrit: Kirata; Hindi: Kirayat; Bengali: Kalmegh; Tamil: Nelavemu; English: Creat,

Occurrence and Distribution: Common in shady places, wastelands and roadsides throughout warmer parts of India.

Botany of Plant: Family: Acanthaceae. An erect annual, about 80 cm high. Stems quadrangular, much branched. Leaves glabrous, dark green, lanceolate. Flowers borne in axillary and terminal, panicled racemes, sepals linear-lanceolate, pubescent corolla two-lipped for at least half of its length, hairy, white, spotted rose purple ovary and base of style subglabrous or thinly hairy. Fruits almost linear-oblong capsules. Seeds subquadrate or oblong. Flowers and fruits during August-February.

Useful Parts: Whole plant, leaves and root.

Medicinal Uses: Whole plant: anodyne, antifebrile, anthelmintic, alexipharmic, antidysenteric, astringent, useful in bronchitis, consumption, diabetes, dyspepsia, gonorrhoea, influenza, in intermittent and remittent fevers (combined with arsenic); itches, jaundice, liver troubles, piles, swellings, major constituent of the Ayurvedic drug Switradilapa effective in treating vertilago; Leaves and root: alterative, anthelmintic, antipyretic, cholagogue and tonic, infusion/decoction of leaves useful in dysentery, general debility, dyspepsia, sluggish liver, neuralgia; stomachic; pills made with expressed juice in combination with cardamom, clove and cinnamon found beneficial for digestive disorders in children; Root: tincture is gently aperient, stimulant and tonic; decoction/concentrated infusion of root stalks is a household anthelmintic, febrifuge and bitter tonic; useful in intermittent fevers.

Chemical Constituents: Andrographolide, a furanoid diterpene (leaves, root, whole plant); caffeic, chlorigenic, dicaffeoylaunic and myristic acids; carvacrol. eugeol, hentriacontane, tritriacontane; andrographone deoxyandrographolide, α, β-unsaturated lactone; β-sitosterol glucoside (leaves); apigenin-7,4'-di-o-methylether, andrographin (a monohydroxy trimethylflavone), 5-hydroxy-7,8-flavanone, 5-hydroxy-7,8-2',3' tetramethoxyflavone, flavanone glucoside, andrographidine A and flavone glucosides andrographidines B, C, D, E and F, 5'-hydroxy-3, 7, 8, 2' tetramethoxyflavone, mono-o-methylurthin, 7-0-methylwogonin; β-sitosterol (root): andrographiside, andropanoside (ninadrographolide), 14-deoxy-andrographolide, oroxylin A, wogonin from the plant.

BACOPA MONNIERI (L.) PENN.

Vernacular Names: Sanskrit, Hindi and Bengali: Brahmi; Tamil: Nirbrahmi; English: Thyme-leafed Gratiola.

Occurrence and Distribution: Common in moist places throughout India.

Botany of Plant: Family Scrophulariaceae. A glabrous, punctate herb, rather succulent, leaves sessile, obovate or spathulate, entire. Flowers solitary, axillary, white; peduncles usually longer than the leaves; bracteoles linear. Fruits ovoid, acute capsules included in the persistent calyx. Flowers and fruits almost throughout the year but chiefly during February-April.

Useful Parts: Whole plant and leaves.

Medicinal Uses: Whole plant: Astringent, bitter, cardiotonic, cooling, diuretic, brain tonic; used for the treatment of asthma, epilepsy, hoarseness, insanity; an important ingredient of various Ayurvedic formulations. Leaves: aperient, diuretic and improves memory; juice prescribed to children in bronchitis and diarrhoea; paste externally applied as a remedy for rheumatism.

Chemical Constituents: Ascorbic acid, nicotinic acid, carbohydrates, fat and protein (leaves, tender stalks); brahmine, herpestine, nicotine, alanine, aspartic acid, glutamic acid, serine; d-mannitol, dotriacontane, hentriacontane, heptacosane, nonacosane, octacosane, triacontane; 3-Formyl-4-hydroxy-2H-pyran, apigenin-7-glucuronide, luteolin and its 7-glucuronide, luteolin-7-glucoside. Saponis: monnierin, hersaponin, bacosides A and B, the mixture of which on hydrolysis yields rabinose, glucose and four sapogenins, namely, bacogenins A1-A4: 3, 18-dihydroxy-20, 25-epoxy-22 (or 23)-methyl-24-nor-dammar-22-en-16-one (bacogenin A1); and its 20-R-epimer (bacogenin A2), bacogenin A3, ebelin lactone (bacogenin A4), betulic acid, stigmasterol and its esters, β sitosterol from the herb.

BERBERIS ARISTATA DC.

Vernacular Names: Sanskrit: Daruharidra; Hindi: Darhald; Bengali: Darhaldi; English: Indian barberry.

Occurrence and Distribution: Found in the Himalayas (1,829-3,048 metres) and the Nilgiri Hills.

Botany of Plant: Family Berberidaceae. An erect, glabrous, spinescent shrub, 3-6 metres in height. Leaves acute to obtuse, entire or toothed, elliptic to obovate. Flowers yellow, borne in corymbose racemes. Fruits ovoid or oblong-ovoid, bright red. Flowers and fruits from August-October.

Useful Parts: Fruits, stem and root bark.

Medicinal Uses: Paste of root bark finds external application for healing ulcers. Extract prepared from root bark is used as a local application in affected parts of the eyelids and in chronic ophthalmia. The tincture of the root is used against intermittent fever and considered to be advantageous over quinine and cinchona since it does not produce deafness or cardiac depression. The decoction is particularly useful in the enlargement of liver and spleen associated with malarial fever. It is also used for fever accompanied by diarrhoea. Root combined with opium, rock salt and alum is considered to be an useful anti-inflammatory agent. In bleeding piles, application of powdered root mixed with butter is beneficial. 'Rasaut' of the root (extract prepared with milk) is found useful in stomatitis and leucorrhoea. Decoction of stem mixed with that of *Curcuma longa* is recommended in gonorrhoea. Bark juice is useful in jaundice. Fruits are edible and prescribed as a mild laxative for children.

Chemical Constituents: The plant contains berberine, oxyberberine, berbamine, aromoline, karachine, palmatine, oxyacanthine and taxlamine.

CASSIA AUGUSTIFOLIA VAHL.

Vernacular Names: Sanskrit: Kalyani; Hindi: Sona-ka-pat; Bengali: Sona-mukhi; Tamil: Nila virai; English: Indian senna.

Occurrence and Distribution: Cultivated mainly in South India, particularly Tamil Nadu, Karnataka and Andhra Pradesh.

Botany of Plant: Family: Leguminosae (Fabaceae)-Caesalpinioideae. A small shrub, 61-91 cm in height. Leaves paripinnate; leaflets in 7-8 pairs, glabrous, yellowish-green, 2.5-5.1 cm × 0.4-1.3 cm. Flowers yellow. Pods greenish brown to dark brown, 3.4-6.8 cm long and 1.9 cm broad. Seeds 5-7, obovate, smooth, dark brown. Flowers and fruits almost throughout the year.

Useful Parts: Fruits and leaves.

Medicinal Uses: Fruits and Leaves: Laxative and purgative; Leaves (powder): admixed with vinegar applied externally to cure skin diseases.

Chemical Constituents: The pods contain sennosides A and B, (-) Serinidin-8, 8'-diglucoside (Sennoside A1), glycosides of rhein and chrysophanic acid, aloe-emodia, its dianthrone diglucoside and emodin glucoside. Occurrence of oxymethyl-anthraquinone has been reported from the fruits. Leaves contain flavonols, isorhamnetin, kaempferol, rhein, emodin and sennosides A, B, C and D.

COLEUS FORSKOHLII (WILLD.) BRIG.
SYN. *COLEUS BARBATUS* BENTH.

Vernacular Names: Hindi: Gurmal; English: Kaffir potato.

Occurrence and Distribution: Found wild in dry and barren hills of subtropical Himalayas including Kumaon and Nepal ascending to 2,700 metres and in the Deccan Peninsula, Gujarat and Bihar; cultivated in Baroda and Maharashtra.

Botany of Plant: Family Lamiaceae. A perennial, branched, aromatic herb, about 30-62 cm high with a thick root. Stem stout, villous with long hair, ascending. Leaves narrowed into the petioles, ovate or obtuse, crenate villous or hispid. Flowers borne in racemes, stout, upper calyx-lip rounded-ovate, acute; corolla pale blue. Fruits nutlets. Flowers and fruits during August-October.

Useful Parts: Aerial part and root.

Medicinal Uses: Aerial part: spasmolytic; Root: hypotensive, spasmolytic and given to children in constitution; decoction as tonic and in the treatment of worms. Paste to allay burning in festering boils; mixed with mustard oil, powdered root internally applied to eczema and skin diseases.

Forskolin, isolated from the roots, is a bronchodilator, cardiotonic in the treatment of congestive heart failure, glaucoma therapy, anti-hypertensive, remedy for mitastatic condition and thrombosis.

Chemical Constituents: Allylroyleanone, barbatusin, 3 β-hydroxy-3-deoxybasbatusin, coleons E and F, cyclobutatusin, plectrin, 16(R), plectrinon A, plectrinon B (leaves), barbatusol, 20-

deoxocarnasol (stem); 1-acetoxycoleosol, coleol, coleonol=forskolin, B, C, D, F, coleonone, coleosol, deoxycoleonol.

COMMIPHORA WIGHTII (ARNOTT) BHANDARI
SYN. *COMMIPHORA MUKUL* (HOOK EX-STOCKS) ENGL.

Vernacular Names: Sanskrit: Guggulu; Hindi and Bengali: Guggul; Tamil: Maishakshi; English: Indian Bdellium tree.

Occurrence and Distribution: Found in the arid and rocky zones in certain parts of south-west and north-western regions of India including Mysore and Rajasthan.

Botany of Plant: Family: Burseraceae. A small tree or shrub with spinescent branches. Leaves usually unifoliolate, alternate or crowded at the end of short branches, cuneate-obovate, rhomboidal or oval, acute, deeply serrate, smooth and shining. Flowers small, subsessile, 2-3 together, unisexual. Males with ovary short and barren; females with short stamens and imperfect anthers. Calyx cylindrical. Petals 4-5, strap-shaped, brownish-red, lips curled back. Fruit red drupes, ovate, acuminate, separating into two fleshy valves, leaving the nut enveloped by a 4-cleft yellow pulp. Nuts ovoid, acute, splitting into two, each 1-celled. Flowers in March-April and fruits later.

Part Used: Gum.

Medicinal Uses: Gum: Alterative, anti-inflammatory, antiseptic, antispasmodic, antisuppurative, aperient, aphrodisiac, appetising, astringent, carminative, diaphoretic, diuretic, ecbolic, emmenagogue, expectorant; useful in amenorrhoea, anaemia, endometritis, leucorrhoea, menorrhagia, nervous diseases, rheumatism, scrufulous, affections and skin diseases, particularly applied in indolent ulcer and bad wounds; specially recommended in the treatment of lipid and urinary disorders, obesity, in marasmus of children and in rheumatoid arthritis; inhalation of the fumes of burnt guggul beneficial in chronic bronchitis, acute and chronic nasal catarrh; laryngitis and tuberculosis.

Guggulipid, the ethylacetate extract of the gum, has recently been established as an effective hypolipidaemic as well as an anti-inflammatory agent in certain types of hypercholesterolaemia.

Chemical Constituents: Linoleic, oleic, palmitic and stearic acids; campesterol, cholesterol, β-sitosterol and stigmasterol (seed oil). Quercetin, its 3-O-α-L-ara-binoside-, 3-O-β-D-galactoside, 3-O-α-L-rhamnoside- and 3-O-β-D-glucoronide, ellagic acid and pelargonidin 3,5-di-O-glucoside (flowers); the lignans, sesamin pluviatilol, guggullignans I and II, myricyl alcohol, β-sitosterol, series of long-chain polyol esters derived from homologous tetrols (guggultetrols) and ferulic acid (D-xylo-guggultetrol-16 to 22 ferulate), monocyclic diterpenoids, namely, α-camphorene, cembrene, cembrene A, 2-hydroxy-4,8,12-trimethyl 1-1-isopropyl-3, 7, 11-cyclodecatrine (mukulol; allylcembrol), cholesterol, three C-27 guggulsterols I, II and III and several pregnane derivatives, z-guggulsterol, guggulsterol VI, two hypolipaemic agents, namely, Z- and E-guggulsterones, 20-α- and 20-β-hydroxy-4-pregnen-3-one, 16 β-hydroxy-4, 17 (20)-Z-pregnatien-3-one and 16α -hydroxy-4-pregnen-3-one (gum); z-guggulsterone (oleoresin), amino acids, namely, alanine, arginine, aspartic acid, cystine, glutamic acid, histidine, isoleucine, leucine, lysine, proline, serine, threonine, tryptophan, tyrosine and valine were detected in the plant.

***EMBLICA OFFICINALIS* GAERTN**
SYN. *PHYLLANTHUS EMBLICA* L.

Vernacular Names: Sanskrit and Bengali: Amalakee; Hindi: amla; Tamil: Nelli; English: Indian gooseberry.

Occurrence and Distribution: Wild or cultivated throughout tropical India from the foot of the Himalayas.

Botany of Plant: Family: Euphorbiaceae. A large deciduous tree with greenish-grey or red bark, peeling of into scales and long strips. Leaves pinnate, distichously close-set, linear-oblong, obtuse. Flowers densely fascicled along the branchlets, yellowish; males on slender pedicels, females sub-sessile, few. Fruits depressed, globose, succulent, yellow or pink when ripe, obscurely 6-lobed. Seeds trigonous. Flowers during February-May and fruits during October-April.

Useful Parts: Fruits, seeds, flowers, leaves, bark and root.

Medicinal Uses: Fruit: astringent, antidiarrhoeal, antidysenteric, antiscorbutic, carminative, cooling, stomachic and tonic; beneficial in urinary troubles; prescribed in anaemia, jaundice and dyspepsia in combination with iron. Seeds: used as a collyrium in eye complaints; infusion useful in asthma, bronchitis and fever; Flowers: aperient and refrigerant; Leaves: juice applied externally to ulcers; infusion mixed with fenugreek seeds useful in chronic dysentery; Bark and root: astringent.

Chemical Constituents: A good source of vitamin C; carotene, nicotinic acid, riboflavin, D-glucose, D-fructose, myoinositol and a pectin with D-galacturonic acid, D-arabinosyl, D-xylosyl, L-rhamnosyl, D-glucosyl, D-mannosyl and D-galactosyl residues; embical, mucic and phyllemblic acids, phyllembin and fatty acids (seed oil); leucodelphinidin, procyanidin, 3-O-gallated prodelphinidin and tannin (bark); ellagic acid, lupeol, oleanolic aldehyde and O-acetyl oleanolic acid from root.

***GLYCYRRHIZA GLABRA* L.**

Vernacular Names: Sanskrit: Yashti-madhu; Hindi: Jethi-madhu; Bengali: Jashtimadhu; English: Liquorice.

Occurrence and Distribution: Cultivated in Jammu and Kashmir, Punjab and sub-Himalayan tracts.

Botany of Plant: Family: Fabaceae-Papilionoideae. A hardy herb or undershrub, attaining a height of 1.8 metres. Roots thick, having many branches with red or lemon-colour outside and yellowish or pale yellow inside. Leaves imparipinnate; leaflets in 4-7 pairs, ovate-lanceolate, smooth. Flowers borne in axillary spikes, papilionaceous, lavender to violet in colour. Pods compressed. Seeds 2-5, reniform, flat, deep grey. Flowers in March and fruits in August.

Useful Part: Root.

Medicinal Uses: Root (powder): prescribed in coughs, hoarseness and in respiratory troubles; mixed with citrus juice efficacious in catarrhal affections and with honey in jaundice; in combination with ginger and milk acts as a good tonic during convalescence; infusion, decoction or extract is laxative and an useful medicine in urinary diseases, bronchial and gastric troubles.

Chemical Constituents: Glycyrrhizin isolated from the root is the principal sweetening constituent. Glycyrrhizic and glycyrrhetinic acids, liquiritin, isoliquiritin, neoisoliquiritin, liquiritigenin, isoliquiritigenin, rhamnoliquiritin, glabrine, glabranine, formonenetin, licuraside, licochalcones A and B, hispaglabridin A and B, licoricidin, glabrene, pinocembrin, prunetin, saponaretin (isovitexin), II-deoxoglycyrrhetic, liquiritic and 18α-hydroxyglycyrrhetic acids, 24-hydroxy-11-deoxyglycyrrhetic and 24-hydroxyglycyrrhetic acids, 24-hydroxyliquiritic and liquiridiolic acids, glyzarin, glyzaglabrin, licoisoflavones A, B, glycrin, sugars and aspargin are reported from this plant.

GYMNEMA SYLVESTRE R.BR.

Vernacular Names: Sanskrit: Meshasringi; Hindi: Gur-mar; Bengali: Mera-sringi; Tamil: Cherukuringa.

Occurrence and Distribution: Common in the hills of Bihar, Orissa, Madhya Pradesh and the Deccan Peninsula.

Botany of Plant: Family: Asclepiadaceae. A large stout woody climber, with densely appressed hairy branchlets. Leaves rarely pubescent above, thinly coriaceous, elliptic or obovate-acute. Flowers small in crowded umbelliform cymes; corolla sub-rotate with thick lobes and fleshy coronal processes on the throat. Fruits slender follicles, glabrous. Seeds narrowly ovoid-oblong, flat with a broad thin wing, pale brown. Flowers during July-September and fruits during October-December.

Useful Parts: Whole plant, seeds, leaves and root.

Medicinal Uses: Whole Plant: antiperiodic, diuretic and stomachic; Seeds: emetic and remedy for cold. Leaves: hypoglycaemic; useful in cough, fever and in the management of maturity onset diabetes; important ingredient in the Ayurvedic formulations for diabetes, mixed with castor oil applied externally to swollen glands and to enlarged spleen, powder diuretic and stimulant. Root: astringent, emetic, expectorant, refrigerant, stomachic and tonic.

Chemical Constituents: Alanine, γ-aminobutyric acid, isoleucine, valine, adenine, choline, betaine, gymnamine (alkaloid), hentriacontance, nonacosane, pentatriacontane, tritriacontane, conduritol A; inositol, d-quercitol, α and β-chlorophylls; butyric, formic and tartaric acids; β-amyrin, lupeol; stigmasterol; gymnamosaponins; D-glucosides of 3 β, 16 β, 23, 28-tetrahydroxyolean-12-ene, dammarane type saponins-gimnemasides (I-VII), gymnemagenin and gymnemic acids.

NARDOSTACHYS GRANDIFLORA DC.
SYN. *NARDOSTACHYS JATAMANSI* DC.

Vernacular Names: Sanskrit, Hindi and Bengali: Jatamansee; Tamil: Jatamanshi; English: Indian nard

Occurrence and Distribution: Found in Alpine Himalayas from Kumaon to Sikkim, ascending up to 6,000 metres altitude.

Botany of Plant: Family: Valerianaceae. Rootstock woody, long, covered with fibres from the petioles of withered leaves; erect perennial herbs. Radical leaves elongated, spathulate and narrowed into the petiole; Cauline leaves oblong or subovate. Flowers capitate. Calyx-limb 5-lobed, enlarged in fruit. Corolla-tubular-companulate, lobes five, spreading, rosy. Fruit and seed obovate and compressed. Flowers and fruits during April-October.

Useful Parts: Rhizomes and root.

Medicinal Uses: Rhizomes and root: antiseptic, antispasmodic, aromatic, bitter, deobstruent, diuretic, emmenagogue, laxative, stomachic, tonic; infusion given in chorea, epilepsy, hysteria, palpitation of heart, fresh root used as an adjunct in the preparation of medicinal oils, as an important ingredient in many useful Ayurvedic formulations; spikenard oil antiarrhythmic, hypotensive, having distinct depressant action on central nervous system; promotes appetite and digestion, growth and darkness of hair; useful in leprosy and jaundice; tincture of rhizomes given for intestinal colic and flatulence.

Chemical Constituents: Actinidine; carotene, aristolen-1-α-O1, 1 (10)-aristolen-2-one; calarene, calorenol, 9-dyhdroaristolene, 1(10)-dehydroaristolene, elemol, erythro-1-2-propan-1-01, n-hexacosane n-hexacosanol, n-hexacosanylarachidae and isovalerate, 2-β maleine, β-maliene, α- and β-pinenes, Jatamols A and B, jatamansic acid, jatamansone, nardol, nardostachnol, nardostachone, patchouli alcohol, α and β-patchouleness.

***OCIMUM SANCTUM* L.**

Vernacular Names: Sanskrit: Tulasi; Hindi and Bengali: Tulsi; Tamil: Thulasi; English: Sacred basil.

Occurrence and Distribution: Cultivated, also found wild in waste places throughout India ascending up to 2,000 metres in the Himalayas.

Botany of Plant: Family: Lamiaceae. Much-branched, highly aromatic herb, sometimes woody, branches ascending, softly patently hairy. Leaves oblong or ovate-oblong, obtuse or acute, entire or subserrate. Flowers very small, borne in terminal and axillary racemes. Fruits subglobose or broadly oblong nutlets. Flowers and fruits almost throughout the year but chiefly during September-February.

Useful Parts: Whole plant, seeds, leaves and root.

Medicinal Uses: The plant, as a whole, is an important ingredient in many Ayurvedic formulations. Whole plant: antibacterial, antiperiodic, demulcent, expectorant, insecticidal and mosquito repellent, stomachic; decoction useful in bronchitis, catarrh and diarrhoea; Seeds: demulcent, used in genito-urinary disorders; Leaves: expectorant, cures dysentery and dyspepsia, chronic fever, haemorrhage; dried leaves used as snuff in myiosis and ozoena; juice is antiperiodic, diaphoretic, expectorant and stimulant; checks vomiting and destroys intestinal worms; useful for colds, bronchitis, catarrh, influenza, and remedy for earache; infusion beneficial in hepatic affections and also given to gastric disorders of children; fresh leaves, stems and roots bruised and applied externally for curing ringworm and other skin diseases; Root: aphrodisiac, decoction used as diaphoretic in malarial fever.

Chemical Constituents: Bornyl acetate, cadinene, camphene, camphor, carvacrol, β-caryophyllene, 1:8-cineole, decylaldehyde, eugenol, eugenol methyl ether, humelene, limonene, methylchavicol, nerol, α- and β- pinenes, γ-selinene, terpen-4-ol; linoleic, oleic, palmitic and stearic acids (oil); ascorbic acid; β-carotene, apigenin and its 7-0-glucuronide, luteolin and its 7-0-glucoronide, molludistin, oreantin, ursolic acid in leaves.

PHYLLANTHUS NIRURI SENSU HOOK F.
PHYLLANTHUS AMARUS

Vernacular Names: Sanskrit: Bhudhatri; Hindi: Jar-amla; Bengali: Bhiun-amla; Tamil: Keelanelli.

Occurrence and Distribution: Common throughout the hotter parts of India in waste places and shady gardens.

Botany of Plant: Family: Euphorbiaceae. An annual herb, 10-30 cm high. Leaves subsessile, elliptic-oblong or linear-oblong. Flowers axillary, yellowish, greenish or whitish; male flowers 1-3, females solitary. Capsules depressed, globose, smooth. Seeds trigonous, pale brown with 6-7 straight longitudinal ribs. Flowers and fruits from April-September.

Useful Parts: Whole plant, leaves, shoots and root.

Medicinal Uses: Whole plant: antipyretic, antiseptic, astringent, cooling, deobstruent, diuretic; beneficial in dropsy, gastro-intestinal troubles like colic, diarrhoea, dysentery, dyspepsia, gonorrhoea, menorrhagia and other genital diseases and in jaundice; Leaves: diuretic, mixed with salt applied locally to skin affections, swelling and ulcers in the form of poultice; decoction used as a refrigerant for the scalp; the latex is beneficial in indolent ulcer; mixed with oil used in opthalmia. Shoots: infusion of young tender leaves is given in chronic dysentery. Fresh leaves and root: efficacious in jaundice.

Chemical Constituents: Enantiomer of norsecurinine, 4-methoxy securinine, 4-methoxy-norsecurinine, nirphyllin and phyllinirubin, phyllantheol, phyllanthenol, phyllanthenone and 3,7,11,15,19,23-hexamethyl 2z, 6z, 10z, 14E, 18E, 22E-tetracosahexen-1-01 (aerial part); lintetralin, niranthin, nirletsalin, phyllanthin, hypophyllanthin, phyltetsalin (leaves); phyllochrysine alkaloids (leaves, stem); lupa-20 (29)-ene-3-ol, 3,5,7-trihydroxyflavonal-4'-O-α-L (-)-rhamnopyranoside, 5, 3', 4'-trihydroxy-8 flavone-5-O-rutinoside (root); estradiol (bark, root); cartilagin, ellagic acid, gallic acid, geranin, an angiolensin converting enzyme inhibitor, and the flavonoids- FG 1 and FG 2 have also been reported from the plant.

PICRORRHIZA KURROA ROYLE EX BENTH.

Vernacular Names: Sanskrit: Katuka; Hindi: Kuru; Bengali: Katki; Tamil: Katukarogani.

Occurrence and Distribution: Found in alpine Himalayas at an altitude of 3,000-5,000 metres.

Botany of Plant: Family: Scrophulariaceae. A low hairy herb with perennial bitter rootstock. Leaves subradical, spathulate, serrate. Flowering branch longer than the leaves. Flowers borne in many-flowered spikes. Fruits ovoid capsules. Flowers and fruits during October-December.

Useful Parts: Rhizome and root.

Medicinal Uses: Rhizome and root: valuable bitter tonic. Comparable to gentian; cholagogue;

prescribed in hepatic disorders; antipyretic; antiperiodic, effective in malaria, stomachic used in dyspepsia, in small doses the powdered root acts as anthelmintic and laxative; in large doses it is cathartic and used in dropsy. Combined with liquorice effective in heart diseases and hiccups. Used in scorpion sting.

Chemical Constituents: D-mannitol, kutkiol, kutkisterol, 4-hydroxy-3-methoxyacetophenone (apocyanin); vanillic acid, cinnamoyl-α and 6-cinnamoyl-β-D-glucopyranose; phenol glucosides; androsin and picein iridoid, glycosides; 6-feruloylcatalpol, kutkin, kutkoside, picroside-II, III; minecoside, picrorhizin, veronicoside; cucurbitacin glycosides, arvenin III.

PIPER LONGUM L.

Vernacular Names: Sanskrit: Pippali; Hindi: Piplamul; Bengali: Pipul; Tamil: Tippili; English: Long pepper.

Occurrence and Distribution: Occurs in the hotter parts of India from the Central Himalayas to Assam, Khasi and Mikir Hills, lower hills of West Bengal and evergreen forests of the Western Ghats from Konkan to Kerala. Also recorded from Car Nicobar Islands.

Botany of Plant: Family: Piperaceae. An aromatic slender climber, stems creeping, jointed and become attached to other plants. Leaves 5-9 cm long and 3-5 cm wide, subacute, entire, glabrous, cordate with broad rounded lobes at the base. Spikes pedunculate and upright, male larger and slender; female 1.3-2.5 cm long and 4-5 mm diam. Fruits yellowish orange, ovoid, sunk in fleshy spike. Flowers in the rainy season and fruits in the autumn.

Useful Parts: Fruits and root.

Medicinal Uses: The plant is an age-old Ayurvedic drug. Both roots and the fruits are attributed with various medicinal properties and as such, find applications in diseases of the respiratory tract, dysentery, skin disease (leucoderma), as cholagogue in obstruction of bile duct and gall bladder; analgesic, Old long pepper is considered to be more useful than fresh one. Powdered long pepper, mixed with honey is efficacious in cold, cough, asthma and hiccups. It is an important ingredient in the preparation of medicated oil used externally in sciatica and paraplegia. A mixture of long pepper, long pepper root, black pepper and ginger (in equal parts) is an useful preparation in colic, flatulence, cough, coryza and hoarseness. Long pepper in combination with black pepper, is used in the preparation of irritating snuff which is recommended in coma and drowsiness. Long pepper in the form of powder is suspended in warm water and given to women after parturition to check haemorrhage and fever. As vermifuge, it is prescribed for colic in children.

Chemical Constituents: The plant contains essential oil consisting of long chain hydrocarbons, mono- and sequiterpenes, caryophyllene being the main product. Other constituents are piperine, piplartine, piperlongumine, piperlonguminine and its dihydro-derivative, pipernonaline, piperundecalidine, pipercide and guineesine, sesamin, dieudesmin, β sitosterol and dihydrostigmasterol. Four aristolactams and five 4,5-dioxoaporphines, quinoline-4-5- its 6-demethyl-4H-dibenzo (de, g) quinoline-4-5-(6H)-dione, its 6-demethyl derivative and amino acids.

PLANTAGO OVATA FORSK.

Vernacular Names: Sanskrit: Ishadgola; Hindi: Isabgol; Bengali: Ishabgul; Tamil: Iskolvirai; English: Blond psyllum.

Occurrence and Distribution: Cultivated in parts of North Gujarat, Punjab and Uttar Pradesh.

Botany of Plant: Family: Plantaginaceae. A stem-less annual herb, softly hairy or woolly. Leaves filiform or narrowly linear, entire or distantly toothed. Flowers borne in cylindrical or ovoid spikes. Fruits ellipsoid capsules, 8 mm long, obtuse, the upper half coming off as a blunt conical lid; membranous, glabrous, seeds ovoid-oblong, 3 mm long, boat shaped, smooth, yellowish brown. Flowers and fruits during January-April.

Useful Parts: Seeds.

Medicinal Uses: Seed husk: anti-inflammatory; used in gastrointestinal and genito-urinary disorders; astringent (mild), demulcent, diuretic, emollient and laxative, used in chronic cases such as constipation of varied aetiology, diarrhoea, specially of hill origin and of children, dysentery of amoebic and bacillary origin; in piles, decoction in cough and cold. Seeds: in febrile condition and affections of bladder. Kidneys and uretha; poultice applied to glandular swellings and rheumatism.

Chemical Constituents: Planteose, raffinose, stachyose, sucrose (also in stem, root); fructose, glucose, mucilage containing arabinose, galactose, galacturonic acid, rhamnose and xylose, aucubin (glucoside); ascorbic acid; DL alanine, L (-) asparagine, L-cystine, glutamic acid, glycine, L-lysine, DL-norleucine, tyrosine, Dl-valine, g-hydroxyoctadec-cis-12-enoic acid, g-oxooctadec-cis.

RAUVOLFIA SERPENTINA BENTH EX KURZ.

Vernacular Names: Sanskrit and Bengali: Sarpagandha; Hindi: Chhotachand; Tamil: Chivanmelpodi; English: Serpentina.

Occurrence and Distribution: Grows in waste places and in shady forests in different parts of India from Punjab eastwards to Nepal, Sikkim, Bhutan and Assam; also in certain parts of Central India and the Western Ghats.

Botany of Plant: Family: Apocyanaceae. Glabrous undershrub. Leaves in whorls of 3 or 4, rarely opposite, shining green above, pale beneath, elliptic-lanceolate or obovate acute or acuminate. Inflorescence many-flowered cymes. Corolla salver-shaped, tube cylindrical, white with red tinge, mouth constricted, throat usually hairy within. Fruits obliquely ovoid drupes, purple-black when ripe, seeds ovoid. Flowers and fruits almost throughout the year but chiefly during February-May.

Useful Parts: Leaves and root.

Medicinal Uses: Leaves: Juice applied to remove corneal opacities. Root: Decoction employed to increase uterine contractions and for expulsion of foetus in difficult cases. The extract is particularly used for intestinal disorders; it is anthelmintic, bitter tonic and febrifuge; the total alkaloidal extract of the root induces bradycardia, hypotension, sedation and produces tranquillising effect; used in hypochondria, neuropsychiatric disorders, psychosis and schizophrenia.

Reserpine (an indole alkaloid) was found to be the most active principle responsible for the antihypertensive and tranquillising properties of the plant; the other alkaloids, namely, ajmalicine, deserpidine, rescinnamine and serpentine also show similar properties with reduced activity. Ajmaline, in combination with other hypotensive agents, is used in the treatment of hypertension complicated with arrhythmia.

Chemical Constituents: Arachidic, behenic, lauric, linoleic, myristic, oleic, palmitic, stearic acids (seeds); the isolation of reserpine, the well-known hypotensive and tranquillising drug from *Rauvolfia serpentina,* triggered an intense research and led to the isolation of a number of indole and dihydroindole alkaloids of considerable biogenetic and therapeutic interest from the root.

SANTALUM ALBUM L.

Vernacular Names: Sanskrit: Srikhanda; Hindi: Safed Chandan; Bengal: Chandan; Tamil: Chandanam; English: Sandalwood tree.

Occurrence and Distribution: Found in hedge-rows and dry open scrub forests. Occurs from Vindhya mountains southward, particularly in Karnataka and Tamil Nadu and ascending to an altitude of 1,200 metres. Reportedly introduced into Rajasthan, Uttar Pradesh, Madhya Pradesh and Orissa where it has become naturalised.

Botany of Plant: Family: Santalaceae. A small or medium sized evergreen semi-parasitic tree, with slender branches, sometimes attaining a height of 18 metres and a girth of 2.4 metres. Bark dark grey or nearly black or reddish, rough, with deep vertical cracks on old trees. Sapwood unscented and whitish yellow to white, but heartwood scented and light yellowish brown (when freshly cut) or dark brown, reddish brown (upon exposure and ageing). Leaves elliptic-ovate or ovate-lanceolate, glabrous, thin, 1.5-8.0 cm $\times$1.6-3.2 cm or larger. Flowers brownish purple, violet or straw-coloured, unscented, borne in axillary and terminal paniculate cymes. Drupes purple-black, globose 1.3 cm diam., with hard ribbed endocarp. Seeds globose or ovoid. Flowers from rainy to winter season.

Useful Parts: Wood and sandalwood oil.

Medicinal Uses: Both the sandalwood and oil (derived from heartwood) are considered to be cooling, diaphoretic, diuretic and expectorant. A paste of the wood finds applications in burns, headache, fever, skin diseases and to allay heat and pruritis. Decoction of the wood, mixed with that of dried ginger, is beneficial in haemorrhoids. Sandalwood oil is valued in the treatment of gonorrhoea. It is also used in the symptomatic treatment of dysuria. Sandalwood oil, mixed with its double the quantity of mustard oil, finds useful application for pimples on the nose.

Chemical Constituents: Sandalwood oil contains a-santatol, santene, a- and B- santalences, santenol, teresantalol, a- and B-santalic acids. The leaves, fruits and seeds contain santalbic acid, palmitic acid, oleic acid, linoleic acid, glucose, fructose, sucrose, palmitone and 10-hydroxypalmitone.

SARACA ASOCA (ROXB.) DE WIDE
SYN. *SARACA INDICA* AUCT. NON L.

Vernacular Names: Sanskrit, Hindi and Bengali: Ashoka; Tamil: Asogam; English: Asoka.

Occurrence and Distribution: Grows wild along streams or in shady evergreen forests up to an altitude of 750 metres in the central and eastern Himalayas as well as in the Khasi, Garo and Lushai hills, abundant in South India.

Botany of Plant: Family Leguminosae-Caesalpinideae. A small evergreen, 6-9 metres in height. Bark with warty surface, dark-brown to grey or almost black. Leaves paripinnate, 15-20 cm long, leaflets 6-12, rigidly subcoriaceous, oblong or oblong-lanceolate, 7.5-22.5 cm × 1.3 cm. Flowers borne in dark axillary corymbs, very fragrant, orange or orange-yellow, finally turning vermilion-red. Pods, flat, oblong, woody 7.6-25.4 ×3.8-5.1 cm. Seeds 4-8, ellipsoid-oblong, compressed. Flowers in March-April and fruits in August-September.

Useful Parts: Seeds, flowers and stem-bark.

Medicinal Uses: Seeds: diuretic; Flowers: effective in blood dysentery; Stem bark: reputed to cure colic, dysentery, dyspepsia, piles, ulcers and uterine troubles, in particular menorrhagia due to uterine fibroids, leucorrhoea and menstrual pain.

Chemical Constituents: The flowers contain fatty acids and gallic acid, apigenin-7-0-β-D-glucoside, cyanidin-3-5-diglucoside, kaempferol-3-0-β-D-glucoside, pelargonidin-3-5-diglucoside, quercetin and its 3-0-β-D-glucoside and sitosterol. Bark yields alkanes, esters and primary alcohols.

SAUSSUREA COSTUS (FALC.) LIPSCH.
SYN. *SAUSSUREA LAPPA* (DECNE) SCH-BIP.

Vernacular Names: Sanskrit: Kushta; Hindi and Bengali: Kut; Tamil: Kostum; English: Kuth.

Occurrence and Distribution: Apparently endemic in the valley of Kashmir at 2,500-3,000 metres; cultivated in Kashmir and neighbouring regions like Lahaul in Himachal Pradesh and Garhwal in Uttar Pradesh at 2,700-4,000 metres.

Botany of Plant: Family: Asteraceae. A tall, stout, perennial herb with tuberous roots having a characteristic smell. Radical leaves with long, lobately winged stalks up to 1 metre long; cauline leaves membranous, scaberulous above, glabrate beneath, irregularly toothed. Flowers dark-blue, purple or almost black in colour, borne in stalk-less subglobose heads. Fruits compressed achenes with narrow tips. Flowers and fruits during September-November.

Useful Part: Root.

Medicinal Uses: Root: alterative, antiseptic, antispasmodic, anthelmintic, astringent, carminative, diuretic, narcotic when smoked, prophylactic, sedative, aromatic, stimulant, tonic; infusion with a little cardamom found useful in asthma, cough, fever, dyspepsia, chronic rheumatism, skin diseases; useful in dropsy and jaundice; powdered root and tincture are expectorant in bronchial asthma especially those of vagotonic type; used as an ingredient in stimulating mixtures for cholera, powdered root is applied locally to wounds, severe ulceration; powdered root mixed with mustard oil is applied to the scalp in prurigo.

Chemical Constituents: Saussurine (also in root), α-amyrin stearate, β-amyrin palmitate, lupeol palmitate, taraxasterol and its acetate (leaves); costic, linoleic, oleic, palmitic acids; amino acids, betulin, friedelin, β-sitosterol, stigmasterol and its 22, 23-dihydro derivatives from root oil/root.

SOLANUM NIGRUM L.

Vernacular Names: Sanskrit: Kakamachi; Hindi: Makoi; Bengali: Kakmachi; Tamil: Manatakali; English: Black nightshade.

Occurrence and Distribution: Common in waste places, roadsides and along railway tracks throughout India.

Botany of Plant: Family Solanaceae. A glabrous or sparingly pubescent annual herb. Leaves ovate or oblong, sinuate toothed or lobed. Peduncles extra-axillary; pedicels subumbelled. Calyx teeth small, obtuse. Corolla white, nearly glabrous, ovary glabrous, style-base hairy. Berry globose, red or black, sometimes yellow. Seeds smooth or nearly so. Flowers and fruits almost throughout the year, but chiefly during February-July.

Useful Parts: Whole plant, berries, flowers and leaves.

Medicinal Uses: All parts: alterative, diuretic and laxative; Whole plant: anodyne, antidysentric, antiseptic, diaphoretic, expectorant, hydragogue, sedative; useful in cardalgia and gripe, fresh extract employed in dropsy, gonorrhoea, haemoptysis, piles, enlargement of liver and spleen; decoction antispasmodic and narcotic; Berries: antidiarrhoeal, antipyretic, tonic, beneficial in *anasarca*, eye trouble and heart diseases; decoction of berries and flowers prescribed in cough and colds; Leaves: applied with benefit to painful and swollen testicles; paste used as poultice in gout and rheumatic joints; skin diseases; fresh juice produces dilation of pupils.

Chemical Constituents::α, β and γ-carotenes, lutein, lycopene, cryptoxanthin and vitamin C (also in leaves): glucose, fructose, caffeoyl glucose; caffeic, chlorogenic, iso-and neo-chlorogenic acids; uttronin A, uttrosides A and B. solasodine, tomatidenol and figogenin (also in leaves, stem, root). Solanergine and solasonine (also in leaves), five steroidal glycosides (fruits); palmitic, stearic, oleic, linoleic and linolenic acids (seeds).

SWERTIA CHIRAYITA (ROXB. EX FLEM). KARST.
SYN. _SWERTIA CHIRAYITA_ (WALL) CL; _SWERTIA TONGLUENSIS_ BURKILL

Vernacular Names: Sanskrit: Kirata; Hindi: Chirayita: Bengali: Chirata; Tamil: Nilavembu: English: Chiretta.

Occurrence and Distribution: Found in the temperate Himalayas ascending to an altitude of about 1,350-3,350 metres from Kashmir to Bhutan and in the Khasi Hills in Meghalaya at 1,200-1,500 metres.

Botany of Plant: Family Gentianaceae. Stem about 5-13 cm high, subterete, cauline leaves subsessile, elliptic acute, five-nerved, the lower often much larger, sometimes petioled. Flowers borne in many flowered, leafy, large panicles, often fascicled. Corolla lurid-green-yellow, near the base of each lobe 2 glandular depressions, each terminated by long hair. Fruits sessile, ovate capsules. Seeds polyhedral, smooth. Flowers and fruits in August-October.

Useful Part: Whole plant.

Medicinal Uses: Whole Plant: Used as powder, infusion or as an extract; antidiarrhoel, antimalarial, anthelmintic, astringent, bitter, laxative, stomachic and tonic; used as a special remedy for bronchial asthma and liver disorders; beneficial in cough, dropsy, dyspepsia, melancholia, sciatica and skin diseases; given with sandal wood paste to stop internal haemorrhage in the stomach; taken daily in the morning on an empty stomach to keep fit and healthy.

Chemical Constituents: Rich in protein (15.45 per cent); amarogentin, gentiopicrin; isobellicifolin, swertianin, swertinin and the dimeric xanthone, chiratanin; enicoflavine, gentianine, gentiocrucine; cerolic, oleic, ophelic, palmitic and stearic acids.

***TINOSPORA CORDIFOLIA* (WILLD.) MIERS EX HOOK F. AND THOMAS**

Vernacular Names: Sanskrit: Guruchi; Hindi: Amrita; Bengali: Gulancha; Tamil: Amudom.

Occurrence and Distribution: Found throughout tropical India; ascending to an altitude of 300 metres.

Botany of Plant: Family Menispermaceae. A large glabrous climbing shrub. Stems rather succulent with long filiform; aerial roots arising from branches. Bark warty, creamy-white or grey-brown, wood soft, perforated, leaves membranous, cordate with broad sinus blade 5.1 -10.2 cm and petiole 3.8-7.6 cm long. Flowers unisexual, greenish; male fascicled and female usually solitary. Drupes ovoid, succulent, lustrous, red, pea sized. Seeds curved. Flowers during the summer and fruits during the winter.

Useful Parts: Leaves and stem.

Medicinal Uses: Stem juice is valued in high fever and also given in jaundice either alone or mixed with honey. Decoction of the stem is used for rheumatic fever and vomiting due to excessive bile secretion; slow fever associated with cough is arrested by the administration of its decoction mixed with *Piper longum* (fruits) and honey. General dose of extract is 0.35-1.05 g/day. Stem paste with a little ginger is prescribed in urticaria. In combination with the stem of *Piper nigrum* and honey, it is useful to control heart palpitation due to flatulency; stem juice found beneficial in elephantiasis when administered in combination with sweet oil. A kind of starch called 'Palo' is prepared from the aqueous extract of dried stem and is considered to have antacid, antidiarrhoeal and antidysenteric properties (dose: 0.7 to 2.10 g/day). Leaves of the plant are rich in protein, calcium and phosphorus with no toxic effect and as such prescribed in fever. Aqueous extract of the plant is a febrifuge.

Chemical Constituents: The plant contains tinosporin, columbin, chasmanthin, palmarin, herberine, tinosporon, tinosporic acid, tinosporol, giloin, giloinisin, substituted pyrrolidine, a diterpenoid furanolactone, 18-norclerodane diterpene-O-glucoside, an aryltetrahydrofuranolignan, octacosanol, nonacosan-15 one and β sitosterol.

***WITHANIA SOMNIFERA* DUNAL**

Vernacular Names: Sanskrit, Hindi and Bengali: Ashwagandha; Tamil: Achuvagandi.

Occurrence and Distribution: Throughout the dry and subtropical parts of India.

Botany of Plant: Family Solanaceae. An erect undershrub, about 0.5-2 metres high, slightly woolly. Leaves entire, ovate, subacute. Flowers axillary, sessile or shortly pedicelled, fascicled or solitary, hermaphrodite, calyx campanulate, acutely 5-6 toothed. Fruit-calyx inflated, papery, larger than the berry. Corolla campanulate; lobes 3-6 short, greenish or lurid yellow. Stamens attached near the base of the corolla, ovary 2-celled, stigma shortly 2-fid. Fruits globose berries. Seeds many discoid. Flowers and fruits during November-February.

Medicinal Uses: Fruits and Seeds: diuretic; Leaves: antipyretic, anthelmintic and bitter; Leaves and root: emphysematous dyspnea; Bruised leaves and ground root: Locally applied in carbuncles, scabies, painful swellings and ulcers: Root: adaptogenic, alternative, aphrodisiac, deobstruent; diuretic and tonic; useful in cough, dropsy, hiccups, leucorrhoea and menstrual troubles, restores loss of memory; used in cases of nervous exhaustion, spermatorrhoea and senile debility; powder with equal parts of ghee and honey beneficial in impotency or seminal debility; decoction boiled with milk and ghee promotes nutrition; an important ingredient in various Ayurvedic formulations (Ashwagandha Ghrita, Ashwagandharista and Narayana Taila) prepared from Aswagandha is prescribed as aphrodisiac, galactogogue, invigorating and also in lumbago and rheumatism.

Chemical Constituents: Proteins and amino acids (all aerial parts); Withaferin-A, Withanone (also in leaves), Withanolide WS-1 (in seeds); Withanolide C, chlorohydrin of Withanolide D, isowithanolide E, Withanolide F, Withanolide G, H, I, J, K, L, M, N, O, P, Q, R, S, T, U, Y; Somnisol, Somnitol (leaves); Withasomniferin A from aerial parts; anatygrine, anaferine and its dl-form, cuscotygrine, hygrine, nicotine, pseudotropine, tropine, solasodine, Withasomnine, Visamine; dulcitol, hentriacontane, sominone, sominolide.

CONCLUSION

That human beings are still dependent on nature for remedies is well apparent from the fact that all the major systems of medicine, for example, Ayurveda, Unani and Homeopathy, are largely based on drugs of plant origin. Undoubtedly, we have a vast, promising and yet unexplored repository of medicinal plants, some of which are already in wide clinical use as crude drug preparations or formulations. Effort must, therefore, continue to re-evaluate the therapeutic efficacy of Ayurvedic drugs and standardise the preparations by chemical and biochemical assays to ensure the consistency of active principles in each dose. The seasonal variations of the active components, their efficacy and appropriate methods of storage need to be carefully assessed. We must also be able to harness Ayurveda for modern drug development through investigations of single drug plant. Modern science demands meticulous work on the drugs on a rational basis to make them more acceptable for the benefit of mankind.

REFERENCES

Ambasta, S. P., Ramachandran, K., Kashyapa, K. and Chand, R. *The Useful Plants of India.* New Delhi: CSIR, 1986.

Atal, C. K. and Kapur, B. M. *Cultivation and Utilisation of Medicinal and Aromatic Plants.* Jammu-Tawi: CSIR, 1977, 1982.

Barton, D. H. R. and Ollis, W. D. *Advances in Medicinal Phytochemistry.* London: John Libbey Eurotex Ad., 1986.

Chatterjee, A. and Pakrashi, S. C. *The Treatise of Indian Medicinal Plants.* vols. I-V. New Delhi: National Institute of Science Communication (CSIR), 1991.

Chopra, R. N. *Indigenous Drugs of India.* 2nd edn. Kolkata: Academic Publishers, 1982.

Chopra, R. N., Badhwar, R. L. and Ghosh, S. *Poisonous Plants of India.* Jaipur: Academic Publishers, 1984.

Chopra, R. N., Chopra, I. C. and Varma, B. S. *Supplement to Glossary of Indian Medicinal Plants*. New Delhi: CSIR, 1969.

CSIR. *The Wealth of India-Raw Materials*. Vols. I-XI, 1948-1976. Revised edition, vol. IA (1985), vol. 2B (1988). New Delhi: CSIR.

Kirtikar, K. R. and Basu, B. D. Revised by Blatter, E., Caius, J. F. and Mhaskar, K. S. vols. I-IV, 2nd edn. Allahabad: L. M. Basu, 1935.

Kochhar, S. L. *Economic Botany in the Tropics*. Chennai: Macmillan India Ltd., 1981.

Ray, P., Gupta, H. and Roy, M. *Susruta Samhita*. New Delhi: Indian National Science Academy, 1980.

Satyavati, G. V., Gupta, A. K. and Tandon, N. (Eds.). *Medicinal Plants of India*, vol. 1 (1976), vol. II (1987). New Delhi: Indian Council of Medical Research, 1976, 1987.

Singh, U., Wadhwani, A. M. and Johri, B. M. *Dictionary of Economic Plants in India*, 2nd edn. New Delhi: Indian Council of Agricultural Research, 1983.

Swain, T. *Plants in the Development of Modern Medicine*. Cambridge: USA: Harvard University Press, 1972.

Watt, G. A. *A Dictionary of the Economic Products of India*. vols. I-VI. Reprinted edition. New Delhi: Cosmo Publication, 1972.

Willis, J. C. *A Dictionary of the Flowering Plants and Ferns*. 8th edn. London: Cambridge University Press, 1973.

—oo(O)oo—

21

Medicinal Plant Solutions to Asthmatic Problems

Gayatri K. Vaidya and Vincent J. Braganza S.J.

ASTHMA

Modernization has brought in its wake an evident increase in many environment related diseases. Asthma is one such common chronic disease. In simple words, Asthma can be understood as the disease in which the lungs don't get enough air to breathe. Its most debilitating factor manifests as bronchoconstriction, a result of various environmental, physical, biological and immunological factors. These factors are known as triggers. A range of triggers have been identified till date for asthma.

In recent years, asthma has become a global phenomenon. Genetic predisposition is one of the factors that accounts for increased prevalence in children. However, urbanisation triggers like air pollution and environmental tobacco smoke contribute more significantly. Children exposed to urbanized life styles and thereby exposed to pollutants show more prevalence of the disease (Paramesh, 2002).

With the number of asthma patients rising continuously, the focus of concern is on paediatric asthma, i.e. asthma in children. In its 121st report the committee on Science & Technology, Environment & Forests in the Rajya Sabha, has expressed concerns about the sharply rising numbers of asthmatic patients in all age groups as well as different strata of society. The committee has recommended an ASTHMATIC & ALLERGIC DISORDERS MITIGATION MISSION to check this rise through grassroots level research, including early phase detection of the disease, to be carried out by various institutes in India (Committee on Science and Technology, Environment & Forests report, 2004).

The Indian scenario is only a reflection of the global phenomenon. Globally, over 180,000 people die of asthma each year. India has approximately 15-20 million asthmatics. The prevalence and incidence is higher amongst the affluent stratum. New evidence points to the ever-increasing role of environmental factors and triggers. The increasing trends in childhood asthma continue to haunt researchers and parents.

In general, symptoms of asthma commonly include coughing, wheezing, shortness of breath and tightness in chest. Fig. 1 explains in detail various triggers, their mode of action and symptoms of asthma.

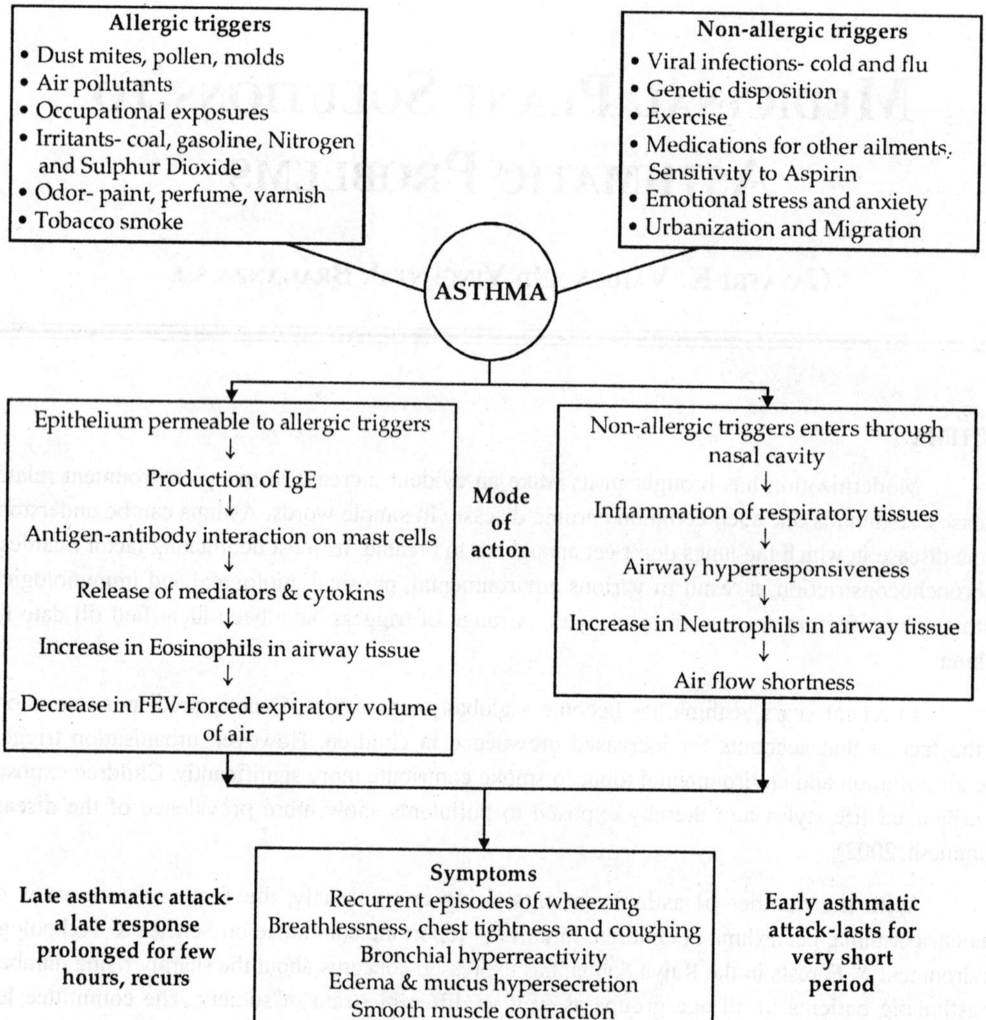

Fig. 1.

Asthma can roughly be divided into two categories. In the first category asthma is associated with atopy, while the second category comprises the non-atopic asthmatics. The majority of patients have atopic asthma, characterized by an elevation of total and allergen- specific IgE in serum (Jeffery *et al*, 1989). Non- atopic asthmatics are skin test negative to common allergens and there is no evidence of allergen-specific serum IgE (Humbert *et al*, 1999). Amin and coworkers in the recent past showed that besides the difference in serum IgE levels, atopic and non-atopic patients had different pathological changes present in their airways despite their similar clinical respiratory symptoms (Amin *et al*, 2000).

The overall understanding of the various effects of the triggers leading to a host of symptoms has been explored by a range of workers in the field. Their findings (Sekkadde *et al*, 1994; Roche, 1991; Mori *et al*, 1995; Meeusen, 1999; Cerwenka & Swain, 1999; Kraneveld *et al*, 1998; Garssen *et al*, 1989; Askenase *et al*, 1983; Friedman-Jimenez *et al*, 2000) have been summarized further by us in a diagrammatic form in fig. 1, thus giving an overview of asthma at one glance.

MAST CELLS

Mast cells are widely distributed throughout the body in connective tissues, particularly around blood vessels and nerves (Botchkarev *et al*, 1997). They are abundant in the submucosa of the digestive tract (Wershil & Galli, 1991), oral and nasal mucosa (Otsuka *et al*, 1985), respiratory mucosal surfaces (Kaliner, 1987) and skin (Botchkarev *et al*, 1997; Arizono *et al*, 1990; Scholzen *et al*, 1998).

Mast cells are involved in the regulation of their own overall tissue cell mass since mast cell degranulation leads to an overall increase in mast cells (Marshall *et al*, 1990). A range of scientific explorations reveal a lot about mast cells, their characteristics and functions, their role in asthma and the mediators that they release. (Valent, 1995; Rottem *et al*, 1994; Galli, 1990; Befus *et al*, 1987; Galli, 1993; Ramirez-Romero *et al*, 2000; Kraneveld *et al*, 1998; Vallinga *et al*, 1997; Redegeld *et al*, 2002; Van Loveren *et al*, 1983; Garssen *et al*, 1994; Johnson and Krenger, 1992; Ogasawara *et al*, 1997; Emadi-Khiav *et al*, 1995; Mousli *et al*, 1994; Mousli *et al*, 1990; Combrink *et al*, 1998; Krumins and Broomfield, 1993, Ansel *et al*, 1993). Mast cells are versatile cells capable of synthesis of a large number of pro- and anti-inflammatory mediators including cytokines, products of arachidonic acid metabolism, serotonin, histamine and growth factors including NGF (Nerve Growth Factor) and SCF (Stem Cell Factor). These mediators are pre-stored or can be newly synthesized upon stimulation. Pre-stored mediators, such as histamine, serine proteases like tryptase, proteoglycans, sulfates and TNF-± are released within minutes after degranulation of the cell. After this primary response a second wave of newly synthesized mediators are released and include PGD2 (Prostaglandin D2), LTC4 (Leukotriene C4), LTD4 (Leukotriene D4) and LTE4 (Leukotriene E4). On later exposures, cytokines like IL-4, IL-5, IL-6, IL-8, IL-13 (Interleukins) are secreted (Church & Levi-Schaffer, 1997).

BIOCHEMISTRY OF ASTHMA

In the past two decades considerable attention has been focused on two molecules found in mast cells, which have a role in asthma i.e. tryptase and histamines.

Role of Tryptase

Tryptase is a tetrameric serine proteinase that constitutes approximately 20% of the total protein within human mast cells and is responsible for at least 95% of the trypsin-like activity in lysates of mast cells derived from lung and skin tissue (Wenzel *et al*, 1990). It is stored in the secretory granules in a catalytically active form (Glenner and Cohen, 1960) and is secreted along with histamine, heparin and other mast cell granule products on mast cell degranulation (Schwartz *et al.*, 1981). Because it is stored almost exclusively in mast cells (Shaoheng *et al*, 1990), this proteinase has attracted particular attention as a marker for mast cells and for mast cell activation. Relatively high concentrations of tryptase have been detected in the serum from cases of systemic anaphylaxis (Wenzel *et al*, 1987); in bronchoalveolar lavage fluid from patients with bronchial asthma or interstitial lung disease (Buckley *et al*, 1991); in nasal lavage fluid of patients with allergic rhinitis (Jarjour *et al.*, 1991); in skin blister fluid from subjects with allergic contact dermatitis (Brockow *et al.*, 1996), and in synovial fluid from patients with arthritis (Buckley *et al*, 1997). Evidence is emerging that this major secretory product of the human mast cell may be a key mediator of allergic inflammation and a promising target for therapeutic intervention (Walls, 1995). In seeking to determine the contribution of tryptase in acute inflammatory responses it is especially important to consider the early cellular events. Studies of human tryptase function in animal models have suggested that some of the effects noted may depend on the ability of tryptase to activate mast cells. The increase in microvascular permeability induced by tryptase in guinea pig skin can be abrogated by pretreatment of guinea pigs with histamine H1 and H2 receptor antagonists (He and Walls, 1997). Moreover, addition of tryptase to dispersed guinea pig lung and skin tissue can provoke the release of histamine by a noncytotoxic mechanism *in vitro*. Although not investigated directly, the finding that both skin microvascular leakage and bronchoconstriction (Molinari *et al.*, 1996) stimulated by tryptase in sheep could also be blocked by a histamine antagonist provides evidence that this human proteinase may induce the activation of mast cells in this species also. Several proteinases have been characterized as secretagogues for mast cells. Thus the degranulation of rodent mast cells may be stimulated by bovine pancreatic trypsin, thrombin (Razin and Marx, 1984), ±-chymotrypsin or rat mast cell chymase (Schick *et al.*, 1984). In addition, certain broad-spectrum proteinase inhibitors can reduce IgE-dependent histamine release from chopped guinea pig (Austen & Brocklehurst, 1961) or human lung tissue (Kaliner & Austen, 1973), and inhibitors of chymase reduce IgE-dependent histamine release from human tonsil mast cells (Dietze *et al.*, 1990). However, the actions of human tryptase on human mast cells have not been investigated, and the potential of inhibitors and substrates of tryptase to act as mast cell stabilizers is not known. In the present study, the ability of human tryptase to stimulate histamine release from dispersed human skin and tonsil cells and to modulate histamine release by other stimuli were observed and investigated. The findings suggest that tryptase released from degranulated mast cells has the capacity to activate certain mast cell populations.

Role of Histamine

Histamine is a biogenic amine, which is synthesized and stored mainly in mast cells and basophils and plays a very important role in the pathophysiology of inflammatory diseases like asthma and utricaria. (White, 1990; Greaves & Sabroe, 1998; Friedmann, 1999). Several immunologic and non-immunologic stimuli induce the release of histamine from mast cells and basophils and it then diffuses rapidly into the surrounding tissues and exerts its effects, and is excreted in the urine (White *et al*, 1987). In experimental asthma induced by allergen or exercise challenge, it has been demonstrated that the levels of histamine are increased in the circulation and implicated in bronchoconstriction (Barnes & Brown, 1981; Howarth *et al*, 1985; Busse & Swenson, 1989). Apart from the classical activities of histamine, there is an increasing body of evidence that histamine also elicits pro-inflammatory and immune-modulatory effects, having more critical role in allergic disease than is considered presently.

RECENT DEVELOPMENTS IN THE FIELDS OF ASTHMA CURE

In asthma, both genetic and environmental factors contribute to the development of the disease, which can vary in the same patient through time.

The first step in achieving long-term control of asthma is avoiding triggers. More than two thousand irritants are found indoors where we may spend as much as 90 percent of our time. To optimally protect us from getting exposed to indoor and outdoor irritants maintenance of hygienic conditions becomes mandatory.

The second step in managing asthma involves use of medications according to the severity of the disease. Bronchodilation is promoted by cAMP. Sympathomimetics and methylxanthines (Fanta *et al,* 1986) are used in direct relaxation of airway smooth muscle. Sympathomimetic agents that have been widely used in the treatment of asthma include steroidal compounds like epinephrine, ephedrine, isoproterenol and selected ^{2}2-agents (Rochat, 1994; Djukanoviâc, 1997). These adrenoreceptor agonists relax airway smooth muscle, inhibit release of some bronchoconstricting substances from mast cells and increase mucociliary transport. As in other tissues, ^{2}-agonists facilitate adenylyl cyclase and catalyze the formation of cAMP in the airway tissues (Vulliemoz *et al,* 1975; Colasanti & Trotter, 1981). Not all sympathomimetic drugs promisingly provide treatment solely for all asthmatic patients. Because epinephrine and ispproterenol cause more cardiac stimulation, they should be reserved for special situations. Epinephrine can cause tachycardia, arrhythmias, and worsening of angina pectoris. Compared to epinephrine, ephedrine has a longer duration, oral activity, more pronounced central effects, and much lower potency. Isoproterenol is a potent bronchodilator. High dose of inhaled isoproterenol is believed to give rise to asthma mortality resulting from cardiac arrhythmias (Wyser, 1997). At present, ^{2}2-selective adrenoceptor agonist drugs are the most widely used sympathomimetics for the treatment of asthma. They are effective after inhaled or oral administration and have long effective duration. Albuterol and terbutaline inhalation offers greatest efficacy without systemic toxicity. They give less cardiac stimulation (Wolfe *et al*, 1985).

Methylxanthine drugs also play important role in treating asthma. Agents include theophylline, theobromine, and caffeine (Nakahara, 1996). They can be found in tea, cocoa, and coffee, respectively. Inhibition of phosphodiesterase by theophylline can increase and stimulate cAMP production. cAMP, in turn, promotes bronchodilation. From the clinical perspective, theophylline is the most effective bronchodilator of the xanthines. It has been shown repeatedly both to relieve airflow obstruction in acute asthma and to reduce the severity of symptoms. Theophylline is effective when taken orally. It improves long-term control of asthma when taken as the sole maintenance treatment or when added to inhaled corticosteriods. For oral therapy, the usual dose is 3-4 mg/kg of theophylline every 6 hours. Overuse of theophylline will develop adverse effects (Barnes, 2006).

Inflammation of the bronchial system leading to asthma has not stopped researchers studying the prevention of further worsening conditions. Glucocorticosteroids are fundamental to the treatment of asthma, but they should be used as part of an overall plan of treatment that includes reduction in allergen exposure. Corticosteroids may potentiate effects of β-receptor agonists

(Woolcock, 1981; Reynisdottir, 1995; Ikuta, 1996). Primary effect is inhibition of the eosinophilic airway mucosal inflammation in asthmatic airway, via increased lipocortin, decreased activity of phospholipase A, decreased arachidonic acid and metabolites. Corticosteroid use is preferred by inhalation rather than by system intake and aerosol treatment is the most effective way to decrease the systemic adverse effects of corticosteroid. Chronic use of inhaled corticosteroids effectively reduces symptoms and improves pulmonary function in patients with mild asthma as well as reducing the use of oral corticosteroids in patients with more severe forms of the disease. Another approach to the treatment of asthma is the use of cromolyn sodium to prevent mast cell degranulation. Cromolyn sodium prevents antigen-induced release of mediators from mast cells. It prevents release of granules by blocking transmembrane influx of calcium provoked by IgE antibody-antigen interactions. Clinically, Cromolyn sodium is used prophylactically. During pretreatment, it blocks the bronchoconstriction caused by antigen inhalation, by exercise, by aspirin and by a variety of causes of occupational asthma, including toluene diisocyanate, wood dusts, etc. Cromolyn is also effective in reducing the symptomatic severity and the need for bronchodilator medications in patients with perennial asthma. It is effective in asthma only when inhaled directly into the airways (Barnes, 2006).

Muscarinic antagonists known as parasympatholytics, can also be used to inhibit brochoconstriction. Muscarinic antagonists have been used in treating asthma for hundreds of years. They competitively inhibit the effect of acetylcholine at muscarinic receptors. In the airway, efferent endings of the vagus nerves release acetylcholine. At the same time, muscarinic antagonists can effectively block the contraction of airway smooth muscles and the increase in secretion of mucus that occurs in response to vagal activity. High concentrations are required to inhibit the response of airway smooth muscle to nonmuscarinic stimulation. Ipatropium given by aerosol leads to bronchodilation and minimizes systemic effects. Anti-muscarinic agents appear to be of significant value in chronic obstructive pulmonary disease. They are useful as alternative therapies for patients intolerant of β-adrenoceptors agonists. When muscarinic antagonists are used for long-term treatment, they appear to be effective bronchodilators (Gosens, 2006).

Leukotriene involvement in many inflammation diseases has also led to the studies of leukotriene pathway inhibitors (O'Byrne, 1997; Mèannistèo, 1997). A study of the effect of treatment with zileuton has shown that a three-month of 5-lipoxygenase inhibition produced a significant improvement in asthma control (Isreal *et al*, 1996). Leukotrienes originate from the action of 5-lipoxygenase on arachidonic acid and are synthesized by eosinophils, mast cells, macrophages, and basophils. Leukotriene B4 is a potent neutrophil chemoattractant, and LTC4 and LTD4 is known to contribute to bronchoconstriction, increased bronchial reactivity, mucosal edema, and mucus hypersecretion. Inhibition of 5-lipoxygenase might be one of the possibilities in preventing leukotriene synthesis. Zileuton has been known to be the 5-lipoxygenase inhibitor, and zafirlukast is an LTD4-receptor antagonist. Both have the advantage of being effective when taken orally, and both have been shown to be effective when taken regularly in outpatient clinical trials (Holgate *et al*, 1996).

Besides the basic pharmacology of agents exclusively used in the treatment of asthma, other drugs in the treatment of asthma are also under serious consideration. With the knowledge of role of calcium in muscle contraction, contraction of airway smooth muscle, secretion of various mediators, and transmission along airway nerves, all depend on some degree of the calcium movement into cells. Calcium channel blockers significantly inhibit the airway narrowing that is induced by various stimuli. Nifedipine and verapamil inhaled greatly inhibit the bronchoconstriction induced by exercise, methacholine, or antigen, but to a lesser extent than of inhaled albuterol. Nitric oxide donors also relax airway smooth muscle. It can be inhaled as a gas in acute asthma and dilate the pulmonary blood vessels (Barnes, 2006).

Managing asthma can be challenging when the asthmatics fall into a state where they are convinced of the uselessness of medications. Immunotherapy, however, is one of the alternatives in treating asthma. For those who cannot control symptoms by avoiding triggers and using medications, immunotherapy can help them get better. In this treatment, tiny amounts of the trigger substance are injected in progressively larger doses to increase the asthmatic tolerance. In some cases, immunotherapy can help prevent development of airway inflammation and the resulting hyperreactivity. Immunotherapy seems to work best for allergies to dust mites, pollen and cat dander. Life-threatening reactions to immunotherapy are rare but can occur. An adverse reaction typically occurs within 20 minutes (A position paper of the Thoracic Society of Australia and the Asutralasian Society of Clinical Immunology and Allergy, 1997).

Inhibitors of immunomodulators

Many inhibitors have been developed and tested to control asthmatic attacks in patients. These inhibitors are mainly inhibitory to the immunomodulatory substances released by the mast cells on antigen-induced early and late responses. However, much attention is focused on the development of highly potent and selective tryptase inhibitors for the treatment of allergic and inflammatory diseases, including asthma (Burgess *et al*, 1999; Bisacchi *et al*, 2001; Combrink *et al*, 1998; Jackson *et al*, 1998). B-Tryptase, a serine protease, enzymatically active only as a heparin-stabilized tetramer, is the predominant protein of human lung mast cells and is thought to be involved in the pathogenesis of asthma and other allergic and inflammatory disorders (Caughey *et al*, 1997). Stimulation of mast cells with antigens or other stimuli results in the release of active tryptase into the extracellular environment (Wright *et al*, 1999). The enzyme is resistant to all known endogenous proteinase inhibitors. In the airways of asthmatic patients tryptase levels are elevated (Wenzel *et al*, 1988). *In vivo*, the known tryptase inhibitor APC-366 reduces the acute airway response in a pig model (Sylvin *et al*, 2001) and also in a sheep model of allergen-induced asthma, but was only poorly effective in asthma patients. Several concepts in the design of potent tryptase inhibitors are currently under investigation Dener *et al*, 2001; Rice *et al*, 1998). Findings of Hallgren *et al* show heparin antagonists as the potent inhibitors for mast cell tryptase. (Hallgren *et al*, 2001).

The unique tetrameric architecture (Pereira *et al*, 1998; Sommerhoff *et al*, 1999) explains many of tryptases distinct biochemical properties and provides a basis for the rational design of bifunctional tryptase inhibitors being highly selective against other serine proteases (Figure 1). In a study two inhibitors of tryptase, APC 366 [N-(1-hydroxy-2-naphthoyl)-L-arginyl-L- prolinamide hydrochloride] and BABIM [bis(5-amidino-2- benzimidazolyl)methane], which though showed inhibitory effects immediately, showed complete inhibition of tryptase after 24 hours. (Clark *et al*, 1995).

A group of scientists created efficient syntheses of potent and selective bifunctional tryptase inhibitors containing pyran moieties and aryl diynes as scaffolds. The compounds tested showed *in vitro* potencies between 1 μM (26) and 1.3 nM (15) with selectivities against other serine proteases in the range of 1,000 to 100,000. Continuing biological screening studies *in vivo* are currently under investigation (Martin, 2001).

The ability of tryptase and inhibitors of tryptase modulate histamine release from human lung mast cells and the potential contribution of proteinase-activated receptor 2 (PAR2) were investigated. The tryptase inhibitor APC366 [*N*-(1-hydroxy-2-naphthoyl)-L-arginyl-L-prolinamide hydrochloride] was highly effective at inhibiting histamine release stimulated by anti-IgE antibody or calcium ionophore from enzymatically dispersed human lung cells. A concentration of APC366 as low as 10 μM was able to inhibit anti-IgE-dependent histamine release by some 50%. Addition of leupeptin or the tryptic substrate *N*-benzoyl-D,L-arginine-*p*-nitroanilide also inhibited IgE-dependent histamine release. Purified tryptase in the presence of heparin stimulated a small but significant release of histamine from lung cells, suggesting that tryptase may provide an amplification signal from activated cells that may be susceptible to proteinase inhibitors. Trypsin was also able to induce histamine release apparently by a catalytic mechanism. Moreover, pretreatment of cells with metabolic inhibitors or with pertussis toxin reduced responses, indicating a noncytoxic pertussis toxin-sensitive G proteinmediated signaling process. Addition to cells of the PAR2 agonists SLIGKV-NH_2 or tc-LIGRLO-NH_2 or appropriate control peptides were without effect on histamine release, and PAR2 was not detected by immunohistochemistry in tissue mast cells. The potent actions of tryptase inhibitors as mast cell-stabilizing agents could be of value in the treatment of allergic inflammation of the respiratory tract, possibly by targeting the non-PAR2-mediated actions of tryptase.

In the recent past tryptase has been purified from various species. An efficient expression/purification procedure was developed which allowed the production of pure, biologically active recombinant leech- derived tryptase inhibitor (rLDTI), originally found in the leech *Hirudo medicinalis*. The purified protein was tested for its ability to inhibit tryptase and trypsin *in vitro* and to interfere with the tryptase-induced proliferation of human fibroblasts and keratinocytes (Shaoheng *et al*, 2004). Braganza & Simmons were the first ones to purify it to homogeneity from rat skin (Braganza & Simmons, 1991).

IgE dependent tryptase release from colon mast cells was inhibited by up to approximately 37%, 40% and 36.6% by chymase inhibitors Z-Ile-Glu-Pro-Phe-CO_2Me (ZIGPFM), N-tosyl-L-phenylalanyl-chloromethyl ketone (TPCK), and '-1-antitrypsin, respectively. Similarly, the inhibitors of tryptase leupeptin, N-tosyl-L-lysine chloromethyl ketone (TLCK) and lactoferrin were also able to inhibit anti-IgE induced tryptase release by a maximum of 39.4%, 47.6% and 36.6%, respectively (Elrod *et al*, 1997).

Shao-Heng and his team showed that the heparin antagonists Polybrene and protamine are potent inhibitors of both human lung tryptase and of recombinant mouse tryptase. Protamine inhibited tryptase in a competitive manner whereas Polybrene showed noncompetitive inhibition kinetics. Treatment of tetrameric, active tryptase with Polybrene caused dissociation into monomers, accompanied by complete loss of enzymatic activity. The present report thus suggests that heparin antagonists potentially may be used in treatment of mast cell-mediated diseases such as asthma.

Another tryptase inhibitor was designed named as CRA-2059: HT² interaction were defined in this study. Bivalent inhibition was demonstrated by this inhibitor HT², 24% or 53% inhibited by preincubation with an irreversible inhibitor. (Sekwood *et al*, 2005).

Certain inhibitors to other mediators have also been worked on (Devillier, 1997).

While there are numerous scientific investigations carried out to establish a synthetic chemical inhibitor for tryptase, there are no reports on natural Tryptase inhibitors, which is yet to be explored using the alternative systems like, Ayurveda, Siddha and Unani systems of medications.

AYURVEDA AND ASTHMA

The alternative systems like Ayurveda, Siddha and Unani are becoming popular amongst the patients. This is because of the versatile approach of Ayurveda in addressing the root cause of the problem and its belief in preventing the disease rather than treating it.

In Ayurveda, Asthma is known as 'Swas Roga'. The pathogenesis, known as Samprapti is that the vitiated 'Pranvayu' combines with deranged 'Kapha dosha' in the lungs causing obstruction in the 'Pranavaha srotasa' (Respiratory passage). This results in gasping and laboured breathing.

However, Ayurvedic texts define five types of Swasa Roga (asthma):

1. Maha-shwas
2. Urdhva-shwas
3. Chinna-shwas
4. Tamak-shwas
5. Kshudra-shwas

The first three types are said to be incurable types while the last two are curable.75% of the patients fall in the category of last two types.

Ayurvedic plants having anti-asthmatic properties

Ayurveda is the most ancient scripture that offers herbal remedies for various ailments. The practitioners of Ayurveda, Ayurvaidyas have gathered and catalogued information in form of various books and compendia like Wealth of India. A book by T. Pullaiah highlights important Indian medicinal plants, which are believed to possess anti-asthmatic activity (Anonymous, 1946; Pullaiah, 2002).

Using this data available in alternative medicinal systems, over past few years, pharmacological data have been generated on various medicinal plants. Many groups of scientists are actively working on scrutinizing the claims made in ayurveda or other Complementary and Alternative medical systems using modern scientific methodologies. As a result of these scientific interventions many plant species have been identified and confirmed to possess anti-asthmatic activity *in vivo* as well as *in vitro*. Table-1 is the result of extensive literature review of such work, which enlists plant reported to possess anti-asthmatic activity.

Phytochemicals responsible for anti-asthmatic activity

Though significant work has been done in scrutinizing anti-asthmatic plants, it is to be noted that very few reports on the bioactive compounds are seen. Most of the work that is reported

TABLE 1

Reported Antiasthmatic Studies in Different Plant Species

No.	Plant Name	Part Used	Research Done	References
1.	*Actinidia polygama*	Fruits	Extract showed a deep inhibitory effect on airway inflammation and hyperresponsiveness in murine model modulating the relationship between Th1/ Th2 cytokine imbalance.	Lee *et al*, 2006
2.	*Saururus chinensi*	Whole plant	The ethanol extract of S. chinensis inhibited cyclooxygenase-2 dependent phases of prostaglandin D(2) and Leukotriene C(4) in bone marrow-derived mast cells in a concentration-dependent manner.	Lee *et al*, 2006
3.	*Argemone platyceras*	Leaves and Fruits	Methanol extracts of leaves and flowers, subsequent organic and aqueous extraction phases, and silica gel chromatography fractions were assayed on the carbachol-induced response, and/or on ovalbumin antigenic challenge, and on leukotriene D(4)-induced response of tracheae from sensitized and non-sensitized guinea-pigs which showed curative effects.. Isoquercitrin and rutin were the main compounds found to be responsible for curing asthma.	Fernandez *et al*, 2005
4.	*Red Wine*	Red skin	Resveratrol found in red-skinned fruit, may act as an anti-inflammatory agent useful in the treatment of COPD and corticosteroid-resistant asthma.	Donnelly *et al*. 2004
5.	*Asystasia gangetica*	Leaves	The hexane, ethyl acetate and methanol extracts inhibited the contraction evoked, relaxed histamine-	Akah *et al*, 2003

Continued ...

... Continued

No.	Plant Name	Part Used	Research Done	References
			precontracted tracheal strips. the phytochemical screening showed the presence of carbohydrates, proteins, alkaloids, tannins, steroidal aglycones, saponins, flavonoids, reducing sugars, and triterpenoids.	
6.	*Passiflora incarnata*	Leaves	The methanol extract of the leaves was evaluated for its antiasthmatic effects against acetylcholine chlorideinduced bronchospasm in guinea-pigs at doses of 50, 100 and 200 mg/kg.	Dhawan *et al*, 2003
7.	*Crinum glaucum*	Fresh Bulbs	Aqueous extract administered in guinea pigs showed reduction in histamine-induced contractions as well antigen induced mediator release from lung tissues.	Okpo & Adeyemi, 2002
8.	*Typhonium flagelliforme Blune*	Whole plant	All water, alcohol and ester extracts showed effects of relieving a cough, eliminating expectoration, anti-asthmatic, analgesia, anti-inflammation and sedation.	Zhong *et al*, 2001
9.	*Radix Codonopsis* *Folium eriobotryae* *Radix cynanchi* *Radix glycyrrhizae* *Armenicacae amarae* *Mori radicis* *Cudrania cochinensis* *Fructus amomi* *Datura metel L* *Ficus simplicissima*	Whole plant	Analysis of CPM (Chinese Pulmonary medicine) for the presence of codein (opioid alkaloid), which acts as a cough depressant.	*S.Y. Liu et al*, 2000

Continued ...

... *Continued*

No.	Plant Name	Part Used	Research Done	References
10.	*Sida cordifolia L*	Roots	The aqueous extract showed a significant inhibition of arrageenin-induced rat paw edema on oral administration.	Franzotti *et al*, 2000
11.	*Solanum xanthocarpum*	Fruits and whole plants	Relief from the symptoms of bronchial asthma produced by bronchodilator effect, reduction in the bronchial mucosal edema, and reduction in the	Govindan *et al*, 1999
	Solanum trilobatum	Stems & buds	secretions within the airway lumen in the humans.	
12.	*Cissampelos sympodialis Eichl.*	Roots	An aqueous fraction of the ethanol extract of the leaves inhibited N-formyl-Met-Leu-Phe (fMLP)-induced release of lysozyme and myeloperoxidase from human neutrophils.	Thomas *et al*, 1999
13.	*Curcuma longa*	Tubers	The volatile oil was significantly active in removing sputum, relieving cough and preventing asthma.	Li *et al*, 1998
14.	*Cultispecies sichuan*	Bulbs	The ethanol extracts from the cultured bulb were proved similar to the wild one in treating coughing in mice, expectoration in rats, asthma in guinea pigs, bronchodilation of isolated lungs in mice, and cyclic nucleotide(cAMP, cGMP) in the plasma and lungs of mice.	Mo *et al*, 1998
15.	*Boswellia serrata*	Gum resin	In a double-blind, placebo-controlled study forty patients treated with a preparation of gum resin for a period of 6 weeks showed improvement of disease evident by disappearance of physical and clinical symptoms.	Gupta *et al*, 1998

Continued ...

... *Continued*

No.	Plant Name	Part Used	Research Done	References
16.	*Ginkgo biloba*	Leaves & seeds	In contrast to placebo group, GLC significantly reduced airway hyperreactivity and improved clinical symptoms, pulmonary functions of the asthmatic patients.	Li *et al*, 1997
17.	*Cynanchum komarovii*	Whole plant	The water and ethanol extracts could increase secretion of repiratory tract and promote expectoration, alleviate asthma induced by histamine and acetylcholing chloride in guinea pigs.	Lu *et al*, 1997
18.	*Ephedra sinica* *Prunus armeniaca Linne* *Magnolia obovata Thunberg* *Citrus unshiu Markovich* *Glycyrrhiza uvalensis Fischer* *Bupleurum falcatum L.* *Perilla frutescens Britton var. Acuta Kudo*	Stalk Seeds Bark Fruit peel Root Root Leaf	Formulation of these herbs can act in the treatment of bronchial asthma byInhibiting the biosynthesis of LTC 4 and LTB 4.	Hamasaki *et al*, 1997
19.	*Umbelliferae Bupleurum falcatum L.*	Root	Inhibits the A23187-stimulated production of cLTs and LTB4 in intact RBL-1 cells.	Kobayashi *et al*, 1995
	Araceae Pinellia ternata Breitenbach Root	Root		
	Polyporaceae Poria cocos Wolf	Sclerotium		
	Labiatae Sculellaria baicalensis Georgi	Root		

Continued ...

... Continued

No.	Plant Name	Part Used	Research Done	References
	fructus Rhamnaceae Zizyphus jujuba Miller var. inermis	Fruit		
	Araliaceae Panax ginseng C.A. Meyer	Root		
	radix Leguminosae Glycyrrhiza uvalensis Fischer	Root		
	Zingiberaceae Zingiber officinale Roscoe	Root		
20.	*Desmodium adscendens*	Aerial parts	Different concentrations of a hot water extract showed inhibition of histamine-induced ileal contraction and caused a dose-dependent reduction in the amount of spasmogens released anaphylactically and in anaphylactic-induced contraction of ileal muscle.	Addy & Dzandu, 1986
21.	*Allium cepa*	Bulbs	Inhibitory effects of crude ethanolic onion extracts on allergic skin reactions in allergen-induced bronchial asthma in man and guinea-pigs by Isothiocyanate found to be the compound responsible.	Dorsch *et al*, 1984
22.	*Tylophora asthmatica*	Whole plant	Patients given extracts of T. asthmatica for at least two years showed marked improvement.	Thiruvengadam *et al*, 1978
23.	*Cannabis sativa*	Leaves, stems, seeds	Delta1-Tetrahydrocannabinol proved to be a drug against glaucoma and asthma.	Mechoulam & Carlini, 1978
24.	*Scutellaria baicalensis Georgi*	Root	S. baicalensis showed anti-asthmatic activity.	Koda *et al*, 1972

in Table 1 is on crude extracts of various plant parts. Very few scientists have been successful in going up to purification of a single responsible compounds for anti-asthmatic activity. However, there are reported anti-asthmatic compounds and the species that contain them. Table-2 highlights such compounds with the plant names (Duke, 1992).

TABLE 2

Putative Anti-asthmatic Compounds with the Plant Species and Plant Part

No.	Compound	Plant Name	Plant Part
1.	4-TERPINEOL	*Agathosma betulina*	Leaf
		Barosma betulina	Leaf
		Camellia sinensis L.	Leaf
		Carica papaya L.	Fruit
		Thymus vulgaris L	Thyme
		Satureja thymbra L.	Shoot
		Psoralea corylifolia L.	Seed
		Origanum vulgare subsp. Hirtum	Shoot
		Origanum onites L.	Shoot
		Coridothymus capitatus L. Reichb.F.	Shoot
		Citrus aurantium L.	Plant
2.	ALLYL-ISOTHIOCYANATE	*Alliaria petiolata* BIEB. Cavara & Grande	Plant
		Brassica oleracea **var**. *gemmifera*	Seed
		Brassica oleracea **var**. *capitata l.* **var**. *capitata* L.	Leaf
		Brassica oleracea **var**. *botrytis l.* **var**. *botrytis* L	Leaf
		Brassica nigra L. W. D. J. Koch	Seed
		Brassica juncea L. Czernj. & Cosson	Seed
		Armoracia rusticana Gaertn. *et al.*	Root
3.	ALPHA-BOSWELLIC-ACID, BETA- BOSWELLIC ACID	*Boswellia sacra*	Latex exudate
4.	ANDROSIN	*Apocynum androsaemifolium* L.	Root
5.	ATROPINE	*Anisodus tanguticus* Maxim. Prasher	Plant
		Atropa bella-donna L.	Root
		Solanum dulcamara L.	Seed
		Scopolia carniolica Jacq.	Rhizome
		Mandragora officinarum L.	Root
		Latua pubiflora (GRIS.) Phil.	Stem

Continued ...

... *Continued*

No.	Compound	Plant Name	Plant Part
		Hyoscyamus niger L.	seed
		Datura stramonium L.	plant
		Datura metel L.	Seed
		Datura innoxia Mill.	Plant
		Datura candida (Pers) Saff	Root
		Brugmansia amesianum Schultes	Plant
6.	AVENANTHRAMIDES	*Avena sativa* L.	Seed
7.	BAICALEIN & BAICALIN	*Scutellaria sp*	Leaf
		Scutellaria galericulata L.	Plant
		Scutellaria baicalensis Georgi	Root
		Plantago major L.	Leaf
8.	BENZYL-BENZOATE	*Cinnamomum aromaticum* Nees	Plant
		Vaccinium macrocarpon Aiton	Fruit
		Telosma cordata	Flower
		Sideritis scardica Griseb	Shoot
		Polianthes tuberosa L.	Flower
		Peumus boldus Molina	Leaf
		Myroxylon balsamum L. Harms	Gum
		Jasminum officinale L.	Flower
		Hyacinthus orientalis L.	Flower
		Cinnamomum verum J.	Bark
		Cananga odorata (Lam.) Hook. F. & Thomson	Flower
9.	BENZYL-ISOTHIOCYANATE	*Tropaeolum majus* L.	Seed & Shoot
		Alliaria petiolata (Bieb.) Cavara & Grande	Essential oil
		Allium cepa L.	Bulb
		Brassica oleracea **var**. *capitata l.* **var**. *capitata* L.	Leaf
		Carica papaya L.	Fruit
		Lepidium sativum L.	Plant
10.	CORILAGIN	*Geranium thunbergii* Sieb. & Zucc	Leaf
		Punica granatum L.	Leaf
		Ricinus communis L.	Leaf

Continued ...

... Continued

No.	Compound	Plant Name	Plant Part
		Terminalia catappa L.	Fruit
		Terminalia chebula Retz.	Fruit
11.	CURCUMIN	*Zingiber officinale*	Plant
		Curcuma zedoaria (Christm) Roscoe	Rhizome
		Curcuma longa L.	Rhizome
		Curcuma xanthorrhiza Roxb.	Rhizome
12.	EPHEDRINE	*Taxus baccata* L.	Plant
		Sida rhombifolia L.	Root
		Ephedra sinica Stapf	Plant
		Ephedra nevadensis S. Wats.	Plant
		Ephedra gerardiana Wall.	Plant
		Catha edulis Vahl.	Leaf
		Aconitum napellus L.	Root
13.	ESCIN	*Aesculus hippocastanum* **L.**	Seed
		Panax quinquefolius L.	Plant
14.	FORSKOLIN	*Coleus barbatus* Benth	Tuber
		Coleus forskohlii	Tuber
15.	GERANIIN	*Spondias pinnata* L.	Leaf
		Geranium thunbergii Sieb. & Zucc	Leaf
		Erythroxylum coca var. *coca*	Leaf
16.	GINKGOLIDE-A GINGKOLIDE-B GINGKOLIDE- C	*Ginkgo biloba* L.	Root
17.	GLYCYRRHETIC-ACID, GLYCYRRHETINIC-ACID, GLYCYRRHIZIN	*Glycyrrhiza glabra* L.	Plant & Root
		Glycyrrhiza uralensis Fisch. Ex DC	Root
		Abrus precatorius L.	Root
		Glycyrrhiza uralensis Fisch. Ex DC	Root
		Polypodium vulgare L.	Rhizome
18.	HORDENINE	*Zea mays* L.	Fruit
		Tamarindus indica L.	Bark
		Selenicereus grandiflorus	Plant
		Pancratium maritimum L.	Shoot
		Lophophora williamsii	Plant
		Hordeum vulgare L.	Seedling

Continued ...

... *Continued*

No.	Compound	Plant Name	Plant Part
		Citrus sinensis	Fruit
19.	KHELLIN	*Ammi visnaga* (L.) Lam.	Seed
		Ammi majus L.	Plant
20.	L-ALPHA-TERPINEOL	*Jasminum officinale* L.	Flower
		Ephedra sinica Stapf.	Plant
		Artemisia cina Berg.	Bud
21.	LIGUSTILIDE	*Cnidium officinale* Makino.	Rhizome
		Apium graveolens L	Essential oil
		Angelica sinensis (Oliv.) Diels	Root
		Angelica archangelica L.	Plant
22.	LOBELINE	*Lobelia tupa* L.	Plant
		Lobelia inflata L.	Plant
23.	METHYL-GALLATE	*Rosa multiflora* Thunb. ex Murray	Fruit
		Prunus persica L.	Flower
		Lagerstroemia indica L.	Flower
		Aleurites fordii Hemsl.	Petiole
		Acacia farnesiana (L.) Willd.	Fruit
24.	NIGELLONE	*Nigella sativa* L.	Plant
25.	OXYMATRINE	*Sophora subprostrata* Chun & Chen	Root
		Sophora pachycarpa Schrenk.	Plant
		Sophora angustifolia Ait.	Root
26.	PAPAVERINE	*Rauvolfia serpentina* (L.) Benth. ex Kurz	Root
		Papaver somniferum L.	Fruit
		Papaver bracteatum L.	Plant
27.	SCOPOLAMINE	*Scopolia carniolica* Jacq.	Root
		Mandragora officinarum L.	Root
		Latua pubiflora (Gris.) Phil.	Plant
		Hyoscyamus niger L.	Seed
		Duboisia myoporoides R. Br.	Leaf
		Datura stramonium L.	Seed
		Datura metel L.	Whole plant
		Datura innoxia Mill.	Whole plant
		Datura candida (Pers.) Saff.	Plant
		Brugmansia amesianum (Schultes) D'Arcy	Plant

Continued ...

... *Continued*

No.	Compound	Plant Name	Plant Part
		Atropa bella-donna L.	Root
		Anisodus tanguticus (Maxim.) Prasher	Plant
28.	STROPHANTHIDIN	*Strophanthus kombe*	Seed
		Strophanthus hispidus A. DC.	Seed
		Corchorus olitorius L.	Plant
		Convallaria majalis L.	Plant
29.	TETRAMETHYL-PYRAZINE	*Glycyrrhiza glabra* L.	Root
		Glycine max (L.) Merr.	Seed
		Capsicum annuum L.	Fruit
		Camellia sinensis L.	Leaf
30.	THEOBROMINE	*Theobroma cocao* L.	Seed
		Theobroma bicolor HBK.	Plant
		Theobroma angustifolium	Seed
		Paullinia cupana Kunth ex HBK	Seed
		Ilex paraguariensis St. Hil.	Leaf
		Cola acuminata (P. Beauv.) Schott & Endl.	Seed
		Coffea arabica L.	Seed
		Camellia sinensis (L.) Kuntze	Leaf
31.	THEOPHYLLINE	*Theobroma cocao* L.	Seed & testa
		Theobroma bicolor HBK.	Seed & testa
		Theobroma angustifolium	Seed & testa
		Paullinia cupana Kunth ex H.B.K.	Seed
		Ilex paraguariensis St. Hil.	Leaf
		Coffea arabica L.	Seed
		Camellia sinensis (L.) Kuntze	Leaf & Seed
32.	THYMOQUINONE	*Satureja montana* L.	Plant
		Nigella sativa L.	Seed
		Monarda fistulosa L.	Essential oil
33.	VASICINONE	*Peganum harmala* L.	Seed
		Justicia adhatoda L.	Plant
34.	VISNADIN	*Ammi visnaga* (L.) Lam.	Seed
35.	Z-LIGUSTILIDE	*Apium graveolens* L.	Plant
		Anethum graveolens L.	Root

There are a range of other phytochemicals like β-Carotene, Ascorbic acid, Phylline, caffeine, Gallic acid, HCN, Menthol, Piperitone, Quercetin, Scopoletin, solanine, Terpinen-4-ol, Terpineol and Trans-Carveol, which are found commonly in medicinal plants and are proved to have anti-asthmatic effects in certain concentrations.

WORK ON NATURAL INHIBITORS TO TRYPTASE

In preliminary work done in our laboratory, a range of plants known to have antiasthmatic effects are being tested against tryptase, purified from rat (Braganza & Simmons, 1991). The work has been summarized in Table 3. The data need to be corroborated further.

TABLE 3

Preliminary Work on Establishing Natural Inhibitors to Tryptase

No.	Project Title	Findings	Investigators
1.	Ethnobotanical plant based protease inhibitor- A possible cure for asthma	PE and Chloroform extract of *Euphorbia hirta, Cassia fistula, Calotropis procera, Curcuma domestica* showed little inhibitory activity on tryptase like enzymes	Rashi Priya & Vincent Braganza
2.	Tryptase cures asthma - An analysis of the correlation between tryptase, trypsin and asthma	Plant like *Adhatoda vasica, Tamarindus indica, Boerhavia diffusa, toori rough, toori smooth, satavari* were tested for inhibitory effect on tryptase like enzyme and showed slight inhibition	Purvi Gaglani & Vincent Braganza
3.	Isolation and inhibition studies on tryptase	Tryptase was recovered from the rat skin at a very low recovery percentage and inhibition studies of various polar and apolar solvent extracts of *Cassia fistula* and *Calotropis procera* which was 70% and 49% with water extracts respectively	Rohini Kohli & Vincent Braganza

Continued ...

... *Continued*

No.	Project Title	Findings	Investigators
4.	Investigations into tryptase for anti-allergic response	Chloroform extracts of *Calendula* flowers and PE extract of Borasalli showed inhibitory effects upto 79% and 65%	Vineeta Tripathi & Vincent Braganza
5.	Investigating the activation profile of tryptase	Incremental effects on the activity of enzyme was observed with plants *Aloe vera* and *Vitex negundo*	Anirvan Dutt Chaudhari & Vincent Braganza
6.	Study of Tryptase II: A partial physical characterization	Tryptase was isolated from rat skin and inhibitory effect of *Vitex negundo* was studied on enzyme activity. However, in these preliminary studies no inhibitory activity was observed	Shital Tripathi, Parimal Sheth & Vincent Braganza
7.	Study of putative anti-inflammatory effect of vitex extract on rat tryptase enzyme	PE extract of *Vitex* showed decrease in enzyme activity which could be because of an inhibitor present in the extract	Maulika Shroff & Vincent Braganza

FUTURE PROSPECTS

As reviewed here in this chapter, asthma is a complex disease and has multifactorial origin. However, the immunohistopathology of the disease remains the same in all the cases.

Various inhibitors have been established mainly against the tryptase enzyme, which is one of the key immunomodulators released by the mast cells in the response to the allergen attack; however natural inhibitors still remain unexplored. While these synthetic inhibitors might not be readily acceptable by our system and cause side effect, herbal alternatives can be envisaged as a safer and cheaper option. For, this the plants that have been reported to possess anti-asthmatic activities in ethnic medicinal systems or in established alternative systems like Ayurveda, Siddha and Unani need to be scrutinized till the level of obtaining a bioactive compound or formulation having the optimum activity.

There needs to be taken an integrative approach to mitigate the disease, which is creeping into the urbanized system slowly, becoming a very evident ailment.

Associated efforts by phytotherapists, ayurvaidyas, phytochemists and pharmacologists in a holistic manner can give rise to a complete cure for asthma.

REFERENCES

121st Report on Action taken by The Department of Scientific & Industrial Research on the Recommendations contained in the 113th Report of The Department related Parliamentary standing committee on Science and Technology, Environment & Forests on the demands for Grants (2003-04) of the Department of Scientific and Industrial Research by Committee on Science and Technology, Environment & Forests. 2004.

Addy, M. E. and Dzabdu, W. K. Dose-response effects of *Desmodium adscendens* aqueous extract on histamine response, content and anaphylactic reactions in the guinea pig. *J. Ethnopharmacol.* 18(1): 13-20, 1986.

Akah, P. A., Ezike, A. C., Nwafor, S. V., Okoli, C. O. and Enwerem, N. M. Evaluation of the anti-asthmatic property of *Asystasia gangetica* leaf extracts. *J. Ethnopharmacol.* 89(1): 25-36, 2003.

Amin, K., Ludviksdottir, D., Janson, C., Nettelbladt, O., Bjornsson, E., Roomans, G. M., Boman, G., Seveus, L. and Venge, P. Inflammation and structural changes in the airways of patients with atopic and nonatopic asthma. *Am J Respir Crit Care Med* 162: 2295, 2000.

Anonymous. Wealth of India. CSIR Publications. New Delhi, 1946.

Ansel, J. C., Brown, J. R., Payan, D. G. and Brown, M. A. Substance P selectively activates TNF-alpha gene expression in murine mast cells. *J Immunol* 150: 4478, 1993.

Arizono, N., Matsuda, S., Hattori, T., Kojima, Y., Maeda, T. and Galli, S. J. Anatomical variation in mast cell nerve associations in the rat small intestine, heart, lung, and skin. Similarities of distances between neural processes and mast cells, eosinophils, or plasma cells in the jejunal lamina propria. *Lab Invest.* 62: 626, 1990.

Askenase, P. W., Rosenstein, R. W. and Ptak, W. T cells produce an antigen-binding factor with in vivo activity analogous to IgE antibody. *J Exp Med.* 157: 862, 1983.

Austen, K. F. and Brocklehurst, W. E. Anaphylaxis in chopped guinea pig lung. I. Effect of peptidase substrates and inhibitors. *J Exp Med* 113: 521-239, 1961.

Barnes, P. J. and Brown, M. J. Venous plasma histamine in exercise- and hyperventilation-induced asthma in man. *Clin Sci.* 61: 159-162, 1981.

Barnes, P. J. Drugs for asthma. *Br J Pharm.* 147: s297-s303, 2006.

Befus, A., Dyck, D. N., Goodacre, R. and Bienenstock, K. Mast cells from the human intestinal lamina propria. Isolation, histochemical subtypes, and functional characterization. *J Immunol.* 138: 2604, 1987.

Bisacchi, G. S., Roberts, D. G. M., Stanley, P. and Seiler, S. M. Potent selective nonpeptidic inhibitors of human lung tryptase. *J. Med. Chem.* 15: 8348-8352, 1998.

Bisacchi, G. S., Bolton, S. A., Gaitonde, D., Hartl, K. S., Huang, M. H., Jacobs, G., Ogletree, M. L., Pi, Z., Schumacher, W. A., Slusarchyk, W. A., Sutton, J., Treuner, U. Zhang, Z., Zhao, G., Zahler, R., Seiler, S. M ACS MEDI 22 (Abs), San Diego, 2001.

Botchkarev, V. A., Eichmuller, S., Peters, E. M., Pietsch, P., Johansson, O., Maurer, M. and Paus, R. A simple immunofluorescence technique for simultaneous visualization of mast cells and nerve fibers reveals selectivity and hair cycle. dependent changes in mast cell. Nerve fiber contacts in murine skin. *Arch Dermatol Res.* 289-292, 1997.

Braganza, V. J. and Simmons, W. H. Tryptase from rat skin: purification and properties. *Biochemistry*. 30: 4997-5007, 1991.

Brockow, K., Ring, J. and Abeck, D. The therapeutic concept of patient management in atopic eczema. *Allergy*. 51(4): 206-215, 1996.

Burgess, L. E., Newhouse, B. J., Ibrahim, P., Rizzi, J., Kashem, M. A., Hartman, A., Brandhuber, B. J., Wright, C. D., Thomson, D. S.,Vigers, G. P. A. and Koch, K. *Proc. Natl. Acad. Sci.* 96: 8348-8352, 1996.

Busse, W. W. and Swenson, C. A. The relationship between plasma histamine concentrations and bronchial obstruction to antigen challenge in allergic rhinitis. *J Allergy Clin Immunol.* 84: 658–666, 1989.

Caughey, G. H. Of mites and men: trypsin-like proteases in the lungs. *Am. J. Respir. Cell. Mol. Biol.* 16: 621-628, 1997.

Cerwenka, A. and Swain, S. L. TGF-beta1: immunosuppressant and viability factor for T lymphocytes. *Microbes Infect.* 1: 1291, 1999.

Church, M. K. and Levi-Schaffer, F. The human mast cell. *J Allergy Clin Immunol.* 99: 155, 1997.

Clark, J. M., Abraham, W. M., Fishman, C. E., Forteza, R., Ahmed, A., Cortes, A., Warne, R. L., Moore, W. R. and Tanaka, R. D. Tryptase inhibitors block allergen-induced airway and inflammatory responses in allergic sheep. *Am. J. Respir. Crit. Care Med.* 152(6): 2076-2083, 1995.

Colasanti, B. K. and Trotter, R. R. Effects of selective beta 1- and beta-2 adenoreceptor agonists and antagonists on intraocular pressure in the rat. *Invest Opth Vis Sci.* 20: 69-76, 1981.

Combrink, K. D., Gülgeze, H. B., Meanwell, N. A., Pearce, B. C., Zulan, P., Cooke, H. J. P. Fox, L., Alferes, C. C. Fox, and S. A. Wolfe, Jr. Presence of NK1 receptors on a mucosal-like mast cell line, RBL-2H3 cells. *Can J Physiol Pharmacol* 76: 188, 1998.

Dener, J. M., Rice, K. D., Newcomb, W. S., Wang, V. R., Young, W. B., Gangloff, A. R., Kuo, E. Y. L., Cregar, L., Putnam, D. and Wong, M. *Biorg. Med. Chem. Lett.* 11: 1629-1633, 2001.

Devillier, P. Leukotriene antagonists: a new approach in the treatment of asthma. *Revue des Maladies Respiratoires.*14(3): 159-70, 1997.

Dhawan, K., Kumar, S., Sharma, A. Antiasthmatic activity of the methanol extract of leaves of *Passiflora incarnata*. *Phytother. Res.* 17(7): 821-822, 2003.

Dietze, S. C., Sommerhoff, C. P. and Fritz, H. Inhibition of histamine release from human mast cells *ex vivo* by natural and synthetic chymase inhibitors. *Biol Chem Hoppe Seyler.* 371: 75-79, 1990.

Djukanoviâc, R. The effect of treatment with oral corticosteroids on asthma symptoms and airway inflammation. *Am. J. Respir. Crit. Care Med.* 155(3): 826-32, 1997.

Duke, J. A. Handbook of phytochemical constituents of GRAS herbs and other economic plants. Boca Raton, FL. CRC Press, 1992.

Elrod, K. C., Moore, W. R., Abraham, W. M. and Tanaka, R. D. Lactoferrin, a Potent Tryptase Inhibitor, Abolishes Late-Phase Airway Responses in Allergic Sheep. *Am. J. Respir. Crit. Care Med.* 156(2): 375-381, 1997.

Emadi-Khiav, B., Mousli, M., Bronner, C. and Landry, Y. Human and rat cutaneous mast cells: involvement of a G protein in the response to peptidergic stimuli. *Eur J Pharmacol.* 272: 97, 1995.

Fanta, C. H., Rossing, T. H. and McFadden, E. R. Jr. Treatment of acute asthma. Is combination therapy with sympathomimetics and methylxanthines indicated? *Am J Med.* 80(1): 5-10, 1986.

Fernandez, J., Reyes, R., Ponce, H., Oropeza, M., Vancalsteren, M. R., Jankowski, C., Campos, M. G. Isoquercitrin from *Argemone platyceras* inhibits carbachol and leukotriene D4-induced contraction in guinea-pig airways. *Eur. J. Pharmacol.* 522(1-3):108- 115, 2005.

Franzotti, E. M., Santos, C. V., Rodrigues, H. M., Mourao, R. H., Andrade, M. R., Antoniolli, A. R. Anti-inflammatory, analgesic activity and acute toxicity of *Sida cordifolia* L. *J. Ethnopharmacol.* 72(1-2): 273-277, 2000.

Friedman-Jimenez, G. W. S., Beckett, J., Szeinuk, and Petsonk, E. L. Clinical evaluation, management, and prevention of work-related asthma. *Am J Ind Med.* 37: 121, 2000.

Friedmann, P. S. Assessment of urticaria and angio-oedema. *Clin Exp Allergy.* 29: 109-112, 1999.

Galli, S. J. New insights into the riddle of the mast cells: microenvironmental regulation of mast cell development and phenotypic heterogeneity. *Lab Invest.* 62: 5, 1990.

Galli, S. J., Gordon, J. R., Wershil, B. K. Cytokine production by mast cells and basophils. *Curr Opin Immunol.* 3: 865-873, 1991.

Galli, S. J. New concepts about the mast cell. *N Engl J Med.* 328: 257, 1993.

Garssen, J., Nijkamp, F. P., Wagenaar, S. S., Zwart, A., Askenase, P. W. and Van Loveren, H. Regulation of delayed-type hypersensitivity-like responses in the mouse lung, determined with histological procedures: serotonin, T-cell suppressor-inducer factor and high antigen dose tolerance regulate the magnitude of T-cell dependent inflammatory reactions. *Immunology* 68: 51, 1989.

Garssen, J., Nijkamp, F. P., Van Vugt, E., Van der Vliet, H. and Van Loveren, H. T cell-derived antigen binding molecules play a role in the induction of airwayhyperresponsiveness. *Am J Respir Crit Care Med.* 150: 1528, 1994.

Glenner, G. G. and Cohen, L. A. Histochemical demonstration of a species-specific trypsin-like enzyme in mast cells. *Nature* 185: 846-847, 1960.

Gosens, R., Zaagsma, J., Meurs, H. and Halayko, A. J. Muscarinic receptor signaling in the pathophysiology of asthma and COPD. *Resp Res.* 9: 7-73, 2006.

Greaves, M. W. and Sabroe, R. U. Allergy and the skin- Urticaria. *Br Med J.* 316: 1147-1150, 1998.

Gupta, I., Gupta, V., Parihar, A., Gupta, S., Ludtke, R., Safayhi, H. and Ammon, H. P. Effects of *Boswellia serrata* gum resin in patients with bronchial asthma: results of a double-blind, placebo-controlled, 6-week clinical study. *Eur. J. Med Res.* 3(11): 511-514, 1998.

Holgate, S. T., Bodey, K. S., Janezic, A., Frew, A. J., Kaplan, A. P. and Teran, L. M. Release of rantes, MIP-1alpha and MCP-1 into asthmatic airways following endobronchial allergen challenge. *Am. J. Respir. Crit. Care Med.* 156(5): 1377-1383, 1997.

Howarth, P., Durham, S., Lee, T., Kay, B., Church, M. and Holgate, S. Influence of albuterol, cromolyn sodium and ipratropium bromide on the airway and circulating mediator responses to allergen provocation in asthma. *Am Rev Respir Dis.* 132: 986-992, 1985.

Humbert, M., Menz, G., Ying, S., Corrigan, C. J., Robinson, D. S., Durham, S. R. and Kay, A. B. The immunopathology of extrinsic (atopic) and intrinsic (non-atopic) asthma: more similarities than differences. *Immunol Today* 20: 528, 1999.

Ikuta, N. Effect of long-term treatment with an inhaled corticosteroid on bronchial hyper- responsiveness and clinical asthma in asthmatic subjects. *Japanese Journal of Allergology.* 45(12): 1231-6, 1996.

Isreal, E. Effect of treatment with zileuton, a 5-lipoxygenase inhibitor, in patients with asthma. *Jama*. 275(12): 931-936, 1996.

Jackson, D. S., Fraser, S. A., Ni, L. M., Kam, C. M., Winkler, U., Johnson, D. A., Froelich, C. J., Hudig, D. and Powers, J. C. Synthesis and evaluation of diphenyl phosphonate esters as inhibitors of the trypsin-like granzymes A and K and mast cell tryptase. *J. Med. Chem.* 41: 2289-2301, 1998.

Jarjour, N. and Enhorning, G. Antigen-induced airway inflammation in atopic subjects generates dysfunction of pulmonary surfactant. *Am. J. Respir. Crit. Care Med.* 160(1): 336-341, 1999.

Jeffery, P. K., Wardlaw, A. J., Nelson, F. C., Collins, J. V. and Kay, A. B. Bronchial biopsies in asthma. An ultrastructural, quantitative study and correlation with hyperreactivity. *Am Rev Respir Dis* 140: 1745, 1989.

Jenny Hallgren, Sergio Estrada, Ulrika Karlson, Kjell Alving, and Gunnar Pejler. Heparin Antagonists Are Potent Inhibitors of Mast Cell Tryptase. *Biochemistry*, 40(24), 7342-7349, 2001.

Johnson, D. and Krenger, W. Interactions of mast cells with the nervous system. recent advances. *Neurochem Res.* 17: 939, 1992.

Kaliner, M. and Austen, K. F. Cyclic AMP, ATP, and reversed anaphylactic histamine release from rat mast cells. *J Immunol.* 112(2): 664-674, 1974.

Kraneveld, A. D., Muis, T., Koster, A. S. and Nijkamp, F. P. Role of mucosal mast cells in early vascular permeability changes of intestinal DTH reaction in the rat. *Am J Physiol* 274: G832, 1998.

Krumins, S. A. and Broomfield, C. A. C-terminal substance P fragments elicit histamine release from a murine mast cell line. *Neuropeptides*. 24: 5, 1993.

Lee, E., Haa, K., Yook, J. M., Jin, M. H., Seo, C. S., Son, K. H., Kim, H. P., Bae, K. H., Kang, S. S., Son, J. K. and Chang, H. W. Anti-asthmatic activity of an ethanol extract from *Saururus chinensis*. *Biol. Pharm. Bull.* 29(2): 211-215, 2006.

Lee, Y. C., Kim, S. H., Seo, Y. B., Roh, S. S. and Lee, J. C. Inhibitory effects of *Actinidia polygama* extract and cyclosporine A on OVA-induced eosinophilia and bronchial hyperresponsiveness in a murine model of asthma. *Int. Immunopharmacol.* 6(4): 703-713, 2006.

Li, C., Li, L., Luo, J. and Huang, N. Effect of turmeric volatile oil on the respiratory tract. *Zhongguo Zhong Yao Za Zhi.* 23(10): 624-625, 1998.

Li, M. H., Zhang, H. L. and Yang, B. Y. Effects of ginkgo leave concentrated oral liquor in treating asthma. *Zhongguo Zhong Xi Yi Jie He Za Zhi.* 17(4): 216- 218, 1997.

Lu, Y., Liang, Z., Song, J. and Liu, W. The antibechic, expectorant and antiasthmatic actions of *Cynanchum komarovii. Zhong Yao Cai.* 20(2): 88-90, 1997.

Marshall. J. S., Stead, R. H., McSharry, C., Nielsen, L. and Bienenstock, J. The role of mast cell degranulation products in mast cell hyperplasia. I. Mechanism of action of nerve growth factor. *J Immunol.* 144: 1886, 1990.

Martin, A. J. The natural history of childhood asthma to adult life. *British Medical Journal.* 280(6229): 1397-1400, 1980.

Mèannistèo, J. New drugs in asthma treatment. Leukotriene receptor blockers and leukotriene synthesis inhibitors. *Nordisk Medicine*. 112(4): 122-5, 1997.

Mechoulam, R. and Carlini, E. A. Toward drugs derived from *Cannabis*. *Naturwissenschaften* 65(4): 174- 179, 1978.

Meeusen, E. N. Immunology of helminth infections, with special reference to immunopathology. *Vet Parasitol* 84: 259, 1999.

Mo, Z., Tang, X., Sun, Z. and Li, W. Comparison of pharmacological effects between cultispecies Sichuan Fritillary bulb (*F. wabueasis, F. mellea*) and wild Sichuan Fritillary bulb (*F. unibracteata*). Zhongguo Zhong Yao Za Zhi. 23(1): 14-16, 61, 1998.

Molinari, M., Dell'Anna, M. E., Rausell, E., Leggio, M. G., Hashikawa, T. and Jones, E. G. Auditory thalamocortical pathways defined in monkeys by calcium-binding protein immunoreactivity. *J Comp Neurl.* 362(2): 171-194, 1995.

Mori, L., Kleimberg, J., Mancini, C., Bellini, A., Marini, M. and Mattoli, S. Bronchial epithelial cells of atopic patients with asthma lack the ability to inactivate allergens. *Biochem Biophys Res Commun* 217: 817-824, 1995.

Mousli, M., Bronner, C., Bockaert, J., Rouot, B. and Landry, Y. Interaction of substance P, compound 48/80 and mastoparan with the alpha-subunit C-terminus of G protein. *Immunol Lett.* 25: 355, 1990.

Mousli, M., Hugli, T. E., Landry, Y. and Bronner, C. Peptidergic pathway in human skin and rat peritoneal mast cell activation. *Immunopharmacology*. 27: 1, 1994.

Nakahara, Y. Significance of the therapeutic range of serum theophylline concentration in the treatment of an attack of bronchial asthma. Biological and Pharmaceutical Bulletin. 19(5):710-5, 1996.

O'Byrne, P. M. Antileukotrienes in the treatment of asthma. *Annals of Internal Medicine*. 127(6): 472-80, 1997.

Ogasawara, T., Murakami, M., Suzuki-Nishimura, T., Uchida, M. K. and Kudo, I. Mouse bone marrow-derived mast cells undergo exocytosis, prostanoid generation, and cytokine expression in response to G protein-activating polybasic compounds after coculture with fibroblasts in the presence of c-kit ligand. *J Immunol.* 158: 393, 1997.

Otsuka, H., Denburg, J., Dolovich, J., Hitch, D., Lapp, P., Rajan, R. S., Bienenstock, J. and Befus, D. Heterogeneity of metachromatic cells in human nose: significance of mucosal mast cells. *J Allergy Clin Immunol* 76: 695), respiratory mucosal surfaces, 1985.

Paramesh, H. Epidemiology of asthma in India. Indian Journal of Paediatrics. 69(4): 309-312, 2002.

Pereira, P. J. B., Bergner, A., Macedo-Rebeiro, S., Huber, R. Matschiner, G., Fritz, H., Sommerhoff, C. P. and Bode, W. R. *Nature*. 392: 306-311, 1998.

Platts-Mills, Thomas. Asthma: causes and mechanisms of this epidemic inflammatory disease. Boca Raton: Lewis Publishers, 1999.

Pullaiah, T. Medicinal Plants in India. Regency Publications. New Delhi, 2002.

Ramirez-Romero, R., Gallup, J. M., Sonea, I. M. and Ackermann, M. R. Dihydrocapsaicin treatment depletes peptidergic nerve fibers of substance P and alters mast cell density in the respiratory tract of neonatal sheep [In Process Citation]. *Regul Pept.* 91-97, 2000.

Redegeld, F. A., Van Der Heijden, M. W., Kool, M., Heijdra, B. M., Garssen, J., Kraneveld, A. D., Loveren, H. V., Roholl, P., Saito, T., Verbeek, J. S., Claassens, J., Koster, A. S. and Nijkamp, F. P. Immunoglobulin-free light chains elicit immediate hypersensitivity-like responses. *Nat Med* 8: 694, 2002.

Reynisdottir, S. Effect of glucocorticosteroid treatment on beta-adrenoceptor subtype function in adipocytes from patients with asthma. *Clinical Science*. 85(2): 237-244, 1995.

Rochat, T. Long-acting beta-2-agonists in the treatment of asthma. *Journal Suisse de Medicine*. 124(39): 1714-1719, 1994.

Roche, W. R. Fibroblasts and asthma. *Clin Exp Allergy*. 21: 545-548, 1991.

Rottem, M., G., Hull and Metcalfe, D. D. Demonstration of differential effects of cytokines on mast cells derived from murine bone marrow and peripheral blood mononuclear cells. *Exp Hematol* 22: 1147, 1994.

Schick, B., Austen, K. F. and Schwartz, L. B. Activation of rat serosal mast cells by chymase, an endogenous secretory granule protease. *The Journal of Immunology*. 132(5): 2571-2577, 1998.

Scholzen, T., Armstrong, C. A., Bunnett, N. W., Luger, T. A., Olerud, J. E. and Ansel, J. C. Neuropeptides in the skin: interactions between the neuroendocrine and the skin immune systems. *Exp Dermatol*. 7: 81, 1998.

Sekkadde, K. Betelnut chewing causes bronchoconstriction in some asthma patients. *Papua New Guinea Medical Journal*. 37(2): 90-99, 1994.

Selwood, T., Elrod, K. C, Schechter, N. M. Potent Bivalent Inhibition of Human Tryptase-^{2} by a Synthetic Inhibitor. *Biological Chemistry*, 384(12): 1605-1611, 2005.

Shaoheng He, Ahmed Aslam, Marianna D. A. Gaça, Yongsong He, Mark G. Buckley, Morley D. Hollenberg, and Andrew F. Walls. Inhibitors of Tryptase as Mast Cell-Stabilizing Agents in the Human Airways: Effects of Tryptase and Other Agonists of Proteinase-Activated Receptor 2 on Histamine Release. *JPET* 309: 119-126, 2004.

Shao-Heng He, Hua, Xie. Inhibition of tryptase release from human colon mast cells by protease inhibitors. *R World J Gastroenterol*. 10(3): 332-336, 2004.

Sommerhoff, C. P., Bode, W., Pereira, P. J., Stubbs, M. T., Sturzebecher, J., Piechottka, G. P., Matschiner, G. and Bergner, A. *Proc. Natl. Acad. Sci*. 96(20): 10984-10991, 1999.

Specific allergen immunotherapy for asthma. A position paper of the Thoracic Society of Australia and the Asutralasian Society of Clinical Immunology and Allergy. *Med J Australia*: 167: 540-544, 1997.

Sylvin, H., Stensdotter, M., van der Ploeg, I. and Alving, K. ATS. D31 (Poster K33), San Francisco, U.S.A., 2001.

Thiruvengadam, K. V., Haranath, K., Sudarsan, S., Sekar, T. S., Rajagopal, K. R., Zacharian, M. G., Devarajan, T. V. *Tylophora indica* in bronchial asthma (a controlled comparison with a standard anti-asthmatic drug). *J. Indian Med. Assoc*. 71(7): 172- 176, 1978.

Thomas, G., Solak, M. and Henson, P. M. Effects of the aqueous fraction of the ethanol extract of the leaves of *Cissampelos sympodialis* Eichl. in human nutrophils. *Phytother. Res*. 13(1): 9-13, 1999.

Thomas J. Martin. Synthesis Of Bifunctional Inhibitors Against Human Mast Cell-Tryptase: A Potential Approach To Attack Asthma. *In:* Fifth International Electronic Conference on Synthetic Organic Chemistry (ECSOC-5), 2001.

Valent, P. Cytokines involved in growth and differentiation of human basophils and mast cells. *Exp Dermatol.* 4: 255, 1995.

Van der Molen. Starting with a higher dose of inhaled corticosteroids in primary care asthma treatment. *Am J Respir Crit Care Med.* 158(1): 121-5. Rottem, 1998.

Van Loveren, H., Meade, R. and Askenase, P. W. An early component of delayed type hypersensitivity mediated by T cells and mast cells. *J Exp Med.* 157: 1604, 1983.

Van Loveren, H., Meade, R. and Askenase, P. W. An early component of delayed-type hypersensitivity mediated by T cells and mast cells. *J Exp Med* 157: 160, 1983.

Vulliemoz, Y., Verosky, M. and Triner, L. Effect of albuterol and terbutaline, synthetic beta adrenergic stimulants, on the cyclic 3'-5'-adenosine monophosphate system in smooth muscle. *J Pharmacol Exp Ther.* 195(3): 549-56, 1975.

Walker, C. The immunology of extrinsic and intrinsic asthma. *Agents Actions Suppl* 43: 97, 1993.

Wenzel, S. E., Fowler, A. A. III., Schwartz, L. B. *Am. Rev. Respir.* Dis. 137: 1002-1008. 1988.

Wershil, B. K. and Galli, S. J. Gastrointestinal mast cells. New approaches for analyzing their function in vivo. *Gastroenterol Clin North Am.* 20: 613, 1991.

White M. V., Slater, J. and Kaliner, M. Histamine and asthma. *Am Rev Respir Dis.* 135: 1165-1176, 1987.

White, M. V. The role of histamine in allergic diseases. *J Allergy Clin Immunol.* 86: 599-605, 1990.

Wolfe, J. D., Yamate, M., Biedermann, A. A. and Chu, T. J. Comparison of the acute cardiopulmonary effects of oral albuterol, metaproterenol and terbutaline in asthmatics. *J Am Med As.* 253(14): 2068-2072, 1985.

Woolcock, A. J. Use of corticosteroids in treatment of patients with asthma. *Journal of Allergy and Clinical Immunology.* 84 (6 Pt 1): 975-8, 1981.

Wright, C. D., Havill, A. M., Middleton, S. C., Kashem, M. A., Dripps, D. J., Abraham, W. M., Thomson, D. S. and Burgess, L. E. *Biochem. Pharm.* 58: 1989-1996, 1999.

Wyser, C. New aspects in the treatment of bronchial asthma and chronic obstructive lung disease. *Journal Suisse de Medecine.* 127(21): 885-90, 1997.

Zhong, Z., Zhou, G., Chen, X. and Huang, P. Pharmacological study on the extracts from *Typhonium flagelliforme* Blume. *Zhong Yao Cai.* 24(10): 735- 738, 2001.

—oo(O)oo—

22

BIOTECHNOLOGICAL ADVANCES IN SOME ETHNOMEDICINAL PLANT SPECIES

KIRTI D'SOUZA

FORESTS are one of the earth's most important and valuable renewable natural resources. More than half of the world's tropical forest area has been destroyed since the beginning of this century. The sustainability of forest species to provide wood and other products depends on the maintenance and management of these resources.

Therefore research on conservation, protection and sustainable development of existing forests to conserve biodiversity is a priority.

India has probably the oldest, richest and most diverse cultural traditions in the use of medicinal plants. Over 7500 species of plants are used by several ethnic communities (Katwal *et al.*, 2003).

The renewed interest in "alternative" medicines has resulted in an increase in the demand for medicinal plants. Collecting naturally occurring medicinal plants is not sustainable as 70% of such collections involve destructive harvesting (Report of Task Force on Conservation and Sustainable use of Medicinal Plants, 2000). This has serious implications on the survival of plant species many of which are under threat of becoming extinct, because of the rapid loss of natural habitats and overexploitation of plants from the wild.

Wild harvesting of medicinal plants can not only be problematic in terms of biodiversity loss, but may also lead to potential variation in medicinal plant quality, and occasionally, improper plant identification with potential tragic consequences (Briskin, 2000).

Despite enormous threats of extinction there is no systematic cultivation of medicinal plants and with fast disappearing forests we stand to lose a wealth of traditional knowledge handed down over generations.

Commercial cultivation of medicinal plants will help in conserving endangered species in their natural habitat, permit production of uniform materials, provide good income to the farmers and a continuity of supply as well as contribute towards a better environment through utilizing waste and unproductive lands. However, there are several constraints in cultivation of medicinal plants; these include biotic, abiotic, technological as well as socioeconomic factors which lead to poor yield and quality of materials (Chapman and Chomchalow, 2005).

Modern biotechnology provides tools that can be used as complements to conventional technologies to overcome some of these constraints. Biotechnology utilizes fundamental discoveries in the field of plant tissue culture for clonal forestry, gene transfer techniques, molecular biology and genomics.

Several reviews have covered the role of biotechnology in forestry, its economic benefit and role in conservation, ecological issues and in recent innovative techniques in improvement (Sedjo, 2001, 2003, 2006; Nehra *et al.*, 2005).

Clonal propagation by tissue culture offers an alternate to conventional vegetative practices and provides an extended platform for improvement of traits. Where vegetative propagation is difficult, low-cost cloning techniques are a pre-requisite for genetic engineering to be commercially viable. However, genetic modification will become a reality only for particularly novel and valuable traits in short-rotation species in intensively managed plantations (Yanchuk, 2001).

Biotechnological approaches are also found to have potential as a supplement to traditional agriculture in the industrial production of bioactive plant metabolites, and particularly, in possibly altering them by means of tissue culture technology (Balandrin *et al.*, 1985; Briskin, 2000;Vanisree *et al.*, 2004). Cell suspension systems could be used for the large-scale culturing of plant cells from which secondary metabolites can be extracted.

The Dediapada forests in the South of Gujarat are a part of the Shoolpaneshwar Wildlife Sanctuary. This area has assumed greater significance in recent times as it forms the major portion of the Sardar Sarovar Submergence area. This biodiversity rich area is inhabited by Vasava tribals who possess a wealth of knowledge on the use of many plant species in herbal medicines. A recent study has led to the documentation of over 250 plant species belonging to 75 families, of ethnomedicinal importance, several having novel uses (D'Cruz, 2002). Since some of these species are rare (Shah, 1978) or have been listed in the Threatened Biodiversity of Gujarat: Baseline Information (GEC, 2001) (Table 1) there is an urgent need to restore them in their natural habitat. However no concerted efforts are being made towards their conservation as threatened species like *Derris scandens* (Roxb) Benth., *Desmodium heterocarpon* (L.) DC, *Ceropegia fantastica* Sedgw. to name a few have not been worked upon. This article provides an overview of the achievements and advances in the application of plant tissue culture technology namely clonal propagation and secondary metabolite production of 22 species, reported elsewhere, these have been selected on the basis of their ethno medicinal significance with reference to the Dediapada forests (Table 1). The work on some of these species in our laboratory has used resource material from the Dediapada forests.

CLONAL PROPAGATION OF PLANTS OF THE LEGUMINOSAE FAMILY

Table 2 summarizes the reported data in clonal propagation of some ethno medicinal species.

TABLE 1

Clonal Propagation and Conservation Status of Some Ethno Medicinal Species of the Dediapada Forests

No.	Plant Species	Family/Subfamily	Medicinal Part	Conservation Status	Clonal Propagation
1.	*Acacia nilotica var indica* (Benth)	Leguminosae/ Mimosaceae	Roots	Not threatened	Direct organogenesis, Somatic embryogenesis, Triploid production
2.	*Albizia lebbeck*(L.) Willd.	Leguminosae/ Mimosaceae	Bark	Not threatened	Direct, Indirect organogenesis, Somatic embryogenesis
3.	*Albizia procera* (Roxb.) Bth.	Leguminosae/ Mimosaceae	Bark , roots	Not threatened	Direct, Indirect organogenesis
4.	*Bauhinia vahlii* Graham	Leguminosae/ Caesalpineae	Roots	Threatened	Direct organogenesis
5.	*Cassia fistula*	Leguminosae/ Caesalpineae	Bark, leaves, roots	Not threatened	Indirect organogenesis
6.	*Pterocarpus marsupium* Roxb. var. *acuminata* Prain	Leguminosae/ Papilionaceae	Bark, gum, roots	Rare	Direct, Indirect organogenesis
7.	*Butea monosperma* (Lam.) Taub.	Leguminosae/ Papilionaceae	Bark, roots, flowers, seeds	Rare	Direct, Indirect organogenesis somatic embryogenesis
8.	*Uraria picta* Desv.	Leguminosae/ Papilionaceae	Roots	Not threatened	Direct, indirect organogenesis
9.	*Vigna calcaratus* (Roxb.) Kurz	Leguminosae/ Papilionaceae	Roots	Rare	Direct organogenesis

Continued ...

... Continued

No.	Plant Species	Family/Subfamily	Medicinal Part	Conservation Status	Clonal Propagation
10.	*Costus speciosus* (Koenig ex Retz.) Sm	Zingiberaceae	Rhizome, tubers	Threatened	Direct, Indirect organogenesis
11.	*Curcuma amada* Roxb.	Zingiberaceae	Rhizome, tubers	Common	Direct, Indirect organogenesis
12.	*Ceropegia bulbosa* Roxb.	Asclepiadaceae	Tubers	Vulnerable	Direct organogenesis, Somatic embryogenesis
13.	*Tylophora fasciculata* Ham. ex Wight	Asclepiadaceae	Leaves, roots	Threatened	Direct organogenesis
14.	*Tylophora rotundifolia* Ham. ex Wight	Asclepiadaceae	Roots.	Threatened	No reports
15.	*Anogeissus latifolia* Roxb Wall. ex Bedd	Combretaceae	Roots, stem bark	Frequent	Direct organogenesis
16.	*Terminalia arjuna* Roxb W. & A	Combretaceae	Stembark	Occasional	Direct organogenesis, Somatic embryogenesis
17.	*Terminalia bellirica* (Gaertn.) Roxb.	Combretaceae	Leaves, stem bark, twigs	Common	Direct organogenesis
18.	*Adina cordifolia* Benth & Hook.	Rubiaceae	Leaves, stembark	Occasional	Direct organogenesis

Continued ...

... *Continued*

No.	Plant Species	Family/Subfamily	Medicinal part	Conservation status	Clonal Propagation
19.	*Mitragyna parvifolia* (Roxb.) Korth	Rubiaceae	Stem bark	Frequent	Direct organogenesis
20.	*Buchanania lanzan* Spreng.	Anacardiaceae	Stem bark	Vulnerable	Direct organogenesis, Somatic embryogenesis
21.	*Corallocarpus conocarpus* (Dalz. & Gibbs) Hook	Cucurbitaceae	Roots	Rare	Direct organogenesis, Callus induction
22.	*Tecomella undulata* (sw.) Seem.	Bignoniaceae	Stembark	Threatened	Direct, Indirect organogenesis

TABLE 2

Clonal Propagation of Some Ethno Medicinal Species of the Dediapada Forests

Plant Species	Explant	Basal Medium	Plant Growth Regulators and/ or Additives (mg/l) Shoot/Callus Induction	Shoot Multiplication	Rooting	Reference
Acacia nilotica	Immature endosperm	MS	2,4-D, BA + CH.	*Glutamine + CH + CW.	-	Garg *et al.*,(1996)
A. nilotica	*In vitro*-grown Seedlings	B_5	BA+ CW	-	NAA/IAA + CW	Gupta and Agrawal, (1992)
A. nilotica	Cotyledonary node	B_5	1.5 BA	1.5 BA	2.0 IAA	Dewan *et al.*, (1992)
A. nilotica	Stem	MS	0.5–1.0 IAA	-	-	Marthur and Chandra, (1983)
Albizia lebbeck	Cotyledon node	MS	2.0-2.5 BA +0.2 NAA	2.5 BA+0.2 NAA	-	Mamun *et al.*, (2004)
			2.5 BA+0.5 NAA	-	1.0 IBA	
	In vitro node		2.0 BA + 0.2 NAA			
	In vitro internode		2.0BA + 0.5 NAA	2.5 BA + 0.2 NAA	-	
A. lebbeck	Leaf	*MS	0.4 BA + 0.25 K + CM12% (v/v)	8.0 BA + 0.25 IAA + CM 8% (v/v)	-	Ghosh *et al.*, (2001)
A.lebbeck	Leaf	B5	4.5 K + 0.05 IBA + 300 CH + 1.5g/l Ads	-	-	Ghosh *et al.*, (1998)
		MS	6.0 BA + 0.25 IBA + CM 12% (v/v) + 70 CH	-	-	
A. lebbeck	Stem, Petiole,	B5	1.0 BA + 0.5 IAA or 0.5 BA + 2.0 NAA.	-	0.1 IAA	Gharyal and Maheshwari, (1990)
A. lebbeck	Hypocotyl	MS	0.1K +1.0 NAA	-	-	Ramawat and Arya, (1982)

Continued ...

... *Continued*

Plant Species	Explant	Basal Medium	Plant Growth Regulators and/ or Additives (mg/l) Shoot/Callus Induction	Shoot Multiplication	Rooting	Reference
Albizia procera	Epicotyl, hypocotyl Axillary bud Shoot tip	½ MS	0.003 BA	0.002 GA	0.006 IBA + 500 AC	Swamy *et al.*, (2004)
A.procera	Leaflets	MS	2.25 BA + 0.2 NAA.	0.002 BA + 0.2 NAA.	* IBA 0.4	Kumar *et al.*, (1998)
Bauhinia vahlii	Cotyledonary nodes	MS	0.22 TDZ + 0.21 K	-	0.2 NAA	Bhatt and Dhar, (2000)
B. vahlii	Nodes	MS	0.55 K+ 100 Ads	-	a. * 2.0 NAA+ 2.05 IBA (pulse) b. no pgrs	Dhar and Upreti, (1999)
B. vahlii	Cotyledonary nodes	MS	0.22 TDZ	0.2 2 TDZ	*0.2 NAA	Upreti and Dhar, (1996)
Cassia fistula	Stem	B5	0.5 IAA + 1.0 BA or 2.0 NAA + 0.5 BA.	-	-	Gharyal and Maheshwari, (1990)
Pterocarpus marsupium	Cotyledonary nodes	MS	1.15 BA	-	a. 40.8 IBA + phenolic acid (pulse)b.0.1IBA	Anis *et al.*, (2005)
P. marsupium	Cotyledonary nodes	MS	1.0 BA + 0.05 NAA	-	2.0 IBA	Chand and Singh (2004)
P. marsupium	Nodes	MS	No PGRS/ 0.2 IBA	-	-	Tiwari *et al.*, (2004)
P. marsupium	Mesocotyl,	B5	2.0 BA	-	-	Pullaiah, (1999)
Butea monosperma	Cotyledonary nodes	½ (WP)	5.0 BA + 10.0 fructose	-	-	Kulkarni and D'Souza,(2000)

Continued ...

... Continued

Plant Species	Explant	Basal Medium	Plant Growth Regulators and/ or Additives (mg/l) Shoot/Callus Induction	Shoot Multiplication	Rooting	Reference
B. monosperma	Nodes	WP	2.5 BA	-	-	Kulkarni *et al.*, (1997)
	Cotyledonary nodes	½ WP	10.0 BA + 10.0 fructose	-	-	
	Cotyledonary segments	MS	5.0 K	5.0 K	_	
	Cotyledonary segments	MS	5.0 BA	5.0 BA		
	Hypocotyl	MS	K + phloroglucinol	BA+phloroglucinol	-	
Uraria picta	Axillary nodes	MS	1.0 BA + 0.5 NAA	0.45 AdS	-	Anand *et al.*, (1998)
	Node callus		1.0 BA + 0.5 NAA	0.03 BA	*No pgrs	
Vigna calcaratus	Nodes	MS	3.0 BA	3.0 BA	-	Vaidya and Braganza, (2006)
Costus speciosus	Rhizome	B_5	0.005 TRIA.	-	0.002 TRIA.	Malabadi *et al.*, (2005)
C. speciosus	Rhizome	* B_5	4.0 TDZ	-	1.0 NAA.	Malabadi *et al.*, (2004)
C. speciosus		B_5	1.0 BA + NAA 1.11	-	-	Malabadi, (2002)
C. speciosus	Zygotic embryos	SH	BA/K+NAA/IBA/ IAA/2,4 -D+ Ads + 250 CA	-	-	Roy and Pal, (1991)
C. speciosus	Mature embryo	SH	0.1K + 0.1IBA	-	-	Pal and Roy, (1991)
C. speciosus	Shoot tips	*SH	0.5 BA or K + 15 Ads+ 1.0 IAA	-	1.0 IAA	Chaturvedi, *et al.*, (1983)
Curcuma amada	Rhizome	MS	1.0 BA + 0.2 NAA	-	1.0 BA + 0.2 NAA	Prakash *et al.*, (2004)

Continued ...

... Continued

Plant Species	Explant	Basal Medium	Plant Growth Regulators and/ or Additives (mg/l) Shoot/Callus Induction	Shoot Multiplication	Rooting	Reference
C. amada	Shoot buds	MS	3.0 BA + 0.5 NAA	3.0 BA + 0.5 NAA	-	Nayak, (2002)
	In vitro shoot	MS		-	* 5.0 BA	
Ceropegia bulbosa	Nodes	B_5	3.0 BA + 0.05NAA	3.0 BA + 0.05NAA	2.0 IBA /2.0 IBA = 0.05 K	Britto *et al.*, (2003)
C. bulbosa	Nodes	*MS	2.0 BA	0.5BA	5.0 BA+5.0 K	Patil (1998)
	Shoots	MS	2.0 2,4 –D	0.5 BA	-	
Tylophora fasciculata	Nodes	MS	(0.5-5 BA) + (0.1-1.0) NAA	-	-	D'Souza et al.,(2005)
Tylophora rotundifolia	Leaf	MS	1.0 BA + 0.1 2,4-D	-	-	D'Souza, (unpub. data)
Anogeissus latifolia	seeds	MS	No pgrs.	1.0 BA + 1.0 IAA + CH 100 + AA 50	0.4 IAA + 0.5 IBA	Saxena and Dhawan, (2001)
A. latifolia	Cotyledonary node, epicotyl	MS	1.5 BA + 0.1 IAA + additives	BA 1.0	a. IBA or b. 100 IBA + 100 NOA (pulse)	Shekhawat *et al.*, (2000)
Terminalia arjuna	Cotyledonary nodes	*MS	0.5 BA	0.5 BA	a. 1.0 IBA (pulse) b. * no pgrs	Pandey and Jaiswal, (2002)
T. arjuna	Leaves	MS	5.0 2,4-D + 0.01 K	-	No pgrs.	Nishi kumari et al., (1998)
Terminalia bellirica	Nodal (seedlings)	MS	1.0 -5.0 BA	1.0 BA	* 1.0 IBA	Sadanandam *et al.*, (2004)
Adina cordifolia	Apical buds (3yr)	MS	0.5 BA + 0.5 NAA	0.5 BA + 0.5 NAA	0.5 BA + 0.5 NAA	Dubey *et al.*, (2004)
	Apical buds (30yr)	MS	1.0 NAA	1.0 NAA	3.0 IBA	

Continued ...

... Continued

Plant Species	Explant	Basal Medium	Plant Growth Regulators and/ or Additives (mg/l) Shoot/Callus Induction	Shoot Multiplication	Rooting	Reference
Mitragyna parvifolia	Shoot apice	MS	1.0 BA	-	* three auxins	Roy *et al.*, (1988)
Buchanania lanzan	Decoated seeds	MS	5.0 BA + 1.0 NAA	-	5.0 K	Shende and Rai, (2005)
B. lanzan	Immature zygotic embryos	MS	1.0 2, 4-D + 1.0 NAA + 1.0 BA.	2.75 ABA	-	Sharma *et al.*, (2005)
Corallocarpus conocarpus	Nodes	MS	2.0 BA+ 0.01 NAA	-	-	D'Souza *et al.*, (2005)
Tecomella undulata	*In vitro* shoots	MS	BA 1.0-1.5	-	-	Nandwani *et al.*, (1996)
T. undulata	Cotyledonary nodes	MS	2.5 BA + IAA 0.05	-	* 5 each IAA+ IBA+NAA (pulse)	Nandwani *et al.*, (1995)
T.undulata	Seedling shoots	WP	1.0 BA	-	0.3 IBA	Bhansali, (1993)
T. undulata	Node	MS	2.0 BA + 0.05 IAA	1.0 BA +0.01 IAA	*a. 2.5 IBA b. no pgrs	Rathore *et al.*, (1991)

*- modified basal medium

MS, Murashige and Skoog (1962) medium;B5, Gamborg (Gamborg *et al.*,1968);SH,Schenk and Hildebrandt (1972) medium;WP,Woody plant medium (Llyod and McCown 1980;BA, Bezyladenine;K, Kinetin; GA,Giberillic acid;TDZ,thiadiazuron;TRIA, Triancontal; IAA, Indole acetic acid; NAA, 1-napthaleneacetic acid; IBA, Indole butyric acid; 2,4-D,2,4-dichlorophenoxyacetic acid; NOA, 2-naphthyloxyacetic acid. CH,activated charcoal; CW, Coconut water; CM, Coconut milk; Ads, Adenine sulphate; AA, Ascorbic acid; CA, Casamino acids.

Species of Mimosaceae subfamily

Beck and Dunlop (2001) have reviewed micro propagation work in acacia species and found the use of juvenile plant material was most successful for *in vitro* propagation.

In *Acacia nilotica,* seedling explants responded on Gamborg's (B_5) Medium (Gamborg et al. 1968) in the presence of Benzyladenine (BA) in combination with Indole acetic acid (IAA) or 1-napthaleneacetic acid (NAA) (Dewan *et al.,* 1992; Gupta and Agrawal, 1992). This is in accordance with most reports of other acacia species.

Similarly, establishment of *in vitro* cultures using juvenile tissues of *A. lebbeck* has been successful (Gharyal and Maheshwari,1983;Ramawat and Arya,1982;Mamun *et al.,* 2004) and of *A. procera* (Kumar *et al.,* 1998) on either Murashige and Skoog (MS) (Murashige and Skoog, 1962) or B_5 media supplemented with BA along with either NAA or Indole butyric acid (IBA). Swamy et al. (2004) found BA more efficacious in inducing *de novo* shoots from callus derived from seedling explants on half strength MS medium.

Establishment of *in vitro* cultures from mature tissue in acacia species has been reported to be difficult, with reports of shoot bud formation and *in vitro* bud break in *A. nilotica* (Marthur and Chandra, 1983; Singh *et al.,* 1993) and *A.lebbeck* (Gharyal and Maheshwari, 1990; Roy, 1992; Mamun *et al.,* 2004). Callus from explants from mature trees was found to be non-morphogenic in *A. procera.*

Garg et al. (1996) succeeded in inducing somatic embryogenesis in immature embryos to obtain triploid plantlets of *A.nilotica* by using a combination of 2,4-dichlorophenoxyacetic acid (2,4-D) and BA, whereas Ghosh et al. (1998, 2001) obtained embryos of *A.lebbeck* in leaf-derived calli on media supplemented with BA and Kinetin (K) singly or in combination, along with IBA and additives.

IBA was found to be more effective in inducing roots in regenerated shoots in *Albizia* species whereas IAA or NAA were used in *Acacia* species.

Successful transfer to soil of *in vitro* plantlets of these tree legumes has been achieved however there is a paucity of reports of large scale plantations using such plantlets.

Species of Caesalpineae subfamily

Unlike the plant species of the Mimosaceae subfamily both the species of this subfamily were successfully put in culture using explants from mature trees.

Cotyledonary nodes and those from mature trees of *Bauhinia vahlii* responded in MS medium fortified with K and Thiadiazuron (TDZ) singly and in combination (Upreti and Dhar,1996; Dhar and Upreti,1999; Bhatt and Dhar,2000) while , the combination of BA with IAA or NAA in B_5 medium was used to regenerate *in vitro* shoots from stem explants of *Cassia fistula.* (Gharyal and Maheshwari, 1990).

Rooting was obtained in *B.vahlii* on half-strength and one-fourth strength MS medium either supplemented with NAA or after a pulse treatment with a combination of NAA and IBA indicating that this species is amenable to root in low salt media.

Rooted plantlets were acclimatized and established *ex vitro* however the successful field transfer of tissue cultured plantlets was not reported.

Species of Papilionaceae subfamily

Considerable success has been reported on the tissue culture of leguminous ethno medicinal species belonging to this subfamily.

Most of the experiments in *Pterocarpus marsupium* have used seeds or seedling explants to initiate cultures (Pullaiah, 1999; Chand and Singh, 2004; Anis *et al.*, 2005) as in *Butea monosperma* (Kulkarni *et al.*, 1997; Kulkarni and D'Souza, 2000) demonstrating the efficacy of juvenile tissues.

Various media compositions were employed to establish cultures of *P. marsupium* of which MS seemed most efficacious as Tiwari et al. (2004) were able to induce shooting on hormoneless medium.

Shoots from cotyledonary nodes of *P. marsupium* were also regenerated on medium fortified with BA singly or in combination with NAA (Chand and Singh, 2004; Anis *et al.*, 2005) whereas nodal segments required IBA supplemented medium. This points out to the possibility that the hormone requirement may depend on the age of the explants.

Efficacy of BA supplemented MS media in regenerating multiple shoots from nodal explants of *Vigna calcaratus* (Vaidya and Braganza, 2006) and in *Uraria picta (*Anand *et al.*, 1998) have also been reported. Nodal Callus of the leguminous herb *U. picta* was morphogenic and required only cytokinin to stimulate shooting.

On the contrary, cotyledonary nodes of *B. monosperma* regenerated shoots on half-strength Lloyd and McCown (WP) medium (Lloyd and McCown 1980) supplemented with BA. The morphogenic response of callus induced from cotyledon segments was dependent on the growth regulator used, wherein somatic embryogenesis was induced on MS medium supplemented with BA whereas K induced shoots. Hypocotyl developed tubers when K was added along with phloroglucinol, which regenerated shoots when subcultured to WP medium supplemented with BA and phloroglucinol.

Rooting of shoots was reported to be difficult in *B. monosperma*; limited success was obtained when shoots were planted in moist sand supplemented with $MnSO_4$ and IBA.

Conflicting reports are available on studies on rooting of micro shoots of *P. marsupium.*

While Chand and Singh, (2004) indicated the efficacy of IBA supplemented half strength MS medium for rooting, Anis *et al.*, (2005) have reported no rooting but callusing occurred at the base of shoots on rooting medium containing different concentration of MS salts and different auxins. The latter study found a pulse treatment of IBA and phenolic acid for 5 days followed by culture on half-strength MS medium supplemented with low levels of the auxin more efficacious in inducing rooting. The difference in results obtained could be due to the carry over effect of plant growth regulators as the earlier study used a combination of cytokinin and auxin for shoot induction as compared to single cytokinin by the latter.

Most reports on tissue culture of the leguminous species of ethno medicinal significance have employed MS medium supplemented with a combination of BA and NAA for shoot induction and IBA has been used most frequently for the induction of rooting.

CLONAL PROPAGATION OF SPECIES FROM THE ZINGIBERACEAE FAMILY

Various basal media and plant growth regulators have been successfully used to induce organogenesis from different explants of plants from this family.

Shoot regeneration occurred from mature embryos of *Costus speciosus* on Schenk and Hildebrandt (1972) (SH) medium (Roy and Pal, 1991; Pal and Roy, 1991) supplemented with a combination of cytokinin and auxins. Optimum Rhizome formation was observed on medium fortified with Casamino acids.

Shoot tips regenerated adventitious shoots on modified SH medium supplemented with either BA or K with AdS along with IAA (Chaturvedi *et al.,* 1983).

On the other hand thin rhizome sections were used as explants on B_5 medium supplemented with either BA and NAA (Malabadi, 2002) or TDZ (Malabadi 2004) or Triacontanol (TRIA) (Malabadi 2005) to induce shoots. Use of TRIA was found to be most efficient for the proliferation of shoots of *C. speciosus* as well as for rooting.

These studies indicate that various explants of this threatened species and a wide variety of plant growth regulators can be used successfully to establish *in vitro* cultures.

Similarly, various explants of another Zingiberaceae species *Curcurma amada,* namely, vegetative buds (IISR 2005), rhizome, and leaf sheath and *in vitro* shoots (Nayak, 2002) have been used to initiate cultures. Direct organogenesis (shoots and rhizomes) occurred on MS medium fortified with BA and NAA. Prakash et al. (2004) induced callus formation in leaf sheath explants on MS medium containing 2, 4 –D which regenerated shoots on subculture to medium to which BA and NAA were added.

Rooting or rhizome formation of this species has been reported to require the presence of cytokinin in the medium. *In vitro* plantlets or micro rhizomes where successfully transferred to soil.

CLONAL PROPAGATION OF PLANTS FROM THE ASCLEPIADACEAE FAMILY

Nodes of *Ceropegia bulbosa* responded by multiple axillary branching when half-strength basal medium (MS) was supplemented with BA. Multiple shooting occurred upon subculture to medium supplemented with low levels of BA whereas micro tubers were induced on medium fortified with a combination of BA and K at high concentrations. Callus induced from shoots on media containing 2,4-D was embryogenic and when sub cultured to medium containing BA embryoids were obtained (Patil, 1998).

In another study, nodes responded in B_5 medium in the presence of a combination of BA and NAA along with AdS. Shoots obtained flowered *in vitro* when sub cultured onto medium containing a combination of BA with Giberillic acid (GA_3). Shoots formed roots on medium supplemented with IBA while micro tubers were obtained if kinetin was added to the rooting medium (Britto *et al.,* 2003).

Preliminary work on *Tylophora fasciculata* in our laboratory has indicated the effectiveness of BA supplemented MS medium in the establishment of shoot cultures from nodal explants. The presence of NAA resulted in enhanced axillary shooting. Callusing was induced at the base of nodal explants on medium containing kinetin singly or in combination with 2, 4-D. Further work in establishing a protocol for efficient clonal propagation is in progress.

Callus induction in leaf explants of *T. rotundifolia* required the presence of auxin (unpub. data); investigations are underway to induce organogenesis.

CLONAL PROPAGATION OF PLANTS FROM THE COMBRETACEAE FAMILY

Juvenile explants of species of this family seem to be amenable to establish shoot cultures. Saxena and Dhawan, (2001) induced multiple shoots from seeds of *Anogeissus latifolia* cultured on hormone free MS medium. Further multiplication occurred on medium supplemented with a combination of BA with IAA along with additives.

On the contrary, multiple shoots were obtained from seedling explants using lower concentrations of auxin in induction medium and only cytokinin in the shoot multiplication medium (Shekhawat *et al.*, 2000).

A combination of two auxins in half-strength MS medium was found to induce rooting in *in vitro* shoots in both reports. However, the latter study found a pulse treatment followed by *ex-vitro* root induction more efficient in acclimatizing the plantlets.

In both the *Terminalia* species the juvenile explants proliferated shoots on medium to which cytokinin BA alone was added (Sadanandam *et al.*, 2004; Pandey and Jaiswal, 2002). IBA was found to be efficacious in inducing rooting in the medium or in a pulse treatment.

Nishi Kumari et al. (1998) has reported somatic embryogenesis from mature tree leaf derived callus which required the presence of 2, 4-D along with kinetin. Conversion of the embryoids to plantlets occurred on hormone free MS medium.

Tissue cultured plantlets of this family have been reported to have been successfully established in the field.

CLONAL PROPAGATION OF PLANTS BELONGING TO RUBIACEAE FAMILY

In vitro propagation of species of this family has been reported using explants from mature trees.

Mature tree shoot apices of *Mitragyna parvifolia* responded to MS medium supplemented with BA (Roy *et al.*, 1988).

The response of apical buds of *Adina cordifolia* from younger (3yr.) mother plants on medium supplemented with BA along with NAA was better in comparison to those from older plants which responded to NAA alone. (Dubey *et al.*, 2004).

This study indicates the interrelation of the age of the mother plant and plant growth regulator requirements in establishment of shoot cultures.

In vitro shoots of species from this family were rooted on low strength medium supplemented with auxins.

CLONAL PROPAGATION OF PLANTS BELONGING TO OTHER FAMILIES

Buchanania lanzan: Anacardiaceae

Tissue cultures of this fruit tree have been initiated using juvenile tissues.

Decoated seeds were used to establish shoot cultures on MS medium supplemented with BA and NAA. (Shende and Rai, 2005).

Unlike other species wherein auxins are used to induce rooting, the *in vitro* shoots of *B. lanzan* rooted on MS medium supplemented with cytokinin Kinetin.

On the other hand when 2, 4-D was added to MS medium along with BA and NAA, embryogenic callus from immature embryos was induced. Maturation and conversion of somatic embryos of *B.lanzan* occurred on MS medium supplemented with ABA (Sharma *et al.,* 2005).

Corallocarpus conocarpus: Cucurbitaceae

Attempts at establishing *in vitro* cultures of this cucurbit have indicated the efficacy of BA in induction of axillary shooting in nodal explants. Experiments to initiate shoot cultures on media supplemented with various cytokinins singly and in combination with auxins revealed that higher concentrations of auxins caused callus formation. Axillary shooting was obtained on MS medium supplemented with BA along with low levels of NAA. Optimization of protocols is underway in our laboratory.

Tecomella undulata: Bignoniaceae

Various tissues have been used to establish cultures of this species namely, juvenile explants, (Nandwani *et al.,* 1995; Bhansali, 1993) nodes, (Rathore *et al.,*1991) and *in vitro* shoots (Nandwani *et al.,*1996).MS or WP media fortified with BA has been found to be effective in these reports. *In vitro* shoots or seedling required only cytokinin whereas nodes of mature trees responded on combination of BA and NAA as did callus.

Rooting of the regenerated shoots was induced on half-strength or full strength MS or WP medium fortified with auxins or on basal medium without PGRs after a pulse treatment.

SECONDARY METABOLITE PRODUCTION FROM CELL SUSPENSION CULTURES OF SOME ETHNO MEDICINAL PLANTS

The beneficial medicinal effects of plant materials result from the combinations of secondary products present in the plant. Plants are rich in a wide variety of secondary metabolites, such as tannins, terpenoids, alkaloids, and flavonoids and many more. The content of bioactive phytochemicals can be altered qualitatively and quantitatively, by various factors like stress, physical and chemical stimuli. Raskin et al (2002) have observed that elicitation-induced reproducible increases in bioactive molecules should significantly improve reliability and efficiency of plant resources in drug discovery while at the same time preserve wild species and their habitats. Of the 22 species selected in this article secondary metabolites isolation has been reported from only two species. Bahorun *et al.* (2005) have reviewed the primary and secondary metabolite composition of various parts of *Cassia fistula* and the cell cultures thereby derived. There is an urgent need to work in this direction as indicated by the paucity of data available on secondary metabolite production of ethno medicinal plants.

Table 3 summarizes the results reported using cell suspension cultures of these ethno medicinal species.

TABLE 3
Summary of Work Done Using Cell Suspension Cultures of Some Ethno Medicinal Plants

No.	Plant species	Result Obtained	Reference
1.	*Costus speciosus*	Increased biomass and sitosterol production	Kartosentono *et al.*, (2002)
2.	*C. speciosus*	Biotransformation of diosgenin	Indrayanto *et al.*, (2001)
3.	*C. speciosus*	Diosgenin production	Rathod and Khanna, (1978)
4.	*Cassia fistula*	Proanthocyanidin synthesis	Neergheen *et al.*, (2002)
5.	*C. fistula*	Polyphenolic production, biomass production, Proanthocyanidins synthesis	Chisolm and Steinberg, (2000)
6.	*C. fistula*	Production of Chrysophanol and physcion	Ahuja *et al.*, (1988)
7.	*C. fistula*	Bioconversion	Ahuja *et al.*, (1984)
8.	*C. fistula*	Production of an interferon-like antiviral factor	Babbar and Madan, (1981)
9.	*C. fistula*	Polyphenol production	Shah *et al.*, (1976)
10.	*C. fistula*	Polyphenol synthesis	Subbaiah *et al.*, (1974)

CONCLUSION

The contribution of plants to disease treatment and prevention is enormous and they remain an important source for the discovery of novel pharmacologically active compounds. It is believed that the majority of plant derived natural products remain undiscovered or unexplored for their biological activity (Gentry, 1993; Mendelson and Balick, 1995).

Only a few decades remain to survey the chemical constituents of a large part of the plant kingdom, given the threatened status of many ethno medicinal species. Advances in plant cell and tissue culture and genetic manipulation could provide new means for economic production of ethno medicinal plants and the chemicals that they produce and will thus serve to enhance their continued usefulness.

REFERENCES

Ahuja, A., Parshad, R. and Grewal, S. Bioconversion of vasicine by plant cell cultures. *Indian Journal of Pharmaceutical Sciences* 46(1): 17-9, 1984.

Ahuja, A., Parshad, R. and Kaushik, J. P. Anthraquinones from callus cultures of *Cassia fistula. Fitoterapia* 49: 496-500, 1988.

Anand, A., Rao S. C., Latha, R., Josekutty, P. C. and Balakrishna, P. Micropropagation of *Uraria picta*, a medicinal plant, through axillary bud culture and callus regeneration. *In Vitro Cellular and Developmental Biology - Plant*: 34: 136-140, 1998.

Anis, M., Husain, M. K. and Shahzad, A. *In vitro* plantlet regeneration of *Pterocarpus marsupium* Roxb., an endangered leguminous tree. *Current Science* 88(6): 25, 2005.

Babbar, O. P. and Madan, A. R. Studies on the possibilities to infect the cells of callus of *Cassia fistula* by an animal virus and induce production of interferon-like antiviral factor(s). *Indian Journal of Experimental Biology* 18: 349-355, 1981.

Bahorun, T., Neergheen, V. S. and Aruon, O. I. Phytochemical constituents of *Cassia fistula. African Journal of Biotechnology* 4(13): 1530-1540, 2005.

Balandrin, M. F., Klocke, J. A., Wurtele, E. S. and Bollinger, W. H. Natural plant chemicals: Sources of industrial and medicinal materials. *Science* 228: 1154-60, 1985.

Beck, S. L. and Dunlop, R. W. Micropropagation Of The *Acacia* Species: A Review. *In Vitro Cellular and Development Biology – Plant* 37(5): 531-538(8), 2001.

Bhansali, R. R. Bud culture for shoot multiplication and plantlet formation of *Tecomella undulate* (Rohida) a wood tree of arid zone. *Tropical Science* 33: 1-8, 1993.

Bhatt, I. D. and Dhar, U. Combined effect of cytokinins on multiple shoot production from cotyledonary node explants of *Bauhinia vahlii. Plant Cell Tissue and Organ Culture* 62(1): 79-83, 2000.

Briskin, D. P. Medicinal Plants and Phytomedicines Linking Plant Biochemistry and Physiology to Human Health. *Plant Physiology* 124: 507-514, 2000.

Britto, J. S., Natarajan, E. and Arockiasamy, D. I. *In Vitro* Flowering and Shoot Multiplication from Nodal Explants of *Ceropegia bulbosa* Roxb. var. bulbosa *Taiwania*, 48(2): 106-111, 2003.

Chand, S. and Singh, A. K. In vitro shoot regeneration from cotyledonary node explants of a multipurpose leguminous tree, *Pterocarpus marsupium* Roxb. *In Vitro Cellular and Development Biology – Plant* 40(5) 464-466(3), 2004.

Chapman, K. and Chomchalow, N. Production of Medicinal Plants in Asia. Proc. WOCMAP III, Vol. 5: Quality, Efficacy, Safety, Processing & Trade in MAPs Eds. E. Brovelli, S. Chansakaow, D. Farias, T. Hongratanaworakit, M. Botero Omary, S Vejabhikul, L.E. Craker and Z.E. Gardner .Acta Hort. 679, ISHS 2005 http://www.pubhort.org/members/showdocument?booknrarnr=679-6, 2005.

Chisholm, G. M. and Steinberg, D. The oxidative modification hypothesis of atherogenesis: an overview. *Free Radical Biology and Medicine* 28: 1815-1826, 2000.

D'Cruz, L. Phytochemical and Biochemical studies of some Ethnomedicinal plants of Dediapada forests. Ph.D. Thesis. Gujarat University, Ahmedabad, 2002.

D'Souza, K. J., Christian G., D'Cruz, L. and Braganza, V. B. *In vitro* conservation of some ethno medicinal species of the Dediapada Forests of South Gujarat. Abstract Proceedings: National Symposium on Plant Biotechnology: New Frontiers. CIMAP, Lucknow.18-20 November 2005. p. 87, 2005.

Dewan, A., Nanda, K. and Gupta, S. C. *In vitro* micropropagation of *Acacia nilotica* subsp. indica Brenan via cotyledonary nodes. *Plant Cell Reports* 12(1): 18-21, 1992.

Dhar, U. and Upreti, J. *In Vitro* Regeneration of a Mature Leguminous Liana (*Bauhinia vahlii* Wight & Arnott). *Plant Cell Reports* 18(7-8) 664-669, 1999.

Dubey, D., Koche, V. and Mishra, S. K. *In vitro* plant regeneration from apical buds of *Adina cordifolia* (Hook). p:72-77.In: Recent Trends in Biotechnology/edited by M.K. Rai, N.J. Chikhale, P.A. Wadegaonkar, P.V. Thakare and A.P. Ramteke. Jodhpur, Scientific, 2004.

Gamborg, O. L., Miller, R. A. and Ojjrima, K. Nutrients requirements of suspension cultures of soyabean root cells. *Experimental Cell Research* 50: 151-158, 1968.

Garg, L., Bhandari, N. N., Rani, V. and Bhojwani, S. S. Somatic embryogenesis and regeneration of triploid plants of *Acacia nilotica. Plant Cell Reports* 15: 855-858, 1996.

Gentry, A. H. Tropical forest biodiversity and the potential for new medicinal plants. ACS Symposium Series Washington, *DC American Chemical Society* 534, 13-20, 1993.

Gharyal, P. K. and Maheshwari, S. C. Differentiation in explants from mature leguminous trees. *Plant Cell Reports* 8: 550-553, 1990.

Gharyal, P. K. and Maheshwari, S. C. *In vitro* differentiation of plantlets from tissue cultures of *Albizia lebbeck* L. *Plant Cell Tissue Organ Culture* 2: 49-53, 1983.

Ghosh, N., Chatterjee, A. and Smith, D. W. Regeneration of *Albizia lebbeck* via somatic embryogenesis in suspension culture and study on the karyotype and growth_behavior._AIBS annual meeting, Baltimore Convention Center, Baltimore, Maryland.August 2-6, 1998. http://www.ou.edu/cas/botany-micro/bsa-abst/section10/abstracts/, 1998.

Ghosh, N., Chatterjee, A. and Smith, D. W. *Albizia lebbeck* Benth.: *In vitro* regeneration via embryogenesis, karyotypic analysis and SEM studies. "Botany 2001 Abstracts," published by Botanical Society of America. http://www.botany2001.org/section2/abstracts/45.shtml, 2001.

Gupta, S. C. and Agrawal, V. P. Micropropagation of woody taxa and plant productivity. In: Prasad, B. N., Ghimire, G. P. S., Agrawal, V. P., Eds. Role of biotechnology in agriculture. New York: International Science Publisher; pp. 37-52, 1992.

Indian Institute of Spice Research. Abstracts of M.Sc. and Ph.D Dissertations on spice crops. Calicut. Thomas J. Callus induction and *in vitro* regeneration from rhizome buds of *Curcuma amada* and *Curcuma aromatica* (PR 69). M.Sc Dissertation. Mahatma Gandhi University, 2005.

Indrayanto, G., Zumaroh, S., Syahrani, A. and Wilkins, A. L. C-27 and C-3 glucosylation of diosgenin by cell suspension cultures of *Costus speciosus. Journal of Asian Natural Products Research* 3(2): 161-8, 2001.

Jain, M., Rathore A. K. and Khanna P. Influence of kinetin and auxins on the growth and production of diosgenin by *Costus speciosus* (Koen) Sm. callus derived from rhizome. *Agricultural and Biological Chemistry* 48: 529, 1984.

Kartosentono, S., Suryawati, S., Indrayanto, G. and Zaini, N. C. Accumulation of Cd^2+ and Pb^2+ in the suspension cultures of *Agave amaniensis* and *Costus speciosus* and the determination of the culture's growth and phytosteroid content. *Biotechnology Letters* 24(9): 687-690(4), 2002.

Katwal, R. P. S., Srivastva, R. K., Kumar, S. and Jeeva, V. *State of Forest Genetic Resources Conservation and Management in India.* Forest Genetic Resources Working Papers, Working Paper FGR/65E. Forest Resources Development Service, Forest Resources Division. FAO, Rome, 2003.

Kulkarni , K. R. and D'Souza, L. Control of *in vitro* shoot tip necrosis in *Butea monosperma. Current Science* 78(2): 25, 2000.

Kulkarni, K. R., Hegde S. and D' Souza, L. Micropropagation of *Butea monosperma* (Lam) Taub In: Trends in Plant Tissue Culture and Biotechnology. (Ed) L. K. Pareek. Agro Botanical Publishers, Bikaner. 291-293, 1997.

Kumar, S., Sarkar, A. K. and Kunhikannan, C. Regeneration of plants from leaflet explants of tissue culture raised safed siris (*Albizia procera*). *Plant Cell, Tissue and Organ Culture* 54(3): 137-143, 1998.

Lloyd, G. and McCown, B. H. Commercially feasible micropropagation of mountain laurel, *Kalmia latifolia* by use of shoot tip cultures. *Proc. Intl Plant Prop. Soc.*, 30: 421-427, 1980.

Malabadi, R. B. *In vitro* propagation of spiral ginger (*Costus speciosus* (Koen.) Sm. *Indian Journal of Genetics and Plant Breeding.* 62: 277-278, 2002.

Malabadi, R. B., Mulgund, G. S. and Nataraja, K. Effect of triacontanol on the micropropagation of *Costus speciosus* (Koen.) Sm. using rhizome thin sections. *In Vitro Cellular and Developmental Biology - Plant*: 41(2): 129-132, 2005.

Malabadi, R. B., Mulgund, G. S. and Nataraja, K. Thiadiazuron induced shoot regeneration of *Costus speciosus* (Koen.) Sm using thin rhizome sections. *South African journal of Botany* 70(2): 255-278, 2004.

Mamun, A. N. K., Matin, M. N., Bari, M. A., Siddique, N. A., Sultana, R. S., Rahman, M. H. and Musa, A. S. M. Micropropagation of woody legume (*Albizia lebbeck*) through tissue culture. *Pakistan Journal of Biological Sciences* 7(7): 1099-1103, 2004.

Marthur, I. and Chandra, N. Induced regeneration in stem explants of *Acacia nilotica. Current Science* 52: 882-883, 1983.

Mendelson, R. and Balick, M. J. The value of undiscovered pharmaceuticals in tropical forests. *Econ. Bot.* 49, 223-228, 1995.

Murashige, T. and Skoog, F. A revised medium for rapid growth and bioassays with tobacco tissue cultures *Physiologia Plantarum* 15: 473-497, 1962.

Nandwani, D., Mathur, N. and Ramawat, K. G. *In vitro* shoot multiplication from cotyledonary node explant of *Tecomella undulata. Gartenbauwissenschaft –Munchen* 60: 65-68, 1995.

Nandwani, D., Sharma, R. and Ramawat, K. G. High frequency regeneration in callus cultures of a tree *Tecomella undulata. Gartenbauwissenschaft -Munchen* 61: 147-150, 1996.

Nayak, S. High frequency *in vitro* production of microrhizomes of *Curcuma amada. Indian Journal of Experimental Biology* 40: 230-232, 2002.

Neergheen, V. and Bahorun, T. Optimisation of growth and polyphenolic production in *Cassia fistula* callus cultures. *Asian Journal of Microbiology Biotechnology and Environmental Science* 4: 181-185, 2002.

Nehra, N. S., Becwar, M. R., Rottmann, W. H., Pearson, L., Chowdhury, K., Chang, S., Wilde, D. H., Kodrzycki, R. J., Zhang, C., Gause, K. C., Parks, D. W. and Hinchee, M. A. Invited review: Forest biotechnology: innovative methods, emerging opportunities. *In Vitro Cellular and Development Biology—Plant* 41: 701-717, 2005.

Nishi Kumari, Jaiswal, U. and Jaiswal, V. S. Induction of somatic embryogenesis and plant regeneration from leaf callus of *Terminalia arjuna* Bedd.*Current Science* 75(10): 1052-1055, 1998.

Pal, A. and Roy, A. Embryo culture of *Costus speciosus* (Koen.) Sm. to regenerate variable diosgenin yielding clones. *Plant Cell Reports* 10(11): 65-568, 1991.

Pandey, S. and Jaiswal, V. S. Micropropagation of *Terminalia arjuna* Roxb. from cotyledonary nodes. *Indian Journal of Experimental Biology* (8): 950-3, 2002.

Patil, V. M. Micropropagation studies in Ceropegia spp. *In Vitro Cellular and Developmental Biology - Plant* 3: 240-243, 1998.

Prakash, S., Elangomathavan, R., Seshadri, S., Kathiravan, K. and Ignacimuthu, S. Efficient regeneration of *Curcuma amada* Roxb. plantlets from rhizome and leaf sheath explants. *Plant Cell, Tissue Organ Culture* 78(2): 59-165, 2004.

Pullaiah, T. In Vitro Propagation Of *Pterocarpus Marsupium* Roxb Abstract Proceedings XVI International Botanical Congress. Abstract Number: 5119,Poster No. = 1624, 1999.

Ramawat, K. G. and Arya, H. C. Differentiation in hypocotyls explants of *Alibizia lebbeck. Comparative Physiology and Ecology* 7: 240-242, 1982.

Raskin, I., Ribnicky, D. M., Komarnytsky, S., Ilic, N., Poulev, A., Borisjuk, N., Brinker, A., Moreno, D. A., Ripoll, C., Yakoby, N., O'Neal, J. M., Cornwell, T., Pastor, I. and Fridlender, B. Plants and human health in the twenty-first century. *TRENDS in Biotechnology* 20(12): 522-531, 2002.

Rathore, A. K. and Khanna, P. Production of diosgenin from *Costus speciosus* (Koen.) Sm. and *Solanum nigram* L. suspension cultures. *Current Science* 47: 870-871, 1978.

Rathore, T. S., Singh, R. P. and Shekhawat, N. S. Clonal propagation of desert teak (*Tecomella undulata*) through tissue culture. *Plant Science.* 79: 217-222, 1991.

Report of the Task Force on Conservation and Sustainable use of Medicinal Plants. Planning Commission Government of India New, Delhi.p27. http://planningcommission.nic.in/aboutus/taskforce/tsk_medi.pdf, 2000.

Roy, A. T. *In vitro* propagation of *Albizia lebbeck* using axillary and apical buds. In: Dhawan V., Ganapathy P.M.and Khurana D.K. _Eds_, Tissue culture of forest species: recent researches in India. Proc. of National Workshop on mass propagation of tree species through *in vitro* methods. New Delhi, India. pp. 9-17, 1992.

Roy, A. and Pal, A. Propagation of *Costus speciosus* (Koen.) Sm. through *in vitro* rhizome production. *Plant Cell Reports* 10(10): 525-528, 1991.

Roy, K. S., Rahman, S. L. and Datta, P. C. *In Vitro* Propagation of *Mitragyna parvifolia* Korth. *Plant Cell, Tissue and Organ Culture* 12(1) 75-80, 1988.

Sadanandam, A., Ramesh, M., Umate, P. and Rao, V. Micropropagation of *Terminalia bellirica* Roxb. – a sericulture and medicinal plant. *In Vitro Cellular and Developmental Biology - Plant*: 41(3): 320-323, 2004.

Saxena , S. and Dhawan, V. Large-scale production of *Anogeissus pendula* and *A. latifolia* by micropropagation. *In Vitro Cellular and Developmental Biology - Plant* 37(5): 586-591(6), 2001.

Saxena, S. and Dhawan, V. Large-scale production of *Anogeissus pendula* and *A.latifolia* by micropropagation. *In Vitro Cellular and Development Biology - Plant* 7: 586-591, 2001.

Schenk, R. U. and Hildebrandt, A. C. Medium and techniques for induction and growth of monocotyledonous and dicotyledonous plant cell cultures. *Canadian Journal of Botany* 50: 199-204, 1972.

Sedjo, R. Toward Commercialization Of Genetically Engineered Forests: Economic And Social Considerations. RFF Report. March, 2006.

Sedjo, R. A. Biotechnology's potential contribution to global wood supply and forest conservation (Discussion Paper 01-51). Washington, DC: Resources for the Future, 2001.

Sedjo, R. A. Biotech and planted trees: Some economic and regulatory issues. *AgBioForum*, 6(3):113-119, 2003.

Shah, G. L. Flora of Gujarat State (part I& II) Sardar Patel University Publication, Vallabh Vidyanagar p:319,431, 1978.

Shah, R. R., Subbaiah, K. V. and Mehta, A. R. Hormonal effect on polyphenol accumulation in Cassia tissues cultured *in vitro*. *Canadian Journal of Botany* 54: 1240-1245, 1976.

Sharma, P., Koche, V., Quraishi, A. and Mishra, S. K. Somatic Embryogenesis In *Buchanania Lanzan* Spreng. *In Vitro Cellular and Development Biology - Plant*, 41(5): 645-647(3), 2005.

Shekawat , N. S., Yadav, J., Arya, V. and Singh, R. P. Micropropagation of *Anogeissus latifolia* (Roxb. Ex DC.) Wall. ex Guill. & Perr.-A Tree of Fragile Ecosystems. *Journal of Sustainable forestry* 11: 4, 2000.

Shende, S. and Rai, M. Multiple shoot formation and plant regeneration of a commercially useful tropical plant, *Buchanania lanzan* (Spreng). *Plant Biotechnology* 22(1): 59-61, 2005.

Singh, H. P., Singh, S., Saxena, R. P. and Singh, R. K. *In vitro* bud break in axillary nodal segments of mature trees of *Acacia nilotica*. *Indian Journal Plant Physiology* 36: 21-24, 1993.

Subbaiah, K. V., Mehta, A. R. and Shah, R. R. Studies on polyphenolcontent in tissue cultures of Datura and Cassia grown on defined medium. In: 3rd International congress of plant tissue culture, Leicester, pp.181, 1974.

Swamy, S. L., Ganguli, J. L. and Puri, S. Regeneration and multiplication of *Albizia procera* Benth. through organogenesis. *Agroforestry Systems* 60(2):113-121, 2004.

Threatened Biodiversity of Gujarat:Baseline Information. Gujarat Ecological Society, Maharaja Sayajirao University of Baroda, Gujarat Institute of Desert Ecology, 2001.

Tiwari, S., Shah, P. and Singh, K. In vitro propagation of *Pterocarpus marsupium* Roxb.:an endangered medicinal tree. *Indian journal of biotechnology*. 3: 422-425, 2004.

Upreti, J. and Dhar, U. Micropropagation of *Bauhinia Vahlii* Wight & Arnott A Leguminous Liana. *Plant Cell Reports* 16: 250-254, 1996.

Vaidya, G. K. and Braganza, V. J. Direct organogenesis and qualitative phytochemical analysis of *Vigna calcaratus* Roxb.: An *in vitro* study. *Journal of Cell and Tissue Research* Vol. 6(1): 541-544. 2006.

Vanisree, M., Lee, C. Y., Lo, S. F., Nalawade, S. M., Lin, C. Y. and Tsay, H. S. Studies on the production of some important secondary metabolites from medicinal plants by plant tissue cultures. *Botanical Bulletin of Academia Sinica*. 45: 1-22, 2004.

Yanchuk, A. D. The role and implication of biotechnological tools in forestry. *Unasylva* 204(52): 53-61, 2001.

—oo(O)oo—

23

CATHARANTHUS ROSEUS (PERIWINCKLE) : A POTENTIAL DRUG SOURCE FOR CANCER CHEMOTHERAPY AND BIOTECHNOLOGICAL INTERVENTIONS

C.C. GIRI, ARCHANA GIRI AND M. LAKSHMI NARASU

INTRODUCTION

Botanicals have been used for the treatment of diseases for centuries. Some of nature's most complicated chemistry takes place in the shoots and leaves of the plants. Plants can be considered as nature's most gifted chemists. Chemical analysis of plants with a suitable history for the treatment of cancer has resulted in the isolation of active principles with antitumour activity. Cancer is characterized by an uncontrollable rate of cell division and has been known for 3,500 years. The most successful plant material used for cancer chemotherapy, are the alkaloids of *Catharanthus roseus*. vincaleucoblastine (vinblastine) and leurocristine (vincristine). These compounds are extracted commercially from *C. roseus* and used alone or in combination with other therapies for the treatment of cancer. Vincristine is used to treat hodgkin's disease (a cancer of lymphatic system) and vinblastine is used to treat pediatric leukemia, a cancer of bone marrow and other blood cell producing organs. Both vinblastine and vincristine destroy cells by inhibiting cell division, and mitosis is halted during metaphase by affecting formation of microtubules. Therefore, for quite some time the plant material of *C. roseus* is successfully used as a source of drug for managing cancer by chemotherapy. In folklore, it has been reported as an oral hypoglycemic agent. Initially, the research group of Noble, Beer and Cults at the University of Western Ontario observed a peripheral granulocytopenia and bone marrow depression in rats produced by certain selected extracted fractions of *C. roseus* (Noble 1990). Investigations on these active fractions resulted in the isolation of the dimeric indole alkaloids vincaleukoblastine (VLB) as the sulfate salt (Svobodo,

1975). A number of dimeric indole alkaloids showing antileukemic activity have subsequently been isolated in due course of time.

Three distinct pharmacological activities that have been reported with a number of these alkaloids isolated from *C. roseus* are hypoglycemic, diuretic and having antitumour property. Six of the twenty-three reported dimeric alkaloids from this plant possess experimental oncolytic activity and two of these vincaleukoblastine and leurocristine have found extensive applications in the treatment of human neoplasmas. Podophyllotoxin from the Himalayan plant *Podophyllum hexandrum* is also an equally important source for chemotherapy for the management of cancer (Giri *et al.*, 2002).

Amid more than 90 alkaloids isolated from *C. roseus*, antimitotic bisindole alkaloids vinblastine and vincristine are of greatest clinical value. The plant material of *C. roseus* is the sole natural source of these important alkaloids and the yield of these alkaloids from plants is very low, thereby making the cost of these life saving drugs very expensive. Vinblastine was first isolated in 1959, and vincristine one year later. The compounds are structurally very similar and are well known to understand biochemically.

C. roseus produces vinblastine and vincristine in very small quantities which is less than 0.002 percent by weight. Pharmaceutical companies isolating vincristine charge upto $1 million per kilogram and for vinblastine it is $ 3.5 million per kilogram. Use of the drugs has been restricted because of their high price. Vinblastine and vincristine are now extracted commercially from *C. roseus* and used alone or in combination with other therapies for the treatment of cancer. Although a minor difference exists in the structure of vinblastine and vincristine but a significant difference has been observed in the spectrum of human neoplasmas, which respond to these alkaloids. However, it would be even more difficult (and expensive) to synthesize vinblastine in the laboratory. The synthesis of vinblastine is currently most elegantly worked out, but it's not cost-effective, so industry does not currently use synthesis to make vinblastine. Recently MIT researchers in USA have emphasized the importance of this important plant and have now figured out how to manipulate those complicated biosynthetic pathways to produce novel compounds, some of which could have pharmacological benefits (MIT, USA News Office, November 15, 2006).

Alkaloid chemistry of many members has been characterized. Among these vinblastine and vincristine are of particular interest because of their worldwide use in cancer chemotherapy. These alkaloids are produced *in vivo* by the condensation / dimerization of vindoline and catharanthine. It has long been known that plants are rich sources of important pharmaceuticals. But in many cases, compounds found in plants are produced at such a low levels that supply is limited and isolating even small amounts can cost millions, making them less than ideal for commercial exploitation. The pharmaceutical value of dimeric alkaloids, their low abundance and cost of production has promoted to search an alternative pathway. Since last one decade extensive efforts to generate cost effective high yielding cell and organ cultures of *C. roseus* is being undertaken as an alternative route to production of these valuable compounds.

Alkaloids accumulate as mostly as salts with organic acids in vacuoles of only some cells in a cluster, termed alkaloid cells. It has been argued that differentiation of storage compartments, such as laticiferous cells, are essential for alkaloid production. Dimeric indole alkaloids of *Catharanthus* are biosynthesized in specifically differentiated tissues (De Luca *et al.*, 1987, Endo *et al.*, 1987). It was established that the alkaloid metabolism is restricted to certain tissues and it is modulated by different developmental and environmental mechanisms. The expression of the enzymes involved in the late steps of vindoline biosynthesis, an important intermediate are under strong developmental control and modulated by tissue specific and light dependent factors (Aerts and De Luca 1992). Dimeric indole alkaloids have been detected in the light induced green callus, leaf organ cultures and multiple shoot cultures (Endo *et al.,* 1987, Loyola –Vargas *et al.,* 1986, Miura *et al.,* 1988 and Hirata *et al.,* 1991, 1992).

Transport of vacuolar strictosidine to the cytoplasm is essential for further alkaloid biosynthesis. Further, in addition to this the differentiation of chloroplast is also essential for vindoline biosynthesis. Therefore, differentiation and maturation of the tissues are the preconditions for the biosynthesis of more complex dimeric alkaloids (Datta and Srivastava 1997). Cell cultures of *C. roseus* accumulates high levels of monoterpinoid alkaloids, however, dimeric alkaloids are generally and routinely not produced by cell suspension cultures. This is because of the inability of these cultures to produce vindoline which is an important intermediate of biosynthetic pathway leading to dimeric alkaloid. Recently it has been found that vindoline biosynthesis is transcription-ally locked in *C. roseus* suspension cultures (Vazquez-Flota *et al.,* 2002). The surprising ability of transformed cultures to accumulate vindoline raises the possibility for its exploitation and the dimeric alkaloids have been detected in light induced green callus, leaf, organ cultures and transformed multiple shoot cultures.

ABOUT THE DRUG FROM *C. ROSEUS*: PREPARATION, ADMINISTRATION, TOXICITY, SIDE EFFECTS, PHARMACOGNOSY AND MODE OF ACTION

Drug preparations and uses:

Vincristine: Oncovin, VCR (317) 276-2000

Manufacturer : Elililly customer Service,Lilly corporate Center

Indianapolis, Indiana 46 285

Vincristine is clinically more important than vinblastine and is used for the treatment of childhood leukemias and is main component of several highly successful combination regimens. It is used mainly in combination therapy for the induction of remission in childhood acute leukemias. Vincristine along with prednison is the main therapy for induction of acute lymphatic leukemia. Complete remissions are obtained in 80- 90% of patients. It is also used for the treatment of Hodgkins and non- hodgkins lymphoma and vincristine is very successful here.

Unlike most other antineoplastic agents vincristine does not cause significant bone marrrow suppression. Therefore, it is often found in combination therapies with other drugs that are mylosuppressive. Other alkaloids cause bone marrow depression, mylosuppression (neutropenia) is major toxicity of vincristine. Vincristine is used alone or in combination with other antineopolastic medications for the treatment of many types of cancers including leukemia (cancer of white blood cells), lymphoma (cancer of lymph cells), malignant melanoma, breast cancer, lung cancer, cancer of uterine cervix, colorectal cancer and wilms tumour.

Vinblastine

Other names : Velbe, velban, VBL

Vinblastine is a drug used in the treatment of cancer. It interferes with the multiplication of cancer cells and slows or stops their growth and spread in the body.

Velban is one of the older chemotherapy drugs, which has been used and around for many years. Velban, when prepared for use becomes a clear and colorless liquid and is given by intravenous route only. It is most commonly used in the treatment of following cancers:

- Lymphomas
- Hodgkin's Disease
- Gestational throphoblastic disease
- Testis
- Breast Cancer

Velban is normally given once every 1-2 weeks. It is mainly useful in the treatment of Hodgkin's disease (cancer affecting the lymph glands, spleen and liver). Most important use of vinblastine is in the therapy of metastatic testicular tumour where it is combined with bleomycin and cisplastine. It has also been used for Hodgkin's and non Hodgkin's lymphoma.. In hodgkins disease it has been used in place of vincristine providing similar antitumour activity with less neuotoxicity.

Vindesine

It is the newest vinca alkaloid having significant activity in the treatment of acute leukemia, blast cris (chronic myelogenous leukemia) and Hodgkin's and non-Hodgkin's lymphoma. Vinblastine has been structurally modified to form desacetyl vinblastine amide (vindesine), which is used for the treatment of acute lymphoid leukemia in children. Vinorelbine is an anhydroderivative of 5'-norvinblastine. It is a semisynthetic derivative with broder anticancer activity and lower side-effects than vinblastine and vincristine. Lymphopenia is dose limiting toxicity of vindesine.

Toxicity

Peripheral neuropathy and other neurological toxicities:

The most common symptom is depressed achelles tendon reflex followed by parenthesis. Autonomic neuropathy occurs early in course of therapy resulting in abdominal pain, constipation, paralytic ileus, urinary retention and orthostatic hypotension. About 30-40 % of patients will respond to these drugs, and most responses are temporary. Vincristine is given at a dose of 1-2 mg into the vein every week for no more than 4-6 doses. If a permanent response does not occur no further vincristine is given.

Side Effects

Nausea, vomiting, bone marrow depression or decreased blood counts are the common side effects of the drug. It lowers the number of white blood cells, which guard against infection and platelet which prevent bleeding. Sores of mouth (stomatitis) and loss of hair (alopesia) are the common feature, that identifies the patient. This is because hair cells are very fast growing as are the cancer cells and since the drug oncovin is aimed at the very fast growing, it also kills some of the hair cells. Nervous system changes, tingling sensation, muscle weakness, jaw pains, loss of coordination, unsteadiness and constipation are the common side effects.

Pharmacology

Their absorption is unpredictable and they are usually given by i.v. infusion. They are very irritating to tissue. They are rapidly cleared from the plasma and excreted predominately by the liver by a combination of hepatic metabolism and biliary excretion. Vincristine is eliminated much more slowly than vinblastine and vindesine. Despite close similarity in their structure different vinca alkaloids have quite different therapeutic uses.

Mechanism of action

Microtubules are protein polymers responsible for various aspects of cellular shape and movement. Major component of microtubules is polymer tubulin, which is a protein containing two non-identical subunits α and β. Vinblastine and vincristine act by affecting the equilibrium between free tubulin dimers and assembled polymers.

There are slight structural differences between different vinca alkaloids but there is significant difference in their therapeutic uses and toxicity. Vinca alkaloids are cell- specific agents and block cells in mitosis. Their biological activity is explained by their specific binding to tubulin. Upon binding to vinca alkaloids tubulin dimers are unable to aggregate to form microtubules, this decreases the pool of free tubulin dimers available for microtubule assembly resulting in a shift of equilibrium towards disassembly.

They form paracrystalline aggregates which shifts the equilibrium further towards disassembly and microtubule shrinkage. They block mitosis with metaphase arrest. Vinca alkaloids bind to the tubulin dimers on the β subunit and induce a reversible self association into spiral polymers.

Biosynthetic pathway for indole alkaloids and possibilities of manipulation

C. roseus produces a wide range of indole alkaloids as a part of its secondary metabolism. Six alkaloids can be viewed as production targets. Four are obtained commercially from the intact plant and those are mentioned below:

- Powerful antineopolastic agents, vinblastine and vincristine
- Antihypertensive agents ajmalicine and serpentine
- Catharanthine
- Vindoline

The last two can be coupled enzymatically *in vitro* to form vinblastine and vincristine (Kutney *et al.,* 1988,). The low yield of these valuable indole alkaloids in plants has been the major motivation to produce them by cell and tissue cultures. Vinblastine and vincristine could not be produced in an economically viable bioprocess. The absence of vindoline in cell suspension cultures as a production system is the major limitation. Metabolic engineering or the manipulation of metabolic pathway may help in the overproduction of these target alkaloids using *in vitro* cultures. However, the complexity of the genetic, catalytic and transport processes of the terpenoid indole alkaloid pathway, presents a formidable challenge to the metabolic engineering of these compounds. The complexity and the paucity of knowledge on the critical enzymatic steps add more challenges for its manipulation. In addition to the economically important leaf derived alkaloids vincristine and vinblastine in *C. roseus*, root derived alkaloid ajmalicine, used in the treatment of circulatory disorders and hypertension. Secondary metabolites found in *C. roseus* arise from two major metabolic routes:

1. Shikimate pathway
2. Terpenoid pathway

Chorismate leads the shikimate pathway to the biosynthesis of aromatic acids phenylalanine, tyrosine and tryptophan. Monoterpenoid indole alkaloids and phenolic compounds are derived from tryptophan and phenylalanine (tyrosine), respectively. The terpenoid pathway yields secologonin, a second building block of terpenoid indole alkaloids (Fig. 1, Fig. 2). Over about 30 steps are involved in the synthesis of these six alkaloids. Only 16 enzymes have been characterized and cloning of 3 genes has been reported in early 1990s (Meijer *et al.*, 1993). But recently some more information has been added, besides the elucidation of the genes cloned, some regulatory elements are being characterized and could be promising step for the manipulation of this complex pathway (Hilliou *et al.*, 2001, Memelink *et al.*, 2001). Currently the basic peroxidase isozyme has received the designation of anhydrovinblastine (AVLB) synthase and been characterized, which is a immediate precursor of both vinblastine and vincristine (Sottomayor and Ros Barcelo 2003). Sub-cellular compartmentalization of enzymes- tissue specific and developmental control and environmental factors such as light and biotic factors are implicated in the regulation of these pathways.

Catharanthine and vindoline can be coupled enzymatically *in vitro* to form vinblastine and vincristine (Fig 3). The low yield of these valuable indole alkaloids in plants has been the major motivation to produce them by cell and tissue cultures, vinblastine and vincristine could not be produced in an economically viable tissue culture bioprocess. Shikimate and mevalonate pathways from primary metabolism feed the terpenoid indole alkaloid pathways. Tryptamine is produced from tryptophan by the enzyme tryptophan decarboxylase (TDC), which has been cloned (De Luca and Laflamme 2001). Secologanine is formed through the terpenoid pathway and a key enzyme for the flux limitation in this branch is geraniol 10-hydroxylase (G10 H) . Its provacuolar location has made the cloning of this cytochrome P-450 difficult. The co –enzyme of G10 H, NADPH cytochrome P-450 reductase has been cloned (Meijer *et al.*, 1993). The indole and terpenoid pathways converge with the condensation of tryptamine and secologanine to form strictosidine, which is the central precursor of all terpenoid indole alkaloids (Fig. 2). This step is catalyzed by enzyme strictosidine synthase (SSS), which has been cloned (Kutchan 1995, De Luca and Laflamme 2001). The current hypothesis is that the terpenoid branch is more limiting than tryptamine formation (Moreno *et al.*, 1993). Goddijen *et al.*, 1995 further supported this hypothesis, where he reported over-expression of TDC by an oncogenic transformation, without any increase in alkaloid production.

Intermediate branch points leading to the different classes of alkaloids are not well defined. Considerable progress has been done in characterizing the tabersonine to vindoline branch. Metabolic engineering of this branch is most critical for commercial success of vinblastine production in plant cell and tissue culture. Catharanthine and vindoline are coupled by a peroxidase to form vinblastine. Many cell and hairy root cultures produce catharanthine and tabersonine and thus limitation exist in the conversion of tabersonine to vindoline. Five to six enzymes in the tabersonine to vindoline branch have been characterized and reported cloning steps in this pathway (De Carolis and De Luca 1993, St.-Piere and De Luca 1995)

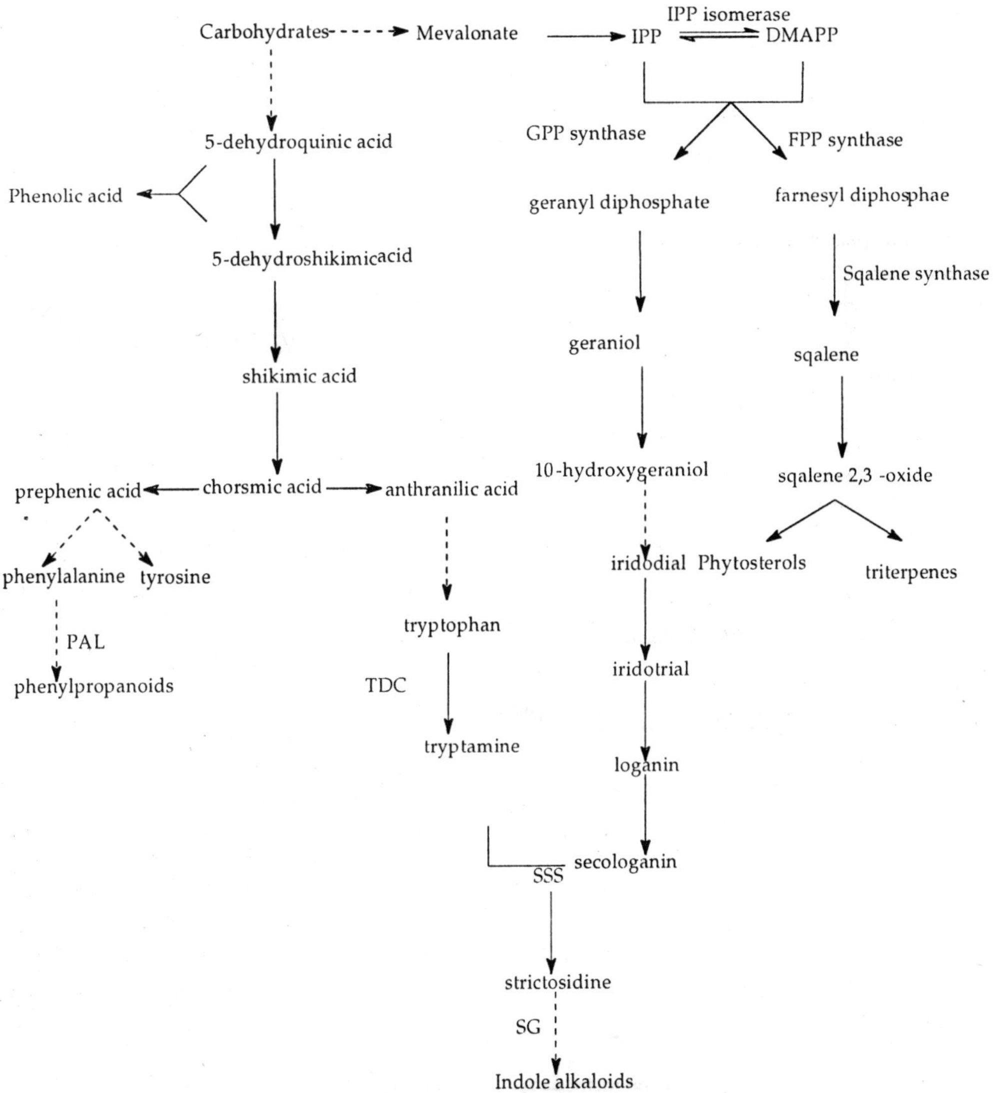

Figure 1. Biochemical pathway leading to the biosynthesis of phenolics, indole alkaloids and terpenes. AS: Anthranilate synthesis ; CM: Chorismate mutase ; FPP: Farnesyl diphosphate ; GPP: Geranyl diphosphate ; G10H: Geraniol -10- hydroxylase ; IPP : Isopentenyl diphosphate isomerase ; PAL: Phenylalanine ammonia lyase ; SG: Strictosidine b-glucosidase ; SSS: Strictosidine synthase ; TDC: Tryptophan decarboxylase

Experiments with leaves of *C. roseus* showed that early stages enzymes (TDC) and (STR) which contribute to the biosynthesis of early central intermediate strictosidine were expressed

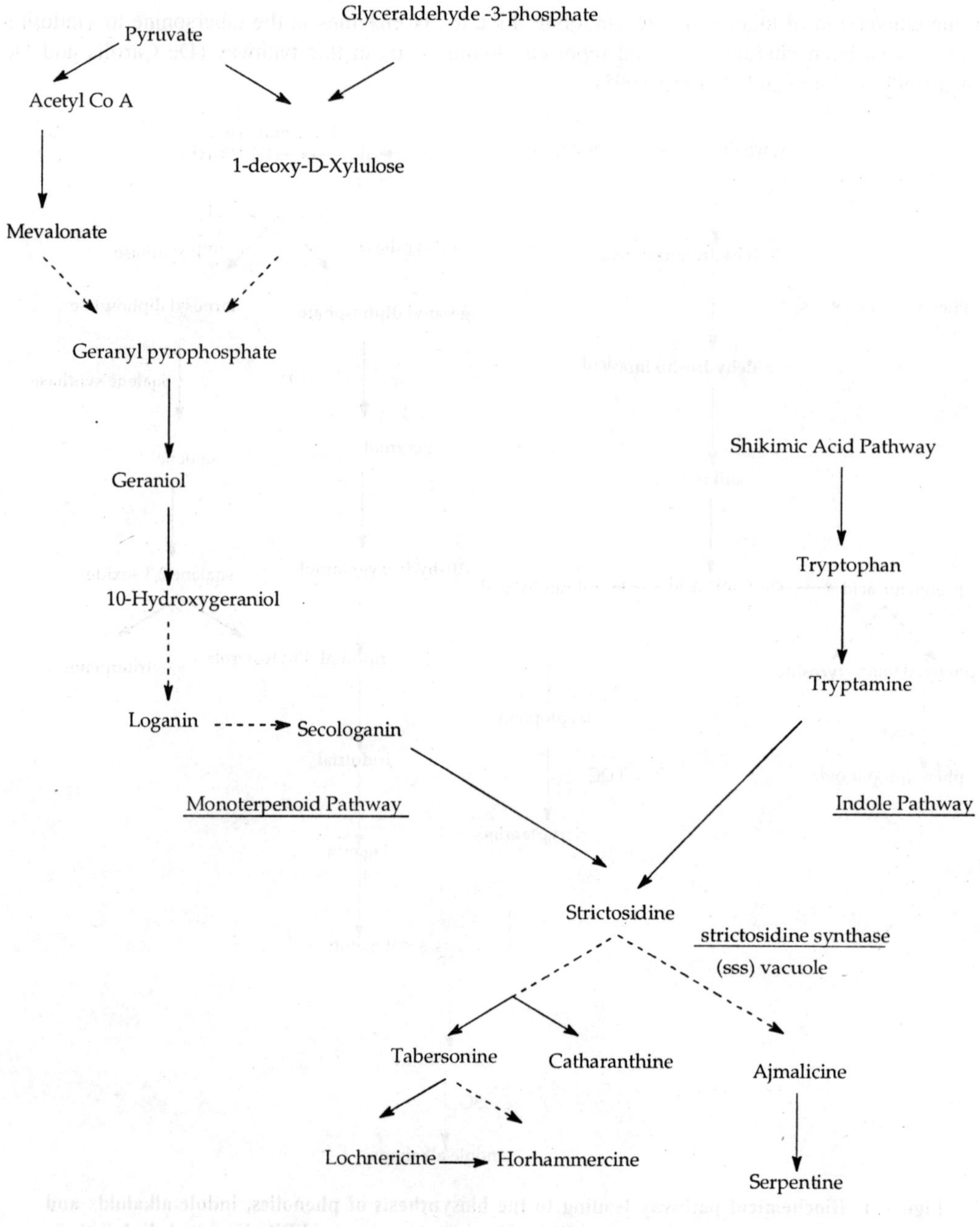

Figure 2. Proposed biosynthetic pathway leading to the indole alkaloids in *Catharanthus roseus.*

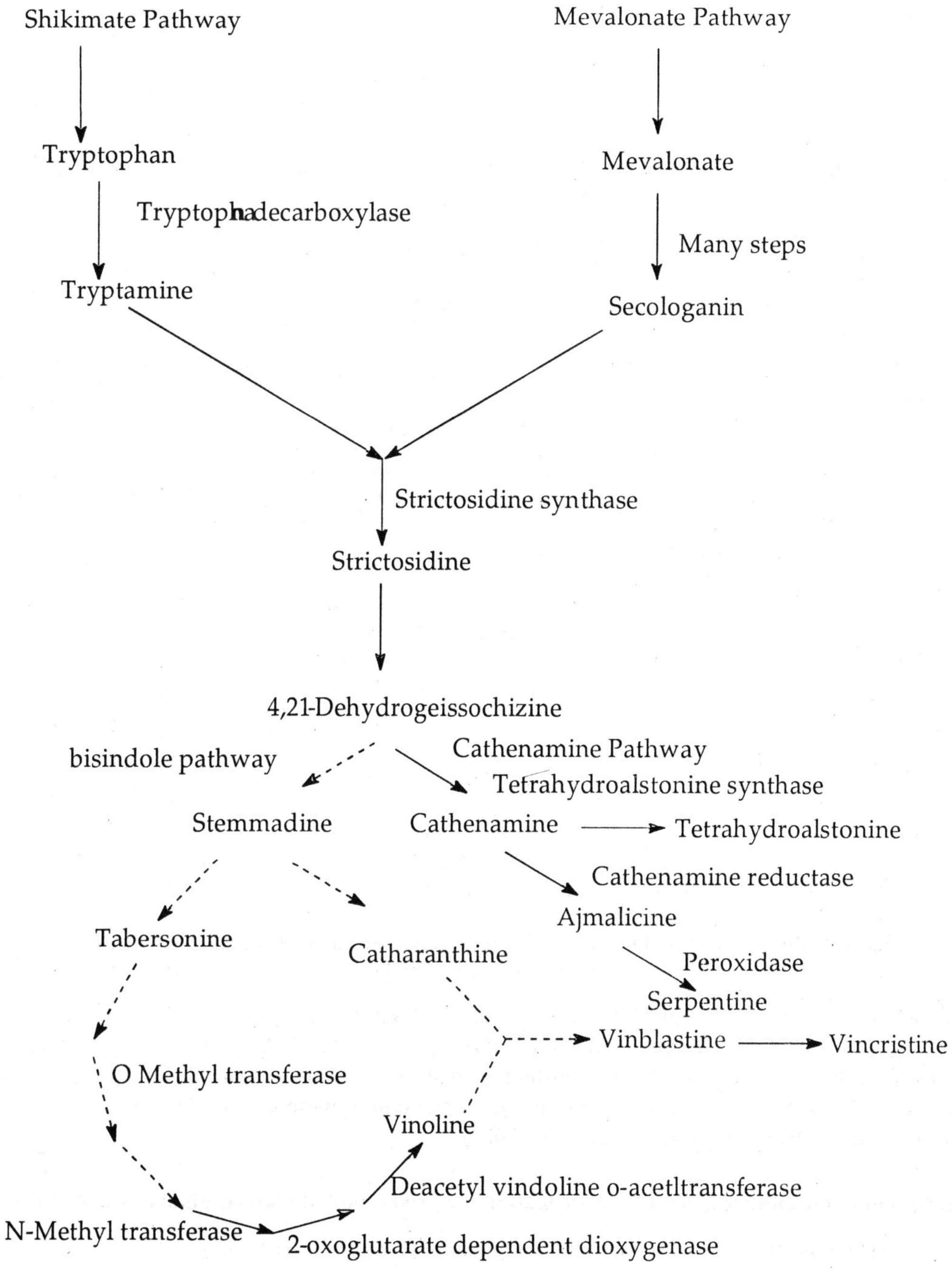

Figure 3. Schematic representation of monoterpenoid indole alkaloid pathway of *Catharanthus roseus*, dashed lines represent hypothesized steps (Shanks and Bhadra 1997).

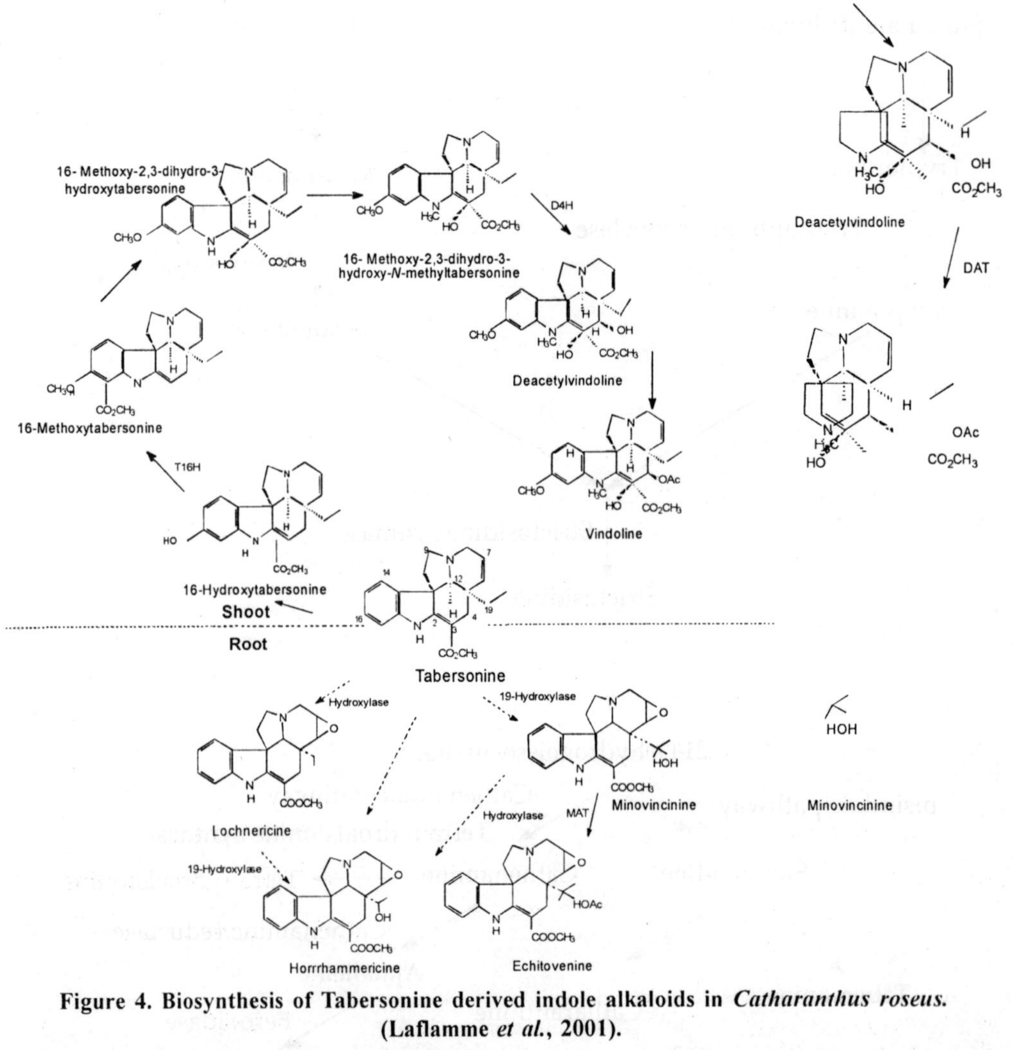

Figure 4. Biosynthesis of Tabersonine derived indole alkaloids in *Catharanthus roseus*. (Laflamme *et al.*, 2001).

specially in upper and lower epidermis of young leaves. Late stage enzymes like deacetoxyvindoline 4-hydroxylase (D4H) and Deacetyl vindoline 4-O-acetyltransferase (DAT), which catalyzes the last two steps in the biosynthesis of highly substituted alkaloid vindoline were localized to laticifer and idioblast cells in the mesophyll of leaves and the expression of these genes is shown to occur in a characteristic basipetal gradient (Irmler *et al.*, 2000).

Studies on tissue culture genetic transformation for production of dimeric alkaloids in *C. roseus*

The production of these valuable compounds in cell and tissue cultures of *C. roseus* may be one potential alternative to the supply source of the drug. Quite recently a study has shown that the demand for herbal remedies is threatening the valuable medicinal plants worldwide. The study carried out by the conservation organization WWF headed by Alan Hamilton warned that between 4,000 and 10,000 plants may be at risk (Source: New Scientist magazine, January, 2004).

Therefore, it becomes obvious and urgent for the production of pharmaceutically important compounds *in vitro* using plant cell and tissue through biotechnological interventions. Plant cell cultures mimicking a plant's natural processes in a laboratory flask when scaled up to the commercial level turns the culture into biochemical reactor. Plant cell cultures of *C. roseus* has received considerable attention and attracted many researchers by manipulating the *in vitro* conditions for enhanced production of indole alkaloids, i,e change in media composition , alteration in light, pH , precursor feeding, elicitation , immobilization and other *in vitro* manipulations (Table 1). Over past 30 years many attempts have been made to produce clinically useful compounds using classical plant cell culture techniques (Verpoorte *et al.,* 2002). Cell and tissue cultures of *Catharanthus roseus* : a literature survey II. Updating from 1988 to 1993 has already been carried out (Moreno *et al.,* 1995).

TABLE 1
Overview of Tissue Culture Studies and Production of Indole Alkaloids from *Catharanthus roseus* During Last One Decade

Culture System	Compounds of Interest	References
Suspension culture	Ajmalicine	Schlatmann *et al.,* 1995a
Two-stage batch process	Ajmalicine	Schlatmann *et al.,* 1995b
High density suspension cells	Ajmalicine	Schlatmann *et al.,* 1995c
Multiple shoots	Indole alkaloids	Mujib *et al.,* 1995
Suspension cells	Indole alkaloids	Jung *et al.,* 1995
Immobilized cell cultures	Indole alkaloids	Takemoto *et al.,* 1996
Elicited cell culture	Indole alkaloids	Moreno *et al.,* 1996
Elicited cell culture	Trytamine and phenols	Garnier *et al.,* 1996a
Callus cultures	Indole alkaloids	Choudhury and Gupta 1996
Elicited suspension culture	Indole alkaloids	Lundberg *et al.,* 1997
Cell culture (chemostat)	Catharanthine	Hong *et al.,* 1997
Cell culture (high density)	Ajmalicine	Schlatmann *et al.,* 1997
Cell suspension (Biotransformation)	Nerol	Hamada *et al.,* 1997
Differentiated cultures	Vinblastine	Datta and Srivastava 1997
Cell suspension	Indole alkaloids	Carpin *et al.,* 1997
Cell suspension	Indole alkaloids	Gantet *et al.,* 1997
Cell suspension	Indole alkaloids	Gantet *et al.,* 1998
Cell suspension	Indole alkaloids	Yahia *et al.,* 1998
Cell cultures	Secologanin, tryptamine	Contin *et al.,* 1998
Cell cultures (Alginate activated)	Key enzymes	Aoyagi *et al.,* 1998

Continued ...

... *Continued*

Culture System	Compounds of Interest	References
Cell suspension (Habituated)	Ajmalicine	Zheng *et al.*, 1999
Callus and cell culture	Indole alkaloids	Zhao *et al.*, 1999
Two-phase-culture (Air-lift reactor)	Indole alkaloids	Yuan *et al.*, 1999
Non-dividing cell culture	Ajmalicine	Schlatmann *et al.*, 1999
Cell aggregate culture	Ajmalicine,tryptamine	Kessler *et al.*, 1999
Suspension culture	Loganin, secologanin	Contin *et al.*, 1999a
Cell suspension (Precursor feeding)	Secologanin	Contin *et al.*, 1999b
Cell suspension culture	Indole alkaloids	Contin *et al.*, 1999c
Shoot cultures	Indole alkaloids	Choudhury and Gupta 1999
Cell cultures	Ajmalicine	Zhao *et al.*, 2000a
Cell culture	Indole alkaloids	Zhao *et al.*, 2000b
Cell suspension (Immobilized)	Ajmalicine, catharanthine	Lee and Shuleer 2000
Suspension culture	Ajmalicine, catharanthine	Zaho *et al.*, 2001 a,b
Suspension culture	Vindoline, serpentine	Zaho *et al.*, 2001c
Cell suspension	Vindoline	Vazquez-Flota *et al.*, 2002
Suspension culture	Indole alkaloids	El-Sayed and Verpoorte 2002
Cell culture	Indole alkaloids	Collu *et al.*, 2002
Cell culture	Anti-infective agents	Khafagi *et al.*, 2003
Shoot cultures	Vindoline	Dominguez *et al.*, 2004
Callus, cell suspension	Indole alkaloids	Kim *et al.*, 2004
Cell culture	Ajmalicine	Lee-Parsons *et al.*, 2004
Suspension culture	Indole alkaloids	El-Sajed *et al.*, 2004
Suspension cells	Catharanthene	Xu *et al.*, 2005a
Suspension cells	Catharanthene	Xu *et al.*, 2005b
Shoot cultures	Indole alkaloids	Hernández-Domínguez *et al.*, 2006
Embryogenic tissue	Indole alkaloids	Junaid *et al.*, 2006
Cell culture	Indole alkaloids	Aoyagi *et al.*, 2006

Irradiation with near-ultraviolet light stimulated dimeric alkaloid accumulation in shoot cultures of *C.* roseus (Hirata *et al.*, 1991, 1992, 1993). The activity of enzymes leading to the alkaloid biosynthesis seemed to be strongly modulated by light dependent factors. Studies on the light adapted cultures of hairy roots of *C. roseus* and indole alkaloid accumulation has been reported (Bhadra *et al.*, 1998).

Due to various biological and technological problems (limitations) in the past *C. roseus* cell cultures could not be commercially used for the production of therapeutically important alkaloids such as vinblastine and vincristine. Ironically the production of these compounds in cell cultures of *C. roseus* is a potential alternative for the supply of these valuable products.

In the next section attempts have been made to understand the possible factors controlling the synthesis of these valuable dimeric alkaloids. Datta and Srivastava (1997) reported traces of vinblastine from callus cultures of immature fruits. In mature seeds of *C. roseus*, vinblastine was absent but in four- week old seedlings the yield was substantial (60% of the mature plants). With further growth and maturity, the vinblastine yield increased, until the plants were 3 months old and the yield became stable at 12μg/g dry wt. In callus induced from the seedling the vinblastine yield decreased sharply and callus produced only 1.6 μ/g dry wt. However, from multiple shoots regenerated from the same callus vinblastine yield increased rapidly. Vinblastine from regenerated shoots was comparable with that of the seedlings of the same age. The amount of vinblastine and regeneration potential decreased with age. Alkaloids accumulate as salts with organic acids in vacuoles of only some cells in a cluster called alkaloid cells. This indicates a link between the morphogenetic and metabolic differentiation. Datta and Srivastava (1997) reported that greening of callus and emergence of shoot buds were the critical steps when vinblastine production showed sharp elevations.

Callus cultures showing emergence of multiple shoots and young seedlings (4- week old) exhibited similar sharp increases in the biosynthesis of vinblastine. They hypothesized that during these early developmental stages key biosynthetic enzymes for final stages of vinblastine production are synthesized and required storage compartments become fully differentiated. Even in callus cultures presence of vinblastine indicates the possible presence of minute patches of differentiated tissues and that vinblastine productivity is quantitatively proportional to the extent of differentiation in the tissues.

Cell cultures accumulated high levels of monoterpenoid alkaloids like serpentine, catharanthine and tabersonine (Table 1). Although, the biosynthesis of many of the monomeric indole alkaloids including ajmalicine and catharanthine has been observed in plant cell cultures, the production of vinblastine and vincristine has not been reproducibly demonstrated in undifferentiated suspension cultures. The inability of cell cultures to accumulate vindoline consistently resulted in the failure to produce important dimeric indole alkaloids. Enzyme and metabolic studies with plants suggested that vindoline biosynthesis is restricted to the aboveground organs and that pathway beyond tabersonine is not expressed in tissue cultures. These studies raised the possibility that cell cultures lacked the cell types required to accommodate the late stages of vindoline biosynthesis. St-Pierre *et al.*, (1999) reported that the formation of vindoline in intact plant involves two separate cell types requiring the translocation of pathway intermediate. *In situ* hybridization and immunolocalization studies confirmed that tryptophan decarboxylase and strictosidine synthase which are involved in the formation of strictosidine were expressed only in the epidermis of aerial tissues and in cortical cells of the root apical meristem. Expression of desacetoxy vindoline-4 hydroxylase (D4 H) and deacetylvindoline-4-O-acetyl transferase (DAT) which catalyze the last two steps in vindoline biosynthesis, occurred exclusively in laticifers and idioblasts of aerial tissues. Recently it has been found that vindoline biosynthesis is transcription-ally locked in *C. roseus* suspension cultures (Vazquez-Flota *et al.*, 2002).

Hairy root cultures appear to be more stable than cell cultures. The plus point of hairy roots for production of alkaloids, have been attributed to their high level of differentiation combined with genetic stability and to the fact that they can be readily transformed (Table 2). Therefore, many studies used hairy root cultures for enhanced yields in general and indole alkaloids in particular (Bhadra *et al.*, 1993, Giri *et al.*, 1997, Giri *et al.*, 2001a, Giri *et al.*, 2001b, Giri *et al.*, 2003). Rijhwani and Shanks (1998a) investigated hairy root cultures for their ability to produce secondary metabolites. They reported tabersonine, lochnericine and horhammericine are major products in addition to ajmalicine and serpentine but not vindoline (Shanks *et al.*, 1998). The biosynthesis and accumulation of specific metabolites are influenced by tissue type rate limitations in hairy roots are different in hairy roots than in cell suspension cultures. O' Keefe *et al.*, (1997) reported low levels of vindoline in hairy root cultures transformed with *Agrobacterium rhizogenes.* Hairy root cultures of *C. roseus,* with their apparent genetic stability, differentiation and amenability to genetic transformation have been investigated for the production of indole alkaloids (Rhijhwani and Shanks 1998 a,b). In addition, suspension cultures established after leaf disc transformation with either *A. rhizogenes* or *Agrobacterium tumefaciens* accumulated catharanthine as well as low levels of vindoline and showed deacetylvindoline -o- acetyltransferase activity which catalyzes last step in vindoline biosynthesis. The surprising ability of transformed cultures to accumulate vindoline raises the possibility that the differential cell type specific expression required for this to occur in leaves and stem may not be absolutely needed under all circumstances. Therefore, hope still persists that the plant cell cultures can be engineered rather than whole plants to produce targeted therapeutic compounds in higher quantities and lower cost. Biotransformation of valuable indole alkaloids using cell and organ culture can be useful for the production of dimeric alkaloids (Giri *et al.*, 2001c). In callus vinblastine accumulation is very low, however from multiple shoots regenerated from callus vinblastine yield increased rapidly. Dimeric alkaloids have been detected in light induced green callus, leaf organ cultures and multiple shoot cultures.

TABLE 2

Studies on Genetic Transformation, Isolation of Gene for Key Enzyme and Expression of Genes for Production of Indole Alkaloids from *Catharanthus roseus*

Culture System Candidate Genes	Compounds of Interest	References
Hairy roots/cell suspension	Indole alkaloids	Jung *et al.*, 1995
Crown gall	Tryptamine	Goddijn *et al.*, 1995a
Tryptophan decarboxylase(OE)	Terpenoid indole alkaloids	Goddijn *et al.*, 1995b
Hairy root	Indole alkaloids	Bhadra and Shanks 1995
Callus/ipt	Indole alkaloids	Garnier *et al.*, 1995
Transgenic tissue	Indole alkaloids	Garnier *et al.*, 1996b
Transgenic tissue	Indole alkaloids	Garnier *et al.*, 1996c
Deacetoxyvindiline-	Vindoline	Vazquez *et al.*, 1997

Continued ...

... *Continued*

Culture System Candidate Genes	Compounds of Interest	References
4-hydroxylase,a2-oxoglutarate dependent-dioxygenase	biosynthesis	
Transformed tissue	Indole alkaloids	Carpin *et al.*, 1997
Hairy root	Indole alkaloids	Bhadra and Shanks 1997
Methyljasmonate activated transgenic callus	Indole alkaloids	Dymov *et al.*, 1997
Tryptophan decarboxylase, Strictosidine synthase	Strictosidine	Godoy and Loyola 1997a
Tumour suspension culture	Indole alkaloids	Godoy and Loyola 1997b
Transgenic cell line	Indole alkaloids	Whitmer *et al.*, 1998a
Transgenic cell line	Indole alkaloids	Whitmer *et al.*, 1998b
Hairy root/	Indole alkaloids	Rodriguez and
Protein kinase	Hemandez 1998a	
Tyrosine phosphatase/	Indole alkaloids	Rodriguez and Hemandez 1998b
Hairy root	Indole alkaloids	Hemandez 1998b
Hairy root	Indole alkaloids	Rijhwani and Shanks 1998
Transformed root culture	Indole alkaloids	Palazon *et al.*, 1998
Hairy root	Indole alkaloids	Moreno *et al.*, 1998
Strictosidine beta-D glucosidase	Strictosidine	Luijendijk *et al.*, 1998
Tryptophan decarboxylase, Strictosidine synthase	Indole alkaloids	Canel *et al.*, 1998
Hairy root	Indole alkalcdeoids	Bhadra *et al.*, 1998
Transgenic shoots	Indole alkaloids	Zarate *et al.*, 1999
Isochorismate synthase	Indole alkaloids	van *et al.*, 1999
Hairy root	Tabersomine	Morgan and Shanks 1999
Hairy root	Indole alkaloids	Moreno *et al.*, 1999a
Hairy root	Indole alkaloids	Moreno *et al.*, 1999b
ORCA 3a jasmonate responsive transcription factor	No of metabolic links	van *et al.*, 2000
Hairy root	Indole alkaloids	Morgan *et al.*, 2000

Continued ...

... *Continued*

Culture System Candidate Genes	Compounds of Interest	References
Strictosidine beta-D glucosidase	Terpinoid alkalois	Greelings *et al.*, 2000
Hairy root	Indole alkaloids	Morgan *et al.*, 2000
Strictosidine beta-D glucosidase	Terpinoid alkalois	Zarate *et al.*, 2000
Transformed cell Line T22	Indole alkaloids	Whitmer *et al.*, 2002a
Transformed cell Line S1	Indole alkaloids	Whitmer *et al.*, 2002b
Hairy root/ 3-hydroxy-Methyleglutaryl-CoA Reductase	indole alkaloids	Ayora-Talavera *et al.*, 2002
Transformed cell Line S1	Indole alkaloids	Whitmer *et al.*, 2003
Hairy root	Taberosonine	Rodriguez *et al.*, 2003
MEP pathway genes	Indole alkaloids	Burlat *et al.*, 2004
Hairy root	Plant regeneration	Choi *et al.*, 2004
Hairy root	Indole alkaloids	Batra *et al.*, 2004
Hairy root	Tryptamine/Serpentine	Hughes *et al.*, 2004a
Hairy root/ Anthranilate synthase	Indole alkaloids	Hughes *et al.*, 2004b
Terpenoid alkaloid biosynthetic genes	Indole alkaloids	Dutta *et al.*, 2005
Hairy root /	Indole alkaloids	Peebles *et al.*, 2005
Hairy root /	Indole alkaloids	Hong *et al.*, 2006a
Hairy root / Tryptophan decarboxylase	Indole alkaloids	Hong *et al.*, 2006b
Hairy root / Anthranilate synthase	Indole alkaloids	Peebles *et al.*, 2006
Engineered cell cultures	Indole alkaloids	Pasquali *et al.*, 2006
Hairy root/ Kinetic modeling	Indole alkaloids	Leduc *et al.*, 2006

Metabolic engineering of terpenoid indole alkaloid biosynthesis

Genetic engineering of plant cell and tissue cultures for enhanced production of pharmaceutically valuable alkaloids holds promise due to the recent advances in plant molecular, developmental biology and recombinant DNA technology. In addition the metabolic engineering offers potential to enhance the yield of valuable natural products from plants. A growing body of knowledge exists in the cloning of genes from alkaloid biosynthetic pathway, in their expression by sense and antisense techniques, and in gene activation and gene expression studies in response to environmental perturbation such as elicitation and light are the key factors for pathway manipulation (Kutchan, 1995).

The complexity of biosynthetic pathway of indole alkaloids has presented a major challenge for its production and combinations of approaches are essential for enhanced production. However, we cannot overlook the tremendous possibilities for the manipulation of the biosynthetic pathway using *in vitro* cultures with special reference to the transgenic hairy root and transformed shoot culture system. Recently, plant specific issues has been addressed for the metabolic engineering of plants for alkaloid pathway manipulation (Hughes and Shanks 2002). Currently, the finding explaining the jasmonate-induced epoxidation of tabersonine by a cytochrome P-450 in hairy root cultures of *C. roseus* has developed hope for a global metabolic engineering strategy for vindoline production (Rodriguez *et al.,* 2003).

Rational genetic manipulation of an alkaloid producing pathway requires determination of the points in the pathway at which flux is most severely restricted (Shanks *et al.,* 1998). In the beginning only one gene of a key step has been over expressed in *C. roseus,* but indole alkaloid production did not increase (Goddijn *et al.,* 1995). This result must be due to the complex interactions between biosynthetic pathways in which several steps in the network share flux control.

Flux into the alkaloid pathways, diversion of flux at intermediate branches, and lack of final conversion at the end of a specific branch all appear to affect alkaloid production in *C. roseus* cell and tissue culture. Experiments including light adaptation and genetic modification of a single step are useful in gaining information about the pathway. Adding enzyme inhibitors, elicitors, and precursors are useful in trying to pin point rate limiting branches and develop a working model of the pathways and these steps can be pursued for genetic modification (Rajhwani and Shanks 1998b). Recently, quantification of metabolic flux in plant secondary metabolism by biogenetic organizational approach has been emphasized by grouping metabolites of similar biosynthetic origin (Morgan and Shanks 2002). Shank *et al.,* (1998) have reported quantification of alkaloids to identify points of possible flux limitations and challenges in metabolic engineering of *C. roseus* for indole alkaloid production. They have also analyzed responses of the levels of several alkaloids in different branches of the pathway in response to light adaptation, precursor feeding and fungal elicitation.

Genetic engineering of microorganisms is feasible and one can thus consider the possibilities of transferring the production of a plant secondary metabolite into a microorganism. To do this one has to know the biosynthetic pathway of the compound and identify the enzymes involved and the genes coding for the enzymes. Most of the plant secondary metabolites result from a pathway involving a large number of steps (as many genes are involved). For secondary metabolite pathway 10-20 steps and the same number of genes are quite normal. Only a few secondary metabolite pathways are completely known at the level of enzymes, consequently very few genes from secondary metabolism are known (except some genes from flavonoid pathway). In the case of alkaloids only a few isolated steps from the biosynthetic pathway have been studied to the level of genes e.g. strictosidine synthase, tryptophan decarboxylase (Geerlings *et al.,* 2000). Even if all the genes are known, transferring a large number of genes to a microorganism is not feasible, as the enzymes produced have to work in a concerted way. Furthermore, in plants secondary metabolism is often compartmentalized on subcellular or cellular levels. This will be impossible to realize in microorganisms. Genetic engineering of microorganisms does not seem to be a practical approach, exploitation of genetic information of plant cell can pave the way. Plant cells are totipotent i.e. each cell carries all genetic the information for all the plant functions, including the biosynthesis of secondary metabolites. The activity of two enzymes in the late steps of vindoline biosynthesis (NMT) and (DAT) could be detected only the hypocotyls and cotyledons of the seedlings. It was previously found that a part of the vindoline biosynthesis could be localized in chloroplasts of the leaf cells and specifically associated with the thylakoids.

St. Pierre and De Luca (1995) reported detailed investigations on enzymology and of regulation of vindoline biosynthesis. Tabersonine is transformed to vindoline through a sequence of six enzymatic steps. These constitute the late stages of vindoline biosynthesis , which seems to absent from *C. roseus* cell cultures. They reported characterization of an enzyme responsible for conversion of tabersonine 16-hydroxy tabersonine and showed it to be a microsomal cyt P-450 dependent monooxygenase. This enzyme is found in young leaves of intact plants and is developmentally regulated and light regulated in germinating seedlings.

Laflamme *et al.,* (2001) reported cloning and biochemical characterization of minovincine-O- acetyltransferase (MAT). The gene, which is expressed only in roots, is a homolog of DAT that is expressed in idioblasts and laticifers. They have presented the evidence that MAT whose function is to acetylate minovincine and /or horhammericine may also be involved in vindoline biosynthesis in the special circumstances created during plant transformation. The terminal step in the biosynthesis of the monoterpenoid indole alkaloids, vindoline and minovincine are catalyzed by separate acetyl Co-A dependent O- acetyltransferase in *C. roseus.* Laflamme *et al.,* (2001) reported isolation of two genes that had 63% nucleic acid similarity and whose deduced amino acid sequences were 78% identical. All the terpenoids indole alkaloids are derived from a central intermediate strictosidine . Indole portion is derived from tryptamine, which is formed by decarboxylation of tryptophan. The terpenoid portion of strictosidine, secologonine is known to be derived from geranyl pyrophosphate, which is subsequently converted, to geraniol, 10 hydroxygeraniol and loganin by multiple steps (Meijer *et al.,* 1993). Moreno *et al.,* 1993 reported that based on precursor feeding and enzyme activity studies a current hypothesis is that precursors from the terpenoid pathway are a flux limitation in cell suspension cultures.

Contin *et al.,* (1998) reported that mevalonic acid is not the only precursor of strictosine, a novel triose phosphate / pyruvate pathway is implicated as the major provider of carbon for the monoterpenoid pathway leading to the indole alkaloids. The complexity of the indole alkaloid biosynthetic pathways has presented a major challenge for enhancement of secondary metabolite productivity and a combination of approaches will be essential for enhanced production. The secondary metabolite pathway of *C. roseus* has been reviewed in detail by Meijjer *et al.,* (1993). In some findings it has also been reported that conversion of tabersonine into lochnericine and horhammericine possibly diverts the flux away from the tabersonine to vindoline branch.

Advances in cloning of genes in the indole alkaloid pathway indicate that metabolite engineering may be used to eliminate some bottlenecks in the pathways (Kutchan 1995, Hilliou *et al.,* 2001, Memelink *et al.,* 2001, Verpoorte *et al.,* 2002, Rodriguez *et al.,* 2003). Metabolic studies with tools such as fungal elicitation to manipulate flux will be necessary and complimentary to genetic approaches in the advancement of production goal.

CONCLUSION

In future, the majority population of the world will depend on plant derived medicaments and it will remain as the primary source of health care. This is true because, with the increased population and demand for drug the costs and availability of synthetic and gene-based products may not be sufficient. Recently, it is emphasized that a long-term mission with a new vision has to be created by exploiting the natural products from medicinal plants in drug discovery (Cordell 2002). Despite intense efforts using plant cell, tissue and hairy root cultures it has failed to prove itself appropriate for the synthesis of two bisindole alkaloids that are composed of catharanthine and vindoline monomers. Currently many studies have been carried out on the enzymology and regulation of the biosynthesis of theses monomers, which may lead to the development of new strategies for their production. In the recent past several biosynthetic genes involved in the tropane and terpenoid indole alkaloids have now been isolated. Further, the early events of signal perception, transduction and function of gene promoters have been studied in relation to alkaloid metabolism (Facchini 2001). Recently, the inducible promoter system in *C. roseus* hairy roots have been characterized (Hughes *et al.*, 2002). In addition, we have to also attempt to find out the existence of new bioactive chemicals in already studied plants such as *C. roseus*. Over the years in the last two decades the research in the medicinal plants has been the introduction of the simple and productive bioassays for the bio-actively-guided isolation of active principles. Recently, the pharmacognosy and biotechnology of *Catharanthus* alkaloids has been well documented (van Der Heijden *et al.*, 2004). Another important finding has been the development of hyphenated techniques involving HPLC, LC/UV, LC/MS and LC/NMR etc. for the early detection and identification of new compounds in the crude plant extract (Hostettmann and Marston 2002). Keeping in view the limitations in the isolation and characterization of dimeric alkaloids from *in vitro* cultures of *C. roseus*, the above mentioned recent developments would be helpful in the early detection and identification of compounds of interest. This may facilitate the proper exploitation of *in vitro* culture systems such as cell suspension, transgenic hairy roots and shooty teratomas. Recently, micropropagation as a tool for production of high value plant based pharmaceuticals has been emphasized (Debnath *et al.*, 2006). More studies on the real time analysis of the metabolic flux and the pathway in transformed cultures may help in the metabolic engineering. Further, the role of the non-mevalonate pathway in indole alkaloid production by *C. roseus* hairy roots have also been studied (Hong *et al.*, 2003). Therefore, an enhanced understanding of the biochemical pathway, the factors regulating their accumulation especially the morphological and metabolic differentiation may promote the metabolic engineering for the production of pharmaceutically valuable alkaloids from *C. roseus*. Recent developments in the study of gene-to-gene metabolic network, integrated transcript and metabolic profiling and transcriptome analysis in *Catharanthus roseus* has open up enormous possibilities for the could be the bench mark for metabolic engineering efforts and further biotechnological interventions in this important plant (Rischer *et al.*, 2006a, Rischer *et al.*, 2006b, Shukla *et al.*, 2006, McCoy and O'Connor 2006).

REFERENCES

Aerts, R. J. and De Luca, V. Phytochrome is involved in the light regulation of vindoline biosynthesis in *Catharanthus Plant Physiol* 100: 1029-1032, 1992.

Aoyagi, H., Yasuhira, J. and Tanaka, H. Alginate promotes production of various enzymes by *Catharanthus roseus* cells. *Plant Cell Reports* 17: 243-247, 1998.

Aoyagi, H., Sakamoto, Y., Asada, M. and Tanaka, H. Indole alkaloids production by *Catharanthus roseus* protoplasts with artificial cell walls containing of guluronic acid rich alginate gel. *Journal of Fermentation and Bioengineering* 85(3): 306-311, 1998.

Aoyagi, H., Akimoto-Tomiyama, C. and Tanaka, H. Preparation of mixed alginate elicitors with high activity for the efficient production of 52 -phosphodiesterase by *Catharanthus roseus* cells *Biotech Lett* 28: 1567-1571, 2006.

Ayora-Talavera, T., Chappell, J., Lozoya-Gloria, E. and Loyola-Vargas, V. M. Overexpression in *Catharanthus roseus* Hairy Roots of a Truncated Hamster 3-Hydroxy-3-Methylglutaryl-CoA Reductase Gene *Appl Biochem and Biotechnol* 97: 135-145, 2002.

Batra, J., Dutta, A., Singh, D., Kumar, S. and Sen, J. Growth and terpenoid indole alkaloid production in *Catharanthus roseus* hairy root clones in relation to left- and right-termini-linked Ri T-DNA gene integration *Plant Cell Rep* 23: 148-154, 2004.

Aoyagi, H., Yasuhira, J. and Tanaka, H. Alginate promotes production of various enzymes by *Catharanthus roseus* cells. *Plant Cell Reports* 17: 243-247, 1998.

Bhadra, R., Vani, S. and Shanks, J. V. Production of indole alkaloids by selected hairy root lines of *Catharanthus roseus*. *Biotechnol. Bioeng.* 41: 581-592, 1993.

Bhadra, R. and Shanks, J. V. Transient studies of nutrient uptake, growth and indole alkaloid accumulation in heterotrophic cultures of hairy roots of *Catharanthus roseus*. *Biotechnol. Bioeng.* 55: 527-534, 1997.

Bhadra, R., Morgan, J. A. and Shanks, J. V. Transient studies of light-adapted cultures of hairy roots of *Catharanthus roseus*: growth and indole alkaloid accumulation. *Biotechnol. Bioeng.* 60: 670-678, 1998.

Burlat, V., Oudin, A., Courtois, M., Rideau, M. and St-Pierre, B. Co-expression of three MEP pathway genes and geraniol 10-hydroxylase in internal phloem parenchyma of *Catharanthus roseus* implicates multicellular translocation of intermediates during the biosynthesis of monoterpene indole alkaloids and isoprenoid-derived primary metabolites. *Plant J* 38: 131-141, 2004.

Canel, C., Lopes-Cardoso, M. I., Whitmer, S., van der, F. L., Pasquali, G., van der Heijden, R., Hoge, J. H. C. and Verpoorte, R. Effects of over-expression of strictosidine synthase and tryptophan decarboxylase on alkaloid production by cell cultures of *Catharanthus roseus*. *Planta* 205(3): 414-419, 1998.

Choudhury, S. and Gupta, K. Effect of CCC on growth and alkaloid production in *Catharanthus roseus* (L.) G.Don. *Indian Journal of Plant Physiology* 1(3): 163-167, 1996.

Choudhury, S. and Gupta, K. Effect of dikegulac on biomass and alkaloid production in *Catharanthus roseus* (L) G. Don under in vitro condition. *Indian Journal of Experimental Biology* 37(6): 594-598, 1999.

Canel, C., Lopescardoso, M. I., Whitmer, S., Vanderfits, L., Pasquali, G., Vanderheijden, R., Hoge, J. H. C. and Verpoorte, R. Effects of over-expression of strictosidine synthase and tryptophan decarboxylase on alkaloid production by cell cultures of *Catharanthus roseus*. *Planta* 205: 414-419, 1998.

Carpin, S., Garnier, F. *et al.* Changes of both polypeptide pattern and sensitivity to cytokinin following transformation of periwinkle tissues with the isopentenyl transferase gene. *Plant Physiology and Biochemistry* 35(8): 603-609, 1997.

Choi, P. S., Kim, Y. D., Choi, K. M., Chung, H. J., Choi, D. W. and Liu, J. R. Plant regeneration from hairy-root cultures transformed by infection with *Agrobacterium rhizogenes* in *Catharanthus roseus Plant Cell Rep* 22: 828-831, 2004.

Collu, G., Garcia, A. A., van der Heijden, R. and Verpoorte, R. Activity of the cytochrome P450 enzyme geraniol 10-hydroxylase and alkaloid production in plant cell cultures. *Plant Science* 162: 165-172, 2002.

Constable, F., Gaudet-LaPrairie, P., Kurz, W. G. W. and Kutney, J. P. Alkaloid production in *Catharanthus roseus* cell cultures.XII. Biosynthetic capacity of callus from original explants and regenerated shoots. *Plant Cell Rep* 1: 139-142, 1982.

Contin, A., Collu, G., van der Hijden, R., Lefeber, A. W. and Verpoorte, R. The iridoid glucoside secologanin is derived from the novel triose phosphate/pyruvate pathway in a *Catharanthus roseus* cell culture. *FEBS Lett.* 434: 413-416, 1998.

Contin, A., van D. H. R., ten Hoopen, H. J. G. and Verpoorte, R. The inoculum size triggers tryptamine or secologanin biosynthesis in a *Catharanthus roseus* cell culture. *Plant Science* 139: 205-211. 1998.

Contin, A., van der Heijden, R. and Verpoorte, R. Accumulation of loganin and secologanin in vacuoles from suspension cultured *Catharanthus roseus* cells. *Plant Science* 147(2): 177-183, 1999a.

Contin, A., van der Heijden, R. and Verpoorte, R. Effects of alkaloid precursor feeding and elicitation on the accumulation of secologanin in a *Catharanthus roseus* cell suspension culture. *Plant Cell Tissue and Organ Culture* 56(2): 111-119, 1999b.

Contin, A., Collu, G., van der Heijden, R. and Verpoorte, R. The effects of phenobarbital and ketoconazole on the alkaloid biosynthesis in *Catharanthus roseus* cell suspension cultures. *Plant Physiology and Biochemistry* 37(2): 139-144, 1999c.

Cordell, G. A. Natural products in drug discovery – Creating a new vision. *Phytochemistry Reviews* 1: 261-273, 2002.

Datta, A. and Srivastava, P. S. Variation in vinblastine production by *Catharanthus roseus* during *in vivo* and *in vitro* differentiation. *Phytochemistry* 46: 135-137, 1997.

Debnath, M., Malik, C. P. and Bisen, P. S. Micropropagation: a tool for the production of high quality plant-based medicines. *Current Pharmaceutical Biotechnology* 7(1):33-49, 2006.

Decendit, A., Liu, D., Ouelhazi, L., Doireau, P., Merillon, J. M. and Rideau, M. Cytokinin enhanced accumulation of indole alkaloids in *Catharanthus roseus* cell cultures: the factors affecting the cytokinin response. *Plant Cell Reports* 11: 400-403, 1992.

De Luca, V., Balsevich, J., Tyler, R. T., Eilert, U., Panchuk, B. D. and Kurz, W. G. W. Biosynthesis of indole alkaloids: developmental regulation of the biosynthetic pathway from tabersonine to vindoline in *Catharanthus roseus*. *J Plant Physiol* 125: 147-156, 1986.

De Luca, V. and Laflame, P. The expanding universe of alkaloid biosynthesis. *Curr Opinion Plant Biol* 4: 225-233, 2001.

De Carolis, E. and De Luca, V. Purification, characterization, and kinetic analysis of a 2-oxoglutarate-dependent dioxygenase involved in vindoline biosynthesis from *Catharanthus roseus*. *J Biol Chem* 268: 5504-5511, 1993.

Drapeau, D., Blanch, H. W. and Charles, R. W. Ajmalicine, serpentine and catharanthine accumulation in *Catharanthus roseus* bioreactor cultures. *Planta Medica* 53: 373-376, 1987.

Dutta, A., Batra, J. , Pandey-Rai, S., Singh, D., Kumar, S. and Sen, J. Expression of terpenoid indole alkaloid biosynthetic pathway genes corresponds to accumulation of related alkaloids in *Catharanthus roseus* (L.) *G. Don. Planta* 220: 376-383, 2005.

Eilert, U., De Luca, V., Kurtz, W. G. W. and Constable, F. Alkaloid formation by habituated and tumorous cell suspension cultures of *Catharanthus roseus. Plant Cell Reports* 6: 271-274, 1987.

El-Sayed, M. and Verpoorte, R. Effect of phytohormones on growth and alkaloid accumulation by a *Catharanthus roseus* cell suspension cultures fed with alkaloid precursors tryptamine and loganin *Plant Cell Tissue Org. Cult.* 68: 265-270, 2002.

El-Sayed, M., Choi, Y. H., Frédérich, M., Roytrakul, S. and Verpoorte, R. Alkaloid accumulation in *Catharanthus roseus* cell suspension cultures fed with stemmadenine *Biotechnology Letters* 26: 793-798, 2004.

Endo, T., Goodbody, A. and Misawa, M. Alkaloid production in root and shoot cultures of *Catharanthus roseus. Planta Med* 53: 479-482, 1987.

Endo, T., Goodbody, A., Vukovic, J. and Misawa, M. Biotransformation of anhydrovinblastine to vinblastine by a cell- free extract of *Catharanthus roseus* cell suspension cultures. *Phytochemistry* 26: 3233-3234, 1987.

Facchini, P. J. Alkaloid biosynthesis in plants: Biochemistry, cell biology, molecular regulation and metabolic engineering applications. *Ann Rev Plant Physiol & Plant Mol Biol* 52: 29-66, 2001.

Ganapathi, G. and Kargi, F. Recent advances in indole alkaloid production by *Catharanthus roseus* (Periwinkle). *J. Exp. Bot.* 41: 259-267, 1990.

Gantet, P., Imbault, N., Thiersault, M. and Doireau, P. Inhibition of alkaloid accumulation by 2,4 D in *Catharanthus roseus* is overcome by methyl jasmonate. *Acta Botanica Gallica* 144: 501-508, 1997.

Gantet, P., Imbault, N., Thiersault, M. and Doireau, P. Necessity of a functional octadecanoic pathway for indole alkaloid synthsis by *Catharanthus roseus* cell suspensions cultured in an auxin starved medium. *Plant and Cell Physiology* 39: 220-225, 1998.

Garnier, F., Depierreux, C., Petit–Pally, G., Hamdi, S., Chenieux, J. C. and Rideau, M. Induction of the accumulation of tryptamineand phenols by endogenous elicitors by cell suspension cultures of periwinkle. *Plant Physiology* 148: 701-706, 1996a.

Garnier, F., Label, P., Hallard, D., Chenieux, J. C., Rideau, M. and Hamdi, S. Transgenic periwinkle tissues overproducing cytokinins do not accumulate enhanced levels of indole alkaloids. *Plant Cell Tissue Org. Cult.* 45: 223-230, 1996b.

Garnier, F., Carpin, S., Label, P., Creche, J., Rideau, M. and Hamdi, S. Effect of cytokinin on alkaloid accumulation in periwinkle callus cultures transformed with light inducible *ipt* gene. *Plant Sci.* 120: 47-45, 1996c.

Geerlings, A., Ibanez, M. M. I., Memelink, J., Van der Heijden, R. and Verpoorte, R. Molecular cloning and analysis of strictosidine β-D- Glucosidase, an enzyme in terpenoid indole alkaloid biosynthesis in *Catharanthus roseus.* 275: 3051-3056, 2000.

Giri, A., Banerjee, S., Ahuja, P. S. and Giri, C. C. Production of hairy roots in *Aconitum heterophyllum* wall. using *Agrobacterium rhizogenes In Vitro Cell & Dev. Biol. - PLANT* 33: 280-284, 1997.

Giri, A., Ravindra, S. T., Dingra, V. and Lakshmi Narasu, M. Influence of different strains of *Agrobacterium rhizogenes* on induction of hairy roots and artimisinin production in *Artemisia annua Curr. Science* 81: 378-382, 2001a.

Giri, A., Giri, C. C., Dhingra, V. and Lakshmi Narasu, M. Enhanced production of podophyllotoxin from *Agrobacterium rhizogenes* transformed cultures of *Podophyllum hexandrum Natural Product Research* 15(4): 229-235, 2001b.

Giri, A., Dhingra, V., Giri, C. C., Singh, A., Ward, O. P. and Narasu, M. Lakshmi Biotransformation using cell, tissue, organ cultures and enzyme systems: current trend and future prospects. *Biotechnology Advances* 19(3): 175-199, 2001c.

Giri, A., Giri, C. C., Dhingra, V. and Narasu, M. Lakshmi *Podophyllum hexandrum* Royle A potential source for production of clinically useful anticancer drugs. In: Role of Biotechnology In Medicinal Aromatic Plants,(IA Khan & A Khanum Eds.,)Vol.5 (Special Edition on Cancer),Ukaaz Pubs. India. pp.212-220, 2002.

Giri, A., Giri, C. C. and Lakshmi Narasu, M. Recent advances in applications of transgenic hairy roots. In: Plant Genetic Engineering: Improvement of Commercial Plants –II Jaiwal P.K. and Singh R. P. (Eds) Vol. 4 Sci Tech. Pubs. LLC, Houston, USA pp. 23-81, 2003.

Goddjin, O. J. M., Pennings, E. J. M., Van der Helm, P., Schilperrort, R. A., Verpoorte, R. and Hoge, J. H. C. Overproduction of a trytophan decarboxylase cDNA in *Catharanthus roseus* crown –gall calluses results in increased tryptamine levels but not in increased terpenoid indole alkaloids. *Transgenic Res* 4: 315-323, 1995.

Godoy-Hernandez, G. and Loyola, V. V. M. Effect of acetylsalicylic acid on secondary metabolism of *Catharanthus roseus* tumor suspension cultures. *Plant Cell Reports* 16(5): 287-290, 1997.

Godoy-Hernandez, G. C., Vazquez-Flota, F. A. and Loyola-Vargas, V. M. The exposure to trans-cinnamic acid of osmotically stressed *Catharanthus roseus* cells cultured in a 14-l bioreactor increases alkaloid accumulation. *Biotech. Lett.* 22: 921-925, 2000.

Hamada, H., Yasumune, H., Fuchikami, Y., Hirata, T., Sattler, I., Williams, H. J. and Scott, A. I. Biotransformation of geraniol, nerol and (+)- and (-)-carvone by suspension cultured cells of *Catharanthus roseus*. *Phytochemistry* 44(4): 615-621, 1997.

Hasezawa, S., Nagata, T. and Syono. Transformation of *Vinca* protoplasts mediated by *Agrobacterium* spheroplasts. *Mol. Gen. Genet.* 182: 206-210, 1981.

Hernández-Domínguez, E., Campos-Tamayo, F. and Vázquez-Flota, F. Vindoline synthesis in *in vitro* shoot cultures of *Catharanthus roseus*. *Biotech. Lett.* 26: 671-674, 2004

Hernández-Domínguez, E., Campos-Tamayo, F., Carrillo-Pech, M. and Vázquez-Flota, F. *Catharanthus roseus* shoot cultures for the production of monoterpenoid indole alkaloids. *Methods in Molecular Biology* 318: 349-355, 2006.

Hilliou, F., van der Fits, L. and Memelink, J. Molecular regulation of monoterpenoid include alkaloid biosynthesis. In: Romeo JJ, Sunders JA, Mathews BF (eds) Regulation of phytochemicals by molecular techniques. Elsevier, Amsterdam pp. 275-295, 2001.

Hirata, K., Horiuchi, M., Ando, T., Asada, M., Miyamoto, K. and Miura, Y. Effect of near ultra–violet light on alkaloid production in multiple shoot cultures of *Catharanthus roseus*. *Planta Medica* 57: 499-500, 1991.

Hirata, K., Horiuchi, M., Asada, M., Ando, T., Miyamoto, K. and Miura, Y. Stimulation of dimeric alkaloid production by near-ultraviolet light in multiple shoot cultures of *Catharanthus roseus. J Ferm. Bioeng*. 74: 222-225, 1992.

Hirata, K., Asada, M., Yatani, E., Miyamoto, K. and Miura, Y. Effect of near ultra-violet light on alkaloid production in *Catharanthus roseus* plants. *Planta Medica* 59: 46-50, 1993.

Hofmann, W., Kubeczka, K. H. and Czygan, F. C. An improved method of isolation and quantitative determination of vincaleucoblastine from intact plants and tissue cultures of *Catharanthus roseus* G. *Don. Z Naturforsch* 38c: 201-206, 1982.

Hong, J., Lee, J., Lee, H., Kim, D. and Hwang, B. Enhancement of catharanthine production by the addition of paper pulp waste liquors to *Catharanthus roseus* in chemostat cultivation. *Biotechnology Letters* 19(10): 967-969, 1997.

Hong, S. B., Peebles, C. A. M., Shanks, J. V., San, K. Y., and Gibson, S. I. Terpenoid indole alkaloid production by *Catharanthus roseus* hairy roots induced by *Agrobacterium* tumefaciens harbouring rol ABC genes. *Biotechnol. Bioeng*. 93,386-390, 2006a.

Hong, S. B., Peebles, C. A. M., Shanks, J. V., San, K. Y., and Gibson, S. I. Expression of the *Arabidopsis* feedback-insensitive anthranilate synthase holoenzyme and tryptophan decarboxylase genes in *Catharanthus roseus* hairy roots. *J. Biotechnol*. 122, 28-38, 2006b.

Hostettmann, K. and Marston, A. Twenty years of research into medicinal plants: results and perspectives. *Phytochemistry Reviews* 1: 275-285, 2002.

Hughes, E. and Shanks, J. V. Metabolic engineering of plants for alkaloid accumulation. *Metabolic Engineering* 4: 41-48, 2002.

Hughes, E., Hong, S. B., Shanks, J. V., San, K. Y. and Gibson, S. I. Characterization of an inducible promoter system in *Catharanthus roseus* hairy roots *Biotechnol Prog* 18: 1183-1186, 2002.

Hughes, E. H., Hong, S. B., Gibson, S. I., Shanks, J. V. and San, K. Y. Expression of a feedback-resistant anthranilate synthase in Catharanthus roseus hairy roots provides evidence for tight regulation of terpenoid indole alkaloid levels. *Biotechnol. Bioeng*. 86: 718-727, 2004a.

Hughes, E. H., Hong, S. B., Gibson, S. I., Shanks, J. V. and San, K. Y. Metabolic engineering of the indole pathway in Catharanthus roseus hairy roots and increased accumulation of tryptamine and serpentine. *Metab. Eng*. 6: 268-276, 2004b.

Irmler, S., Schroder, G., St.-Pierre, B., Crouch, N. P., Hotze, M., Schmidt, J., Strack, D., Matern, U. and Schroder, J. Indole alkaloid biosynthesis in *Catharanthus roseus*: new enzyme activities and identification of cytochrome P450 CYP72A1 as secologanin synthase. *The Plant Journal* 24: 797-804, 2000.

Islas, I., Loyola-Vargas, V. M. and Miranda-Ham, M.·L. Trytophan decarboxylase activity in transformed roots from *Catharanthus roseus* and its relationship to tryptamine, ajmalicine and catharanthine accumulation during the culture cycle. *In Vitro Cell. Dev. Biol*. 30P: 81-83, 1994.

Junaid, A., Mujib, A., Bhat, M. A. and Sharma, M. P. Somatic embryo proliferation, maturation and germination in *Catharanthus roseus* 84: 325-332, 2006.

Jung, K. H., Kwak, S. S., Choi, C. Y. and Liu, J. R. An interchangeable system of hairy root and cell suspension cultures of *Catharanthus* for indole alkaloid production. *Plant Cell Reports* 15: 51-54, 1995.

Kebler Michael, ten Hoopen, H. J. G. and Furusaki, S. The effect of the aggregate size on the production of ajmalicine and tryptamine in *Catharanthus roseus* suspension culture. *Enzyme and Microbial Technology* 24(5-6): 308-315, 1999.

Khafagi, I., Dewerdar, A. and Amein, M. Opportunities of finding novel anti-infective agents from plant cell cultures. *Current Medicinal Chemistry* 2: 191-211, 2003.

Kim, S. W., In, D. S., Choi, P. S. and Liu, J. R. Plant Regeneration from immature zygotic embryo-derived embryogenic calluses and cell suspension cultures of *Catharanthus roseus*. *Plant Cell Tissue Org. Cult.* 76: 131-135, 2004.

Knobloch, K. H. and Berlin, J. Influence of medium composition on the formation of secondary compounds in cell suspension cultures of *Catharanthus roseus* (L.) *G. Don. Z Naturforsch* 35c: 551-556, 1980.

Kohl, W., Witte, B. and Hofle, G. Alkaloide aus *Catharanthus roseus*-Zellkulturen, III. Z *Naturforsch* 37b: 1346-1351. Ibid, 1982.

Krueger, R. J., Carew, D. P., Lui, J. H. C. and Staba, E. J. Initiation, maintenance and alkaloid production of *Catharanthus roseus* leaf organ cultures. *Planta Med* 45: 56-57, 1982.

Kutchan, T. M. Alkaloid biosynthesis – the basis for metabolic engineering of medicinal plants. *Plant Cell* 7: 1059-1070, 1995.

Kurz, W. G. W., Chatson, K. B., Constable, F., Kutney, J. P., Choi, L. S. L., Kolodziejczyk, P., Sleigh, S. K., Stuart, K. L. and Worth, B. R. Alkaloid production in *Catharanthus roseus* cell cultures. IV. Characterization of the 953 cell line. *Helv Chim Acta* 63: 1891-1896, 1980.

Kurz, W. G. W., Chatson, K. B., Constable, F., Kutney, J. P., Choi, L. S. L., Kolodziejczyk, P., Sleigh, S. K., Stuart, K. L. and Worth, B. R. Alkaloid production in *Catharanthus roseus* cell cultures. VIII. Characterization of the PRL 200 cell line. *Planta Med* 42: 22-31, 1981.

Kutney, J. P., Choi, L. S. L., Kolodziejczyk, P., Sleigh, S. K., Stuart, K. L. and Worth, B. R. Alkaloid production in *Catharanthus roseus* cell cultures. III. Catharanthine and other alkaloids from 200 GW cell line. *Heterocycles* 14: 765-768, 1980.

Kutney, J. P., Choi, L. S. L., Kolodziejczyk, P., Sleigh, S. K., Stuart, K. L. and Worth, B. R. Alkaloid production in *Catharanthus roseus* cell cultues. V. Alkaloids from the 176G. 299Y . 340Y and 951G cell lines. *J Nat Prod* 44: 536-540, 1981.

Kutney, J. P., Choi, L. S. L., Nakano, J., Tsukamoto, H., Mchugh, M. and Boulet, C. A. A highly efficient and commercially important synthesis of the antitumour *Catharanthus* alkaloids vinblastine and leurosidine from catharanthine and vindoline. *Heterocycles* 27: 1845-1853, 1988.

Laflamme, P., St- Pierre, B. and De Luca, V. Molecular and biochemical analysis of a Madagascar periwinkle root-specific minovincinine-19-hydroxy-o-acetyltransferase. *Plant Physiology* 125: 189-198, 2001.

Leduc, M., Tikhomiroff, C., Cloutier, M., Perrier, M. and Jolicoeur, M. Development of a kinetic metabolic model: application to *Catharanthus roseus* hairy root. *Bioprocess and Biosystems Engineering* 28: 295-313, 2006.

Lee-Parsons, C. W. T. and Shuler, M. L. The effect of inoculum density and conditioned medium on the production of ajmalicine and catharanthine from immobilized *Catharanthus roseus* cells. *Biotechnology and Bioengineering*. 67(1): 61-71, 2000.

Lee-Parsons, Ç. W. T., Ertürk, S., Tengtrakool, J. Enhancement of ajmalicine production in *Catharanthus roseus* cell cultures with methyl jasmonate is dependent on timing and dosage of elicitation *Biotech Letters* 26: 1595-1599, 2004.

Luijendijk, T. J. C., Stevens, L. H. and Verpoorte, R. Purification and characterisation of strictosidine beta-D-glucosidase from *Catharanthus roseus* cell suspension cultures. *Plant Physiology and Biochemistry* 36(6): 419-425, 1998.

Lundberg, P., Voge, H. J. and Brodelius, P. E. A phosphorus-31 nuclear magnetic resonance study of elicitor-mediated metabolic changes in *Catharanthus roseus* suspension cultures. *In Vitro Cellular and Developmental Biology Plant* 33(4): 301-305, 1997.

McCoy, E. and O'Connor, S. E. Directed Biosynthesis of Alkaloid Analogs in the Medicinal Plant *Catharanthus roseus*. *J. Am. Chem. Soc.*, 128 (44), 14276-14277, 2006.

Meijer, A. H., Verpoorte, R. and Hoge, H. C. Regulation of enzymes and genes involved in terpenoid indole alkaloid biosynthesis in *Catharanthus roseus*. *J. Plant Res. Special Issue* 3: 145-164, 1993.

Memelink, J., Verpoorte, R. and Kijne, J. W. ORCAnization of jasmonate responsive gene expression in alkaloid metabolism. *Trends Plant Sci* 6: 212-219, 2001.

Miura, Y., Hirata, K., Kurano, N., Miyamoto, K. and Uchida, K. Formation of vinblastine in multiple shoot cultures of *Catharanthus roseus*. *Planta Medica* 54: 18-20, 1988.

Moreno, P. R. H., Van der Heijden, R. and Verpoorte, R. Cell and tissue cultures of *Catharanthus roseus* : a literature survey II. Updating from 1988 to 1993. *Plant Cell Tissue Organ Cult*. 42: 1-25, 1995.

Moreno, P. R. H., Poulsen, C., van der Heijden, R. and Verpoorte, R. Effects of elicitation on different metabolic pathways in *Catharanthus roseus* (L.)G. Don cell suspension cultures. *Enzyme and Microbial Technology* 18(2): 99-107, 1996.

Moreno-Valenzuela, O. A., Galaz-Avalos, R. M., Minero-García, Y., Loyola-Vargas, V. M. Effect of differentiation on the regulation of indole alkaloid production in *Catharanthus roseus* hairy roots. *Plant Cell Reports* 18(1-2): 99-104, 1998.

Moreno-Valenzuela, O., Coello-Coello, J., Loyola-Vargas, V. M. and Vázquez-Flota, F. Nutrient consumption and alkaloid accumulation in a hairy root line of *Catharanthus roseus*. *Biotechnology Letters*. 21(11): 1017-1021, 1999.

Moreno, V. O. A., Monforte, G. M. *et al.* Effect of macerozyme on secondary metabolism plant product production and phospholipase C activity in *Catharanthus roseus* hairy roots. *Journal of Plant Physiology. Oct*. 155(4-5): 447-452, 1999.

Moreno-Valenzuela, O. A., Minero-García, Y., Chan, W., Mayer-Geraldo, E., Carbajal, E. and Loyola-Vargas, V. M. Increase in the indole alkaloid production and its excretion into the culture medium by calcium antagonists in *Catharanthus roseus* hairy roots. *Biotechnology Letters* 25: 1345-1349, 2003.

Morgan, J. A. and Shanks, J. V. Inhibitor studies of tabersonine metabolism in *Catharanthus roseus* hairy roots. *Phytochemistry* 51: 61-68, 1999.

Morgan, J. A., Barney, C. S., Penn, A. H. and Shanks, J. V. Effects of buffered media upon growth and alkaloid production of *Catharanthus roseus* hairy roots. *Applied Microbiology and Biotechnology*. 53(3): 262-265, 2000.

Morgan, J. A. and Shanks, J. V. Determination of metabolic rate-limitations by precursor feeding in *Catharanthus roseus* hairy root cultures. *Journal of Biotechnology* 79: 137-145, 2000.

Morgan, J. A. and Shanks, J. V. Quantification of metabolic flux in plant secondary metabolism by a biogenetic organizational approach. *Metabolic Engineering* 4: 257-262, 2000.

Morgan, J. A., Barney, C. S., Penn, A. H. and Shanks, J. V. Effect of buffered media upon growth and alkaloid production of *Catharanthus roseus* hairy roots. *Appl Microbiol Biotechnol* 53: 262-265, 2000.

Noble, R. L. The discovery of the *Vinca* alkaloids-chemotherapeutic agents against cancer. *Biochem Cell Biol* 68: 1344-1351, 1990.

O'Keefe, B. R., Mahady, G. B., Gills, J. J. and Beecher, C. W. W. Stable vindoline production transformed cell cultures of *Catharanthus roseus*. *J. Nat. Prod.* 60: 261-264, 1997.

Parr, A. J., Peerless, A. C. J., Hamill, H. D., Walton, N. J., Robins, R. J. and Rhodes, M. J. C. Alkaloid production by transformed root cultures of *Catharanthus roseus. Plant Cell Rep* 7: 309-312, 1988.

Pasquali, G., Porto, D. D. and Fett-Neto, A. G. Metabolic engineering of cell cultures versus whole plant complexity in production of bioactive monoterpene indole alkaloids: recent progress related to old dilemma. *Journal of Biosciences and Bioengineering* 101(4): 287-296, 2006.

Peebles, C. A. M., Hong, S. B., Gibson, S. I., Shanks, J. V. and San K. Y. Transient effects of over-expressing anthranilate synthase? and ß subunits in *Catharanthus roseus* hairy roots. *Biotech. Prog.* 21, 1572-1576, 2005.

Peebles, C. A. M., Hong, S. B., Gibson, S. I., Shanks, J. V., and San, K. Y. Effects of terpenoid precursor feeding on *Catharanthus roseus* hairy roots over-expressing the alpha or the alpha and beta subunits of anthranilate synthase. *Biotechnol Bioeng* 93, 534-540, 2006.

Petiard, V., Gueritte, F., Langlois, N. and Potier, P. Presence de (-)- tabersonine dans une souche de cultures de tissues de *Catharanthus roseus* G. *Don. Physiol Veg* 18: 711-720, 1980.

Potier, P. Synthesis of the antitumor dimeric indole alkaloids from *Catharanthus* species (vinblastine group). *J Nat Prod* 43: 72-85, 1980.

Rijhwani, S. K. and Shanks, J. V. Effect of subculture cycle on growth and indole alkaloid accumulation by *Catharanthus roseus* hairy root cultures. *Enzyme Microb. Tech.* 22: 606-611, 1998a.

Rijhwani, S. and Shanks, J. V. Effect of elicitor dosage and exposure time on biosynthesis of indole alkaloids by *Catharanthus roseus* hairy root cultures. *Biotechnol. Prog.* 14: 442, 1998b.

Rischer, H., Oresic, M., Seppänen-Laakso, T., *et al.* Gene-to-metabolite networks for terpenoid indole alkaloid biosynthesis in *Catharanthus roseus* cells. Proceedings of the *National Academy of Sciences* (U S A) 103(14): 5614-5619, 2006a.

Rischer, H., Goossens, A., Oreši, M., Inzé, D. and Oksman-Caldentey, K. M. Integrated transcript and metabolite profiling of the medicinal plant *Catharanthus roseus. Planta Med* 72(11): 949790, 2006b.

Rodriguez, Z. L. C. and Hernandez, S. S. M. T. Detection of tyrosine phosphatase activity in *Catharanthus roseus* hairy roots. *Plant Physiology and Biochemistry* 36(10): 731-735, 1998.

Rodriguez, Z. L. C. and Hernandez, S. S. M. T. Evidence of protein-tyrosine kinase activity in *Catharanthus roseus* roots transformed by *Agrobacterium rhizogenes. Planta Heidelberg* 204(1): 70-77, 1998.

Rodriguez, S., Compagnon, V., Crouch, N. P., St-Pierre, B. and De Luca, V. Jasmonate- induced epoxidation of tabersonine by a cytochrome P-450 in hairy root cultures of *Catharanthus roseus. Phytochemistry* 64: 401-409, 2003.

Schlatmann, J. E., Koolhaas, C. M. A. *et al.* The role of glucose in ajmalicine production by Catharanthus roseus cell cultures. Biotechnology and Bioengineering 47(5): 525-534. {a} Biotechnol. Sci. Delft Leiden, Sector Ind. Plant Biotechnol., Dep. Biochem. Eng., Delft Univ. Technol., Julianalaan 67, 2628 BC Delft, Netherlands, 1995a.

Schlatmann, J. E., Moreno, P. R. H. *et al.* Two-stage batch process for the production of ajmalicine by Catharanthus roseus: The link between growth and production stage. Biotechnology and Bioengineering 47(1): 53-59. {a} Dep. Biochem. Eng., Delft Univ. Technol., Julianalaan 67, 2628 BC Delft, Netherlands, 1995b.

Schlatmann, J. E., Vinke, J. L. *et al.* Relation between dissolved oxygen concentration and ajmalicine production rate in high-density cultures of Catharanthus roseus. Biotechnology and Bioengineering 45(5): 435-439. {a} Biotechnol. Sci. Delft Leiden, Sector Ind. Plant Biotechnol., Dep. Biochem. Eng., Delft Univ. Technol., Julianalaan 67, 2628 BC, Delft, Netherlands, 1995c.

Schlatmann, J. E., Moreno, P. R. H., Vinke, J. L., ten Hoopen, H. J. G., Verpoorte, R. and Heijnen, J. J. Gaseous metabolites and the ajmalicine production rate in high density cell cultures of Catharanthus roseus. *Enzyme and Microbial Technology* 20(2): 107-115, 1997.

Schlatmann, J. E., ten Hoopen, H. J. G. and Heijnen, J. J. A simple structured model for maintenance, biomass formation, and ajmalicine production by nondividing *Catharanthus roseus* cell. *Biotechnology and Bioengineering* 66(3): 147-157, 1999.

Schroeder, G. and Schroeder, J. CDNAs for S-adenosyl-L-methionine decarboxylase from Catharanthus roseus, heterologous expression, identification of the proenzyme-processing site, evidence for the presence of both subunits in the active enzyme, and a conserved region in the 5' mRNA leader. *European Journal of Biochemistry* 228(1): 74-78. {a} Univ. Freiburg, Inst. Biol. II, Schaenzlestr. 1, D-79104 Freiburg, Germany, 1995.

Scott, A. I., Mizukami, H., Hirata, T. and Lee, S. L. Formation of catharanthine, akuammicine and vindoline in *Catharanthus roseus* suspension cultures. *Phytochemistry* 19: 488-489, 1980.

Serap Whitmer[1], Camilo Canel[2], Robert van der Heijden[1] and Verpoorte, R. Long-term instability of alkaloid production by stably transformed cell lines of *Catharanthus roseus Plant Cell Tissue and Organ Culture* 74: 73-80, 2003.

Shanks, J. V., Bhadra, R., Morgan, J., Rijhwani, S. and Vani, S. Quantification of metabolites in the indole alkaloid pathways of *Catharanthus roseus*: Implications for metabolic engineering. *Biotech. Bioeng.* 58: 333-338, 1998.

Shukla, A. K., Shasany, A. K., Gupta, M. M. and Khanuja, S. P. S. Transcriptome analysis in *Catharanthus roseus* leaves and roots for comparative terpenoid indole alkaloid profiles. *Journal of Experimental Botany* 57(14): 3921-3932, 2006.

Sim, S. S., Chang, H. N., Liu, J. R. and Jung, K. H. Production and secretion of indole alkaloids in hairy root cultures of *Catharanthus roseus*: effects of *in situ* adsorption, fungal elicitation and permeabilization. *J. Ferm. Bioeng.* 78: 229-234, 1994.

Sottomayor, M. and Ros Barcelo, A. Peroxidase from *Catharanthus roseus* (L.) G. Don and the biosynthesis of α-3',4'- anhydrovinblastine: a specific role for a multifunctional enzyme. *Protoplasma* 222: 97-105, 2003.

Stockight, J. and Soll, H. J. Indole alkaloids from cell suspension cultures of *Catharanthus roseus* and *C. ovalis*. *Planta Med* 40: 22-30, 1980.

St-Pierre, B. and De Luca, V. A cytochrome P-450 monooxygenase catalyzes the first step in the conversion of tabersonine to vindoline in *Catharanthus roseus*. *Plant Physiol.* 109: 131-1139, 1995.

St-Pierre, B., Vazquez-Flota, F. A. and De Luca, V. Multicellular compartmentation of *Catharanthus roseus* alkaloid biosynthesis predicts intercellular translocation of a pathway intermediate. *Plant Cell* 11: 887-900, 1999.

Svoboda, G. H. and Blake, D. A. The phytochemistry and pharmacology of *Catharanthus roseus* (L.) G. Don. In: Taylor WI, Farnsworth NR (Eds) The *Catharanthus* alkaloids , Marcel Dekker Inc., New York. pp. 45-83, 1975.

Takemoto, M., Kazuo, A., Stoynov, N., Chen, D. and Kutney, J. P. Synthesis of optically active alpha-phenylpyridylmethanols by immobilized cell cultures of *Catharanthus roseus. Phytochemistry* 42(2): 423-426, 1996.

Toivonen, L., Balsevich, J. and Kurz, W. G. W. Indole alkaloid production by hairy root cultures of *Catharanthus roseus. Plant Cell Tissue Organ Cult* 18: 79-93, 1989.

Toivonen, L., Ojala, M. and Kauppinen, V. Indole alkaloid production by hairy root cultures of *Catharanthus roseus*: growth kinetics and fermentation. *Biotechnol. Lett.* 12: 519-524, 1990.

Toivonen, L., Ojala, M. and Kauppinen, V. Studies on the optimization of growth and indole alkaloid production by hairy root cultures of *Catharanthus roseus. Biotechnol. Bioeng.* 37: 673-680, 1991.

Van der Heijden, R., Verpoorte, R. and Ten Hoopen, H. J. G. Cell and tissue cultures of *Catharanthus roseus* (L.) G. Don:a literature survey. *Plant Cell Tissue Org. Cult.* 18: 231-280, 1989.

van Der Heijden, R., Jacobs, D. I., Snoeijer, W., Hallard, D. and Verpoorte, R. The *Catharanthus* alkaloids: pharmacognosy and biotechnology. *Current Medicinal Chemistry* 11(5):607-628, 2004.

Van Tellingen, O., Sips, J. H. M., Beijnen, J. H., Bult, A. and Nooijen, W. J. Phamacology, bio-analysis and pharmacokinetics in the *Vinca* alkaloids and semisynthetic derivatives (review). *Anticancer Res* 12: 1699-1716, 1992.

van Tegelen, L. J. P., Moreno, P. R. H., Croes, A. F., Verpoorte, R. and Wullems, G. J. Purification and cDNA cloning of isochorismate synthase from elicited cell cultures of Catharanthus roseus. *Plant Physiology* 119(2): 705-712, 1999.

van der, F. L. and Memelink, J. ORCA3, a jasmonate-responsive transcriptional regulator of plant primary and secondary metabolism. *Science* 289(5477): 295-297, 2000.

Vasquez-Flota, F., Moreno-Valenzuela, O., Miranda–Ham, M. L., Coello-Coello, J. and Loyola-Vargas, V. M. Catharanthine and ajmalicine synthesis in *Catharanthus roseus* hairy root cultures. Medium optimization and elicitation. *Plant Cell Tissue Organ Cult.* 38: 273-279, 1994.

Vazquez-Flota, F., De Carolis, E., Anne-Marie, A. and De Luca, V. Molecular cloning and characterization of desacetoxyvindoline-4-hydroxylase, a 2-oxoglutarate dependent-dioxygenase involved in the biosynthesis of vindoline in *Catharanthus roseus* (L.) G. Don. *Plant Molecular Biology* 34(6): 935-948, 1997.

Vazquez-Flota, F., De Luca, V., Carrillo-Pech, M., Canto-Flik, A. and Miranda-Ham, M. D. L. Vindoline biosynthesis is transcriptionally locked in *Catharanthus roseus* cell suspension cultures. *Molecular Biotechnology* 22: 1-8, 2002.

Verpoorte, R., Contin, A. and Memelink, J. Biotechnology for the production of plant secondary metabolites. *Phytochemistry Reviews* 1: 13-25, 2002.

Whitmer, S., Canel, C., Hallard, D., Goncalves, C. and Verpoorte, R. Influence of precursor availability on alkaloid accumulation by transgenic cell line of *Catharanthus roseus. Plant Physiology* 116: 853-857, 1998a.

Whitmer, S., Verpoorte, R. and Cane, C. Influence of auxins on alkaloid accumulation by a transgenic cell line of *Catharanthus roseus. Plant Cell Tissue and Organ Culture* 53(2): 135-141, 1998b.

Whitmer, S., van der Heijden, R. and Verpoorte, R. Effect of precursor feeding on alkaloid accumulation by a strictosidine synthase over-expressing transgenic cell line S1 of *Catharanthus roseus.* 69: 85-93, 2002a.

Whitmer, S., van der Heijden, R. and Verpoorte, R. Effect of precursor feeding on alkaloid accumulation by a tryptophan decarboxylase over-expressing transgenic cell line T22 of *Catharanthus roseus. J Biotechnol* 96: 193-203, 2002b.

Xu, M. and Dong, J. Elicitor-induced nitric oxide burst is essential for triggering catharanthine synthesis in *Catharanthus roseus* suspension cells *Appl. Micro. Biotechnol.* 67: 40-44, 2005a.

Xu, M. and Dong, J. O_2^{-} from elicitor-induced oxidative burst is necessary for triggering phenylalanine ammonia-lyase activation and catharanthine synthesis in *Catharanthus roseus* cell cultures. *Enzyme and Microbial Technology* 36: 280-284, 2005b.

Yahia, A., Kevers, C., Gaspar, T., Chénieux, J. C., Rideau, M. and Crèche, J. Cytokinins and ethylene stimulate indole alkaloïds accumulation in cell suspension cultures of *Catharanthus roseus* by two distinct mechanisms. *Plant Science* 133: 9-15, 1998.

Zaho, J., Zhu, W. H. and Hu, Q. Promotion of indole alkaloid production in *Catharanthus roseus* cell cultures by rare earth elements. *Biotech. Lett.* 22: 825-828, 2000a.

Zaho, J., Zhu, W. H., Hu, Q. and He, X. W. Improved alkaloid production in *Catharanthus roseus* cell suspension cultures by various chemicals. *Biotech. Lett.* 22: 1221-1226, 2000b.

Zaho, J., Zhu, W. H., Hu, Q. and He, X. W. Enhanced indole alkaloid production in suspension compact callus clusters of *Catharanthus roseus*: impact of plant growth regulators and sucrose. *Plant Growth Regulation* 33: 33-41, 2001a.

Zaho, J., Zhu, W. H. and Hu, Q. Effects of light and plant growth regulators on the biosynthesis of vindoline and other indole alkaloids in *Catharanthus roseus* callus cultures. *Plant Growth Regulation* 33: 43-49, 2001b.

Zaho, J., Zhu, W. H. and Hu, Q. Enhanced catharanthine production in *Catharanthus roseus* cell cultures by combined elicitor treatment in shake flasks and bioreactors. *Enzyme and Microbial Technology* 28: 673-681, 2001c.

Zaho, J., Zhu, W. H. and Hu, Q. Selection of fungal elicitors to increase indole alkaloid accumulation in *Catharanthus roseus* suspension cell culture. *Enzyme and Microbial Technology* 28: 666-672, 2001d.

Zarate, R., Memelink, J., van der Heijden, R. and Verpoorte, R. Genetic transformation via particle bombardment of *Catharanthus roseus* plants through adventitious organogenesis of buds. *Biotechnology Letters.* 21(11): 997-1002, 1999.

Zarate, R., Bonavia, M., Geerlings, A., van der Heijden, R. and Verpoorte, R. Expression of strictosidine b-D-glucosidase cDNA from *Catharanthus roseus*, involved in the monoterpene indole alkaloid pathway, in a transgenic suspension culture of *Nicotiana tabacum. Plant Physiology and Biochemistry* 39 763-769, 2001.

Zheng, Z. G., Liu, D. and Hu, Z. B. Comparison of cell growth and alkaloid production of *Catharanthus roseus* cells cultured in shake flask and in bioreactor. *Acta Botanica Sinica* 40: 51-55, 1998.

—oo(O)oo—

24

Role of Secondary Metabolites in Defence Mechanism of Plants

Renu Sarin and Mala Agarwal

PLANT cells produce a vast amount of secondary products. Many of these are highly toxic and are often stored in specific vesicles or in the vacuole. Several studies indicate that this kind of storage functions on one hand as a detoxification of the plant itself and generates on the other hand a reservoir of nitrogen-rich molecules. In contrast to animals, plants do not excrete them. Some secondary plant products can be reversibly degraded and are fed into the basic metabolism while others cannot. Although secondary plant products are very common, this does not mean that every plant can produce every product. Some compounds are restricted to single species, others to related groups. But they are nearly always found only in certain specific plant organs, often in just one type of cell (and they're again only in a certain compartment). Also, they are often generated only during a specific developmental period of the plant. Secondary compounds can also be used as features of classification.

Many secondary compounds have signalling functions. They influence the activities of other cells, control their metabolic activities and co-ordinate the development of the whole plant. Other substances like the flower colours serve to communicate with pollinators or protect the plants from feeding by animals or infections. Some plants, for example, produce specific phytoalexines after fungi infection that inhibits the spreading of the fungi mycelia within the plant. A number of substances is secreted and influences the existence of other species. Especially with algae but with fungi, too, the communication of the cells is stimulated or kept upright by extracellular substances. These substances may be of consistencies ranging from gas to jelly-like. Small-excreted molecules have large losses due to diffusion though a wide range of action also marks them. Many of them are antibiotic i.e. they inhibit the existence of competing species in the surrounding of their producer thus safeguarding its ecological niche.

The mutual influence of plants by secretion is called allelopathy. It occurs not only in algae but also in higher plants. Allelopathic substances may damage the germination, growth and development of other plants. Their influence is only rarely stimulating. Insects (and other animals) have developed defence strategies against the insecticide effects of some secondary plant products. During evolution, at first detoxification mechanisms, later even dependencies on certain plant products were developed. Some species, for example, need starting compounds for their steroid synthesis that were originally meant to be a plant defence. They are slightly modified within the animal and get thus a simpler structure.

Since centuries, many plant compounds have an outstanding role in medicine. They're pharmacological - and consequently also their economical - value has lost nothing of its importance until today. They are used either directly or after chemical modification. It should be mentioned that some plant products have psychopharmacological effects and morphine or mescaline is even counted among the 'hard' drugs.

Some secondary compounds are not only found in phylogenetically related species (or families) but also in species that are not directly linked. Similar products (in these case naphthoquinone derivatives) can be obtained from very different starting substances and can be synthesized *via* different intermediates (Harborne, 1977): e.g. synthesis of plumbagin (*Plumbago*, Plumbaginaceae) by acetate-malonate pathway, synthesis of juglon (*Juglans*, Juglandaceae) by shikimate pathway, synthesis of chimaphylline (*Chimaphila*, Pyrolaceae) by homogentisate pathway, synthesis of alkannin (*Plagiobothrys*, Boraginaceae) by hydroxybenzoate pathway.

A number of mutants are unable to synthesize certain products due to a blocked metabolism. A classic example is the white-flowering varieties of species which otherwise coloured, often red flowers. Perhaps, it is indeed a feature of some synthetic pathways of the secondary metabolism that genetic defects are permissible and that their carrier has often a large probability to survive under natural conditions. The chemical structure of secondary plant products is more complex than that of primary products. Many of them are derived from amino acids or nucleotides. Most of the compounds found in plants belong to rather few families of substances. Only small chemical modifications like methylations, hydroxylations, intercalations with metal ions, etc. lead to a wide spectrum of functionally different substances. These substances are often glycosylated (certain sugar residues have been added) so that their water solubility is increased. The sugar-free part of such a substance is called an aglycon.

During the last 20 to 30 years, the analysis of secondary plant products has progressed a lot. The use of modern analytical techniques like chromatography (in all its variations), electrophoresis, isotope techniques and enzymology succeeded in the elucidation of exact structural formulas and the most important biosynthetic pathways.

Secondary plant products may be classified into three major groups-

(1) Nitrogen containing secondary compounds e.g.alkaloids, non-protein amino acids.

(2) Isoprenoid compounds or terpenes e.g.essential oils, steroids, rubber etc.

(3) Phenolic compounds e.g. lignins, tannins, flavonoids etc.

ALKALOIDS

Alkaloids are a group of nitrogen-containing bases. Most of them are drugs. Only a few (like caffeine) are derived from purines or pyrimidines, while the large majority is produced from amino acids. Some of the examples are given below:

Ornithine derivatives: Ornithine is a precursor of the cyclic pyrrolidines that occur in the alkaloids of tobacco (nicotine, nornicotine) and other Solanaceae. Nicotine is a starting compound of numerous further tobacco alkaloids. During the biosynthesis of tropane, intermediates are produced that are at the same time starting compounds for cocaine and hyoscamine. Ornithine form starting point for the synthesis of tropane, methylornithine is the first intermediate.

Lysine derivatives: Lysine is the precursor of piperidine that forms the skeleton of several alkaloids. Among them are the bitter principles of the lupine, lupinine and lupanine.

Phenylalanine derivatives: The most important are:

***Ephedra*-alkaloids:** ephedrine, pseudoephedrine,alkaloids gained from micro-organisms: cytochalasine B and D,the *Taxus*-alkaloids: taxine,the *Lunaria*-alkaloids: lunarine and lunaridine,alkaloids of the Lythraceae.

Tyrosine derivatives: Tyrosine is the starting product of a large family of alkaloids. The first important intermediate is dopamine, which is the starting product of the biosyntheses of berberine, papaverine and morphine, too. Two tyrosine rings condense and form the basic structure of morphine that is subsequently modified.

Tryptophane derivatives (Indole alkaloids): The Apocynaceae, Loganiaceae and Rubiaceae families are characterized by a broad range of indole alkaloids of which the *Vinca-*, *Rauvolfia-* and *Catharanthus* - alkaloids are examples. Coupling iridoids generates them; very common compounds derived from monoterpenes to indole that is based on tryptophane. A lot of well-known fungi poisons belong to this group. Among the tryptophane-derivatives is d-tubocurarine, one of the active components of curare, the arrow poison used by South American Indians.

Isoprene derivatives: Gentianine as well as further toxic compounds like, for example aconitine obtained from *Aconitum* and *Delphinium* belong to this group. An important sub-group is formed by the *Solanum-* alkaloids that can be found in nearly all organs of *Solanum-* (potato) and *Lycopersicon* (tomato) - species but occur also in very different taxa (lilies and Asclepiadaceae).

ISOPRENOIDS/TERPENES

Polymeric isoprene derivatives are a large family of substances of little functional and structural common ground: steroids, carotenoids, gibberelic acid are just some of its members. Several thousand different types of molecules from very different plant groups have been isolated and characterized. Despite their varied structures, only a few pathways synthesize all of them.

The starting product of all the different groups of compounds shown in the illustration above is mevalonic acid that is transformed into a phosphorylated isoprene upon phosphorylation. This isoprene polymerizes subsequently. In the course of polymerization, the number and position of the double bonds are fixed. All green plants are able to generate linear isoprenoids in this way.

While terpenes with more than five isoprene units are quite universal, many of the simpler terpenes are restricted to certain plant groups. Sequestiterpenes, for example, are common in mosses but occur in higher plants, too. They can be found with Magnoliales, but not with Ranunculales. This example shows why the presence of certain secondary plant products has proven to be a useful taxonomical feature. The same is also true for monoterpenes (iridoid compounds, iridians). Among the diterpenes are the gibberellins, a group of phytohormones.

Steroids are triterpenes or triterpenoids. Triterpenes are a group of molecules that contain 30 C-atoms and are generated by the polymerization of six isoprene units although a number of derivatives, some with more but most with less C-atoms are also counted among this group. Steroid molecules consist of four rings marked A, B, C and D that have a number of additional residues R. It is of some importance whether two of these are in a cis- (i.e. at the same side of the cyclic system) or in a trans-position (at opposite sites). Steroids have been shown to occur both in gymnosperms and in angiosperms.

Carotenoids are very common both in the plant and the animal kingdom though they are always of plant origin. All of them are tetraterpenes; i.e. they contain 40 C-atoms in eight isoprene residues.They are formally derived by the subsequent hydration, dehydration, ring formation, shifting of double bonds and / or methyl groups, chain elongation or shortening and the incorporation of oxygen into a non-cyclic $C_{40}H_{56}$ compound. Carotenoids can be further classified into carotenes(pure carbohydrates without additional groups) and the xanthophylls(carotenoids containing oxygen).

Members of both groups are components of the pigment systems (the light traps) of chloroplasts and are involved in the primary light absorption and the photon canalization of photosynthesis. Moreover, they also function as light receptors in a number of further light-induced plant processes. Some representative absorption spectra are shown below. The yellow colour of many flowers is caused by carotenoid-containing chromoplasts that are usually devoid of chlorophyll. Carotenoids are also common in fruits. The red colour of ripe tomatoes and of pepper is caused by the presence of lycopene. It is a linear molecule with 13 double bonds, 11 of which are conjugated. Many carotenes (and xanthophylls) are cyclic at their termini and loose as a consequence the terminal double bond(s).

Beta-carotene is best-known as the pigment of the carrot (*Daucus carota*). It occurs mostly as a crystal. One of its most important derivatives is vitamin A (a precursor of visual purple). Xanthophylls like the common xanthophyll of green leaves or lutein are derived from carotenes. Violaxanthin, for example, is a derivative of *alpha*-carotene. The yellow pigment of corn, zeaxanthin is a *beta*-carotene derivative. Fucoxanthin, the brownish pigment of brown algae and diatoms, is another xanthophyll. Among the catabolic products of xanthophyll is the pigment of saffron, the crocetin

RUBBER-LIKE POLYMERS / POLYISOPRENES

Rubber is a carbohydrate consisting of high molecular weight chains of 1,4 - polyisoprene residues in cis-configuration (caoutchouc). The main source is *Hevea brasiliensis*. Gutta-percha consists of 1,4 - polyisoprene residues in trans-configuration. Its molecular weight is far below that of rubber. The main source is *Palaquium gutta*. A similar substance, balata, is obtained from

*Mimosops balata.*Chicle (obtained from *Achras sapota*), finally, is a polymer containing both cis- and trans-bonds (in the ratio 1:2). It is the basic substance of bubble gum. Altogether, more than 1800 plant polyisoprenes have been identified. Their cellular concentrations are usually small, and their molecular weights are relatively low. Polyisoprenes occur in certain plant cells as small latex particles. They can be seen in the electron microscope as clearly defined, cytoplasmatic inclusions specific for the respective species.

PHENOLIC COMPOUNDS

This group consists of a large number of molecules of heterogeneous structure. Their common feature is the presence of at least one hydroxyl-substituted aromatic ring system.

TABLE 1
The Most Important Classes of Phenolic Compounds in Plants

n	**$(C_6 - C_3)_n$** **$(C_6)_n$** **$(C_6 - C_3 - C_6)_n$**	**Lignins** **Catecholmelanine** **(condensed tannins)**
Number of C-Atoms	**Basic Skeleton**	**Class**
6	C_6	simple phenols, benzoquinones
7	$C_6 - C_1$	phenolic acids
8	$C_6 - C_2$	acetophenone, phenylacetic acid
9	$C_6 - C_3$	hydroxycinnamic acid, polypropene, coumarin, isocoumarin
10	$C_6 - C_4$	naphtoquinone
13	$C_6 - C_1 - C_6$	xanthone
14	$C_6 - C_2 - C_6$	stilbene, anthrachinone
15	$C_6 - C_3 - C_6$	flavonoids, isoflavonoids
18	$(C_6 - C_3)_2$	lignans, neolignans
30	$(C_6 - C_3 - C_6)_2$	biflavonoids

The starting product of the biosynthesis of most phenolic compounds is shikimate. Phenols are acidic due to the dissociability of their -OH group. They are rather reactive compounds and as long as no steric inhibition due to additional side chains occurs, they form hydrogen bonds. Consequently, many flavonoids have intramolecular bonds. Another important feature is their ability to form chelate complexes with metals. Also, they are easily oxidized and, if so, form polymers (dark aggregates). The darkening of cut or dying plant parts is caused by this reaction. They have usually an inhibiting effect on plant growth. Among the phenylpropanol derivatives of lower molecular weight are a number of scents like the coumarins, cinnamic acid, sinapinic acid, the coniferyl alcohols and others. These substances and their derivatives are at the same time intermediates of the biosynthesis of lignin.

Flavonoids

In 1975, the number of identified flavonoids was estimated to be larger than 2000. Some important representatives and their biological significance are listed in the table 2 below.

TABLE 2

The Most Important Classes of Flavonoids and their Biological Significance

Class	Number of Known Members	Biological Significance (so far as Known)
Anthocyanin(s)	250	red and blue pigments
Chalcons	60	Yellow pigments
Aurones	20	Yellow pigments
Flavones	350	cream-coloured pigments of flowers
Flavonols	350	feeding repellents (?) in leaves
Dihydrochalcons	10	some taste bitter
Proanthocyanidins	50	Astringent substances
Catechins	40	some have properties like those of tannins
Biflavonoids ?	65	?
Isoflavonoids	15	oestrogen effect, toxic for fungi

Nach J. B. Harborne, 1980

The basic structure of flavonoids is derived from the C_{15} body of flavone. They differ from other phenolic substances in the degree of oxidation of their central pyran ring. And, very fundamentally, also in their biological properties. While some classes (the flavonones, for example) are colourless, the members of other classes (the anthocyanes, for example) are always coloured and known as pigments of flowers or other plant parts. Anthocyanes are normally red or yellow, their colour is pH-dependent. Blue pigments are achieved by chelate formation with certain metal ions (Fe^{III} or Al^{III}, for example).

The variability of the flavonoids is largely based on the hydroxylation and/ or methylation pattern of the three ring systems. A correlation between two flavonoids points often to a relationship between the producing plant species. They have therefore proven to be suitable traits for the study of the phylogenetic relations between higher plants. The quinones are another group of phenolic compounds. We have already met some of its members that function as co-factors. Accordingly, they do not actually belong to the secondary plant products but have to be counted among those of the basic metabolism. As has been mentioned before, phenolic compounds occur usually not unbound within plant tissues. They are mostly coupled to other molecules, often to glucosyl residues, but to sulphate- or acetyl-residues, too. One of the reasons may be that they are toxic when in a free state and are detoxified, at least partially, if coupled. Many low molecular weight compounds, for example thymol, are used in medicine as antiseptics due to their toxicity. Different types of bonds between flavonoids (for example anthocyanes) and a glycosyl residue lead to different derivatives that increase the range of flower colours (and colour shades). The glycosylation of flavonoids has an additional, ecologically not less important function. It has been brought into connection with pest protection and protection against other animals. Based on their biological functions, phenolic compounds can be classified as follows:

TABLE 3
The Ecological Meaning of Some Phenolic Compounds for Plants

Function	Group	Example(s) and Plant Species Where the Effect was Studied
Flower pigments	Anthocyanines	cyanidin-3,5-diglucosid in *Rosa*
	Chalconni	coreopsin in *Coreopsis tinstoria*
	Aurones	aureusin in *Anthirrhinum majus*
	Yellow flavonoids	gossypetine-7-glucoside in *Gossypium*
	Flavones	apigenin-7-glucoside in *Bellis perennis*
Fruit pigments	Anthocyanines	petunidin glucoside in *Atropa belladonna*
	Isoflavones	osajin in *Maclura pomifera*
	Chalcons	ocanin in *Kyllingi brevifolia*
Allelopathic substances	Quinones	juglon in *Juglans regia*
	Phenols	hydroquinone in *Arctostaphylos*
	Phenolcarboxylic acids	sialic acid in *Quercus falcata*
		ferulic acid in *Adenostoma*
	Hydrocinnamic acid	
Protection against pests	Quinones	juglon in *Carya ovata*
	Tannines	gallotannine in *Quercus robur*
	Flavonols	quercitine-glycosids in *Gossypium*
Fungicide	Isoflavones	luteon in *Lupinus*
	Phenolcarboxylic acids	protocatechunic acid in *Allium*
		phloridcine in *Malus pumila*
	Dihydrochalones	
Phytoalexins	Stilbens	reservatrol in *Arachis hypogaea*
	Phenylanthrenes	orchinol in *Orchis militaris*
	Isoflavanes	vestitiol in *Lotus corniculatus*
	Pterocarpanes	pisatin in *Pisum sativum*
	Phenylpropanoids	coniferyl alcohol in *Linum usitiltissimum*
	Fucocoumarins	psoralen in *Petroselinum crispum*

According to J. B. Harborne, 1980

RARE AMINO ACIDS

The term rare amino acids is misleading in some respects. It refers to all those amino acids that are not incorporated into proteins. We already got to know some of them like ornithine or citrulline that are rather common intermediates of the basic metabolism. Roughly 220 different structures are known, most of which occur in plant cells in a free state though glutamate-, oxalate- or acetyl- derivatives can also sometimes be found.

In some fungi, rare amino acids are polymerized to small, sometimes also cyclic polypeptides like in phalloidine or the amanitins, the toxins of the amanita.

Derivatives of nearly all well-known 20 amino acids have been isolated and described. A certain rare amino acid occurs often only in one or a few plant species. Of the 220 different types of molecules, only the synthesis of two derivatives of arginine, octopine and nopaline will be shown here. They became known when it was found out that a plasmid of *Agrobacterium tumefaciens*, the pathogen of crown galls, is the carrier of the genetic information necessary for their synthesis.

PLANT AMINES

Plant amines are derivatives of ammonia. Their collective structures are:

Primary amines: NH_2R

Secondary amines: NHRR'

Tertiary amines: NRR'R"

Quaternary amines: $N^+RR'R''R'''(OH^-)$

A wide range of plant amines can be found in most of the plant cells. They are usually generated by the decarboxylation of amino acids or by transamination of aldehydes. The distinction between plant amines and alkaloids is sometimes a little arbitrary. Some, like mescaline, are counted among the alkaloids although in a chemical sense they are amines.

Aliphatic amines are often produced during anthesis, i.e. the opening of a flower or the formation of the fruiting body of certain fungi (like the stinkhorn, for example). They are insect-attractants. A good example of insect attractants is the aliphatic-aromatic amines in Araceae (lords-and-ladies, arum and others).

Among the di- and polyamines are putrescine ($NH_2(CH_2)_4NH_2$), as well as spermidine ($NH_2(CH_2)_3NH(CH_2)_4NH_2$) and spermine ($NH_2(CH_2)_3$ $NH(CH_2)_4$ NH $(CH_2)_3NH_2$). They occur in nearly all eucaryotic cells and interact with the DNA double helix. Among the tryptamines (tryptophane derivatives) are the phytohormone indole-3-acetic acid (IAA) as well as serotonin.

GLYCOSIDES

Cyanogenic glycosides: Few plant species have the ability to produce cyanides. They are strong cytotoxins, competitive inhibitors of the Fe^{III} of the heme group. The cells detoxify them by glycosylation, i.e. by linking them *beta*-glycosidically to sugar residues (usually glucose).

Glucosinolates: are anions that occur only in the cells of a limited number of dicotyledonous families. Glucosinolates are very common in the order Capparales (best-known family: Brassicaceae) where they occur in every species hitherto examined. Among the best-known representatives are the active ingredients of horseradish, radish and mustard. The elimination of aliphatic glucosinolates in rape (isothiocyanate or oxaziolin-2-thione, for example from glucorapiferin; or rhodaninion from glucobrassicines) achieved by cultivation resulted in so-called double zero varieties (00-varieties). The cultivation of simple zero varieties (0-varieties) is based on the elimination of erucid acid, a long-chained unsaturated fatty acid.

TYPES OF PLANT DEFENCES

Plant defences can be categorized into two groups: Performed and Induced.

Performed defences

Performed defences are due to the presence of secondary metabolites in plants. Secondary metabolites have important ecological functions in plants by protecting plants against being eaten by herbivores and against being infected by microbial pathogen (Gershenzon, 2003).

Plant secondary metabolites can be divided into three chemically distant groups; terpenes, phenolics and nitrogen containing compounds.

Terpenes

The terpenes or terpenoids constitute the largest class of secondary products. The diverse substances of this class are generally insoluble in water. They are biosynthesized from acetyl-CoA or glycolytic intermediates. Terpenes are toxins and feeding deterrents to many plant feeding insects and mammals and play defensive role in the plant kingdom (Gershenzan and Croteau, 1992). The monoterpene esters called pyrethroids that occur in the leaves and flowers of *Chrysanthemum* species show very striking insecticidal activity. Both natural and synthetic pyrethroids are popular ingredients in commercial insecticides

In conifers such as pine and fir, monoterpenes accumulate in resin ducts found in the needles, twigs and trunk. These compounds are toxic to numerous insects, including bark beetles (Trapp and Croteau, 2001).

Many plants contain mixtures of volatile mono and sesquiterpenes, called essential oils, that land a characteristic odor to the foliage for example peppermint, lemon, basil and sage.

Essential oils have well known insect repellent properties. They are frequently found in glandular hairs that project outward from the epidermis and serve to 'advertise' the toxicity of the plant, repelling potential herbivores even before they take a trail bite. In corn, cotton, wild tobacco and other species certain monoterpenes and sesquiterpenes are produced and emitted only after insect bite has already begun. These substance repeal ovipositing herbivores and attract natural enemies, including predatory and parasitic insects, that kill plant feeding insects and so help minimize further damage (Turling *et al.*1995, Kesselar and Baldwin, 2001).

Among the nonvolatile terpene antiherbivore compounds are the limonoids, a group of triterpene (C30) well known as bitter substances in citrus fruits. The most powerful deterrent to insect is azadirachtin, a complex limonoid from the neem tree (*Azadirachta indica*) of Africa and Asia. Azadirachtin is a feeding deterrent to some insects at doses as low as 50 parts per billion, and it exerts a variety of toxic effects (Aerts and Mordue, 1997). It has considerable potential as a commercial insect control agent because of its low toxicity to mammals.

The phytoecdysomes, first isolated from the common fern, *Polypodium vulgare*, are a group of plant steroids that have the same basic structure as insect molting hormones. Ingestion of phytoecdysomes by insect disrupts molting and other developmental processes, often with lethal consequences.

Triterpenes that are active against vertebrate herbivores include cardenolides & saponins.

Phenolic Compounds

Plant produces a large variety of secondary products that contain a phenol group, a hydroxyl functional group on an aromatic ring. These substances are classified as phenolic compounds. Plant phenolics are a chemically heterogeneous group of nearly 10,000 individual compounds against herbivore and pathogens.

The isoflavonoids (isoflavones) are a group of flavonoids in which the position of one aromatic ring (Ring B) is shifted. Isoflavones are found mostly in legumes and have several different biological activities. Rotenoids have strong insecticidal actions; others have anti-estrogenic effects for example ship grazing on clover rich in isoflavonoids often suffer from infertility.

In the past few years, isoflavonoids have become best known for their role in phytoalexins antimicrobial compounds synthesized in responses to bacterial/fungal infection that help to limit spread of the invading pathogen.

Tannins

A second category of plant phenolic polymers with defensive properties is tannins.The tannins are general toxins that significantly reduce the growth and survivorship of many herbivores when added to their diets. In addition, tannins act as feeding repellents to a great diversity of animals. Mammals such as cattle, dear and apes characteristically avoid plants or parts of plants with high tannin contents. Unripe fruits frequently have very high tannin levels, which may be concentrated in the outer cell layers. The defensive properties of most tannin are due to their toxicity, which is generally attributed to their ability to bind proteins nonspecifically. It has long been thought those plant tannin complex proteins in the guts of herbivores by forming hydrogen bonds between their hydroxyl group & electronegative sites on the protein.

Most recent evidences indicate that tannins and other phenolics can also bind to dietary protein in a covalent fashion. The foliage of many plants contain enzymes that oxidize phenolics in there corresponding quinones forms in the gut of herbivores (Felton *et al.* 1989). Quinones are highly reactive electrophilic molecules that readily react with the nucleophilic-NH and-SH groups of protein. By whatever mechanism protein-tannin binding occurs this process has a negative impact on herbivore nutrition. Tannins can inactivate herbivore digestive system and create complex aggregates of tannins and plant proteins that are difficult to digest.

Plant tannins also serve as defenses against microorganisms for example; the non-living heartwood of many trees contains high concentrations of tannins that help in preventing fungal and bacterial decay.

Nitrogen containing compounds

A large variety of plant secondary metabolites have nitrogen in their structure. Included in this category are such well-known anti-herbivore defenses as alkaloids and cyanogenic glycosides, which are of considerable interest because of their toxicity to humans and their medicinal properties.

The alkaloids are a large family of more than15000 nitrogen containing secondary metabolites found in approximately 20% of the species of vascular plants. Most alkaloids believed to function as defense against predators, especially mammals, because of their general toxicity and deterrence capacity (Hartmann, 1992). Large number of livestock deaths is caused by the ingestion of alkaloid containing plants. Nearly all alkaloids are also toxic to humans when taken in sufficient quantity for example strychnine; atropine and conine (from poison hemlock) are classic poisoning agents. At lower doses, many are useful pharmacologically. Morphine, codeine and scopolamine are just a few of plant alkaloids currently used in medicine. Other alkaloids, including cocaine, nicotine and caffeine, enjoy widespread non-medical use as stimulants or sedatives.

Cyanogenic glycosides release the poison HCN. Two group of nitrogenous compounds cyanogenic glycosides and glucosinolates are not in themselves toxic but are readily broken down to give off volatile poisons when the plant is crushed. Cyanogenic glycosides release the well-known poisons gas hydrogen cyanide (HCN). The breakdown of cyanogenic glycosides in plants is a two step enzymatic process In the first step the sugar is cleaved by aglycosidase, an enzyme that separates sugars from other molecules to which they are linked the resulting hydrolysis product called anhydroxynitrile or cyanohydrin can decompose spontaneously at a low rate to liberate HCN. This second step can be accelerated by an enzyme hydroxynitrite lyase.

Cyanogenic glycosides are normally not broken down in the intact plant because the glycoside and the degradative enzymes are spatially separated, in different cellular compartments or in different tissues. In sorghum the cyanogenic glycoside dhurrin is present in the vacuoles of epidermal cells while the hydrolytic enzymes are found in the mesophyll (Poulton, 1990). Under ordinary conditions the compartmentation prevent decomposition of the glycoside. When the leaf is damaged, as during herbivore feeding, the cell contents of different tissue mix and HCN form. Cyanogenic glycosides are widely distributed in plants and are frequently encountered in legumes, grasses and species of rose family.

Considerable evidences indicate that cyanogenic glycosides have protective function in certain plants. HCN is a fast acting toxin that inhibits melloproteins, such as the ion-containing cytochrome oxidase, a key enzyme of mitochondria respiration. The presence of cyanogenic glycosides deters feeding by insects and others herbivores, such as snails and slugs. As with other classes of secondary metabolite, although some herbivores have adapted to feed on cyanogenic plants and can tolerate large doses of HCN.

Glucosinolates release volatile toxins

A second class of plant glycosides called the glucosinolates, or mustard oil glycosides, breakdown to release volatile defensive substances.

A hydrolytic enzyme called a thioglucosidase or myrosinase that cleaves glucose from its bond with the sulfur atom catalyzes the release of these mustard-smelling volatiles from glucosinolates. The resulting aglycone, the non sugar portion of the molecule, rearranges either loss of the sulfate to give pungent and chemically reactive products, including isothiocyanates and nitriles, depending on the condition of hydrolysis. These product function in defense as herbivore toxins and feeding repellents. Like cyanogenic glycosides, glucosinolates are stored in the intact plant separately from the enzymes that hydrolyze them, and they are brought into contact with these enzymes only when the plant is crushed.

INHIBITION OF HERBIVORE DIGESTION BY SOME PLANT PROTEINS

Among the diverse components of plant defense arsenals are proteins that interfere with herbivore digestion e.g. some legume synthesize –amylase inhibitors that block the action of starch digesting enzyme -amylase. Other plant species produce lectins, defensive proteins that bind to carbohydrates or carboyhydrate-containing proteins. After being ingested by a herbivore, lectin bind to the epithelial cells lining the digestive tract and interfere with nutrient absorption (Peumans and Van Dainne,1995).

The best known antidigestive proteins in plants are the protein inhibitors found in legumes, tomato and other plants; these substances block the action of herbivore proteolytic enzymes. After entering the herbivore's digestive tract, they hinder protein digestion by binding tightly and specifically to the active site of protein-hydrolyzing enzymes such as trypsin and chymotrypsin. Insects that feed on plants containing proteinase inhibitors suffer reduced rates of growth and development that can be off set by supplemental amino acid in their diet.

The defensive role of proteinase inhibitors has been confirmed by experiments with transgenic tobacco. Plants that have been transformed to accumulate increased level of proteinase inhibitors suffered less damage from insect herbivores than did untransformed control plants (Johnson *et al.* 1989).

INDUCED

This plant resistance includes the activation of diverse defense mechanism. The response involves opening of numerous ion channels, post translation modifications of protein by protein kinases, activation of the enzymes of the synthesis of active oxygen species, synthesis of low molecular weight defense substances called phytoalexines and transcription activation of numerous defense related genes, moreover several signaling molecules are generated to ensure coordination of defense responses.

The most frequently occurring defense and signaling mechanisms are:

1. Hypersensitive reactions as a result of localized cell death.
2. Reactive oxygen species are often produced during the early stage of plant resistance response
3. Production of nitric oxide induced during incomplete interaction in plants.

4. Cell wall fortification with the deposition of callose, lignin, hydroxyproline rich protein.

5. Synthesis of Salicylic acid and jasmonic acid necessary for the induction of some plant defense mechanism.

6. Induction of pathogen related proteins (PR).

7. Synthesis of organic and inorganic secondary metabolites-Phytoalexin.

8. Induction of localized/systemic plant resistance against pathogens.

Hypersensitive reactions

Some defenses are induced by herbivore attack/microbial infection. Defenses that are produced after only initial herbivore damage theoretically require a small investment of plant resources than defenses that are always present, but they must be activated quickly to be effective.

After being infected by a pathogen, Plant deploys a broad spectrum of defense against invading microbes. A common defense is the hypersensitive response, in which cells immediately surrounding the infection site die rapidly, depriving the pathogen of nutrients and preventing its spread. After a successful hypersensitive response, a small region of dead tissue is left at the site of the attempted invasion, but the rest of the plant is unaffected.

Reactive oxygen species are produced during the early stages of plant defense resistance response

The hypersensitive reaction is often preceded by the production of reactive oxygen species. Cells in the vicinity of the infection synthesize a burst of toxic compounds by the reduction of molecular oxygen, including the superoxide anion (O), hydrogen peroxide(H O) and the hydroxyl radical (OH),an NADPH- dependent oxidase located on the plasma membrane is thought to produce O ,which is then converted into O and H O .

The hydroxyl radical is the strongest oxidant of these active oxygen species and can initiate radical chain reaction with a range of organic molecules leading to lipid peroxidation, enzyme inactivation and nucleic acid degradation (Lamb and Dixon, 1997). Active oxygen species may contribute to cell death as part of the hypersensitive response or act to kill the pathogen directly.

Cell wall fortification with the deposition of callose, lignin, hydroxyproline rich protein

Many species react to fungal/bacterial invasion by synthesizing lignin or callose. These polymers are thought to serve as barriers walling of the pathogen from the rest of the plant and physically blocking its spread. A related response in the modification of cell wall proteins. Certain proline rich proteins of the cell wall become oxidatively cross linked with after pathogen attack in an H O –mediated reaction (Bradely *et al.* 1992) This process strengths the walls of the cells in the vicinity of the infection site, increasing their resistance to microbial digestion.

Synthesis of Salicylic acid and Jasmonic acid necessary for the induction of plant defense genes

A number of defenses are not continuously present in plants, but are synthesized only after initial herbivore or pathogen attack. For example in tomato, insect feeding leads to the rapid accumulation of proteinase inhibitor throughout the plant even in the undamaged areas far from the initial feeding site. The systemic production of proteinase inhibitors in young tobacco plants is triggered by a complex sequence of events.

Wounded tobacco leaves synthesize prosystemin, a large (200 amino acid) precursor protein.

Prostemin is proteolytically processed to produce the short (18amino acid) polypeptide called systemin.

Systemin is produced at the site of wounding, released from damaged cells into the apoplast, then transported out of the wounded leaf via phloem, transported with similar rates as sucrose from source to sink. Systemin is cleaved from a larger protein, called prostemin. The regulation of this protease is unknown, but expression of prosystemin is higher after wounding.

Target cells at the plasma membrane perceive systemin and the wall fragments by receptor proteins. The receptor activates the release and chemical modification of particular lipids, starting with linolenic acid (18:3fatty acid). This initiates a cascade of modifications of these lipids, including a step catalyzed by lipoxygenase, leading to the production of JA, a plant growth regulator that has wide ranging effects (Creelman and Mullet, 1997) both wounding and application of systemin cause a transient increase in JA which is the last step known, leading to activation of proteinase inhibitor genes. JA levels rises steeply in response to damage caused by a variety of different herbivores and trigger the formation of many different kind of plant defenses besides proteinase inhibitors, including terpenes and alkaloids.

The structure and biosynthesis of JA have intrigued plant biologists because of the parallels to some eicasanoids that are central to inflammatory responses and other physiological processes in mammals. In plants JA is synthesized from linolenic acid (18:3), which is released from membrane lipids and then converted to JA.

JA is known to induce the transcription of a host of genes involved in plant defense metabolism for example recent research on the *Catharanthus roseus* (madagascar peri winkle), identified a transcription factor that responds to JA by activating the expression of several genes encoding alkaloid biosynthetic genes (Vander fits and Memlink2000). This transcription factor also activates the gene of certain primary metabolic pathways that provide precursors for alkaloid formation.

JA can rapidly convert to methyl jasmonate, which is volatile. Wounding of a plant can lead to the production of methyl jasmonate this can diffuse through the air to a nearby plant and trigger the expression of defense genes, including proteinase inhibitor proteins, interplant signaling can even occur between two species.

Upon invasion by a weak pathogen or a non-pathogen, there is often a process of programmed cell death, which contains the microbe and stops further replication [hypersensitive reaction (HR)]. This response often also includes a rise in salicylic acid (SA) and production of an unknown attack = systemic acquired resistance (SAR). SAR therefore can be induced by rises in the level of SA. Salicylic acid can be converted to methyl salicylate, which is volatile and may diffuse to another plant to produce PR proteins even in the absence of a direct pathogen attack on plant . Some PR proteins are chitinases (can degrade fungal cell walls) or peroxides (can strengthen plant cell walls and produce hydrogen peroxide which may be toxic to microbes).

Thus upon wounding by a chewing insect or invasion by a weak pathogen/non pathogen, JA and SA are produced respectively (by enzymatic process of a membrane lipid) and signals production of proteinase inhibitor proteins (PINS). These proteins are induced systemically the signal is transmitted through the phloem. Proteinase inhibitors disrupt the protein metabolism of insect that feed on leaves after this initial wounding.

Induction of pathogen related proteins

Another defensive response to infection is the formation of hydrolytic enzymes that attack the cell wall of pathogen. An assortment of glucanasis, chitinases and other hydrolyses are induced by fungal invasion. Chitin, a polymer of N-acetylglucosamine residues, is a principal component of fungal cell walls. The hydrolytic enzymes belong to a group of proteins that are closely associated with pathogen infection and so are known as pathogen related (PR) proteins.

PHYTOALEXINS

The best studied response of plants to bacterial or fungal invasion is the synthesis of phytoalexins. They are a chemically diverse group of secondary metabolites with strong antimicrobial activity that accumulate around the site of infection. Phytoalexins production is a common mechanism of resistance to pathogenic microbes in a wide range of plants. Different plant families employ different types of secondary metabolites as phytoalexins for example isoflavonoids are common phytoalexins in legume family, in Solonaceae (Potato, Tomato, Tobacco) various sesquiterpenes are produced as phytoalexins. Before infection the phytoalexins are undetectable in plants, but very rapidly synthesized after microbial attack due to the activation of new biosynthetic pathways. There is the initiation of gene transcription. The plants do not store any of the enzymatic machinery required for phytoalexin synthesis. Soon after the microbial invasion they begin transcripting and translating the appropriate in mRNAs and synthesizing the enzymes de novo.

Phytoalexins accumulate in concentrations that have been shown to be toxic to pathogen in bioassays. The defensive significance of these compounds in intact plants is not fully known. Experiments on genetically modified plants and pathogens have shown the proof of phytoalexin function in vivo. When tobacco was transformed with a gene that catalyze the biosynthesis of the phenylpropanoid phytoalexin reservatrol, it become much more resistant to a fungal pathogen than non-transformed control plants. *Arabidopsis* mutant deficient in the tryptophan derived phytoalexin camelexin was more susceptible than the wild type to a fungal pathogen. In some experiments, pathogens that had been transformed with genes encoding phytoalexin degrading enzymes were then able to infect plants that are normally resistant to them (Kombrink and Somssich, 1995).

Induction of localized/systemic plant resistance against pathogen

When a plant survives the infection of pathogen at one site, it also develops increased resistance to subsequent attacks at sites throughout the plant and enjoys protection against a wide range of pathogen species. This phenomenon known as systemic acquired resistance (SAR), develops over a period of time following initial infection (Ryals *et al* 1996). Systemic acquired resistance (SAR) appears to result from increased level of certain defense compounds, including chitinases and other hydrolytic enzymes. One of the endogenous signals is Salicylic acid. The level of SA (benzoic acid derivative) rises dramatically in the zone of infection after initial attack, and it is thought to establish SAR in other parts of the plant. In addition to SA, its methyl ester, methyl salicylate acts as a volatile SAR inducing signal transmitted to distant parts of the plants and even to neighboring plants (Shulaev *et al.*1997).

GENETIC BASIS OF PLANT DISEASE RESISTANCE

The plant responses to pathogens can be classified into two broad categories. Non-specific resistance (general, non-host or basic resistance) is a response to all races of a particular pathogen, and occurs in all cultivars of a host plant species. In contrast, specific resistance is dependent upon the presence of a particular pathogen race, a particular host plant cultivar, or both. The underlying genetic basis of each type of plant disease resistance differs according to the genetic makeup of both plant and pathogen.

NON-SPECIFIC PLANT DISEASE RESISTANCE

Non-specific plant disease resistance is multi-component, relying upon a foundation of passive plant defences, and usually also involving the activation of active defences by non-specific elicitors of biotic origin . The combination of defences involved in this type of resistance is highly coordinated and similar for all plant-pathogen interactions. However, substantial variation in both the timing and degree of the active component of plant defence and in environmental factors has been shown to be critical to its success. Whilst stronger, more timely non-specific defence responses are responsible for many incompatible plant-pathogen interactions, weaker non-specific defence responses are often overcome by the pathogen in compatible interactions, and have also been observed in symbiotic relationships with endophytic fungi.

The genetic basis underlying non-specific plant disease resistance is complex, and involves multiple genes that encode proteins with a diversity of functions in both partners of the plant-pathogen interaction. These can be divided into pathogenicity genes that determine the ability of the pathogen to cause disease and defence-related genes that enable the plant host to execute defence responses. Both classes of genes contain members that are expressed in a constitutive manner, in addition to genes that are only expressed in response to the interaction of plant and pathogen. Pathogen genes that govern pathogenicity usually encode proteins that have a negative impact on disease resistance. The majority of pathogenicity genes in plant pathogens condition the ability to establish infection, and these include genes that encode proteins with specific roles in adhesion to the plant surface, the formation of penetration structures , cell wall degradation, and the synthesis of toxic compounds. However, a number of pathogenicity genes instead govern the ability of the pathogen to defeat plant defences, such as those encoding proteins involved in the detoxification of phytoalexins . Plant defence-related genes encode proteins that enable the detection of non-specific elicitors and the activation of an intracellular signalling pathway leading to plant defences, as well as those themselves involved in passive and active plant defences.

RECOGNITION OF NON-SPECIFIC ELICITORS

Various pathogen-derived elicitors such as complex carbohydrates from fungal cell walls, microbial enzymes, polypeptides, proteins and lipids can also trigger plant defence responses.

Recognition of these elicitors by plant receptors triggers mitogen activated protein kinase (MAPK) cascades that cause the rapid and transient phosphorylation of specific nuclear, cytosolic and membrane bound proteins (Dietrich *et al.* 1990; Felix *et al.* 1991; Jensen *et al.* 2002; Peck, 2003). The first complete MAPK cascade in plants was shown in *Arabidopsis.* The cascade functions downstream of the flagellin receptor FLS2 to activate two plant specific transcription factors. Transient overexpression of components of this MAPK cascade provided resistance to bacterial and fungal pathogens (Asai *et al.* 2002).

It has been shown that lipopolysaccharide (LPS) (cell-surface components of Gram-negative bacteria) treatment of *Arabidopsis* suspension cells caused the production of nitric oxide (NO) through the activation of a nitric oxide synthase (Atnos1, previously associated with hormonal signalling) (Zeidler *et al.* 2004). To highlight the importance of NO production in response to LPS, Zeidler et al. further showed that selected defence gene expression was almost abolished in LPS treated Atnos1 mutant plants and that these plants were also more susceptible than wild-type to a virulent strain of *P. syringae.*

SPECIFIC PLANT DISEASE RESISTANCE

In contrast to non-specific resistance, specific plant disease resistance appears to be governed by a single gene or a small number of related genes, which encode proteins capable of altering the outcome of an otherwise compatible plant-pathogen interaction. Genes conditioning host-pathogen specificity are found in particular subpopulations of the pathogen, plant host, or both interacting organisms, and specific plant disease resistance can be subdivided into three major categories on this basis.

(a) Race-specific resistance

Race-specific resistance is induced in response to only a particular race of pathogen, but occurs in all cultivars of the host plant. This type of specific disease resistance is dependent upon genetic variation within the pathogen species, and the production of proteins capable of altering the outcome of an otherwise compatible plant-pathogen interaction in only certain pathogen races.

(b) Cultivar-specific resistance

Cultivar-specific resistance is activated only in a specific host plant cultivar, but in reaction to all races of a pathogen species. In a few plant-pathogen systems where non-specific resistance limits the host range of the pathogen to a plant genus, this type of resistance occurs at the level of the host plant species, and is termed species-specific resistance. Cultivar-specific or species-specific resistance relies upon genetic variation within the host plant species or genus, and the production of proteins capable of altering the outcome of an otherwise compatible plant-pathogen interaction in only certain plant cultivars or species.

(c) Race-cultivar-specific (gene-for-gene) resistance

If both pathogen and host specificity are involved, plant disease resistance is termed race-cultivar-specific resistance, since it results only from the interaction of a particular pathogen race with a particular cultivar of the host plant. This type of resistance is usually referred to as gene-for-gene resistance, because in most cases it requires the presence of both a race-specific avirulence (*avr*) gene in the pathogen and one or more corresponding cultivar-specific resistance (*R*) genes in the host plant.

R GENES AND R-GENE-DEPENDENT RESISTANCE

Host recognition of a potential pathogen determined by a 'gene-for-gene' interaction initiates a very rapid defence response in the plant. The gene-for-gene theory is based on the recognition of an avirulence (avr) gene product in the pathogen by a corresponding resistance (R) gene product in the host. In most cases, this interaction occurs under high specificity, and if the plant or pathogen lacks the appropriate R gene or avr gene, respectively, then activation of plant defence responses may be delayed or ineffective (Nimchuk *et al.* 2003). As a result, disease on the host results in what is classified as a compatible reaction. Defence mechanisms are however commonly induced in plants lacking R-gene-mediated recognition, although activation of these mechanisms may occur later such that defences are consequently less effective (Tao *et al.* 2003).

Although the gene-for-gene interaction has generally been considered to be a receptor–ligand model where plant R proteins were direct receptors for pathogen avirulence proteins, this has been found to be the exception rather than the rule, and thus, suggesting a more indirect mode of pathogen recognition (Bonas and Lahaye, 2002; Schneider, 2002). Dangl and Jones (2001) highlighted a 'guard' model where R proteins act as guards by detecting changes in host targets of pathogen elicitors. Recent evidence to support this model comes from studies of the RPM1-interacting protein RIN4 (the R protein RPM1 confers resistance against *Pseudomonas syringae* carrying AvrRpm1 or AvrB avirulence factors). RIN4 interacts with the pathogen elicitors AvrRpm1 and AvrB (which cause RIN4 phosphorylation), and AvrRpt2 (which causes the elimination of RIN4), as well as being able to interact with the R proteins RPM1 and RPS2. RPM1 acts as a guard by monitoring changes in RIN4 caused by AvrRpm1 or AvrB (Mackey et al. 2002). RPS2 also guards RIN4 by detecting the elimination of RIN4 caused by AvrRpt2 (Axtell and Staskawicz, 2003; Mackey *et al.* 2003). Under this scenario, the plant protein (RIN4) can act as a common target of several pathogen elicitors and is guarded by more than one R protein. Therefore, initiation of defence signalling results from changes in host targets of pathogen elicitors rather than by direct binding of elicitors to R proteins. It is suggested that RIN4 is a negative regulator of basal defence responses and that pathogen elicitors may target it in order to increase its activity and suppress the plant's basal immunity (Mackey *et al.* 2002).

R genes have been isolated from *Arabidopsis* as well as solanaceous species (tomato, potato, pepper, and tobacco) and from barley, wheat, maize, rice and flax, although only a few R genes have been cloned from monocots. So far R genes have been isolated that can provide resistance against viral, bacterial and fungal pathogens, as well as to nematodes and insect pests (for a recent review on R proteins see Martin *et al.* 2003).

Despite the wide range of taxa in which R genes have been described, they encode only five main classes of proteins (Martin *et al.* 2003). The majority of R proteins are classified as nucleotide-binding site leucine rich repeat (NBS-LRR) proteins with the *Arabidopsis* genome containing over 150 genes that encode this class of protein (Jones 2001). The NBS-LRR class can be further divided into those that have N terminal homology to the Toll and Interleukin-1 receptor (TIR) genes (TIR-NBS-LRR), a leucine-zipper (LZ-NBS-LRR) or a coiled-coil motif (CC) (CC-NBS-

LRR). Other conserved motifs within isolated R-gene-encoded proteins from diverse plant genera include serine / threonine kinase domains or the possession of a transmembrane domain (Martin *et al.* 2003).

Several classes of mutants have been generated in *Arabidopsis* that involve signalling components downstream of avr-R gene-mediated recognition. Mutants eds1 (enhanced disease susceptibility1), ndr1 (non-race-specific disease resistance1), pbs2 (avrPphB susceptible2), and pad4 (phytoalexin deficient4) have altered resistance responses to several avr signals. The pbs3 mutant compromises resistances so far to all R genes tested (the P. syringae resistance genes RPS5, RPM1, RPS2, and RPS4, and recognition of Peronospora parasitica resistance genes RPP 2, RPP4, RPP6, RPP7, and RPP19). Mutants impaired in R-gene signalling of specific individual R-genes also exist, for example the pbs1 (avrPphB Susceptible 1) mutation completely suppresses resistance mediated by the R gene RPS5, but not to the other R genes tested. It has been shown that the virulence protein AvrPphB proteolytically cleaves the protein kinase PBS1 and that this generates a signal, possibly a cleavage product of PBS1, which activates the R protein RPS5 . Under this scenario, RPS5 guards the virulence target PBS1 as the plant is able to detect this pathogen based on the enzymatic properties of its elicitor rather than elicitor–receptor binding.

At least two signal transduction cascades acting downstream of R genes exist, one, which are NDR1-dependent and the other EDS1-dependent. Other pathways include those that function independently of NDR1 or EDS1. The recent analysis of resistance signalling components RAR1 (required for Mla12 resistance, allelic to PBS2) and SGT1 (suppressor of the G2 allele of skp1) complicates the downstream responses of the different R-gene-mediated signalling pathways, in some cases requiring RAR1 and SGT1 together, singly or neither. Three distinct R gene-mediated signalling pathways were recently analysed with a GeneChip array (covering 1 / 3 of the genome) to compare defence-associated gene expression profiles. Analysis of activated RPP4 (dependent on PAD4, SGT1 and SA accumulation), RPP7 (dependent on SGT1, but not PAD4 or SA accumulation), and RPP8 (independent of PAD4, SGT1 or SA accumulation) pathways revealed that all three pathways could converge to up-regulate common sets of genes, indicating a funnelling effect of defence signalling.

Mechanism of Specific Plant Disease Resistance

The biochemical mechanisms responsible for the induction of specific resistance in plant-pathogen interactions are poorly understood, but are likely to vary with both the type of specific resistance and the plant-pathogen system involved. The three most common mechanisms underlying specific resistance appear to be race-specific elicitors, host-selective toxins and race-specific suppressors, but others, as yet unknown, may also exist.

(a) Race-specific elicitors

The majority of cases of race-specific resistance appear to result from the generation by a pathogen of race-specific elicitors of active plant defences , and the recognition of these by the plant host. Resistance with this biochemical basis is often also cultivar-specific (and thus gene-for-gene), since the elicitor interacts with a corresponding plant receptor that is usually unique to a particular cultivar of the host plant. The recognition of the elicitor by its receptor is proposed to occur at the plant plasma membrane for most fungal pathogens, and within the plant cell for bacterial and viral pathogens. In bacterial biotrophs such as *Xanthomonas* and *Pseudomonas*, which are extracellular plant pathogens, this event is dependent upon a bacterial membrane transport protein that delivers the elicitor into the plant cell, and is encoded by the *hrp* gene complex Link. Interaction of the elicitor and receptor activates a complex signal transduction pathway resulting in the induction of plant defences against pathogen races harbouring the elicitor. The elicitor is generally the protein that is encoded by the avirulence gene, however in some plant-pathogen interactions the elicitor has been found to be the product of a reaction catalyzed by this protein. Resistance genes in some cases directly encode cultivar-specific receptors of race-specific elicitors, and in these cases a direct physical interaction between avirulence and resistance gene products may occur. However resistance proteins are more likely to function by registering interactions between the elicitor and an unknown target protein, or act as unique links in the signalling pathway leading to active plant defences.

(b) Host-selective toxins

Race-cultivar-specific pathogen resistance can also occur due to the production of compounds that are toxic to plants. These host-selective toxins (HSTs) are generated in a race-specific manner, mainly by necrotrophic species of the fungal genera *Alternaria* and *Cochliobolus*. A few of the approximately twenty known host-selective toxins are proteins or peptides that are directly encoded by race-specific pathogen genes. However, most are non-protein compounds of low molecular weight that are synthesized in reactions catalyzed by proteinaceous race-specific gene products. Following transport into the host plant cell via a highly coordinated delivery system, host-selective toxins cause cellular damage, but only in toxin-sensitive cultivars that harbour a single gene conditioning toxin sensitivity. The mode of action of host-selective toxins is highly variable, but appears to always involve either activation or inhibition of a cultivar-specific protein. For example, T-toxin, produced by *C. heterostrophus*, serves to activate a cultivar-specific protein capable of forming destructive membrane pores, whereas HC-toxin from *C. carbonum* inhibits a cultivar-specific version of an enzyme that modifies DNA-bound proteins to cause disturbances in gene expression.

(c) Race-specific suppressors

Race-specific resistance can also result from pathogen production of race-specific suppressors that inhibit a non-specific resistance response. To date, race-specific suppressors have been described for only a few species of biotrophic plant-pathogenic fungi, including *Phytophthora infestans*. In contrast to race-specific elicitors, they are proposed to interfere with elicitor binding, signal transduction, gene expression or plant defences to suppress the non-specific resistance response towards races that harbour them. Race-specific suppressors may be proteins directly encoded by pathogen genes governing race-specificity, or may be non-protein compounds produced by reactions catalyzed by these proteins. Plant disease resistance in cases involving race-specific suppressors may or may not also be cultivar-specific (and thus gene-for-gene), depending on whether or not the actual mechanism of suppression involves a cultivar-specific plant molecule.

THE RELATIONSHIP BETWEEN NON-SPECIFIC AND SPECIFIC RESISTANCE'S

The connection linking non-specific and specific resistance's is rarely considered and thus poorly understood. However, it is likely that the relationship between these two forms of resistance differs depending on the particular type of specific resistance and the biochemical mechanism involved in its induction.

Specific resistance conditioned by race-specific elicitor molecules is generally of a higher intensity and more successful than non-specific plant disease resistance, and also involves an oxidative burst that is diphasic in nature. These observations indicate that this type of specific resistance may be composed of a race-specific component to resistance, which is supplementary to and superimposed upon an unsuccessful non-specific resistance response. A common signalling pathway leading to defence responses may be activated to different degrees by both non-specific elicitors and race-specific elicitors resulting from the same plant-pathogen interaction. The highly conserved nature of plant resistance mechanisms and the observation that different pathogen races can elicit defence responses that differ only in intensity both supports this hypothesis. However, different pathogen races can also induce resistance responses that contain unique defence components. For example, the hypersensitive response Link is rarely induced by non-specific elicitors, but almost always occur during a race-specific resistance response. This indicates that non-specific and race-specific elicitors may activate different signalling pathways, possibly convergent at some point.

CONCLUSION

One of the majors problems concerning the production of economically important crop is the difficulty of controlling plant disease to maintain the high quality and yield which the producer and consumer expect. Chemical insecticides, pesticides have toxic residues harmful to human, to soil and environment as well as many pathogens have developed resistance to the active ingredients of a wide range fungicides, insecticides, pesticides and there is a public perception that pesticides are undesirable.

To avoid these difficulties the need of present day is application of biotechnology to reduce the incidence of disease in economical important crops. One such approach to the control of plant disease is through the induction and enhancement of the plant's own defense mechanism which excludes the application of toxic compounds to plants.

Plant defence mechanism involves many biochemical reactions between plants and plant pathogens.

Plant defences can be broadly classified into two categories (1) performed defences which are structural in the form of cuticle, trichomes, spines, bark as well as chemical in the form of secondary metabolites that function as secondary defence compounds. These compounds protect plant from predators and pathogens on the basis of their toxicity and repellency to herbivores and microbes. There are three major groups of secondary metabolite terpenes, phenolics and nitrogen containing compounds. Terpenes, composed of 5-carbon isoprene units, are toxins and feeding deterrents to many herbivores.

Phenolics, which are synthesized primarily from products of the shikimic acid pathway, have several important roles in plants. Lignin mechanically strengthens cell walls and flavonoid and other phenolic compounds serve as defence against herbivore and pathogens.

Members of third major group, nitrogen containing secondary metabolites are synthesized principally from common amino acids. Compounds such as alkaloids, cyanogenic glycosides, glucosinolates, non-protein amino acids and proteinase inhibitors protect plant from a variety of herbivore animals.

In induced plant disease resistance recognition of pathogen will trigger an array of events, which will induce resistance to pathogenic agents. Thus resistance reactions involves not only performed components but also more importantly, an induced response to infection which includes a 'cascade' of induced responses.

Plant disease resistance is a complex phenomenon that most commonly occurs in a non-specific manner, as a result of multiple genes conditioning the ability of the pathogen to cause disease and enabling the plant host to mount an effective defence response. However, plant disease resistance can also be induced only in response to particular pathogen races (race-specific resistance), only in particular host plant cultivars (cultivar-specific resistance), or only when both a specific pathogen race and plant cultivar interact (race-cultivar-specific or gene-for-gene resistance). This host-pathogen specificity can be attributed to a single gene or a small number of related genes enabling the production of race-specific elicitors, host-selective toxins, or race-specific suppressors in different host-pathogen systems. Specific plant disease resistance resulting from race-specific elicitors is probably superimposed upon a non-specific resistance response that has been overcome in the host range of the pathogen. In contrast, host-selective toxins and race-specific suppressors most likely achieve host-pathogen specificity in disease resistance through the modification or negation of an otherwise successful non-specific resistance response.

The study of these secondary metabolites has many practical applications. By virtue of their own biological activity against herbivores, animals and microbes. Many of these substances are employed commercially as insecticides, fungicides and pharmaceuticals. The breeding of need for certain costly and potentially harmful pesticides increased level of secondary metabolites into economic crops has made it possible to reduce

REFERENCES

Aerts, R. J. and Mordue, A. J. Feeding deterrence and toxicity of neem triterpenoids. *J. Chem.Ecol.* 23: 2117-2132, 1997.

Agrios, G. N. Plant Pathology, 4th edn. Academic Press, San Diego. pp 115-142,1997.

Asai T, Tena, G., Plotnikova, J., Willmann, M. R., Chiu, W. L., Gomez, L., Boller, T., Ausubel, F. M. and Sheen, J. MAP kinase signaling cascade in *Arabidopsis* innate immunity. *Nature* 415: 977-983, 2002.

Atstt, P. R. and O'dowd, D. J. Plant defense guilds. *Science* 193: 24-29, 1997.

Axtell, M. J. and Staskawicz, B. J. Initiation of RPS2 –specific disease resistance in *Arabidopsis* is coupled to the Avr Rpt 2-directed elimination of RIN4. *Cell* 112: 369-377, 2003.

Banthrope, D. V. and Charlwood, B. V. The terpenoids. In: "Secondary plant products" (E. A. Bell and B. V. Charlwood ed.) (Encyclop. Plant. Physiol. Vol. 8). Berlin-Heidelberg New York: Springer Verlag, 1980.

Bell, E. A. and Charlwood, B. V. (eds). Secondary plant products (Encyclop. Plant Physiology, Vol. 8). Berlin-Heidelberg-New York: Springer Verlag, 1980.

Benhamou, N. Elicitor induced Plant-defense pathways. *Trends in Plant Sciences* 1: 233-240, 1996.

Bonas, U. and Lahaye, T. Plant disease resistance triggered by pathogen – derived molecules: refined models of specific recognition. *Current opinions in Microbiology* 5: 44-50, 2002.

Bradley, D. J., Kjellbon, P. and Lamb, C. J. Elicitor and wound induced oxidative cross-linking of a proline-rich plant cell wall protein: A novel, rapid defense response. *Cell* 70: 21-30, 1992.

Bowers, W., Ohta, S. T., Cleere, S. T. and Marsella, P. A. Discovery of insect antijuvenile hormones in plants. *Science* 193, 542-547, 1986.

Creelman, R. A. and Mullet, J. E. Biosynthesis and action of jasmonates in plants. *Ann.Rev. Plant Physiol-Plant Mol.Biol.* 48: 355-381, 1997.

Dangl, J. L. and Jones, J. D. Plant pathogens and integrated defense responses in infection. *Nature* 411: 826-833, 2001.

Dickinson, C. H. and Lucas, J. A. Plant Pathology and Plant Pathogens. Blackwell Scientific Publications, Oxford. pp 168-183, 1982.

Dietrich, A., Mayer, J. E. and Halbrock, K. Fungal elicitor triggers rapid, transient and specific protein phosphorylation in parsley cell suspension cultures. *Journal of Plant Biological Chemistry*, 1990.

Eilert, U. Elicitation: Methodology and aspects of application. In: F Constabel and I.K. Vasil (Eds.). Cell Culture and Somatic Cell Genetics of Plants Cell culture I Phytochemistry, Vol 4.Acedmic Press, New York. pp. 153-186, 1987.

Felix, G., Grosskopf, D. G., Regenass, M. and Boller, T. Rapid changes of protein phosphorylation are involved in transduction of the elicitor signal in plant cells, Proceedings of the National Academy of Sciences USA 88:8831-8834, 1991.

Felton, G. W., Donato, K., Del Vecchio, R. J. and Duffey, S. S. Activation of plant foliar oxidases by insect feeding reduces nutritive quality of foliage for noctuid herbivores. *J.Chem.Ecol.* 15: 2667-2694, 1989.

Gabriel, D. W. Genetics of plant parasite populations and host-parasite specificity. In Kosuge, T. and Nester, E. W. (Eds) Plant-Microbe Interactions: Molecular and Genetic Perspectives, Volume 3. McGraw-Hill, New York, 1989.

Gershenzon, J. Secondary metabolites and plant defense. In: Plant Physiology. Ed. L. Taiz and Zeiger E. Panima publishing corporation, New Delhi, 283-306, 2003.

Gershenzon, J. and Croteau, R. Terpenoids.In herbivores: their interactions with secondary plant metabolites, Vol 1:The Chemical participants, 2nd ed. G. A. Rosenthel and M. R. Berenbaum, eds. Academic press, San Diego, CA, pp. 165-219, 1992.

Harborne, J. B., Marby, T. J. and Marby, H. The flavonoids. London: Chapman and Hall, 1975.

Harborne, J. B. Introduction to ecological biochemistry. London, New York: Academic Press, 1977.

Harborne, J. B. Ökologische Biochemie. Heidelberg-Berlin-Oxford: Spektrum Akad. Verlag, 1995.

Hertmann, Alkaloids.In herbivores: Their interactions with secondary plant metabolites, Vol.1: The chemical participants, 2nded. G. A. Rosenthal and M. R. Berenbaum, Eds. Academic press, San Diego, CA, pp. 79-121, 1992.

Jalali, B. L. and Bhargava, S. Gene expression during host plant and fungal pathogen interactions. *Proceedings of the National Academy of Sciences of India* 72: 235-255, 2002.

Jensen, A., Reventos, D. and Mundy, J. Fusion genetic analysis of jasmonate-signaling mutants in *Arabidopsis*. *The Plant Journal* 29: 595-606, 2002.

Johnson, R., Narvaez, J., An, G. and Ryan, C. Expression of proteinase inhibitors I and II in transgenic tobacco plants effects on natural defense against *Manduca sexta Larva. Proc. Natl. Acad. Sci.*USA 86: 9871-9875, 1989.

Karrer, W. Konstitution und Vorkommen der organischen Pflanzenstoffe. Basel, Stuttgart: Birkhäuser Verlag, (2. Aufl.), 1976.

Kessler, A. and Baldwin, I. T. Defensive function of herbivore –induced plant volatile emissions in nature. *Science* 291: 2141-2144, 2001.

Kindl, H. Aromatische Aminosäuren im Stoffwechsel höherer Pflanzen. *Naturwissenschaften* 58, 554-563, 1971.

Kindl, H. Biochemie der Pflanzen. Berlin-Heidelberg-New York: Springer Verlag (2. Aufl.), 1987.

Kombrink, E. and Somssich, I. E. Defense responses of plants to pathogens. *Adv. Bot. Res.* 21: 1-34, 1995.

Lamb, C. and Dixon, R. A. The oxidative burst in plant disease resistance. *Annu. Rev. Plant Physiol. Plant Mol.Biol.* 48: 251-275, 1997.

Luckner, M. Secondary metabolism in microorganisms, plants, and animals. Berlin-Heidelberg-New York-Tokyo: Springer Verlag, (2. Aufl.), 1984.

Marby, T. J. Betalains, S. 513-533 in: "Secondary plant products" (E. A. BELL, B. V. Charlwood, eds.) Berlin-Heidelberg-New York: Springer Verlag (Encyclop. Plant Physiol., Vol. 8), 1980.

Mackey, D., Holt, B. F., Wiig, A. and Dangl, J. L. RIN4 Interacts with *Pseudomonas syringae* type III effector molecules and is required for RPM1-mediated resistance in *Arabidopsis. Cell* 108: 743-754, 2002.

Mackey, D., Belkhadir, Y., Alonoso, J. M., Ecker, J. R. and Dangl, J. L. *Arabidopsis* RIN4 is a target of the type III virulence effector AvrRpt2 and modulates RPS2-mediated resistance. *Cell* 112; 379-389, 2003.

Martin, G. B., Bogdanove, A. J. and Sessa, G. Understanding the functions of plant disease resistance proteins. *Annual Review of Plant Biology* 54: 23-61, 2003.

Mothes, K. Chemische Muster und Entwicklung in der Pflanzenwelt. *Naturwissenschaften* 52, 571-585, 1965.

Nimchunk, Z., Eulgem, T., Holt, B. F. and Dangl, J. C. Recognition and response in the plant immune system. *Annual Review of Genetics* 37: 579-609, 2003.

Pant, P. and Rastogi, R. P. The triterpenoids, *Phytochemistry* 18, 1095-1108, 1979.

Peck, S. C. Early phosphorylation events in biotic stress. *Current Opinion in Plant Biology* 6: 334-338, 2003.

Peumans, W. J. and Van Damme, E. J. M. Lectins as plant defense proteins. *Plant Physiol.* 109: 347-352, 1995.

Poulton, J. E. Cyanogenesis in plants, *Plant Physiol.* 94: 401-405, 1990.

Ryals, J. A., Neunschwander, U. H., Willits, M. G., Molina, A., Steiner, H. Y. and Hunt, M. D. Systemic acquired resistance. *Plant Cell* 8: 1809-1819, 1996.

SCHLEE, D. Ökologische Biochemie. Berlin, Heidelberg, New York: Springer Verlag, 1986.

Schneider, D. S. Plant immunity and film noir: What gumshoe detectives can teach us about plant-pathogen interactions. *Cell* 109: 537-540, 2002.

Seigler, D. S. Isolation and characterization of naturally occurring cyanogenic compounds. *Phytochemistry* 14, 9-29, 1975.

Shulaev, V., Silverman, P. and Raskin, I. Airborne signaling by methyl salicylate in plant pathogen resistance. *Nature* 385: 718-721, 1997.

Stahl, E. Pflanzen und Schnecken, biologische Studie über die Schutzmittel der Pflanzen gegen Schneckenfraß. *Jenaische Z. Naturwiss.* 15, 557-684, 1888.

Swain, I. (ed.) Comparative phytochemistry. New York, London: Academic Press, 1966.

Tao, Y., Xie, Z., Chen, W., Glazebrook, J., Chang, H. S., Han, B., Zhu, T., Zou, G. and Katagiri, F. Quantitative nature of *Arabidopsis* responses during compatible and incompatible interactions with the bacterial pathogen *Pseudomonas syringe. The Plant Cell* 15: 317-330, 2003.

Tatiana, C., Spollansky, Sandra, I., Pitta-Alvarez and M. Giulietti. Effect of Jasmonic acid and aluminum on production of tropane alkaloids in hairy root cultures of *Brugmansia candida. Electronic J. of Biotech.* 3: 72-75, 2000.

Trapp, S. and Croteau, R. Defensive resin biosynthesis in conifers. Annu. Rev. Plant. Physiol. *Plant mol.Biol.* 52: 689-724, 2001.

Turlings, T. C. J., Loughrin, J. H., McCall, P. J., Rose, U. S. R., Lewis, W. J. and Tumlison, J. H. How caterpillar damaged plants protect themselves by attracting parasitic wasps. *Proc. Natl. Acad. Sci.* USA 92: 4169-4174, 1995.

Vander Fits, L. and Memelink, J. ORCA3, a jasmonate-responsive transcriptional regulator of plant primary and secondary metabolism. *Science* 289: 295-297, 2000.

Wolpert, T. J., Dunkle, L. D. and Ciuffetti, L. M. Host-selective toxins and avirulence determinants: What's in a name? *Annual Review of Phytopathology* 40: 251-285, 2002.

Yamada, Y., Yun, D. J. and Hashimoto, T. Genetic engineering of medicinal plants for tropane alkaloid production. In: Ryu DDY and Furusaki S (eds). Advances in Plant Biotechnology p83-93. Eisevier Science Publishers, Amsterdam, The Netherlands, 1994.

Young, N. D. The genetic architecture of resistance. *Curr.Opin. Plant Biol.* 3: 285-290, 2000.

Zeidler, D., Zahringer, U., Gerber, I., Dubery, I., Hartung, T., Bors, W., Hutzler, P., Durner, J. Innate immunity in *Arabidopsis thaliana:* lipopolysaccharides activate nitric oxide synthase (NOS) and induced defense genes. *Proceedings of the National Academy of Sciences* USA 101: 15811-15816, 2004.

—oo(O)oo—

INDEX

R

S